Index of Variant Human Fibrinogens

1994 Edition

Compiled and Edited by

Ray F. Ebert
Organon Teknika/Biotechnology Research Institute
Rockville, Maryland

CRC Press
Boca Raton Ann Arbor London Tokyo

Library of Congress Cataloging-in-Publication Data

Ebert, Ray F.
Index of variant human fibrinogens, — 1994 ed. / compiled and edited by Ray F. Ebert
p. cm.
Includes bibliographical references.
ISBN 0-8493-8998-4
1. Fibrinogen polymorphisms. 2. Dysfibrinogenemia. I. Ebert, Ray F.
QP93.5.I48 1994
612.1′15—dc20 94-11110
for Library of Congress CIP

International Standard Book Number 0-8493-8998-4
Library of Congress Card Number 94-11110
Printed in the United States of America 1 2 3 4 5 6 7 8 9 0
Printed on acid-free paper

THE EDITOR

Ray F. Ebert received a B.S. degree in biology from Manhattan College in 1973, a M.S. degree in microbiology from Duquesne University in 1975, and a Ph.D. degree in biochemistry from the University of Pittsburgh in 1980. His work in dysfibrinogenemia began in 1980 as a postdoctoral fellow in the Hematology Division, Department of Medicine, at The Johns Hopkins University in collaboration with William R. Bell, M.D. The university presented two awards to Dr. Ebert for his research in this field: The Johns Hopkins School of Medicine Award for Postdoctoral Investigation and the John W. Graham Fund Award for Research.

During 1983 to 1986, as a research assistant in the Department of Medicine, Dr. Ebert received grants from the National Institutes of Health and the American Heart Association in support of dysfibrinogenemia-related studies. His contributions include the characterization of three "Baltimore" variants, among others, and he has developed or improved upon several high-performance liquid chromatography methods for amino acid analysis, peptide mapping, and measurement of fibrinopeptide release from fibrinogen. A long-term interest in computer programming and database management provided the background required for assembling the *Index of Variant Human Fibrinogens*, which was first distributed as a looseleaf version in 1990.

Currently, Dr. Ebert is employed as a Research Scientist Head with Organon Teknika/ Biotechnology Research Institute in Rockville, Maryland. In this capacity he directs an exploratory coagulation research group focused on generating new diagnostic assays for the Thrombosis-Hemostasis product line of Organon Teknika Corporation, Durham, North Carolina. In addition, he is responsible for research and development of KLH-Immune Activator™, an investigational new drug presently in clinical trials for nonspecific immunotherapy of bladder cancer. Professional memberships include the American Society for Biochemistry and Molecular Biology, the American Society of Hematology, the International Society on Thrombosis and Haemostasis, the International Fibrinogen Research Society, the American Chemical Society, and the Johns Hopkins Medical and Surgical Society.

TABLE OF CONTENTS

SECTION 1

BACKGROUND AND REFERENCE INFORMATION

PREFACE TO THE 1994 EDITION

At least 21 new variant fibrinogens have been identified and the literature on dysfibrinogenemia has increased by approximately 57 citations in the three years since the first edition of this book was published. The 1994 edition reviews a total of 263 variants (261 kindreds) and has as its main objective the presentation of a comprehensive compilation of the literature and results on dysfibrinogenemia for the period 1958—93, inclusive.

The positive response to the first edition of this book, both in published reviews[1,2] and from colleagues, has been most gratifying. Whereas the major challenge for that work was the design, assembly, and display of a database encompassing over 30 years of literature, the present edition seeks a better synthesis of that information to render it more comprehensible to the clinician as well as to the basic scientist. Thus, supplemental summaries that will assist in providing a better context for patient diagnosis and management have been added to Tables 3 through 9 (Section 2), and the scope of Section 1 has been broadened modestly to include revised/updated fibrinogen gene and protein sequences, listings of PCR primers and anti-fibrinogen antibodies, a Synopsis for Health Professionals, and expert guidance for the differential diagnosis and treatment of dysfibrinogenemia. Most of these enhancements have been made possible by contributions from other investigators, and sincere appreciation is extended to Dominic Chung, Gerard Connaghan, Harvey Gralnick, Gerd Grieninger, Susan Lord, and John Owen for their generous assistance.

Let me also express a special word of thanks to Dr. Michael G. Hanna, Jr., Chief Operating Officer of Organon Teknika/Biotechnology Research Institute and Sr. Vice-president of Organon Teknika Corporation, for supporting my work in hematology and fostering an environment conducive to exploratory research and timely publishing.

Users of the 1991 Edition will find the Summary Tables and Dysfibrinogen Reports in their familiar forms (Sections 2 and 3, respectively), and a 467-citation bibliography in Section 4. As before, responsibility for completeness and accuracy of this compendium lies with its editor, who has benefitted greatly from the advice and cooperation of several investigators, especially Drs. D.K. Galanakis, F. Haverkate, M. Matsuda, and M.W. Mosesson. Constructive criticisms and comments from all users are welcome and encouraged.

Time found to complete this endeavor represents for the most part time lost with my family: Thank you Mary, Peter, and Catherine, for not complaining about those weekend mornings when I was nowhere to be found. I'll be home soon . . .

Ray F. Ebert, Ph.D.
January, 1994

---

[1]M.W. Mosesson, *Blood Coag. & Fibrinoly.* **2**:681, 1991.
[2]R.G. Malia, SUBIS **8**:1, 1992.

PREFACE TO THE 1991 EDITION

Despite the publication of at least 70 reviews in the 33 years since the first congenitally variant human fibrinogen was recognized, *comprehensive and current* summaries of the literature in this field have not been readily available. This *Index* is offered with the objective of providing scientists and clinicians with a complete, timely, and useful compilation of the literature and results on dysfibrinogenemia.

Aside from formulating yet another answer to the question "How many dysfibrinogens *are* there. . ." several somewhat more important considerations prompted this work:

> The literature on variant fibrinogens continues to expand and shows few signs of abatement. For example, the database used to compile the *Index* contains 391 citations, over one-third of which were published during the past five years. In 1981, the mutations responsible for functional defects were known only for fibrinogens Detroit, Lille, Petoskey and Metz . . . less than 5% of the total. Today, the molecular defects have been identified in at least 77 variants (32% of the present total). The use of high-performance liquid chromatography — exemplified by Higgins and Shafer in 1981 with their determination of the amino acid substitution in fibrinogen Petoskey — has substantially shortened the time required to probe for structural abnormalities. More recently, polymerase chain reaction (PCR) technology was used by Koopman, Haverkate, and colleagues to identify a deletion of two amino acids in the γ-chain of fibrinogen Vlissingen, and by Galanakis, Henschen, and colleagues to identify Aα(16) Arg —> His substitutions in fibrinogens Hershey II and Leogan I. Now that the fibrinogen genes have been sequenced completely (see pp. 13 to 24), this alternate approach also is likely to catalyze the discovery of many more molecular defects.
>
> At the present rate of progress, by the end of this decade fundamental structure-function studies of variant human fibrinogens may well provide new knowledge regarding mutation mechanisms, polymorphism frequencies, protein-protein and protein-metal interactions, and mechanisms of subunit assembly. This information should complement other fields of research, from the Human Genome Project to thrombolytic therapy, but it needs better organization.
>
> Finally, the patients and families who have cooperated with investigators during these first 33 years merit our gratitude and support. They are likely to benefit from the availability of a centralized database from which clinical correlates may be developed.

Will the present pattern of periodic reviews satisfy the information requirements of the nineties? One may divide the many excellent review articles on the subject of dysfibrinogenemia into those that have taken a comprehensive look at the field and those that focussed on particular aspects of the disease (a bibliography is included in Section 4). Only four recent articles (covering 116-144 variants) fall into the former category [Lane & Southan, 1987; Bithell, 1985; Rocha, et al., 1985; and Rupp & Beck, 1984]. I am indebted to these authors, whose efforts provided an excellent foundation for the *Index*. However, it would be most inappropriate to compare this work with theirs: Whereas these and other reviewers compile selected information and choose what to emphasize and interpret, the principal aim of this *Index* is to provide a more comprehensive repository of information from which interpretations and generalizations may be made.

Thus, the *Index* contains 242 "Dysfibrinogen Reports" (Section 3) that are presented in a unified format and in much more detail than has been possible heretofore. The data elements in these reports were first entered into a computer database. From this core of information, tables summarizing related results have been assembled. This approach facilitates cross-comparisons and organizes the results in such a way that they may easily be accessed and understood.

It is important to emphasize that the *Index* should be regarded as a *secondary* source of information, a reference work. The refereed literature remains the appropriate forum for the introduction of new information in this field, and investigators are discouraged from submitting results that have not been published or accepted for publication elsewhere. At first, this stipulation presented a dilemma: Over 10% of known dysfibrinogens have been reported only in abstracts, and at least 5% have not been described in the published literature. Omission of these would have diminished the scope of the *Index*. Therefore, to ensure comprehensiveness without compromising rigor, abstracted or unpublished variants have been flagged with superscripts "Abs" or "Unp" to emphasize their special status, and only a limited amount of unpublished information is accepted (see p. 36).

A looseleaf version of the *Index of Variant Human Fibrinogens* describing 219 variants was first published in 1990. I am particularly grateful to Drs. Dennis K. Galanakis and Frits Haverkate for their advice, encouragement and assistance during the months preceding that publication. I am also indebted to the folks at CRC Press who recognized that this book should be made available to a wider audience, and who have committed to publishing at least two future editions at 18-24 month intervals. This 1991 edition has been slightly revised in format and extensively updated. If warranted by the pace of new discoveries, a pamphlet-sized mid-edition update containing revised tables and new variants will be provided at nominal cost to registered book owners.

In closing, I wish to thank my wife, Mary, and children, Peter and Catherine, for their patience, understanding and support during the preparation of both editions. And finally, let me acknowledge the investigators whose work is presented on these pages. Many of you already have provided reprints and translations of non-English publications. Your comments and constructive criticisms will be welcome always. Collectively, you represent the reviewers of this work; with your continued help, the *Index* will remain a useful and reliable compendium.

Ray F. Ebert, Ph.D.
December, 1990

How to use this *Index* . . .

What's inside: The 1994 *Index of Variant Human Fibrinogens* was compiled from a database that contains information on 263 dysfibrinogens described in the literature between 1958 and 1993. It is divided into four sections. **Section 1** contains general reference information about fibrinogen, dysfibrinogenemia and the database. **Section 2** contains tables summarizing this information, arranged in an order that corresponds to the format of the "Dysfibrinogen Reports." These reports on individual variants are listed alphabetically in **Section 3**. For a comprehensive bibliography of all literature citations in this book, consult **Section 4**.

Superscripts and abbreviations: All numeric superscripts refer to footnotes under **Remarks** at the end of each dysfibrinogen report (Section 3). The abbreviation "n.a." means the result was *not available* from the literature. If the information was available only from published abstracts, the superscript "Abs" appears after the variant name; if the information is unpublished, the superscript "Unp" appears after the variant name. See the "Detailed Description of Fields" (p. 36) for a complete explanation of each entry.

Last update: All entries from the 1991 Edition of this book were given a **Last update** of 1 December 1990. Additions or corrections have been made to 87 of these entries (including 21 new variants), and for this group the "Last update" field has been revised to 10 January 1994.

To locate information on a variant fibrinogen: If unsure of the spelling, or to determine if new information has been entered, locate the variant in Table 1 (p. 44), consult the "Last update" column, and then refer to Section 2 for comparative information or to Section 3 for information on the variant in question.

To compare one variant with others: Choose the characteristic of interest (e.g., abnormal prothrombin time or molecular defect), locate the corresponding table in Section 2 (See list on p. 43), and inspect the table to find all others with similar properties. After generating a list of relevant variants, refer to Section 3 for additional results or bibliographic information.

To find an article or review on dysfibrinogenemia: If the variant name is known, find its report in Section 3 and consult the references at the end. If the first author or publication year is known, consult Section 4, which contains 467 literature citations arranged alphabetically by first author in descending chronological order.

Note: Please consult the **Detailed Description of Fields** (p. 36) for formal definitions and criteria associated with each field in the dysfibrinogenemia database.

Synopsis for Health Professionals

General description. Congenital dysfibrinogenemia may be broadly defined as an inherited disease in which a somatic cell mutation yields a structurally altered form of fibrinogen. Given that the typical fibrinogen half-molecule contains 1497 amino acids, one would expect most of these mutations to be functionally silent and clinically insignificant. However, about 50% of all reported patients with a diagnosis of dysfibrinogenemia have been found to exhibit bleeding or thrombotic complications (p. 73). This apparent overrepresentation of symptomatic patients is due in large part to the process by which the dysfibrinogenemic patient comes to the attention of the clinician/investigator: an abnormal hematology lab result and/or unexplained coagulopathy. This biases the patient population (and correspondingly the literature and summary statistics in this book) in favor of individuals with functional abnormalities of fibrinogen.

For the sake of interpreting clinical signs and laboratory data it is instructive to consider the many functional defects that might be affected by mutation-induced structural changes: (i) The coagulation rate may be delayed by mutations affecting release of fibrinopeptides A and B by thrombin or fibrin monomer polymerization, and since these two processes are interdependent, both of them may be impaired in the same patient. In turn, this may affect patient hemostasis and clot-based assays. (ii) The rate of t-PA-catalyzed conversion of plasminogen to plasmin may be reduced, since fibrin is known to accelerate this reaction, or (iii) the rate of fibrinolysis may be reduced due to abnormal clot structure (See below: Dusart syndrome). In examples (ii) and (iii) a thrombotic tendency may develop. (iv) Fibrin support of platelet aggregation may be disabled. (v) Fibrin stabilization by factor XIIIa may be impaired, leading to inadequate hemostasis or wound dehiscence. (vi) Mutations affecting fibrinogen assembly, secretion, posttranslational modifications or plasma half-life may be responsible for abnormal concentrations in plasma. Unfortunately, given our present state of knowledge, the extent to which the foregoing functional abnormalities may influence the hemostatic system and laboratory analyses is difficult to predict. A more detailed discussion of differential diagnosis and treatment of dysfibrinogenemia by Drs. H.R. Gralnick and G.D. Connaghan begins on page 9.

Laboratory diagnosis. In the vast majority of reported cases, the structural defect inhibits the conversion of fibrinogen to fibrin, either by reducing the rate or extent of thrombin-catalyzed release of fibrinopeptides, or by interfering with fibrin monomer polymerization. Accordingly, clot-based assays such as the prothrombin time, partial thromboplastin time, thrombin time, and Reptilase (or ancrod) time frequently are abnormal (p. 87). Because it is the most sensitive and specific test for dysfibrinogenemia, the thrombin time is an essential component of the laboratory workup. Also useful is a comparison of plasma fibrinogen determinations via coagulation rate-dependent (e.g. von Clauss method) vs. rate-independent (e.g., Ratnoff method or immunoassay) techniques. The former usually yields an apparently subnormal value that falls within normal limits when a rate-independent assay is used (p. 80), except in cases of hypodysfibrinogenemia (see below). Recalcification time, bleeding and euglobulin lysis times, immunoelectrophoresis, and platelet aggregation studies have been less informative (p. 87) and therefore need not be done unless warranted by other clinical findings.

Hypodysfibrinogenemia. About 14% of reported dysfibrinogenemias (32 kindreds) also exhibit hypofibrinogenemia, which should be confirmed with an immunologic method. These patients generally are at much higher risk for abnormal bleeding; hence the importance of determining the true plasma fibrinogen concentration by means of a method that does not depend on the coagulation rate.

Homozygous vs. heterozygous expression. Dysfibrinogenemia is associated with an autosomal dominant inheritance pattern. About 10% (12/126) of families with dysfibrinogenemia have individuals who are homozygous for the phenotype. As expected, the disease is exacerbated among these patients, often with life-threatening consequences. Unfortunately, there are no routine laboratory tests that can distinguish between homo- and heterozygotes. Standard research techniques such as polyacrylamide gel electrophoresis, high-performance liquid chromatography and PCR analyses should be employed early in the course of an investigation since often they are able to elucidate homo- vs. heterozygous expression.

Dusart syndrome. Dysfibrinogenemia patients with thrombotic complications frequently have been found to exhibit impaired rates of fibrinolysis. Collet et al. (1993) have shown that clots generated from fibrinogen Dusart I (p. 176) have an altered structure characterized by shorter, narrower fibers, decreased gel porosity, and increased rigidity. These abnormal clots are resistant to fibrinolysis and consequently more thrombogenic than normal. Further, it was postulated that the risk of emboli in such patients was increased due to increased clot "brittleness." These authors have proposed the term "Dusart syndrome" to describe a dysfibrinogenemic condition characterized by severe, recurrent thrombotic disease associated with reduced fibrinolysis due to abnormal clot architecture.

Dysfibrinogenemia without coagulopathy. Recently, mutations near the C-terminus of the fibrinogen Aα-chain have been associated with hereditary renal amyloidosis, a late-onset disorder characterized by proteinuria, hypertension and azotemia (See fibrinogens Indianapolis I, II, and III; pp. 215-217). Deposits of both normal and variant fibrinogens (patients are heterozygotes) have been identified in kidneys of affected individuals. Importantly, of three different kindreds studied thus far, hematologic assays (including thrombin time) have been normal, and the subjects did not manifest any coagulation abnormalities. Thus, dysfibrinogenemia in association with renal amyloidosis represents a new subgrouping of "Dysfibringenemia without coagulopathy."

Differential Diagnosis and Treatment of Congenital Dysfibrinogenemia

Harvey R. Gralnick and Gerard D. Connaghan
Hematology Service
The National Institutes of Health
Bethesda, Maryland 20892

Differential diagnosis

All potential causes of delayed fibrinogen to fibrin conversion must be considered in the differential diagnosis of congenital dysfibrinogenemia. These can be divided into three major groups: those induced by structural changes in fibrinogen, those attributable to effects of other plasma proteins or drugs on fibrin formation, and those due to decreased plasma fibrinogen concentration.

Fetal fibrinogen circulates in newborns during the first 6 weeks of life. This normal variant exhibits delayed polymerization and a finer fibril network, both of which result from unusual posttranslational modifications including increased sialic acid[1,2] and phosphate[3] content, and missing N-terminal alanine in the Aα subunit.[4] Consequently, fetal fibrinogen often exhibits prolonged thrombin and Reptilase times. Thus, diagnosis of dysfibrinogenemia in the pre- or postnatal period is problematic.

In liver disease, acquired structural changes in fibrinogen often are characterized by an elevated sialic acid content and shortened fibrinogen survival.[5,6,7] The hypofibrinogenemia seen in this situation may reflect increased catabolism due to primary or secondary fibrinolysis, including disseminated intravascular coagulation (DIC), or the inhibitory activity of elevated circulating fibrinogen degradation products on coagulation-based tests.[8] Acquired dysfibrinogenemia also is seen in acute pancreatitis due to the effect of circulating proteases.[9] Finally, acquired dysfibrinogenemias may be associated with tumors, particularly primary or secondary hepatic malignancy, renal cell carcinoma and certain lymphomatous conditions in which elevated circulating sialyltransferase levels have been documented.[10,11,12] Acquired dysfibrinogenemia has been described following administration of Mithramycin to a patient with myeloma,[11] but myeloma itself has been associated with elevated sialytransferase activation in vivo.[12] These acquired dysfibrinogens are often but not exclusively found in association with increased branching of the oligosaccharides in the fibrinogen Bβ and γ chains. It is possible that acquired dysfibrinogens result from ontogenic reversion to fetal forms or altered carbohydrate processing in regenerating or neoplastic liver cells.[13] Family studies will help to distinguish congenital from acquired variants.

Plasma protein inhibitors of fibrin polymerization and stabilization have been described as occurring naturally[14,15] or in the setting of paraproteinemias or plasma cell disorders.[16] Such circulating anticoagulants (autoantibodies) have been described in systemic lupus erythematosus,[16] following drug therapy with isoniazid or procainamide[17,18] and in the settings of cryoglobulinemia,[19] macro-globulinemia[20] and multiple myeloma.[21] The paraprotein in these circumstances typically does not affect fibrinopeptide release, and the circulating fibrinogen concentration usually is normal. These autoantibodies may cause hemorrhage by themselves or may, in concert with other drugs such as heparin, inhibit the hemostatic process and result in bleeding.

In the hospital setting heparin contamination of the plasma sample is the most frequently noted cause of drug-associated prolongation of the thrombin time or activated PTT. This anomaly can be confirmed by the corrective effect of protamine sulfate, Hepa® or toluidine blue on the thrombin time, or by the performance of a Reptilase time, which is insensitive to heparin.[22] Prolonged thrombin *and* Reptilase times may signify either a dysfibrinogen with abnormal fibrinopeptide release or fibrinogen autoantibodies. In this case, plasma mixing experiments in which the thrombin time is corrected supports a diagnosis of dysfibrinogenemia.

Suramin or dermatan sulfate therapy may prolong coagulation tests, but the fibrinogen level usually is normal in this situation.[23] Elevated FDPs associated with DIC or fibrinolytic bleeding also will prolong the screening tests and should be excluded by specific assays. Expect the platelet count and platelet function to be normal in most dysfibrinogenemic states.

Acquired inhibitors of bovine thrombin, which occur in patients previously exposed to this agent during coronary bypass procedures, will spuriously prolong the thrombin time;[24] normalization of this assay when performed with human thrombin suggests this diagnosis. Thrombin time prolongation in the presence of normal fibrinogen has been seen in almost 50% of patients with systemic amyloidosis;[25] a correction to normal will be seen when the thrombin time is performed on the patient's isolated fibrinogen.

Hypofibrinogenemia is differentiated from dysfibrinogenemia by the uniformly subnormal plasma fibrinogen levels in the former, regardless of whether a rate-dependent (e.g., von Clauss) or rate-independent (e.g. immunologic) technique is used. Except in rare cases of hypodysfibrinogenemia, the patient with congenital dysfibrinogenemia will have normal plasma fibrinogen levels if the determination is made with a physical/chemical or immunologic method. Finally, in dysfibrinogenemia there is a greater abnormality in the thrombin time than would be expected relative to the observed fibrinogen concentration.

Drug-induced causes of hypofibrinogenemia, e.g. L-asparaginase[26] or valproic acid,[27] need to be excluded. Hyperfibrinogenemia has been reported in association with acquired neutrophil myeloperoxidase deficiency.[28] Potentially abnormal coagulation due to hyperfibrinogenemia also will be seen during the acute phase reaction[29,30] or associated with interleukin-6 therapy.[31,32]

Therapy and prognosis

Most patients with congenital dysfibrinogenemia are asymptomatic and require no therapy. In affected individuals, treatment typically is confined to the perioperative period or for acute bleeding events, with the objective of obtaining fibrinogen levels adequate for hemostasis and wound healing. Whole blood, fresh frozen plasma, fibrinogen concentrates and cryoprecipitates have been used by various investigators. However, commercial fibrinogen preparations are no longer available due the prohibitive incidence of hepatitis transmission and the risk of exposure to human immunodeficiency virus.

Cryoprecipitate infusions have been effective in patients undergoing major surgery and in stopping significant hemorrhage.[33,34] As the correlation between structural abnormality and clinical behavior is poorly defined for most of the dysfibrinogenemic defects, the patient's personal clinical history most specifically defines the need for replacement therapy, taking into consideration the requirement of a basal circulating (normal) fibrinogen level of approximately 50 mg per deciliter for adequate hemostasis. This recommendation assumes that patient fibrinogen does not inhibit normal fibrin coagulation, a possibility that can be excluded by plasma mixing studies.

Epsilon-aminocaproic acid administration was useful in preventing bleeding and wound dehiscence during surgery in a patient with fibrinogen Cleveland I.[35] In most congenital dysfibrinogenemias associated with thrombosis, anticoagulation with heparin followed by oral anticoagulants has proven efficacious and necessary. Long-term anticoagulation is indicated in those individuals who have repeated venous thrombosis or pulmonary embolization. If patient studies have progressed to the point where the molecular defect or other distinguishing features are known, comparisons with similar variants listed in this book may suggest additional treatment approaches.

References

1. Galanakis D.K. and Mosesson M.W. Evaluation of the role of in vivo proteolysis (fibrinogenolysis) in prolonging the thrombin time of human umbilical cord fibrinogen. *Blood* **48**:109, **1976.**

2. Guillin M. -C. and Ménaché D.: Fetal fibrinogen and fibrinogen Paris I: Comparative fibrin monomer aggregation studies. *Thromb. Res.* **3**:117, **1973.**

3. Seydewitz H.H., Kaiser C., Rothweiler H. and Witt I.: The location of a second in vivo phosphorylation site in the Aα-chain of human fibrinogen. *Thromb. Res.* **33**:487, **1984.**

4. Hasegawa N. and Sasaki S.: A deficiency in Aα chain's N-terminal alanine residue as a major cause of the slow coagulation of fetal fibrinogen. *Thromb. Res.* **54**:595, **1989.**

5. Martinez J., MacDonald V.A. and Palascak J.E.: The role of sialic acid in dysfibrinogenemia associated with liver disease. *Blood* **61**:1196, **1983.**

6. Regañon E., Vila V., Aznar J. et al: Study of the formation of fibrin clots in cirrhotic patients. An approach to study of acquired dysfibrinogenemia. *Thromb. Res.* **46**:705, **1987.**

7. Lipinski B., Lipinska I., Nowak A. et al: Abnormal fibrinogen heterogeneity and fibrinolytic activity in advanced liver disease. *J. Lab. Clin. Med.* **90**:187, **1977.**

8. Martinez J., MacDonald K.A. and Palascak J.E.: Thrombin and plasmin generation in patients with liver disease. *Amer. J. Hematol.* **32**:30, **1989.**

9. Wilde J.T., Thomas W.E.G., Lane D.A. et al: Acquired dysfibrinogenemia masquerading as disseminated intravascular coagulation in acute pancreatitis. *J. Clin. Pathol.* **41**:615, **1988.**

10. Francis J.L.: Acquired dysfibrinogenemia. In: *Fibrinogen, fibrin stabilization and fibrinolysis. Clinical Biochemical and Laboratory Aspects.* J.L. Francis (ed.) Ellis Harwood Publ., London; pp. 128-156, **1988.**

11. Ashby M.A. and Lazarchick J.: Acquired dysfibrinogenemia secondary to Mithramycin Toxicity. *Amer. J. Med. Sci.* **292**:53, **1986.**

12. Cohen A.M., Allalouf D., Bessler H. et al: Sialytransferase activity and sialic acid levels in multiple myeloma and monoclonal gammopathy. *Eur. J. Haematol.* **42**:289, **1989.**

13. Barr R.D., Allardyce M., Brunt P.W. et al: Dysfibrinogenemia and liver cell growth. *J. Clin. Pathol.* **31**:89, **1978.**

14. Marciniak E. and Greenwood M.F.: Acquired coagulation inhibitor delaying fibrinopeptide release. *Blood* **53**:81, **1979.**

15. Ruiz-Arguelles A. Spontaneous reversal of acquired autoimmune dysfibrinogenemia probably due to an anti-idiotypic antibody directed to an interspecies cross reactive idiotype expressed on antifibrinogen antibodies. *J. Clin. Invest.* **82**:958, **1988.**

16. Galanakis D.K., Ginzler E.M. and Fikrig S.M.: Monoclonal IgG anticoagulants delaying fibrin aggregation in two patients with systemic lupus erythematosus. *Blood* **52**:1037, **1978.**

17. Galanakis D.K., Newman J. and Summers D.: Circulating thrombin time anticoagulants in a procainamide-induced syndrome. *JAMA* **239**:1873, **1978.**

18. Otis P.T., Feinstein D.I., Rapaport S.I. et al: An acquired inhibitor of fibrin stabilization associated with isoniazid therapy: Clinical and biochemical observations. *Blood* **44**:771, **1974**.

19. Panzer, S. and Thaler E.: An acquired cryoglobulinemia which inhibits fibrin polymerization in a patient with IgG Kappa myeloma. *Haemostas.* **23**:69, **1993**.

20. Rosenberg R.D., Colman R.W. and Lorand L.: A new hemorrhagic disorder with defective fibrin stabilization and dysfibrinogenemia. *Brit. J. Haematol.* **26**:269, **1974**.

21. Coleman M., Vigilano E.M., Weksler M.E. et al: Inhibition of fibrin monomer polymerization by lambda myeloma globulins. *Blood* **39**:210, **1972**.

22. Funk C., Gmur J., Herold R. and Straub P.W.: Reptilase R - a new reagent in blood coagulation. *Brit. J. Haematol.* **21**:43, **1971**.

23. Horne III M.K., Wilson O.J., Cooper M., et al: The effect of suramin on laboratory tests of coagulation. *Thromb. Haemostas.* **4**:434, **1992**.

24. Lawson J.H., Pennell B.J., Olson J.D., et al: Isolation and Characterization of an acquired antithrombin antibody. *Blood* **76**:2249, **1990**.

25. Gastineau D.A., Gertz M.A., Daniels T.M. et al: Inhibitor of the thrombin time in systemic amyloidosis: A common coagulation abnormality. *Blood* **77**:2637, **1991**.

26. Gralnick H.R. and Henderson E.: Hypofibrinogenemia and coagulation factor deficiencies with L-asparaginase treatment. *Cancer* **27**:1313, **1971**.

27. Majer R.V. and Green P.J.: Neonatal afibrinogenemia due to sodium valproate. *Lancet* **11**:740, **1987**.

28. d'Onofrio G., Mancini R., Vallone R. et al: Acquired neutrophil myeloperoxidase deficiency: an indicator of subclinical activation of blood coagulation? *Blood Cells* **9**:455, **1983**.

29. Schultz D.R. and Arnold P.I.: Properties of four acute phase proteins: C-reactive protein, serum amyloid A protein, α_1-acid glycoprotein, and fibrinogen. *Semin. Arthritis Rheum.* **20**:129, **1990**.

30. Chooi C.C. and Gallus A.S.: Acute phase reaction, fibrinogen level and thrombus size. *Thromb. Res.* **53**:493, **1989**.

31. Amrani D.L.: Regulation of fibrinogen biosynthesis: glucocorticoid and interleukin-6 control. *Blood Coagul. Fibrinol.* **1**:443, **1990**.

32. Strassman G., Fong M., Windsor S. and Neta R.: The role of interleukin-6 in lipopolysaccharide-induced weight loss, hypoglycemia, and fibrinogen production, in vivo. *Cytokine* **5**:285, **1993**.

33. McLeod B., McKenna R. and Sassetti R.J.: Treatment of von Willebrand disease and hypofibrinogenemia with single donor cryoprecipitate from plasma exchange donation. *Amer. J. Haematol.* **32**:112, **1989**.

34. Ness P.M. and Perkins H.A.: Cryoprecipitate as a reliable source of fibrinogen replacement. *JAMA* **241**:1690, **1979**.

35. Forman W.B. and Kraus J. Transurethral resection in a patient with a dysfibrinogen: Fibrinogen Cleveland I. *J. Urol.* **118**:885, **1977**.

Fibrinogen DNA and Protein Sequences

CONTRIBUTED AND REVIEWED BY

Dominic W. Chung, Ph.D.
Department of Biochemistry
University of Washington
Seattle, WA 98195 USA

Gerd Grieninger, Ph.D.
Lindsley F. Kimball Research Institute
The New York Blood Center
310 E. 67th Street
New York, NY 10021 USA

Source publications for nucleotide sequences:

1. Chung, D.W., Harris, J.E. and Davie, E.W. Nucleotide sequences of the three genes coding for human fibrinogen. In: *Fibrinogen, Thrombosis, Coagulation, and Fibrinolysis*, C.Y. Liu and S. Chien. (eds.); Plenum Press, NY; pp. 39-48, **1990**.

2. Fu, Y., Weissbach, L., Plant, P.W., Oddoux, C., Cao, Y., Liang, T.J., Roy, S.N., Redman, C.M. and Grieninger, G. Carboxy-terminal-extended variant of the human fibrinogen α subunit: A novel exon conferring marked homology to β and γ subunits. *Biochem. USA* **31**:11968-11972, **1992**.

Editor's note: *The significant contributions of R.F. Doolittle, A. Henschen and their associates to elucidation of fibrinogen primary structure are respectfully acknowledged.*

DNA and Protein Sequences

Human Fibrinogen Amino Acid Sequences

Aα Chain

NBRF-PIR accession no. A03116

```
      -19  MFSMRIVCLV LSVVGTAWT -1

ADSGEGDFLA EGGGVRGPRV VERHQSACKD SDWPFCSDED WNYKCPSGCR MKGLIDEVNQ DFTNRINKLK NSLFEYQKNN KDSHSLTTNI MEILRGDFSS  100
ANNRDNTYNR VSEDLRSRIE VLKRKVIEKV QHIQLLQKNV RAQLVDMKRL EVDIDIKIRS CRGSCSRALA REVDLKDYED QQKQLEQVIA KDLLPSRDRQ  200
HLPLIKMKPV PDLVPGNFKS QLQKVPPEWK ALTDMPQMRM ELERPGGNEI TRGGSTSYGT GSETESPRNP SSAGSWNSGS SGPGSTGNRN PGSSGTGGTA  300
TWKPGSSGPG STGSWNSGSS GTGSTGNQNP GSPRPGSTGT WNPGSSERGS AGHWTSESSV SGSTGQWHSE SGSFRPDSPG SGNARPNNPD WGTFEEVSGN  400
VSPGTRREYH TEKLVTSKGD KELRTGKEKV TSGSTTTTRR SCSKTVTKTV IGPDGHKEVT KEVVTSEDGS DCPEAMDLGT LSGIGTLDGF RHRHPDEAAF  500
FDTASTGKTF PGFFSPMLGE FVSETESRGS ESGIFTNTKE SSSHHPGIAE FPSRGKSSSY SKQFTSSTSY NRGDSTFESK SYKMADEAGS EADHEGTHST  600
KRGHAKSRPV RGIHTSPLGK PSLSP                                                                                  625
```

$A\alpha_E$ Chain

```
      -19  MFSMRIVCLV LSVVGTAWT -1

ADSGEGDFLA EGGGVRGPRV VERHQSACKD SDWPFCSDED WNYKCPSGCR MKGLIDEVNQ DFTNRINKLK NSLFEYQKNN KDSHSLTTNI MEILRGDFSS  100
ANNRDNTYNR VSEDLRSRIE VLKRKVIEKV QHIQLLQKNV RAQLVDMKRL EVDIDIKIRS CRGSCSRALA REVDLKDYED QQKQLEQVIA KDLLPSRDRQ  200
HLPLIKMKPV PDLVPGNFKS QLQKVPPEWK ALTDMPQMRM ELERPGGNEI TRGGSTSYGT GSETESPRNP SSAGSWNSGS SGPGSTGNRN PGSSGTGGTA  300
TWKPGSSGPG STGSWNSGSS GTGSTGNQNP GSPRPGSTGT WNPGSSERGS AGHWTSESSV SGSTGQWHSE SGSFRPDSPG SGNARPNNPD WGTFEEVSGN  400
VSPGTRREYH TEKLVTSKGD KELRTGKEKV TSGSTTTTRR SCSKTVTKTV IGPDGHKEVT KEVVTSEDGS DCPEAMDLGT LSGIGTLDGF RHRHPDEAAF  500
FDTASTGKTF PGFFSPMLGE FVSETESRGS ESGIFTNTKE SSSHHPGIAE FPSRGKSSSY SKQFTSSTSY NRGDSTFESK SYKMADEAGS EADHEGTHST  600
KRGHAKSRPV RDCDDVLQTH PSGTQSGIFN IKLPGSSKIF SVYCDQETSL GGWLLIQQRM DGSLNFNRTW QDYKRGFGSL NDEGEGEFWL GNDYLHLLTQ  700
RGSVLRVELE DWAGNEAYAE YHFRVGSEAE GYALQVSSYE GTAGDALIEG SVEEGAEYTS HNNMQFSTFD RDADQWEENC AEVYGGGWWY NNCQAANLNG  800
IYYPGGSYDP RNNSPYEIEN GVVWVSFRGA DYSLRAVRMK IRPLVTQ                                                          847
```

Bβ Chain

NBRF-PIR accession nos. B43568; A90469; B90469; A94433; A90437; A94309

```
      -30  MKRMVSWSFH KLKTMKHLLL LLLCVFLVKS -1

QGVNDNEEGF FSARGHRPLD KKREEAPSLR PAPPPISGGG YRARPAKAAA TQKKVERKAP DAGGCLHADP DLGVLCPTGC QLQEALLQQE RPIRNSVDEL  100
NNNVEAVSQT SSSSFQYMYL LKDLWQKRQK QVKDNENVVN EYSSELEKHQ LYIDETVNSN IATNLRVLRS ILENLRSKIQ KLESDVSAQM EYCRTPCTVS  200
CNIPVVSGKE CEEIIRKGGE TSEMYLIQPD SSVKPYRVYC DMNTENGGWT VIQNRQDGSV DFGRKWDPYK QGFGNVATNT DGKNYCGLPG EYWLGNDKIS  300
QLTRMGPTEL LIEMEDWKGD KVKAHYGGFT VQNEANKYQI SVNKYRGTAG NALMDGASQL MGENRTMTIH NGMFFSTYDR DNDGWLTSDP RKQCSKEDGG  400
GWWYNRCHAA NPNGRYYWGG QYTWDMAKHG TDDGVVWMNW KGSWYSMRKM SMKIRPFFPQ Q                                          461
```

γ-Val411 Chain

NBRF-PIR accession no. A03125

```
      -26  MSWSLHPRNL ILYFYALLFL SSTCVA -1

YVATRDNCCI LDERFGSYCP TTCGIADFLS TYQTKVDKDL QSLEDILHQV ENKTSEVKQL IKAIQLTYNP DESSKPNMID AATLKSRKML EEIMKYEASI  100
LTHDSSIRYL QEIYNSNNQK IVNLKEKVAQ LEAQCQEPCK DTVQIHDITG KDCQDIANKG AKQSGLYFIK PLKANQQFLV YCEIDGSGNG WTVFQKRLDG  200
SVDFKKNWIQ YKEGFGHLSP TGTTEFWLGN EKIHLISTQS AIPYALRVEL EDWNGRTSTA DYAMFKVGPE ADKYRLTYAY FAGGDAGDAF DGFDFGDDPS  300
DKFFTSHNGM QFSTWDNDND KFEGNCAEQD GSGWWMNKCH AGHLNGVYYQ GGTYSKASTP NGYDNGIIWA TWKTRWYSMK KTTMKIIPFN RLTIGEGQQH  400
HLGGAKQAGD V                                                                                                 411
```

γ-Pro423 Chain

```
408  VRP EHPAETEYDS LYP  423
```

NBRF-PIR accession no. A03126

γ-Leu427 Chain

```
408  VRP EHPAETEYDS LYPEDDL  427
```

NBRF-PIR accession no. A03126

Editor's note: Consult pp. 17, 21, and 24 for a discussion of polymorphisms in the sequences given above.

DNA and Protein Sequences

Human Fibrinogen Aα-Chain Gene Sequence

GenBank accession no. M64982

```
                                     [-19]Met Phe Ser Met Arg Ile Val Cys Leu Val Leu Ser Val Val Gly Thr Ala Trp[-2]
GTCTAGGAGC CAGCCCCACC CTTAGAAAAG ] ATG TTT TCC ATG AGG ATC GTC TGC CTA GTT CTA AGT GTG GTG GGC ACA GCA TGG        84

[ GTATGGCCCT TTTCATTTTT TCTTCTTGCT TTCTCTCTGG TGTTTATTCC ACAAAGAGCC TGGAGGTCAG AGTCTACCTG CTCTATGTCC TGACAC     180
ACTCTTAGCT TTATGACCCC AGGCCTGGGA GGAAATTTCC TGGGTGGGCT TGACACCTCA AGAATACAGG GTAATATGAC ACCAAGAGGA AGATCTTAGA   280
TGGATGAGAG TGTACAACTA CAAGGGAAAC TTTAGCATCT GTCATTCAGT CTTACCACAT TTTGTTTTGT TTTGTTTTAA AAAGGGCAAG AATTATTTGC   380
CATCCTTGTA CCTATAAAGC CTTGGTGCAT TATAATGCTA GTTAATGGAA TAAAACATTT TATGGTAAGA TTTGTTTTCT TTAGTTATTA ATTTCTTGCT   480
ACTTGTCCAT AATAAGCAGA ACTTTTAGTG TTAGTACAGT TTTGCTGAAA GGTTATTGTT GTGTTTGTCA AGACAGAAGA AAAAGCAAAC GAATTATCTT   580
TGGAAATATC TTTGCAGTAT CAGAAGAGAT TAGTTAGTAA GGCAATACGC TTTTCCGCAG TAATGGTATT CTTTTAAATT ATGAATCCAT CTCTAAAGGT   680
TACATAGAAA CTTGAAGGAG AGAGGAACAT TCAGTTAAGA TAGTCTAGGT TTTTCTACTG AAGCAGCAAT TACAGGAGAA AGAGCTCTAC AGTAGTTTTC   780
AACTTTCTGT CTGCAGTCAT TAGTAAAAAT GAAAAGGTAA AATTTAACTG ATTTTATAGA TTCAAATAAT TTTCCTTTTA GGATGGATTC TTTAAAACTC   880
CTAATATTTA TCAAATGCTT ATTTAAGTGT CACACACAGT TAAGAAATTT GTACACCTTG TCTCCTTTAA TTCTCATAAC AACTCCATAA AATGGGTCCT   980
AGGATTTCCA TTTGAAGATA AGAAACCTGA AGCTTGCCGA AGCCCTGTGT CTGCTCTCCT TAATCTCTGT GAGAGTGCCA TCTCTTCCTG GGGACTTGTA  1080

                                                                              [-1]Thr [+1]Ala Asp Ser Gly Glu
GGCATGCCAC TGTCTCCTCT TCTGGCTAAC ATTGCTGTTG CTCTCTTTTG TGTATGTGAA TGAATCTTTA AAG ]  ACT    GCA GAT AGT GGT GAA  1171

[6]Gly Asp Phe Leu Ala Glu Gly Gly Gly Val Arg Gly Pro Arg Val Val Glu Arg His Gln Ser Ala Cys Lys Asp Ser Asp
   GGT GAC TTT CTA GCT GAA GGA GGA GGC GTG CGT GGC CCA AGG GTT GTG GAA AGA CAT CAA TCT GCC TGC AAA GAT TCA GAC   1252

[33]Trp Pro Phe Cys Ser Asp Glu Asp Trp[41]
    TGG CCC TTC TGC TCT GAT GAA GAC TGG    [ GTAAGCAGTC AGCGGGGGAA GCAGGAGATT CCTTCCCTCT GATGCTAGAG GGGCTCACAG   1339
GCTGACCTGA TTGGTCCCAG AAACTTTTTT AAATAGAAAA TAATTGAATA GTTACCTACA TAGCAAATAA AGAAAAGGAA CCTACTCCCA AGAGCACTGT    1439
TTATTTACCT CCCCAACTCT GGATCATTAG TGGGTGAACA GACAGGATTT CAGTTGCATG CTCAGGCAAA ACCAGGCTCC TGAGTATTGT GGCCTCAATT    1539
TCCTGGCACC TATTTATGGC TAAGTGGACC CTCATTCCAG AGTTTCTCTG CGACCTCTAA CTAGTCCTCT TACCTACTTT TAAGCCAACT TATCTGGAAG    1639
AGAAAGGGTA GGAAGAAATG GGGGCTGCAT GGAAACATGC AAAATTATTC TGAATCTGAG AGATAGATCC TTACTGTAAT TTTCTCCCTT CACTTTCAG ]  1738

                         *
[42]Asn Tyr Lys Cys Pro Ser Gly Cys Arg Met Lys Gly Leu Ile Asp Glu Val Asn Gln Asp Phe Thr Asn Arg Ile Asn Lys
    AAC TAC AAA TGC CCT TCT GGC TGC AGG ATG AAA GGG TTG ATT GAT GAA GTC AAT CAA GAT TTT ACA AAC AGA ATA AAT AAG  1819

[69]Leu Lys Asn Ser Leu Phe Glu Tyr Gln Lys Asn Asn Lys Asp Ser His Ser Leu Thr Thr Asn Ile Met Glu Ile Leu Arg
    CTC AAA AAT TCA CTA TTT GAA TAT CAG AAG AAC AAT AAG GAT TCT CAT TCG TTG ACC ACT AAT ATA ATG GAA ATT TTG AGA  1900

[96]Gly Asp Phe Ser Ser Ala Asn[102]
    GGC GAT TTT TCC TCA GCC AAT A [ GTAAGTATT ACATATTTAC TTCTTTGACT TTATAACAGA AACAACAAAA ATCCTAAATA AATATGATAT  1991
CCGCTTATAT CTATGACAAT TTCATCCCAA AGTACTTAGT GTAGAAACAC ATACCTTCAT AATATCCCTG AAAATTTTAA GAGGGAGCTT TTGTTTTCGT    2091
TATTTTTTCA AAGTAAAAGA TGTTAACTGA GATTGTTTAA GGTCACAAAA TAAGTCAGAA TTTTGGATTA AAACAAGAAT TTAAATGTGT TCTTTTCAAC    2191
AGTATATACT GAAAGTAGGA TGGGTCAGAC TCTTTGAGTT GATATTTTTG TTTCTGCTTT GTAAAGGTGA AAACTGAGAG GTCAAGGAAC TTGTTCAAAG    2291
ACACAGAGCT GGGAATTCAA CTCCCAGACT CCACTGAGCT GATTAGGTAG ATTTTTAAAT TTAAAATATA GGGTCAAGCT ACGTCATTCT CACAGTCTAC    2391
TCATTAGGGT TAGGAAACAT TGCATTCACT CTGGGCATGG ACAGCGAGTC TAGGGAGTCC TCAGTTTCTC AAGTTTTGCT TTGCCTTTTT ACACCTTCAC    2491
AAACACTTGA CATTTAAAAT CAGTGATGCC AACACTAGCT GGCAAGTGAG TGATCCTGTT GACCCAAAAC AGCTTAGGAA CCATTTCAAA TCTATAGAGT    2591
TAAAAAGAAA AGCTCATCAG TAAGAAAATC CAATATGTTC AAGTCCCTTG ATTAAGGATG TTATAAAATA ATTGAAATGC AATCAAACCA ACTATTTTAA    2691
CTCCAAATTA CACCTTTAAA ATTCCAAAGA AAGTTCTTCT TCTATATTTC TTTGGGATTA CTAATTGCTA TTAGGACATC TTAACTGGCA TTCATGGAAG    2791
GCTGCAGGGC ATAACATTAT CCAAAAGTCA AATGCCCCAT AGGTTTTGAA CTCACAGATT AAACTGTAAC CAAAATAAAA TTAGGCATAT TTACAAGCTA    2891
GTTTCTTTCT TTCTTTTTTC TCTTTCTTTC TTTCTTTCTT TCTTTCTTTC TTTCTTTCTT TCTTTCTTTC TTTCTCCTTC CTTCCTTTCT TCCTTTCTTT    2991

                                                                   [103]Asn Arg Asp Asn Thr Tyr Asn Arg Val Ser
TTTGCTGGCA ATTACAGACA AATCACTCAG CAGCTACTTC AATAACCATA TTTTCGATTT CAG ]  AC CGT GAT AAT ACC TAC AAC CGA GTG TCA  3083

[113]Glu Asp Leu Arg Ser Arg Ile Glu Val Leu Lys Arg Lys Val Ile Glu Lys Val Gln His Ile Gln Leu Leu Gln Lys Asn
     GAG GAT CTG AGA AGC AGA ATT GAA GTC CTG AAG CGC AAA GTC ATA GAA AAA GTA CAG CAT ATC CAG CTT CTG CAG AAA AAT  3164

[140]Val Arg Ala Gln Leu Val Asp Met Lys Arg Leu Glu[151]
     GTT AGA GCT CAG TTG GTT GAT ATG AAA CGA CTG GAG    [ GTAAGTATGT GGCTGTGGTC CCGAGTGTCC TTGTTTTTGA GTAGAGGGAA  3250
```

*Denotes a polymorphic site; see Notes, p. 17.

DNA and Protein Sequences

Human Fibrinogen Aα-Chain Gene Sequence (continued)

GenBank accession no. M64982

```
AAGGAAGGCG ATAGTTATGC ACTGAGTGTC TACTATATGC AGAGAAAAGT GTTATATCCA TCATCTACCT AAAAGTAGGT ATTATTTTCC TCACTCCACA  3350
GTTGAAGAAA AAAAAATTCA GAGATATTAA GTAAATTTTC CAACGTACAT AGATAGTAAT TCAAAGCAAT GTTCAGTCCC TGTCTATTCC AAGCCATTAC  3450
ATCACCACAC CTCTGAGCCC TCAGCCTGAG TTCACCAAGG ATCATTTAAT TAGCGTTTCC TTTGAGAGGG AATAGCACCT TACTCTTGAT CCATTCTGAG  3550
GCTAAGATGA ATTAAACAGC ATCCATTGCT TATCCTGGCT AGCCCTGCAA TACCCAACAT CTCTTCCACT GAGGGTGCTC GATAGGCAGA AAACAGAGAA  3650
TATTAAGTGG TAGGTCTCCG AGTCAAAAAA AATGAAACCA GTTTCCAGAA GGAAAATTAA CTACCAGGAA CTCAATAGAC GTAGTTTATG TATTTGTATC  3750

                                 152 Val Asp Ile Asp Ile Lys Ile Arg Ser Cys Arg Gly Ser Cys Ser Arg Ala
TACATTTTCT CTTTATTTTT CTCCCCTCTC TCTAG | GTG GAC ATT GAT ATT AAG ATC CGA TCT TGT CGA GGG TCA TGC AGT AGG GCT  3836

169Leu Ala Arg Glu Val Asp Leu Lys Asp Tyr Glu Asp Gln Gln Lys Gln Leu Glu Gln Val Ile Ala Lys Asp Leu Leu Pro
   TTA GCT CGT GAA GTA GAT CTG AAG GAC TAT GAA GAT CAG CAG AAG CAA CTT GAA CAG GTC ATT GCC AAA GAC TTA CTT CCC  3917

196Ser Arg Asp Arg Gln His Leu Pro Leu Ile Lys Met Lys Pro Val Pro Asp Leu Val Pro Gly Asn Phe Lys Ser Gln Leu
   TCT AGA GAT AGG CAA CAC TTA CCA CTG ATA AAA ATG AAA CCA GTT CCA GAC TTG GTT CCC GGA AAT TTT AAG AGC CAG CTT  3998

223Gln Lys Val Pro Pro Glu Trp Lys Ala Leu Thr Asp Met Pro Gln Met Arg Met Glu Leu Glu Arg Pro Gly Gly Asn Glu
   CAG AAG GTA CCC CCA GAG TGG AAG GCA TTA ACA GAC ATG CCG CAG ATG AGA ATG GAG TTA GAG AGA CCT GGT GGA AAT GAG  4079

250Ile Thr Arg Gly Gly Ser Thr Ser Tyr Gly Thr Gly Ser Glu Thr Glu Ser Pro Arg Asn Pro Ser Ser Ala Gly Ser Trp
   ATT ACT CGA GGA GGC TCC ACC TCT TAT GGA ACC GGA TCA GAG ACG GAA AGC CCC AGG AAC CCT AGC AGT GCT GGA AGC TGG  4160
                                                                                *
277Asn Ser Gly Ser Ser Gly Pro Gly Ser Thr Gly Asn Arg Asn Pro Gly Ser Ser Gly Thr Gly Gly Thr Ala Thr Trp Lys
   AAC TCT GGG AGC TCT GGA CCT GGA AGT ACT GGA AAC CGA AAC CCT GGG AGC TCT GGG ACT GGA GGG ACT GCA ACC TGG AAA  4241
                                    *
304Pro Gly Ser Ser Gly Pro Gly Ser Ala Gly Ser Trp Asn Ser Gly Ser Ser Gly Thr Gly Ser Thr Gly Asn Gln Asn Pro
   CCT GGG AGC TCT GGA CCT GGA AGT GCT GGA AGC TGG AAC TCT GGG AGC TCT GGA ACT GGA AGT ACT GGA AAC CAA AAC CCT  4322

331Gly Ser Pro Arg Pro Gly Ser Thr Gly Thr Trp Asn Pro Gly Ser Ser Glu Arg Gly Ser Ala Gly His Trp Thr Ser Glu
   GGG AGC CCT AGA CCT GGT AGT ACC GGA ACC TGG AAT CCT GGC AGC TCT GAA CGC GGA AGT GCT GGG CAC TGG ACC TCT GAG  4403

358Ser Ser Val Ser Gly Ser Thr Gly Gln Trp His Ser Glu Ser Gly Ser Phe Arg Pro Asp Ser Pro Gly Ser Gly Asn Ala
   AGC TCT GTA TCT GGT AGT ACT GGA CAA TGG CAC TCT GAA TCT GGA AGT TTT AGG CCA GAT AGC CCA GGC TCT GGG AAC GCG  4484

385Arg Pro Asn Asn Pro Asp Trp Gly Thr Phe Glu Glu Val Ser Gly Asn Val Ser Pro Gly Thr Arg Arg Glu Tyr His Thr
   AGG CCT AAC AAC CCA GAC TGG GGC ACA TTT GAA GAG GTG TCA GGA AAT GTA AGT CCA GGG ACA AGG AGA GAG TAC CAC ACA  4565

412Glu Lys Leu Val Thr Ser Lys Gly Asp Lys Glu Leu Arg Thr Gly Lys Glu Lys Val Thr Ser Gly Ser Thr Thr Thr Thr
   GAA AAA CTG GTC ACT TCT AAA GGA GAT AAA GAG CTC AGG ACT GGT AAA GAG AAG GTC ACC TCT GGT AGC ACA ACC ACC ACG  4646

439Arg Arg Ser Cys Ser Lys Thr Val Thr Lys Thr Val Ile Gly Pro Asp Gly His Lys Glu Val Thr Lys Glu Val Val Thr
   CGT CGT TCA TGC TCT AAA ACC GTT ACT AAG ACT GTT ATT GGT CCT GAT GGT CAC AAA GAA GTT ACC AAA GAA GTG GTG ACC  4727

466Ser Glu Asp Gly Ser Asp Cys Pro Glu Ala Met Asp Leu Gly Thr Leu Ser Gly Ile Gly Thr Leu Asp Gly Phe Arg His
   TCC GAA GAT GGT TCT GAC TGT CCC GAG GCA ATG GAT TTA GGC ACA TTG TCT GGC ATA GGT ACT CTG GAT GGG TTC CGC CAT  4808

493Arg His Pro Asp Glu Ala Ala Phe Phe Asp Thr Ala Ser Thr Gly Lys Thr Phe Pro Gly Phe Phe Ser Pro Met Leu Gly
   AGG CAC CCT GAT GAA GCT GCC TTC TTC GAC ACT GCC TCA ACT GGA AAA ACA TTC CCA GGT TTC TTC TCA CCT ATG TTA GGA  4889

520Glu Phe Val Ser Glu Thr Glu Ser Arg Gly Ser Glu Ser Gly Ile Phe Thr Asn Thr Lys Glu Ser Ser Ser His His Pro
   GAG TTT GTC AGT GAG ACT GAG TCT AGG GGC TCA GAA TCT GGC ATC TTC ACA AAT ACA AAG GAA TCC AGT TCT CAT CAC CCT  4970

547Gly Ile Ala Glu Phe Pro Ser Arg Gly Lys Ser Ser Ser Tyr Ser Lys Gln Phe Thr Ser Ser Thr Ser Tyr Asn Arg Gly 573
   GGG ATA GCT GAA TTC CCT TCC CGT GGT AAA TCT TCA AGT TAC AGC AAA CAA TTT ACT AGT AGC ACG AGT TAC AAC AGA GGA  5051
```

*Denotes a polymorphic site; see Notes, p. 17.

DNA and Protein Sequences

Human Fibrinogen Aα-Chain Gene Sequence (continued)

GenBank accession no. M64982

```
574Asp Ser Thr Phe Glu Ser Lys Ser Tyr Lys Met Ala Asp Glu Ala Gly Ser Glu Ala Asp His Glu Gly Thr His Ser Thr
   GAC TCC ACA TTT GAA AGC AAG AGC TAT AAA ATG GCA GAT GAG GCC GGA AGT GAA GCC GAT CAT GAA GGA ACA CAT AGC ACC  5132

601Lys Arg Gly His Ala Lys Ser Arg Pro Val Arg Gly Ile His Thr Ser Pro Leu Gly Lys Pro Ser Leu Ser Pro625 END
   AAG AGA GGC CAT GCT AAA TCT CGC CCT GTC AGA GGT ATC CAC ACT TCT CCT TTG GGG AAG CCT TCC CTG TCC CCC   TAG  5210

ACTAAGTTAA ATATTTCTGC ACAGTGTTCC CATGGCCCCT TGCATTTCCT TCTTAACTCT CTGTTACACG TCATTGAAAC TACACTTTTT TGGTCTGTTT  5310
TTGTGCTAGA CTGTAAGTTC CTTGGGGGCA GGGCCTTTGT CTGTCTCATC TCTGTATTCC CAAATGCCTA ACAGTACAGA GCCATGACTC AATAAATACA  5410
                    ↓
TGTTAAATGG ATGAATGAAT TCCTCTGAAA CTCTATTTGA GCTTATTTAG TCAAATTCTT TCACTATTCA AAGTGTGTGC TATTAGAATT GTCACCCAAC  5510
TGATTAATCA CATTTTTAGT ATGTGTCTCA GTTGACATTT AGGTCAGGCT AAATACAAGT TGTGTTAGTA TTAAGTGAGC TTAGCTACCT GTACTGGTTA  5610
CTTGCTATTA GTTTGTGCAA GTAAAATTCC AAATACATTT GAGGAAAATC CCCTTTGCAA TTTGTAGGTA TAAATAACCG CTTATTTGCA TAAGTTCTAT  5710
CCCACTGTAA GTGCATCCTT TCCCTATGGA GGGAAGGAAA GGAGGAAGAA AGAAAGGAAG GGAAAGAAAC AGTATTTGCC TTATTTAATC TGAGCCGTGC  5810
CTATCTTTGT AAAGTTAAAT GAGAATAACT TCTTCCAACC AGCTTAATTT TTTTTTTAGA CTGTGATGAT GTCCTCCAAA CACATCCTTC AGGTACCCAA  5910
AGTGGCATTT TCAATATCAA GCTATCCGGA TCC
                                                                                                           5943
```

Underlining denotes poly(A) signal. ↓ Denotes poly(A) site.

Notes

★ There are three known polymorphic sites in the Aα chain:

Aα(47) Ser[TCT] ↔ Thr[ACT]
Aα(296) Thr[ACT] ↔ Ala[GCT]
Aα(312) Thr[ACT] ↔ Ala[GCT]

As discussed by Henschen and McDonagh (*Blood Coagulation*, R.F.A. Zwaal & H.C. Hemker (eds.) Elsevier Science Publ., Amsterdam; pp. 205-206, **1986**), all three polymorphic amino acid pairs have been detected by DNA and protein sequencing. However, Baumann and Henschen (*Blood* **82**:2117-24, **1993**), using RFLP of PCR-amplified segments, were able to confirm polymorphisms only at Aα(312) in a sample of 110 healthy subjects. The reported Thr/Ala allele frequency at this site was 0.76/0.24.

DNA and Protein Sequences

Human Fibrinogen Aα_E-Chain Gene Sequence

GenBank accession no. M64982 (Aα); M58569 (Aα_E)

Fu et al. (*Biochem. USA* **31**:11968-11972; **1992**) have described a carboxy-terminal-extended variant of the human fibrinogen Aα chain (Aα_E). Alternative splicing of a bipartite transcript leads to expression of this Aα_E chain, which is identical to the Aα chain through Arg_{611}, but has an additional 236 amino acids that are homologous to C-terminal regions of the Bβ- and γ chains. The extension is encoded by a heretofore unrecognized sixth exon corresponding to a second reading frame of the bipartite transcript. It is estimated that about 1-2% of circulating fibrinogen contains the Aα_E subunit (Fu & Grieninger, *Proc. Natl. Acad. Sci. USA* **91**:2625-2628, **1994**). Presented below is the elongated 3' sequence of the Aα-chain gene showing overlap with the predominant Aα-chain coding region and the intron E splice sites.

```
574Asp Ser Thr Phe Glu Ser Lys Ser Tyr Lys Met Ala Asp Glu Ala Gly Ser Glu Ala Asp His Glu Gly Thr His Ser Thr
   GAC TCC ACA TTT GAA AGC AAG AGC TAT AAA ATG GCA GAT GAG GCC GGA AGT GAA GCC GAT CAT GAA GGA ACA CAT AGC ACC  5132

601Lys Arg Gly His Ala Lys Ser Arg Pro Val Arg611
   AAG AGA GGC CAT GCT AAA TCT CGC CCT GTC AGA G           [ GTAT CCACACTTCT CCTTTGGGGA AGCCTTCCCT GTCCCCCTAG  5210
ACTAAGTTAA ATATTTCTGC ACAGTGTTCC CATGGCCCCT TGCATTTCCT TCTTAACTCT CTGTTACACG TCATTGAAAC TACACTTTTT TGGTCTGTTT  5310
TTGTGCTAGA CTGTAAGTTC CTTGGGGGCA GGGCCTTTGT CTGTCTCATC TCTGTATTCC CAAATGCCTA ACAGTACAGA GCCATGACTC AATAAATACA  5410
TGTTAAATGG ATGAATGAAT TCCTCTGAAA CTCTATTTGA GCTTATTTAG TCAAATTCTT TCACTATTCA AAGTGTGTGC TATTAGAATT GTCACCCAAC  5510
TGATTAATCA CATTTTTAGT ATGTGTCTCA GTTGACATTT AGGTCAGGCT AAATACAAGT TGTGTTAGTA TTAAGTGATG CTTAGCTACC TGTACTGGTT  5610
ACTTGCTATT AGTTTGTGCA AGTAAAATTC CAAATACATT TGAGGAAAAT CCCCTTTGCA ATTTGTAGGT ATAAATAACC GCTTATTTGC ATAAGTTCTA  5710
TCCCACTGTA AGTGCATCCT TTCCCTATGG AGGGAAGGAA AGGAGGAAGA AAGAAAGGAA GGGAAAGAAA CAGTATTTGC CTTATTTAAT CTGAGCCGTG  5810
CCTATCTTTG TAAAGTTAAA TGAGAATAAC TTCTTCCAAC CAGCTTAATT TTTTTTTTAG ]                                           5870

612Asp Cys Asp Asp Val Leu Gln Thr His Pro Ser Gly Thr Gln Ser Gly Ile Phe Asn Ile Lys Leu Pro Gly Ser Ser Lys
    AC TGT GAT GAT GTC CTC CAA ACA CAT CCT TCA GGT ACC CAA AGT GGC ATT TTC AAT ATC AAG CTA CCG GGA TCC AGT AAG  5950

639Ile Phe Ser Val Tyr Cys Asp Gln Glu Thr Ser Leu Gly Gly Trp Leu Leu Ile Gln Gln Arg Met Asp Gly Ser Leu Asn
   ATT TTT TCT GTT TAT TGC GAT CAA GAG ACC AGT TTG GGA GGA TGG CTT TTG ATC CAG CAA AGA ATG GAT GGA TCA CTG AAT  6031

666Phe Asn Arg Thr Trp Gln Asp Tyr Lys Arg Gly Phe Gly Ser Leu Asn Asp Glu Gly Glu Gly Glu Phe Trp Leu Gly Asn
   TTT AAC CGG ACC TGG CAA GAC TAC AAG AGA GGT TTC GGC AGC CTG AAT GAC GAG GGG GAA GGA GAA TTC TGG CTA GGC AAT  6112

693Asp Tyr Leu His leu Leu Thr Gln Arg Gly Ser Val Leu Arg Val Glu Leu Glu Asp Trp Ala Gly Asn Glu Ala Tyr Ala
   GAC TAC CTC CAC TTA CTA ACC CAA AGG GGC TCT GTT CTT AGG GTT GAA TTA GAG GAC TGG GCT GGG AAT GAA GCT TAT GCA  6193

720Glu Tyr His Phe Arg Val Gly Ser Glu Ala Glu Gly Tyr Ala Leu Gln Val Ser Ser Tyr Glu Gly Thr Ala Gly Asp Ala
   GAA TAT CAC TTC CGG GTA GGC TCT GAG GCT GAA GGC TAT GCC CTC CAA GTC TCC TCC TAT GAA GGC ACT GCG GGT GAT GCT  6274

747Leu Ile Glu Gly Ser Val Glu Glu Gly Ala Glu Tyr Thr Ser His Asn Asn Met Gln Phe Ser Thr Phe Asp Arg Asp Ala
   CTG ATT GAG GGT TCC GTA GAG GAA GGG GCA GAG TAC ACC TCT CAC AAC AAC ATG CAG TTC AGC ACC TTT GAC AGG GAT GCA  6355

774Asp Gln Trp Glu Glu Asn Cys Ala Glu Val Tyr Gly Gly Gly Trp Trp Tyr Asn Asn Cys Gln Ala Ala Asn Leu Asn Gly
   GAC CAG TGG GAA GAG AAC TGT GCA GAA GTC TAT GGG GGA GGC TGG TGG TAT AAT AAC TGC CAA GCA GCC AAT CTC AAT GGA  6436

801Ile Tyr Tyr Pro Gly Gly Ser Tyr Asp Pro Arg Asn Asn Ser Pro Tyr Glu Ile Glu Asn Gly Val Val Trp Val Ser Phe
   ATC TAC TAC CCT GGG GGC TCC TAT GAC CCA AGG AAT AAC AGT CCT TAT GAG ATT GAG AAT GGA GTG GTC TGG GTT TCC TTT  6517

828Arg Gly Ala Asp Tyr Ser Leu Arg Ala Val Arg Met Lys Ile Arg Pro Leu Val Thr Gln847 END
   AGA GGG GCA GAT TAT TCC CTC AGG GCT GTT CGC ATG AAA ATT AGG CCC CTT GTG ACC CAA     TAG                     6580

[GCTGAAGAAG TGGGAATGGG AGCACTCTGT CTTCTTTGCT AGAGAAGTGG AGAGAAAATA CAAAAGGTAA AGCAGTTGAG ATTCTCTACA ACCTAAAAAA  6680
TTCCTAGGTG CTATTTTCTT ATCCTTTGTA CTGTAGCTAA ATGTACCTGA GACATATTAG TCTTTGAAAA ATAAAGTTAT GTAAGGTTTT TTTTATCTTT↓ 6780
AAATAGCTCT GTGGGTTTTA ACATTTTTGT AAAGATATAC CAAGGGCCAT TCAGTACATC AGGAAAGTGG CAGACAGAAG CTTCTCTCTG CAACCTTGAA  6880
GACTATTGGT TTGAGAACTT CTCTTCCCAT ACCACCCAAA ATCATAATGC CATTGGAAAG CAAAAAGTTG TTTTATCCAT TTGATTTGAA TTGTTTTAAG  6980
CCAATATTTT AAGGTAAAAC TCACTGAATC TAACCATAGC TGACCTTTGT AGTAGAATTT ACAACTTATA ATTACAATGC ACAATTTATA ATTACAATAT  7080
GTATTTATGT CTTTTGCTAT GGAGCAAATC CAGGAAGGCA AGAGAAACAT TCTTTCCTAA ATATAAATGA AAATCTATCC TTTAAACTCT TCCACTAGAC  7180
GTTGTAATGC ACACTTATTT TTTTCCCAAG GAGTAACCAA TTTCTTTCTA AAACACATTT AAAATTTTAA AACTATTTAT GAATATTAAA AAAAGACATA  7280
ATTCACACAT TAATAAACAA TCTCCCAAGT↓ATTGATTTAA CTTCATTTTT CTAATAATCA TAAACTATAT TCTGTGACAT GCTAATTATT ATTAAATGTA  7380
AGTCGTTAGT TCGAAAGCCT CTCACTAAGT ATGATCTATG CTATATTCAA AATTCAACCC ATTTACTTTG GTCAATATTT GATCTAAGTT GCATCTTTAA  7480
TCCTGGTGGT CTTGCCTTCT GATTTTTAAT TTGTATCCTT TTCTATTAAG ATATATTTGT CATTTTCTCT TGAATATGTA TTAAAATATC CCAAGC↓      7576
```

NOTE: Fu et al. report an additional base (T) in intron E, nucleotide 5589.

Underlining denotes poly(A) signals. ↓ Denotes poly(A) sites.

DNA and Protein Sequences

Human Fibrinogen Bβ-Chain Gene Sequence

GenBank accession no. M64983

```
GAATTCATGC CCCTTTTGAA ATAGACTTAT GTCATTGTCA GAAAACATAA GCATTTATGG TATATCATTA ATGAGTCACG ATTTTAGTGG TTGCCTTGTG   100
AGTAGGTCAA ATTTACTAAG CTTAGATTTG TTTTCTCACA TATTCTTTCG GAGCTTGTGT AGTTTCCACA TTAATTTACC AGAAACAAGA TACACACTCT   200
CTTTGAGGAG TGCCCTAACT TCCCATCATT TTGTCCAATT AAATGAATTG AAGAAATTTA ATGTTTCTAA ACTAGACCAA CAAAGAATAA TAGTTGTATG   300
ACAAGTAAAT AAGCTTTGCT GGGAAGATGT TGCTTAAATG ATAAAATGGT TCAGCCAACA AGTGAACCAA AAATTAAATA TTAACTAAGG AAAGGTAACC   400

                                                                                                      -22Phe His
ATTTCTGAAG TCATTCCTAG CAGAGGACTC AGATATATAT AGGATTGAAG ATCTCTCAGT TAAGTCTACA TGAAAAGGAT GGTTTCTTGG AGC ] TTC CAC 499

                                                                        -1  +1                                 8
Lys Leu Lys Thr Met Lys His Leu Leu Leu Leu Leu Leu Cys Val Phe Leu Val Lys Ser Gln Gly Val Asn Asp Asn Glu Glu
AAA CTT AAA ACC ATG AAA CAT CTA TTA TTG CTA CTA TTG TGT GTT TTT CTA GTT AAG TCC CAA GGT GTC AAC GAC AAT GAG GAG   583

[ GTGAATTTTT TAAAGCATTA TTATATTATT AGTAGTATTA TTAATATAAG ATGTAACATA ATCATATTAT GTGCTTATTT TAATGAAATT AGCATTGCTT   683
ATAGTTATGA AATGGAATTG TTAACCTCTG ACTTATTGTA TTTAAAGAAT GTTTCATAGT ATTTCTTATA TAAAAACAAA GTAATTTCTT GTTTTCTAGT   783
TTATCACCTT TGTTTTCTTA AGATGAGGAT GGCTTAGCTA ATGTAAGATG TGTTTTTCTC ACTTGCTATT CTGAGTACTG TGATTTTCAT TTACTTCTAG   883
CAATACAGGA TTACAATTAA GAGGACAAGA TCTGAAAATC TCACAAACTA TAAAATAATA AAAGAGCAGA ATTTTAAGAT AAAAGAAACT GGTGGTAGGT   983
AGATTGTTCT TTGGTGAAGG AAGGTAATAT ATATTGTTAC TGAGATTACT ATTTATAAAA ATTATAACTA AGCCTAAAAG CAAAATACAT CAAGTGTAAT  1083
GATAGAAAAT GAAATATTGC TTTTTTCAGA TGAAAAGTTC AAATTAGAGT TAGTGTGTAT TGTTATTATT AATAGTTATG AAACACGGTT CAGTCTAATT  1183
TATTTATTTG TAGAACAGTT TGTCCTCAAC TATTATTTTT GCTGACTTAT TGCTGTTAAT TTGCAGTTAC TAAAAATACA GAAATGCATT TAGGACAATG  1283
GATATTTAAG AAATTTAAAT TTTATCATCA AACGTATCAT GGCCAAATTT CTTACATATA GCATAGTATC ATTAAACTAG AAATAAGAAT ACACAATAAT  1383
ATTTAAATGA AGTGATTCAT TTCGGATCAT TATTGAGTTT CAAGGGAACT TGAGTGTTGT ACTTATCAGA CTCTACATGT AAGAACATAT AGTTAATCTG  1483
GTTGTGTGTG TAAAAACATA TGGTTAATCT GGTTAAGTCT GGTTAATCAT ATTAGGTAAG AAAAATGTAA AGAATGTGTA AGACGAAATT TTTGTAAAGT  1583
ACTCTGCAAA GCACTTTCAC ATTTCTGCTT ATCAACTAAA CCTCACAGAG ATAGTTTAAT AGTTTAGGCT TTAAAATGGA TTTTGATTAT TCAACAAGTG  1683
GCCTTCATAA TTTCTTTAAG TGTTTTTCTT TAAGTATATA CTTTCTTTAA ATATTTTTTA AAATTTCCTT TTCTCTAGTA AAGCCAGACC ATCCATGCTA  1783
CCTCTCTAGT GGCACTCTGA AATAAAAAGA AAATAGTTTT CTCTGTTATA ATTGTATTTG TAATAAGCAG ATGAATCACA TTTCTTAAAA TTTGTTTTAG  1883
AGAGGGTAAG CTCTGACTAG GACCATGACT TCAATGTGAA ATATGTATAT ATCCTCCGAA TCTTTACATA TTAAGAATGT ATATAGTCAA CTGGTTAAAC  1983
AGGAAAATCT GGAACAGCCT GGCTGGGTTT TAATCTTAGC ACCATCCTAC TAAATGTTAA ATAATATTAT AATCTAATGA ATAAATGACA ATGCAATTCC  2083
AAATAGAGTT CATCTGATGA CTTCTAGACT CACAAAATTG CAAGAGAGCT CAGTTGTTGC TCAGTTGTTC CAAATCATGT CGTTTGTTAA TTTGTAATTA  2183
AGCTCCAAAG GATGTATAGC TACTGACAAA AAAAAAAATG AGAATGTAGT TAATCCAAAT CAAAACTTTC CTATTGCAAT GCGTATTTTC TGCTTCATTA  2283
TCCTTTAATA TAATATTTTA AGTTAGCAAG TAATTTTAAT TACAATGCAC AAGCCTTGAG AATTATTTTA AATATAAGAA AATCATAATG TTTGATAAAG  2383
AAATCATGTA AGAAATTTCA AGATAATGGT TTAACAAATA ATTTTGTTGA TAGAAGATAA GACTAAAAGT GAAATTCGAA GTGGAGAGGA CACTTAAACT  2483
GTAGTACTTG TTATGTGTGA TTCCAGTAAA AATAGTAATG AGCACTTATT ATTGCCAAGT ACTGTTCTGA GGGTACCATA TGCAATAAGT TATTTAATCC  2583
TTACAATAAT CTTGTAAGGC AGATTCAAAC TATCATTACA CTTATTTTAC AGATGAGAAA ACTGGGGCAC AGATAAAGCA ACTTGCCCAA GGTCTCATAG  2683
CTGTAAGTCA ACCCTACGGT CAAGACCTAC AAGTAGCCGA GCTCCAGAGT ACATTATGAG GGTCAAAGAT TGTCTTATTA CAAATAAATT CCAAGTAGAA  2783
TCAACCTTTA ATAAGTCTTT AATGTCTCTT AAATATGTTT ATATAGGAGT CTAATCACCA ATTCACAAAA ATGAAAGTAG GGAAATGATT AACAATAATC  2883
ATAGGAATCT AACAATCCAA GTGGCTTGAG AATATTCATT CTTCTTGACA GTATAGATTC TTTACAATTT CGTAAGTTCC AATGTATGTT TTAGGAATAT  2983
GAGGTCATTA CTATTCATAA TCTGATACAG CTTTATCCTA AGGCCTCTCT TTAAAAACTA CACTGCATCA TAGCTTTTTT GTGCAGTTGG TCTTTCTACT  3083
GTTACTGAAC AGTAAGCAAC CTACAGATTC ACTATCACCA ACCAGCCAGT TGATGGATCT TAAGCAAATT ATCAAGCTTG TGATAACCTA AATTATAAAA  3183

                                                                                          9Gly Phe Phe Ser Ala Arg Gly
TGAGGGTGTT GGAATAGTTA CATTCCAAAT CTTCTATAAC ACTCTGTATT ATATTTCTGC CTCATTCCTT GTAG ] GGT TTC TTC AGT GCC CGT GGT  3278

16His Arg Pro Leu Asp Lys Lys Arg Glu Glu Ala Pro Ser Leu Arg Pro Ala Pro Pro Pro Ile Ser Gly Gly Gly Tyr Arg
  CAT CGA CCC CTT GAC AAG AAG AGA GAA GAG GCT CCC AGC CTG AGG CCT GCC CCA CCG CCC ATC AGT GGA GGT GGC TAT CGG   3359

43Ala Arg Pro Ala Lys Ala Ala Ala Thr Gln Lys Lys Val Glu Arg Lys Ala Pro Asp Ala Gly Gly Cys Leu His Ala Asp
  GCT CGT CCA GCC AAA GCA GCT GCC ACT CAA AAG AAA GTA GAA AGA AAA GCC CCT GAT GCT GGA GGC TGT CTT CAC GCT GAC   3440

70Pro Asp Leu
  CCA GAC CTG
                                                                                                               3449

[ GTGGGTGCAC TGATGTTTCT TGCAGTGGTG GCTCTCTCAT GCAGAGAAAG CCTGTAGTCA TGGCAGTCTG CTAATGTTTC ACTGACCCAC ATTACCATCA  3549
CTGTTATTTT GTTTGTTTAT TTTGGAAATA AAATTCAAAA CATAAACATA TTGGGCCTTT GGTTTAGGCT TTCTTTCTTG TTTTCTTTGG TCTGGGCCCA  3649
AAATTTCAAA TTAGGATATG TGGGTGCCAC CTTTCCATTT GTATTTTGCC ACTGCCTTTG TTTAGTTGGT AAAATTTTCA TAGCCCAATT ATATTTTTTC  3749
TGGGGTAAGT AATATTTTAA ATCTCTATGA GAGTATGATG ATGACTTTCG AATTTCTGGT CTTACAGAAA ACCAAATAAT AAATTTTTAT GTTGGCTAAT  3849
CGTATCGCTG AATTTTCCTA TGTGCTATTT TAACAAATGT CCATGACCCA AATCCTTCAT CTAATGCCTG CTATTTTCTT TGTTTTTAG ]            3938

73Gly Val Leu Cys Pro Thr Gly Cys Gln Leu Gln Glu Ala Leu Leu Gln Gln Glu Arg Pro Ile Arg Asn Ser Val Asp Glu
  GGG GTG TTG TGT CCT ACA GGA TGT CAG TTG CAA GAG GCT TTG CTA CAA CAG GAA AGG CCA ATC AGA AAT AGT GTT GAT GAG   4019

100Leu Asn Asn Asn Val Glu Ala Val Ser Gln Thr Ser Ser Ser Ser Phe Gln Tyr Met Tyr Leu Leu Lys Asp Leu Trp Gln
  TTA AAT AAC AAT GTG GAA GCT GTT TCC CAG ACC TCC TCT TCT TCC TTT CAG TAC ATG TAT TTG CTG AAA GAC CTG TGG CAA   4100
```

DNA and Protein Sequences

Human Fibrinogen Bβ-Chain Gene Sequence (continued)

GenBank accession no. M64983

```
Lys Arg Gln Lys Gln Val Lys133
AAG AGG CAG AAG CAA GTA AAA G  [ GTAGATATC CTTGTGCTTT CCATTCGATT TTCAGCTATA AAATTGGAAC CGTTAGACTG CCACGAGAAT   4191

GCATGGTTGT GAGAAGATTA ACATTTCTGG GTTAGTGAAT AGCATTCATA CGCTTTTGGG CACCTTCCCC TGCAACTTGC CAGATAAGCA CTATTCAGCT   4291
CTTATTCCCA GTCTGACATC AGCAAGTGTG ATTTTCTATG AAAAATTCTA CTATGACTCC TTATTTTAAG TATACAAGAA ACTTGTGACT CAGAAGATAA   4391
TATTTACAGA GTGGAAAAAA ACCCCTAGCA TTTATAGTTT TAACATTTGA GGTTTTGAAT GAGAGAGTTA TCCATAATAT ATTCAATTGT GTTGTGGATA   4491
ATGACACCTA ACCTGTGAAT CTTGAGGTCA GAATGTTGAG TGCTGTTGAC TTGGTGGTCA GGAAACAGCT AGTGCGTGAG CCTGGCACAG GCATCTCAGT   4591
GAGTAGCATA CCCACAGTTG GAAATTTTTC AAAGAAATCA AAGGAATCAT GACATCTTAT AAATTTCAAG GTTCTGCTAT ACTTATGTGA AATGGATAAA   4691
TAAATCAAGC ATATCCACTC TGTAAGATTG AACTTCTCAG ATGGAAGACC CCAATACTGC TTTCTCCTCT TTTCCCTCAC CAAAGAAATA AACAACCTAT   4791
TTCATTTATT ACTGGACACA ATCTTTAGCG TATACCTATG GTAAATTACT AGTATGGTGG TTAGGATTTA TGTTAATTTG TATATGTCAT GCGCCAAATC   4891
ATTTCCACTA AATATGACTA TATATCATAA CTGCTTGGTG ATAGCTCAGT GTTTAATAGT TTATTCTCAG AAAATCAAAA TTGTATAGTT AAATACATTA   4991

                                                     134Asp Asn Glu Asn Val Val Asn Glu Tyr Ser Ser Glu
GTTTTATGAG GCAAAAATGC TAACTATTTC TACATAATTT CATTTTTCCA G ]  AT AAT GAA AAT GTA GTC AAT GAG TAC TCC TCA GAA     5077
                                                                     *
146Leu Glu Lys His Gln Leu Tyr Ile Asp Glu Thr Val Asn Ser Asn Ile Pro Thr Asn Leu Arg Val Leu Arg Ser Ile Leu
   CTG GAA AAG CAC CAA TTA TAT ATA GAT GAG ACT GTG AAT AGC AAT ATC CCA ACT AAC CTT CGT GTG CTT CGT TCA ATC CTG  5158

173Glu Asn Leu Arg Ser Lys Ile Gln Lys Leu Glu Ser Asp Val Ser Ala Gln Met Glu Tyr Cys Arg Thr Pro Cys Thr Val
   GAA AAC CTG AGA AGC AAA ATA CAA AAG TTA GAA TCT GAT GTC TCA GCT CAA ATG GAA TAT TGT CGC ACC CCA TGC ACT GTC  5239

200Ser Cys Asn Ile Pro Val Val Ser Gly Lys209
   AGT TGC AAT ATT CCT GTG GTG TCT GGC AAA G[ GTAACTGAT TCATAAACAT ATTTTTAGAG AGTTCCAGAA GAACTCACAC ACCAAAAATA   5329
AGAGAACAAC AACAACAACA AAAATGCTAA GTGGATTTTC CCAACAGATC ATAATGACAT TACAGTACAT CATAAAAATA TCCTTAGCCA GTTGTGTTTT   5429
GGACTGGCCT GGTGCATTTG CTGGTTTTGA TGAGCAGGAT GGGGCACAGG TAGTCCCAGG GGTGGCTGAT GTGTGCATCT GCGTACTGGC TTGAACAGAT   5529
GGCAGAACCA CAGATAGATG TAGAAGTTTC TCCATTTTGT GTGTTCTGGG AGCTCATGGA TATTCCAGGA CACAAAAGGT GGAGAAGAGC TTTGTTCATC   5629
CTCTTAGCAG ATAAACGTCC TCAAAACTGG GTTGGACTTA CTAAAGTAAA ATGAAAATCT AATATTTGTT ATATTATTTT CAAAGGTCTA TAATAACACA   5729
CTCCTTAGTA ACTTATGTAA TGTTATTTTA AAGAATTGGT GACTAAATAC AAAGTAATTA TGTCATAAAC CCCTGAACAT AATGTTGTCT TACATTTGCA G ] 5830

210Glu Cys Glu Glu Ile Ile Arg Lys Gly Gly Glu Thr Ser Glu Met Tyr Leu Ile Gln Pro Asp Ser Ser Val Lys Pro Tyr
    AA TGT GAG GAA ATT ATC AGG AAA GGA GGT GAA ACA TCT GAA ATG TAT CTC ATT CAA CCT GAC AGT TCT GTC AAA CCG TAT  5910

237Arg Val Tyr Cys Asp Met Asn Thr Glu Asn Gly247
   AGA GTA TAC TGT GAC ATG AAT ACA GAA AAT GGA G      [ GTAAGCTTTC GACAGTTGTT GACCTGTTGA TCTGTAATTA TTTGGATACC   5994
GTAAAATGCC AGGAAACAAG GCCAGGTGTG GTGGCTCATA CCTGTAATTC CAGCACCTTG GGAGGCCAAA GTGGGCTGAT AGCTTGAGCC TAGGAGTTTG   6094
AAACTAGCCT GGGCAACATA ATGAGACCCT AACTCTACAA AAAAAAAAAA AATACCAAAA AAAAAAAAAA AATCAGCTGT GTTGGTAGTA TGTGCCTGTA   6194
GTCCCAGCTA TCCAGGAGGC TGAGATGGGA GATCACCTGA GCCCACAACC TGGAGTCTTG ATCATGCTAC TGAACTGTAG CCTGGGCAAC AGAGGATAGT   6294
GAGATCCTGT CTCAAAAAAA AAAATTAATT AAAAAGCCAG GAAACAAGAC TTAGCTCTAA CATCTAACAT AGCTGACAAA GGAGTAATTT GATGTGGAAT   6394
TCAACCTGAT ATTTAAAAGT TATAAAATAT CTATAATTCA CAATTTGGGG TAAGATAAAG CACTTGCAGT TTCCAAAGAT TTTACAAGTT TACCTCTCAT   6494
ATTTATTTCC TTATTGTGTC TATTTTAGAG CACCAAATAT ATACTAAATG GAATGGACAG GGGATTCAGA TATTATTTTC AAAGTGACAT TATTTGCTGT   6594

                                      248Gly Trp Thr Val Ile Gln Asn Arg Gln Asp Gly Ser Val Asp Phe Gly
TGGTTAATAT ATGCTCTTTT TGTTTCTGTC AACCAAAG  ] GA TGG ACA GTG ATT CAG AAC CGT CAA GAC GGT AGT GTT GAC TTT GGC      6679

264Arg Lys Trp Asp Pro Tyr Lys Gln Gly Phe Gly Asn Val Ala Thr Asn Thr Asp Gly Lys Asn Tyr Cys Gly Leu Pro289
   AGG AAA TGG GAT CCA TAT AAA CAG GGA TTT GGA AAT GTT GCA ACC AAC ACA GAT GGG AAG AAT TAC TGT GGC CTA CCA G    6758

[ GTAACGAACA GGCATGCAAA ATAAAATCAT TCTATTTGAA ATGGGATTTT TTTTAATTAA AAAACATTCA TTGTTGGAAG CCTGTTTTAG GCAGTTAAGA  6858
GGAGTTTCCT GACAAAAATG TGGAAGCTAA AGATAAGGGA AGAAAGGCAG TTTTTAGTTT CCCAAAATTT TATTTTTGGT GAGAGATTTT ATTTTGTTTT   6958
TCTTTTAG ]                                                                                                     6966
                             *
290Gly Glu Tyr Trp Leu Gly Asn Asp Lys Ile Ser Gln Leu Thr Arg Met Gly Pro Thr Glu Leu Leu Ile Glu Met Glu Asp
    GT GAA TAT TGG CTT GGA AAT GAT AAA ATT AGC CAG CTT ACC AGG ATG GGA CCC ACA GAA CTT TTG ATA GAA ATG GAG GAC  7046

317Trp Lys Gly Asp Lys Val Lys Ala His Tyr Gly Gly Phe Thr Val Gln Asn Glu Ala Asn Lys Tyr Gln Ile Ser Val Asn
   TGG AAA GGA GAC AAA GTA AAG GCT CAC TAT GGA GGA TTC ACT GTA CAG AAT GAA GCC AAC AAA TAC CAG ATC TCA GTG AAC  7127

344Lys Tyr Arg Gly Thr Ala Gly Asn Ala Leu Met Asp Gly Ala Ser Gln Leu Met Gly Glu Asn Arg Thr Met Thr Ile His370
   AAA TAC AGA GGA ACA GCC GGT AAT GCC CTC ATG GAT GGA GCA TCT CAG CTG ATG GGA GAA AAC AGG ACC ATG ACC ATT CAC  7208
```

*Denotes a polymorphic site; see Notes, p. 21.

DNA and Protein Sequences

Human Fibrinogen Bβ-Chain Gene Sequence (continued)

GenBank accession no. M64983

```
371Asn Gly Met Phe Phe Ser Thr Tyr Asp Arg Asp Asn Asp Gly Trp385
   AAC GGC ATG TTC TTC AGC ACG TAT GAC AGA GAC AAT GAC GGC TG  [  GTATGTGTGG CACTCTTTGC TCCTGCTTTA AAAATCACAC  7292
TAATATCATT ACTCAGAATC ATTAACAATA TTTTTAATAG CTACCACTTC CTGGGCACTT ACTGTCAGCC ACTGTCCTAA GCTCTTTATG CATCACTCGA  7392
AAGCATTTCA ACTATAAGGT AGACATTCTT ATTCTCATTT TACAGATGAG ATTTAGAGAG ATTACGTGAT TTGTCCAATG TCACACAACT ACCCAGAGAT  7492
AAAACTAGAA TTTGAGCACA GTTACTTTCT GAATAATGAG CATTTAGATA AATACCTATA TCTCTATATT CTAAAGTGTG TGTGAAAACT TTCATTTTCA  7592
TTTCCAGGGT TCTCTGATAC TAAGGGTTGT AAAAGCTATT ATTCCAGTAT AAAGTAACAA ACACAGTCCC TAGATGGATT GCCACAAAGG CCCAGTTATC  7692
TCTCTTTCTT GCTATAGGGC ACAGGAGGTC TTTGGTGTAT TAGTGTGACT CTATGTATAG CACCCAAAGG AAAGACTACT GTGCACACGA GTGTAGCAGT  7792
CTTTTATGGG TAATCTGCAA AACGTAACTT GACCACCGTA GTTCTGTTTC TAATAACGCC AAACACATTT TCTTTCAG ]                       7870

386Leu Thr Ser Asp Pro Arg Lys Gln Cys Ser Lys Glu Asp Gly Gly Gly Trp Trp Tyr Asn Arg Cys His Ala Ala Asn Pro
 G TTA ACA TCA GAT CCC AGA AAA CAG TGT TCT AAA GAA GAC GGT GGT GGA TGG TGG TAT AAT AGA TGT CAT GCA GCC AAT CCA  7952

413Asn Gly Arg Tyr Tyr Trp Gly Gly Gln Tyr Thr Trp Asp Met Ala Lys His Gly Thr Asp Asp Gly Val Val Trp Met Asn
   AAC GGC AGA TAC TAC TGG GGT GGA CAG TAC ACC TGG GAC ATG GCA AAG CAT GGC ACA GAT GAT GGT GTA GTA TGG ATG AAT  8033
                                *
440Trp Lys Gly Ser Trp Tyr Ser Met Arg Lys Met Ser Met Lys Ile Arg Pro Phe Phe Pro Gln Gln461  END
   TGG AAG GGG TCA TGG TAC TCA ATG AGG AAG ATG AGT ATG AAG ATC AGG CCC TTC TTC CCA CAG CAA     TAG          8102

[ TCCCCAATAC GTAGATTTTT GCTCTTCTGT ATGTGACAAC ATTTTTGTAC ATTATGTTAT TGGAATTTTC TTTCATACAT TATATTCCTC TAAAACTCTC  8202
↓                                                                          ↓  ↓
AAGCAGACGT GAGTGTGACT TTTTGAAAAA AGTATAGGAT AAATTACATT AAAATAGCAC ATGATTTTCT TTTGTTTTCT TCATTTCTCT TGCTCACCCA  8302
AGAAGTAACA AAAGTATAGT TTTGACAGAG TTGGTGTTCA TAATTTCAGT TCTAGTTGAT TGCGAGAATT TTCAAATAAG GAAGAGGGGT CTTTTATCCT  8402
TGTCGTAGGA AAACCATGAC GGAAAGGAAA AACTGATGTT TAAAAGTCCA CTTTTAAAAC TATATTTATT TATGTAGGAT CTGTCAAAGA AAACTTCCAA  8502
                                     ↓  ↓
AAAGATTTAT TAATTAAACC AGACTCTGTT GCAATAAGTT AATGTTTTCT TGTTTTGTAA TCCACACATT CAATGAGTTA GGCTTTGCAC TTGTAAGGAA  8602
GGAGAAGCGT TCACAACCTC AAATAGCTAA TAAACCGGTC TTGAATATTT GAAGATTTAA AATCTGACTC TAGGACGGGC ACGGTGGCTC ACGACTATAA  8702
TCCCAACACT TTGGGAGGCT GAGGCGGGCG GTCACAAGGT CAGGAGTTCA AGACCAGCCT GACCAATATG GTGAAACCCC ATCTCTACTA AAAATACAAA  8802
AATTAGCCAG GCGTGGTGGC AGGTGCCTGT AGGTCCCAGC TAGCCTGTGA GGTGGAGATT GCATTGAGCC AAGATC                            8878
```

*Denotes a polymorphic site; see Notes (below).

Underlining denotes poly(A) signals. ↓ Denotes poly(A) sites.

Notes

There are three known polymorphisms in the Bβ chain:

(1) Bβ(162) Pro[CCA] ↔ Ala[GCA]: DNA sequences for Pro and Ala have been reported [*Biochem. USA* **22**:3244, **1983**]; protein sequencing has detected only Pro [*Hoppe Seyler's Z. Physiol. Chem.* **358**:1643, **1977**; and *Biochem. USA* **18**:68, **1979**].

(2) Bβ(296) Asn[AAT] ↔ Asp[GAT]: DNA sequencing predicts Asn [*Biochem. USA* **22**:3244, **1983**]; protein sequencing has detected only Asp [*Hoppe Seyler's Z. Physiol. Chem.* **358**:1643, **1977**; and *Biochem. USA* **18**:68, **1979**].

(3) Bβ(448) Arg[AGG] ↔ Lys[AAG]: As discussed in *Thromb. Res.* **52**:173, **1988**, DNA and protein sequences for both forms have been reported. However, Baumann & Henschen (*Blood* **82**:2117-24, **1993**), using RFLP of PCR-amplified segments, were able to confirm polymorphisms only at Bβ(448) in a sample of 110 healthy subjects. The reported Arg/Lys allele frequency at this site was 0.85/0.15.

DNA and Protein Sequences

Human Fibrinogen γ-Chain Gene Sequences

GenBank accession nos. X02415; M10014

```
   CTACACA CTTCTTGAAG GCAAAGGCAA TGCTGAAGTC ACCTTTCATG TTCAAATCAT ATTAAAAAGT TAGCAAGATG TAATTATCAG TGTACTATGT   97
AAATCTTTGT GAATGATCAA TAATTACATA TTTTCATTAT ATATATTTTA GTAGATAATA TTTATATACA TTCAACATTC TAAATATAGA AAGTTTACAG  197
AGAAAAATAA AGCCTTTTTT TCCAATCCTG TCCTCCACCT CTGCATCCCA TTCTTCTTCA CAGAGGCAAC TGATTCAAGT CATTACATAG TTATTGAGTG  297
TTAACTACAA CTATGTTAAG TACAGCTATA TATGTTAGAT GCCGTAGCCA CAGAAATCAG TTTACAATCT AATGCAGTGG ATACAGCATG TATACATATA  397
ATATAAGGTT GCTACAAATG CTATCTGAGG TAGAGCTGTT TGAAAGAATA CTAATACTTA AATGTTTAAT TCAACTGACT TGATTGACAA CTGATTAGCT  497
GAGTGGAAAA GATGGATGAG AAAGATTGTG AGACTTAATT GGCTGGTGGT ATGGTGATAT GATTGACAAT AACTGCTAAG TCAGAGAGGG ATATATTAAG  597
GAGGAGAAGA AAAGCAACAA ATCTGGTTTT GATGTGTTCA CTTTGTTATA ATTATTGATT ATTTACTGAA TATGAATATT TATCTTTGTT TTTGAGTCAA  697
TAAATATACC TTTGTAAAGA CAGAATTAAA GTATTAGTAT TTCTTTCAAA CTGGAGGCAT TTCTCCCACT AACATATTTC ATCAAAACTT ATAATAAGCT  797
TGGTTCCAGA GGAAGAAATG AGGGATAACC AAAAATAGAG ACATTAATAA TAGTGTAACG CCCAGTGATA AATCTCAATA GGCAGTGATG ACAGACATGT  897
TTTCCCAAAC ACAAGGATGC TGTAAGGGCC AAACAGAAAT GATGGCCCCT CCCCAGCACC TCATTTTGCC CCTTCCTTCA GCTATGCCTC TACTCTCCTT  997
TAGATACAAG GGAGGTGGAT TTTTCTCTTC TCTGAGATAG CTTGATGGAA CCACAGGAAC AATGAAGTGG GCTCCTGGCT CTTTTCTCTG TGGCAGATGG 1097
GGTGCCATGC CCACCTTCAG ACAAAGGGAA GATTGAGCTC AAAAGCTCCC TGAGAAGTGA GAGCCTATGA ACATGGTTGA CACAGAGGGA CAGGAATGTA 1197
TTTCCAGGGT CATTCATTCC TGGGAATAGT GAACTGGGAC ATGGGGGAAG TCAGTCTCCT CCTGCCACAG CCACAGATTA AAAATAATAA TGTTAACTGA 1297
TCCCTAGGCT AAAATAATAG TGTTAACTGA TCCCTAAGCT AAGAAAGTTC TTTTGGTAAT TCAGGTGATG GCAGCAGGAC CCATCTTAAG GATAGACTAG 1397
GTTTGCTTAG TTCGAGGTCA TATCTGTTTG CTCTCAGCCA TGTACTGGAA GAAGTTGCAT CACACAGCCT CCAGGACTGC CCTCCTCCTC ACAGCAATGG 1497
ATAATGCTTC ACTAGCCTTT GCAGATAATT TTGGATCAGA GAAAAAACCT TGAGCTGGGC CAAAAAGGAG GAGCTTCAAC CTGTGTGCAA AATCTGGGAA 1597
CCTGACAGTA TAGGTTGGGG GCCAGGATGA GGAAAAAGGA ACGGGAAAGA CCTGCCCACC CTTCTGGTAA GGAGGCCCCG TGATCAGCTC CAGCCATTTG 1697
CAGTCCTGGC TATCCCAGGA GCTTACATAA AGGGACAATT GGAGCCTGAG AGGTGACAGT GCTGACACTA CAAGGCTCGG AGCTCCGGGC ACTCAGACAT C ] 1798

-26 Met Ser Trp Ser Leu His Pro Arg Asn Leu Ile Leu Tyr Phe Tyr Ala Leu Leu Phe Leu Ser Ser Thr Cys Val Ala -1
    ATG AGT TGG TCC TTG CAC CCC CGG AAT TTA ATT CTC TAC TTC TAT GCT CTT TTA TTT CTC TCT TCA ACA TGT GTA GCA     1876
 [ GTAAGT GTGCTCTTCA CAAAACGTTG TTTAAAATGG AAAGCTGGAA AATAAAACAG ATAATAAACT AGTGAAATTT TCGTATTTTT TCTCTTTTAG ] 1972

+1 Tyr Val Ala Thr Arg Asp Asn Cys Cys Ile Leu Asp Glu Arg Phe 15
    TAT GTT GCT ACC AGA GAC AAC TGC TGC ATC TTA GAT GAA AGA TTC  [ GTAAGTAGT TTTTATGTTT CTCCCTTTGT GTGTGAACTG 2056
GAGAGGGGCA GAGGAATAGA AATAATTCCC TCATAAATAT CATCTGGCAC TTGTAACTTT TTAAAAACAT AGTCTAGGTT TTACCTATTT TTCTTAATAG 2156

                                                        16 Gly Ser Tyr Cys Pro Thr Thr Cys Gly Ile Ala Asp Phe
ATTTTAAGAG TAGCATCTGT CTACATTTTT AATCACTGTT ATATTTTCAG ]  GGT AGT TAT TGT CCA ACT ACC TGT GGC ATT GCA GAT TTC 2245

29 Leu Ser Thr Tyr Gln Thr Lys Val Asp Lys Asp Leu Gln Ser Leu Glu Asp Ile Leu His Gln Val Glu Asn Lys Thr Ser
   CTG TCT ACT TAT CAA ACC AAA GTA GAC AAG GAT CTA CAG TCT TTG GAA GAC ATC TTA CAT CAA GTT GAA AAC AAA ACA TCA 2326

56 Glu Val Lys Gln Leu Ile Lys Ala Ile Gln Leu Thr Tyr Asn Pro Asp Glu Ser Ser Lys Pro 76
   GAA GTC AAA CAG CTG ATA AAA GCA ATC CAA CTC ACT TAT AAT CCT GAT GAA TCA TCA AAA CCA A [GTGAGAAAA TAAAGACTAC 2409
TGACCAAAAA ATAATAATAA TAATCTGTGA AGTTCTTTTG CTGTTGTTTT AGTTGTTCTA TTTGCTTAAG GATTTTTATG TCTCTGATCC TATATTACAG ] 2509
                                              *
77 Asn Met Ile Asp Ala Ala Thr Leu Lys Ser Arg Ile Met Leu Glu Glu Ile Met Lys Tyr Glu Ala Ser Ile Leu Thr His
   AT ATG ATA GAC GCT GCT ACT TTG AAG TCC AGG ATA ATG TTA GAA GAA ATT ATG AAA TAT GAA GCA TCG ATT TTA ACA CAT  2589

104 Asp Ser Ser Ile Arg 108
   GAC TCA AGT ATT CG   GTAAGGATTT TTGTTTTAAT TTGCTCTGCA AGACTGATTT AGTTTTTATT TAATATTCTA TACTTGAGTG AAAGTAATTT 2683
TTAATGTGTT TTCCCCATTT ATAATATCCC AGTGACATTA TGCCTGATTA TGTTGAGCAT AGTAGAGATA GAAGTTTTTA GTGCAATATA AATTATACTG 2783
GGTTATAATT GCTTATTAAT AATCACATTG AAGAAAGATG TTCTAGATGT CTTCAAATGC TAGTTTGACC ATATTTATCA AAAATTTTTT CCCCATCCCC 2883
CATTTATCTT ACAACATAAA ATCAATCTCA TAGGAATTTG GGTGTTGAAA ATAAAATCCT CTTTATAAAA ATGCTGACAA ATTGGTGGTT AAAAAAATTA 2983
GCAAGCAGAG GCATAGTAAG GATTTTGGCT CCTAAAGTAA ATTATATTGA ATGTGGAGCA GGAAGAAACA TGTCTTGAGA GACTAAGTGT GGCAAATATT 3083
GCAAAGCTCA TATTGATCAT TGCAGAATGA ACCTGCATAG TCTCTTCCCT TCATTTGGAA GTGAATGTCT CTGTTAAAGC TTCTCAGGGA CTCATAAACT 3183
TTCTGAACAT AAGGTCTCAG ATACAGTTTT AATATTTTTC CCCAATTTTT TTTTCTGAAT TTTTCTCAAA GCAGCTTGAG AAATTGAGAT AAATAGTAGC 3283
TAGGGAGAAG TGGCCCAGGA AAGATTTCTC CTCTTTTTGC TATCAGAGGG CCCTTGTTAT TATTGTTATT ATTATTACTT GCATTATTAT TGTCCATCAT 3383
TGAAGTTGAA GGAGGTTATT GTACAGAAAT TGCCTAAGAC AAGGTAGAGG GAAAACGTGG ACAAATAGTT TGTCTACCCT TTTTTACTTC AAAGAAAGAA 3483
CGGTTTATGC ATTGTAGACA GTTTTCTATC ATTTTTGGAT ATTTGCAAGC CACCCTGTAA GTAACTACAA AAGGAGGGTT TTTACTTCCC CCAGTCCATT 3583
CCCAAAGCTA TGTAACCAGA AGCATTAAAG AAGAAAGGGG AAGTATCTGT TGTTTTATTT TACATACAAT AACGTTCCAG ATCATGTCCC TGTGTAAGTT 3683
ATATTTTAGA TTGAAGCTTA TATGTATAGC CTCAGTAGAT CCACAAGTGA AAGGTATACT CCTTCAGCAC ATGTGAATTA CTGAACTGAG CTTTTCCTGC 3783
TTCTAAAGCA TCAGGGGGTG TTCCTATTAA CCAGTCTCGC CACTCTTGCA GGTTGCTATC TGCTGTCCCT TATGCATAAA GTAAAAAGCA AAATGTCAAT 3883
GACATTTGCT TATTGACAAG GACTTTGTTA TTTGTGTTGG GAGTTGAGAC AATATGCCCC ATTCTAAGTA AAAAGATTCA GGTCCACATT GTATTCCTGT 3983
TTTAATTGAT TTTTTGATTT GTTTTTCTTT TTCAAAAAGT TTATAATTTT AATTCATGTT AATTTAGTAA TATAATTTTA CATTTTCCTC AAGAATGGAA 4083
TAATTTATCA GAAAGCACTT CTTAAGAAAA TACTTAGCAG TTTCCAAAGA AAATATAAAA TTACTCTTCT GAAAGGAATA CTTATTTTTG TCTTCTTATT 4183
```

*Denotes a polymorphic site; see Note 2, p. 24.

DNA and Protein Sequences

Human Fibrinogen γ-Chain Gene Sequences (continued)

GenBank accession nos. X02415; M10014

```
                                   109 Tyr Leu Gln Glu Ile Tyr Asn Ser Asn Asn Gln Lys Ile Val Asn Leu Lys Glu
TTTGTTATCT TATGTTTCTG TTTGTAG ]       A TAT TTG CAG GAA ATA TAT AAT TCA AAT AAT CAA AAG ATT GTT AAC CTG AAA GAG    4265

127 Lys Val Ala Gln Leu Glu Ala Gln Cys Gln Glu Pro Cys Lys Asp Thr Val Gln Ile His Asp Ile Thr Gly Lys 151
   AAG GTA GCC CAG CTT GAA GCA CAG TGC CAG GAA CCT TGC AAA GAC ACG GTG CAA ATC CAT GAT ATC ACT GGG AAA G       4341
[ GTAACTGA TGAAGGTTAT ATTGGGATTA GGTTCATCAA AGTAAGTAAT GTAAAGGAGA AAGTATGTAC TGGAAAGTAT AGGAATAGTT TAGAAAGTGG    4439
CTACCCATTA AGTCTAAGAA TTTCAGTTGT CTAGACCTTT CTTGAATAGC TAAAAAAAAC AGTTTAAAAG GAATGCTGAT GTGAAAAGTA AGAAAATTAT   4539
TCTTGGAAAA TGAATAGTTT ACTACATGTT AAAAGCTATT TTTCAAGGCT GGCACAGTCT TACCTGCATT TCAAACCACA GTAAAAGTCG ATTCTCCTTC   4639

     152 Asp Cys Gln Asp Ile Ala Asn Lys Gly Ala Lys Gln Ser Gly Leu Tyr Phe Ile Lys Pro Leu Lys Ala Asn Gln
TCTAG ]    AT TGT CAA GAC ATT GCC AAT AAG GGA GCT AAA CAG AGC GGG CTT TAC TTT ATT AAA CCT CTG AAA GCT AAC CAG       4718

177 Gln Phe Leu Val Tyr Cys Glu Ile Asp Gly Ser Gly Asn Gly Trp Thr Val Phe Gln Lys 196
   CAA TTC TTA GTC TAC TGT GAA ATC GAT GGG TCT GGA AAT GGA TGG ACT GTG TTT CAG AAG     [ GTAATTTTT TCCCCACCAT    4797
GTGTATTTAA TAAATTCCTA CATTGTTTCT GCCATATGGC AGATACTTTT CTAAGCACCT TGTGAACCGT AGCTCATTTA ATCCTTGCAA TAGCCCTAAG   4897
AGGAAGGTAC TTCTGTTACT CCTATTTACA GAAAAGGAAA CTGAGGCACA CAAGGTTAAA TAACTTGCCC AAGACCACAT AACTAATAAG CAACAGAGTC   4997
AGCATTTGAA CCTAGGCAGT ATAGTTTCAG AGTTTGTGAC TTGACTCTAT ATTGTACTGG CACTGACTTT GTAGATTCAT GGTGGCACAT AATCATAGTA   5097
CCACAGTGAC AAATAAAAAG AAGGAAACTC TTTTGTCAGG TAGGTCAAGA CCTGAGGTTT CCCATCACAA GATGAGGAAG CCCAACACCA CCCCCCACCA   5197
CCCCACCACC ATCACCACCC TTTCACACAC CAGAGGATAC ACTTGGGCTG CTCCAAGACA AGGAACCTGT GTTGCATCTG CCACTTGCTG ATACCCACTA   5297
GGAATCTTGG CTCCTTTACT TTCTGTTTAC CTCCCACCAC TGTTATAACT GTTTCTACAG GGGGCGCTCA GAGGGAATGA ATGGTGGAAG CATTAGTTGC   5397
CAGACACCGA TTGAGCAATG GGTTCCATCA TAAGTGTAAG AATCAGTAAT ATCCAGCTAG AGTTCTGAAG TCGTCTAGGT GTCTTTTTAA TATTACCACT   5497
CATTTAGAAT TTATGATGTG CCAGAAACCC TCTTAAGTAT TTCTCTTATA TTCTCTCTCA TGATCCTTGC AGCAACCCTA AGAAGTAACC ATCATTTTTC   5597
CTATTTGATA CATGAGGAAA CTGAGGTAGC TTGGCCAAGA TCACTTAGTT GGGAGTTGAT AGAACCAGTG CTCTGTATTT TTGACAAAAT GTTGACAGCA   5697

                                                                   197 Arg Leu Asp Gly Ser Val Asp Phe Lys Lys
TTCTCTTTAC ATGCATTGAT AGTCTATTTT CTCCTTTTGC TCTTGCAAAT GTGTAATTAG ]    AGA CTT GAT GGC AGT GTA GAT TTC AAG AAA     5787

207 Asn Trp Ile Gln Tyr Lys Glu Gly Phe Gly His Leu Ser Pro Thr Gly Thr Thr Glu Phe Trp Leu Gly Asn Glu Lys Ile
   AAC TGG ATT CAA TAT AAA GAA GGA TTT GGA CAT CTG TCT CCT ACT GGC ACA ACA GAA TTT TGG CTG GGA AAT GAG AAG ATT  5868

234 His Leu Ile Ser Thr Gln Ser Ala Ile Pro Tyr Ala Leu Arg Val Glu Leu Glu Asp Trp Asn Gly Arg Thr Ser 258
   CAT TTG ATA AGC ACA CAG TCT GCC ATC CCA TAT GCA TTA AGA GTG GAA CTG GAA GAC TGG AAT GGC AGA ACC AG          5942

[ GTACTGTTTT GAAATGACTT CCAACTTTTT ATTGTAAAGA TTGCCTGGAA TGTGCACTTT CCAACTATCA ATAGACAATG GCAAATGCAG CCTGACAAAT   6042
GCAAACAGCA CATCCAGCCA CCATTTTCTC CAGGAGTCTG TTTGGTTCTT GGGCAATCCA AAAAGGTAAA TTCTATTCAG GATGAATCTA AGTGTATTGG   6142
TACAATCTAA TTACCCTGGA ACCATTCAGA GTAATAGCTA ATTACTGAAC TTTTAATCAG TCCCAGGAAT TGAGCATAAA ATTATAATTT TATCTAGTCT   6242
AAATTACTAT TTCATGAAGC AGGTATTATT ATTAATCCCA TTTTATAGAT TAACTTGCTC AAAGTCACAT TGCTGATAAG TGGTAGAGGT AGAATTCAGA   6342
CTCAAGTAGT TTAACTTTAG AGCCTGTCCT CTTAACAACT ATCCTGGTTG AAAAGCAAAT ACAGCCTCTT CAGACTTCTC AGTGCCTTGA TGGCCATTTA   6442
TTCTGTCAAA TCATGAGCTA CCCTAAAAGT AAACCAGCTA GCTCTTTTGA TGATCTAGAG GCTTCTTTTT GCTTGAGATA TTTGAAGGTT TTAAGCATTG   6542
TTACCTAATT AAAATGCAGA AAAATATCCA ACCCTCTTGT TATGTTTAAG GAATAGTGAA ATATATTGTC TTCAAACACA TGGACTTTTT TTTATTGCTT   6642
GGTTGGTTTT TAATCCAGAA AGTGCTATAG TCAGTAGACC TTCTTCTAGG AAAGGACCTT CCATTTCCCA GCCACTGGAG ATTAGAAAAT AAGCTAAATA   6742
TTTTCTGGAA ATTTCTGTTC ATTCATTAAG GCCCATCCTT TCCCCCACTC TATAGAAGTG TTGTCCACTT GCACAATTTT TTCCAGGAAA GAATCTCTCT   6842
AACTCCTTCA GCTCACATGC TTTGGACCAC ACAGGGAAGA CTTTGATTGT GTAATGCCCT CAGAAGCTCT CCTTCTTGCC ACTACCACAC TGATTTGAGG   6942
AAGAAAATCC CTTTAGCACC TAACCCTTCA GGTGCTATGA GTGGCTAATG GAACTGTACC TCCTTCAAGT TTTGTGCAAT AATTAAGGGT CACTCACTGT   7042
CAGATACTTT CTGTGATCTA TGATAATGTG TGTGCAACAC ATAACATTTC AATAAAAGTA GAAAATATGA AATTAGAGTC ATCTACACAT CTGGATTTGA   7142
TCTTAGAATG AAACAAGCAA AAAAGCATCC AAGTGAGTGC AATTATTAGT TTTCAGAGAT GCTTCAAAGG CTTCTAGGCC CATCCCGGGA AGTGTTAATG   7242
AGCTGTGGAC TGGTTCACAT ATCTATTGCC TCTTGCCAGA TTTGCAAAAA ACTTCACTCA ATGAGCAAAT TTCAGCCTTA AGAAACAAAG TCAAAAATTC   7342
CAAGGAAGCA TCCTACGAAA GAGGGAACTT CTGAGATCCC TGAGGAGGGT CAGCATGTGA TGGTTGTATT TCCTTCTTCT CAG ]                  7425

259 Thr Ala Asp Tyr Ala Met Phe Lys Val Gly Pro Glu Ala Asp Lys Tyr Arg Leu Thr Tyr Ala Tyr Phe Ala Gly Gly Asp
   T ACT GCA GAC TAT GCC ATG TTC AAG GTG GGA CCT GAA GCT GAC AAG TAC CGC CTA ACA TAT GCC TAC TTC GCT GGT GGG GAT  7507

286 Ala Gly Asp Ala Phe Asp Gly Phe Asp Phe Gly Asp Asp Pro Ser Asp Lys Phe Phe Thr Ser His Asn Gly Met Gln Phe
   GCT GGA GAT GCC TTT GAT GGC TTT GAT TTT GGC GAT GAT CCT AGT GAC AAG TTT TTC ACA TCC CAT AAT GGC ATG CAG TTC  7588

313 Ser Thr Trp Asp Asn Asp Asn Asp Lys Phe Glu Gly Asn Cys Ala Glu Gln Asp Gly Ser Gly Trp Trp Met Asn Lys Cys
   AGT ACC TGG GAC AAT GAC AAT GAT AAG TTT GAA GGC AAC TGT GCT GAA CAG GAT GGA TCT GGT TGG TGG ATG AAC AAG TGT  7669
```

DNA and Protein Sequences

Human Fibrinogen γ-Chain Gene Sequences (continued) *GenBank accession nos. X02415; M10014*

```
340His Ala Gly His Leu Asn Gly Val Tyr Tyr Gln350
   CAC GCT GGC CAT CTC AAT GGA GTT TAT TAC CAA G                                                                 7703

[ GTATGTTTTC CTTTCTTAGA TTCCAAGTTA ATGTATAGTG TATACTATTT TCATAAAAAA TAATAAATAG ATATGAAGAA ATGAAGAATA ATTTATAAAG  7803
ATAGTAGGGA TTTTATCATG TTCTTTATTT CAACTAAGTT CTTTGAAACT GGAAGTGGAT AATACCAAGT TCATGCCTAA AATTAGCCCT TCTAAAGAAA  7903
TCCACCTGCT GCAAAATATC CAGTAGTTTG GCATTATATG TGAAACTATC ACCATCATAG CTGGCACTGT GGGTTGTGGG ATCTCCTTTA GACATACAAC  8003
ATAAATGATC TGGATGGATT AACATTACTA CATGGATGCT TGTTGACACA TTAACCTGGC TTCCCATGAG CTTTGTGTCA GATACACGCA GTGAACAGGT  8103
GTTTGGAGGA ACAGAATAAA GAGAAGGCAA GCACTGGTAA GGGCAGGGGT TTGTGAAAGC TTGAGAGAAG AGACCAGTCT GAGGACAGTA GACACTTATT  8203
TTAGGATGGG GGTTGGATGA GGAGGCTATA GTTTGCTATA AGCTTGGAAT GGTTTGGAAC ACTGGTTTCA CTCACCTACC CAGCAGTTAT GTGTGGGGAA  8303
GCCTTACCGA TGCTAAAGGA TCCATGTTAC AATAATGGCA TTATTTGGAA ATCCCAGTGG TATTCCATGA ATAAAACCAC TATGAAGATA ATCCCACTCA  8403
ACAGACTCTC CGTTGGAGAA GGACAGCAAC ACCACCCTGG GAAAGCCAAA CAGTCAGACC AGACCTGTTT AGCATCAGTA GGACTTCCCT ACCATATCTG  8503
CTGGGTAGAT GAGTGAAACC AGTGTTCCAA ACCACTCCGG GCTTGTAGCA AACCATAGTC TCCTCATCTA CCAAGATGAG CAACCTTACC TCCTGATGTC  8603
CTAGCCAATC ACCAACTAGG AAACTTTGCA CAGTTTATTT AAAGTAACAG TTTGATTTTC ACAATATTTT TAAATTGGAG AAACATAACT TATCTTTGCA  8703
CTCACAAACC ACATAATGAG AAGAAACTCT AAGGGAAAAT GCTTGATCTG TGTGACCCGG GGCGCCATGC CAGAGCTGTA GTTCATGCCA GTGTTGTGCT  8803
CTGACAAGCC TTTTACAGAA TTACATGAGA TCTGCTTCCC TAGGACAAGG AGAAGGCAAA TCAACAGAGG CTGCACTTTA AAATGGAGAC ATAAAATAAC  8903
ATGCCAGAAC CATTTCCTAA AGCTCCTCAA TCAACCAACA AAATTGTGCT TTCAAATAAC CTGAGTTGAC CTCATCAGGA ATTTTGTGGC TCCTTCTCTT  9003
CTAACCTGCC TGAAGAAAGA TGGTCCACAG CAGCTGAGTC CGGGATGGAT AAGCTTAGGG ACAGAGGCCA ATTAGGGAAC TTTGGGTTTC TAGCCCTACT  9103
AGTAGTGAAT AAATTTAAAG TGTGGATGTG ACTATGAGTC ACAGCACAGA TGTTGTTTAA TAATATGTTT ATTTTATAAA TTGATATTTT AGGAATCTTT  9203
GGAGATATTT TCAGTTAGCA GATAATACTA TAAATTTTAT GTAACTGGCA ATGCACTTCG TAATAGACAG CTCTTCATAG ACTTGCAGAG GTAAAAAGAT  9303
TCCAGAATAA TGATATGTAC ATCTACGACT TGTTTTAG ]                                                                   9341

351Gly Gly Thr Tyr Ser Lys Ala Ser Thr Pro Asn Gly Tyr Asp Asn Gly Ile Ile Trp Ala Thr Trp Lys Thr Arg Trp Tyr
     GT GGC ACT TAC TCA AAA GCA TCT ACT CCT AAT GGT TAT GAT AAT GGC ATT ATT TGG GCC ACT TGG AAA ACC CGG TGG TAT9421

378Ser Met Lys Lys Thr Thr Met Lys Ile Ile Pro Phe Asn Arg Leu Thr Ile Gly Glu Gly Gln Gln His His Leu Gly Gly
   TCC ATG AAG AAA ACC ACT ATG AAG ATA ATC CCA TTC AAC AGA CTC ACA ATT GGA GAA GGA CAG CAA CAC CAC CTG GGG GGA9502

405Ala Lys Gln407  408' Val Arg Pro Glu His Pro Ala Glu Thr Glu Tyr Asp Ser Leu Tyr Pro Glu Asp Asp Leu427' END
   GCC AAA CAG          GTC AGA CCA GAG CAC CCT GCG GAA ACA GAA TAT GAC TCA CTT TAC CCT GAG GAT GAT TTG    TAG9574

[ AAAATTAACT GCTAACTTCT ATTGACCCAC AAAGTTTCAG AAATTCTCTG AAAGTTTCTT CCTTTTTTCT CTTACTATAT TTATTGATTT CAAGTCTTCT  9674
ATTAAGGACA TTTAGCCTTC AATGGAAATT AAAACTCATT TAGGACTGTA TTTCCAAATT ACTGATATCA GAGTTATTTA AAAATTGTTT ATTTGAGGAG  9774

                                                       ↓(γLeu427)
ATAACATTTC AACTTTGTTC CTAAATATAT AATAATAAAA TGATTGACTT TATTTGCATT TTTATGACCA CTTGTCATTT ATTTTGTCTT CGTAAATTAT  9874
TTTCATTATA TCAAATATTT TAGTATGTAC TTAATAAAAT AGGAGAACAT TTTAGAGTTT CAAATTCCCA GGTATTTTCC TTGTTTATTA CCCCTAAATC  9974
ATTCCTATTT AATTCTTCTT TTTAAATGGA GAAAATTATG TCTTTTTAAT ATGGTTTTTG TTTTGTTATA TATTCACAG ]                     10053

        408 Ala Gly Asp Val411 END
            GCT GGA GAC GTT     TAA                                                                              10068

[ AAGACCGTTT CAAAAGAGAT TTACTTTTTT AAAGGACTTT ATCTGAACAG AGAGATATAA TATTTTTCCT ATTGGACAAT GGACTTGCAA AGCTTCACTT 10168
CATTTTAAGA GCAAAAGACC CCATGTTGAA AACTCCATAA CAGTTTTATG CTGATGATAA TTTATCTACA TGCATTTCAA TAAACCTTTT GTTTCCTAAG 10268
 ↓(γVal411)
ACTAGATACA TGGTACCTTT ATTGACCATT AAAAAACCAC CACTTTTTGC CAATTTACCA ATTACAATTG GGCAACCATC AGTAGTAATT GAGTCCTCAT 10368
TTTATGCTAA ATGTTATGCC TAACTCTTTG GGAGTTACAA AGGAAATAGC AATTATGGCT TTTGCCCTCT AGGAGATACA GGACAAATAC AGGAAAATAC 10468
AGCAACCCAA ACTGACAATA CTCTATACAA GAACATAATC ACTAAGCAGG AGTCACAGCC ACACAACCAA GATGCATAGT ATCCAAAGTG CAGCTG     10564
```

Underlining denotes poly(A) signals. ↓ Denotes poly(A) sites.

Notes

1. The three types of fibrinogen γ chains differ in carboxyl-terminal sequence. The recommended terminology (Francis and Mosesson, *Thromb. Haemostas.* **62**:813-814, 1989) is γ-Val411 (formerly γ, γ_A, or γ_{50}), γ-Pro423 (formerly γ_{55}) and γLeu427 (formerly γ', γ_B, or $\gamma_{57.5}$). γ-Pro423 occurs after proteolytic cleavage of γLeu427.

2. There is one known polymorphism in the γ chain: As discussed in *Biochem. USA* **24**:2077 (1985), ATA (**Ile**) and AAA (**Lys**) have been found at γ(88). Protein sequencing disclosed only **Lys** in this position.

Fibrinogen Oligonucleotide Primers

CONTRIBUTED BY

Susan T. Lord, Ph.D.
Department of Pathology
The University of North Carolina at Chapel Hill
603 Brinkhous-Bullitt Building
Chapel Hill, NC 27599-7525 USA
E-MAIL: LORD@uncvx1.oit.unc.edu

This list includes oligonucleotide sequences that have been used successfully in our laboratory and by others for amplification and sequence analysis of human fibrinogen genes. The following additional information may be helpful: (1) Before using any of these primers the sequence should be cross-checked with the latest sequence listed elsewhere in this section. (2) Some of these primers were made years ago, and we still use them because they work. However, we know now that it is not necessary to have primers longer than 20 bases for either PCR or sequencing. Often shorter primers are better, not only because they are more easily synthesized but also because they are less expensive. (3) Some of these primers lie within the coding sequence of the gene. Thus, they cannot be used to determine a mutant within the relevant region. (Of course, this also is true of primers anywhere in the gene, but typically variant fibrinogens arise from mutants within exons; a notable exception is fibrinogen Paris I). (4) A typical sequencing gel will read 200 to 300 bases, but a typical sequencing reaction can include many more bases depending upon the conditions. Thus, when two primers are more than 300 bases apart on the PCR fragment it will be necessary to run more than one sequencing gel (or more than one gel tract, loaded at different times) in order to read this number of bases; that is, run one gel for a short time to read bases 20—250 from the primer and a second gel for a longer time to read bases 200—450 from the primer. (5) It is recommended that both strands of DNA from each region be sequenced. However, the primers listed here will not sequence both strands of all the PCR fragments. Additional ones may be necessary. (6) There are no primers listed to sequence exon I of the Bβ gene or to exon VI from the Aα gene.

I thank Dr. Kevin Siebenlist for contributing two γ-chain primers to this list, and would encourage other investigators to communicate similar information so that it may be included in future editions of this book.

Oligonucleotide Primers

Aα Chain

PCR1α and PCR2α amplify an 832bp fragment to sequence exons II and III:

PCR1α.	TGTCTCCTCTTCTGGCTA	forward from Aα 1091
PCR2α.	TATTGGCTGAGGAAAAATCGCC	reverse from Aα 1922

Sequence exon II with primers:

PCR1α.	TGTCTCCTCTTCTGGCTA	forward from Aα 1091
SEQ1α.	GTCTTCATCAGAGCAGAAGGG	reverse from Aα 1276

Sequence exon III with primer:

SEQ2α.	GCTGCATGGAAACATGCA	forward from Aα 1663

PCR3α and PCR4α amplify an 869bp fragment to sequence exon IV

PCR3α.	TTTGCTGGCAATTACAGA	forward from Aα 2992
PCR4α.	CTTCAGATCTACTTCACGAGCTAAAGC	reverse from Aα 3860

Sequence exon IV with primers:

PCR3α.	TTTGCTGGCAATTACAGA	forward from Aα 2992
SEQ3α.	ACCTCCAGTCGTTTCATATCAAC	reverse from Aα 3202

PCR5α and PCR6α amplify an 863bp fragment to sequence within exon V

PCR5α.	CAGGAACTCAATAGACGT	forward from Aα 3715
PCR6α.	GACCAGTTTTTCTGTGTGGTACTC	reverse from Aα 4577

Sequence within exon V with primers:

PCR5α.	CAGGAACTCAATAGACGT	forward from Aα 3715
PCR6α.	GACCAGTTTTTCTGTGTGGTACTC	reverse from Aα 4577
SEQ4α.	GGAAATTTTAAGAGCCAGCTTCAG	forward from Aα 3978
SEQ5α.	GACATGCCGCAGATGAGAATGGAG	forward from Aα 4032

PCR7α and PCR8α amplify an 829bp fragment to sequence within exon V

PCR7α.	TGGGGCACATTTGAAGAGGTGTCA	forward from Aα 4503
PCR8α.	GGAACTTACAGTCTAGCACAAAAACAGACC	reverse from Aα 5331

Sequence within exon V with primers:

PCR7α.	TGGGGCACATTTGAAGAGGTGTCA	forward from Aα 4503
PCR8α.	GGAACTTACAGTCGACCACAAAAACAGACC	reverse from Aα 5331
SEQ6α.	GGTACTCTGGATGGGTTC	forward from Aα 4785
SEQ7α.	CAAATGTGGAGTCTCCTCTG	reverse from Aα 5064
SEQ8α.	CTGTGCAGAAATATTTAACTTAGTCTA	reverse from Aα 5234

Oligonucleotide Primers

Bβ Chain

PCR1β and PCR2β amplify a 931bp fragment to sequence exon II

PCR1β.	GGTGTTGGAATAGTTACATTCC	forward from Bβ 3188
PCR2β.	TACTTGCTTCTGCCTCTTTTGCCACAG	reverse from Bβ 4118

Sequence exon II with primers:

PCR1β.	GGTGTTGGAATAGTTACATTCC	forward from Bβ 3188
SEQ1β.	ATCAGTGCACCCACCAAGTCTGGG	reverse from Bβ3463

PCR3β and PCR4β amplify a 305bp fragment to sequence exon III

PCR3β.	ACAAATGTCCATGACCC	forward from Bβ3882
PCR4β.	CGTGGCAGTCTAACGGTTCC	reverse from Bβ 4186

Sequence exon III with primer:

PCR3β.	ACAAATGTCCATGACCC	forward from Bβ3882
PCR4β.	CGTGGCAGTCTAACGGTTCC	reverse from Bβ 4186

PCR5β and PCR6β amplify a 401bp fragment to sequence exon IV

PCR5β.	CTGCTTGGTGATAGCTCAGTG	forward from Bβ 4922
PCR6β.	GGTGTGTGAGTTCTTCTGGA	reverse from Bβ 5322

Sequence exon IV with primers:

PCR5β.	CTGCTTGGTGATAGCTCAGTG	forward from Bβ 4922
PCR6β.	GGTGTGTGAGTTCTTCTGGA	reverse from Bβ 5322

PCR7β and PCR8β amplify a 1262bp fragment to sequence exons V and VI

PCR7β.	CACACTCCTTAGTAACTTATGT	forward from Bβ 5726
PCR8β.	CATTTCCAAGCCAATATTCAC	reverse from Bβ 6987

Sequence exon V with primers:

PCR7β.	CACACTCCTTAGTAACTTATGT	forward from Bβ 5726
SEQ2β.	CCTGGCATTTTACGGTATCC	reverse from Bβ 6007

Sequence exon VI with primers:

SEQ3β.	ACATTATTTGCTGTTGG	forward from Bβ 6581
SEQ4β.	CCCATTTCAAATAGAATG	reverse from Bβ 6803

PCR9β and PCR10β amplify a 1316bp fragment to sequence exons VII and VIII

PCR9β.	GCAGTTTTTAGTTTCCC	forward from Bβ 6905
PCR10β.	TCACACTCACGTCTGCTTGA	reverse from Bβ 8220

Sequence exon VII with primer:

PCR9β.	GCAGTTTTTAGTTTCCC	forward from Bβ 6905

Sequence exon VIII with primer:

PCR10β.	TCACACTCACGTCTGCTTGA	reverse from Bβ 8220

Oligonucleotide Primers

γ Chain

PCR1γ and PCR2γ amplify a 755bp fragment to sequence exons II, III and IV

PCR1γ.	GCTCTTCACAAAACGTTGTTTAAAATGG	forward from γ 1885
PCR2γ.	CAGTCTTGCAGAGCAAATTAAAACAAAA	reverse from γ 2639

Sequence exons II and III with primer:

PCR1γ.	GCTCTTCACAAAACGTTGTTTAAAATGG	forward from γ 1885

Sequence exons III and IV with primers:

SEQ1γ.	GTGAAGTTCTTTTGCTGT	forward from γ 2436
PCR2γ.	CAGTCTTGCAGAGCAAATTAAAACAAAA	reverse from γ 2639

PCR3γ and PCR4γ amplify a 750bp fragment to sequence exons V and VI

PCR3γ.	GAAAGCACTTCTTAAGAAAATACTT	forward from γ 4094
PCR4γ.	GTATCTGCCATATGGCAGAAACAAT	reverse from γ 4843

Sequence exons V and VI with primers:

PCR3γ.	GAAAGCACTTCTTAAGAAAATACTT	forward from γ 4094
PCR4γ.	GTATCTGCCATATGGCAGAAACAAT	reverse from γ 4843

PCR5γ and PCR6γ amplify a 297bp fragment to sequence exon VII

PCR5γ.	GATAGTCTATTTTCTCCTTTTGCTCTT	forward from γ 5715
PCR6γ.	GATAGTTGGAAAGTGCACATTCCAGGC	reverse from γ 6011

Sequence exon VII with primers:

PCR5γ.	GATAGTCTATTTTCTCCTTTTGCTCTT	forward from γ 5715
PCR6γ.	GATAGTTGGAAAGTGCACATTCCAGGC	reverse from γ 6011

PCR7γ and PCR8γ amplify a 386bp fragment to sequence exon VIII

PCR7γ.	GAAGCATCCTACGAAAGAGGG	forward from γ 7347
PCR8γ.	AACTTGGAATCTAAGAAAGGAAAACATACC	reverse from γ 7732

Sequence exon VIII with primers:

PCR7γ.	GAAGCATCCTACGAAAGAGGG	forward from γ 7347
PCR8γ.	AACTTGGAATCTAAGAAAGGAAAACATACC	reverse from γ 7732

PCR9γ and PCR10γ amplify an 883 bp fragment to sequence exons IX and X

PCR9γ.	CTTCATAGACTTGCAGAG	forward from γ 9276
PCR10γ.	TTGCAAGTCCATTGTCCAATAGGAAAAATA	reverse from γ 10158

Sequence exon IX with primers:

PCR9γ.	CTTCATAGACTTGCAGAG	forward from γ 9276
SEQ2γ.	ATGTACATCTACGACTTGTTTTAG	forward from γ 9317

Sequence exon X with primer:

PCR10γ.	TTGCAAGTCCATTGTCCAATAGGAAAAATA	reverse from γ 10158

Oligonucleotide Primers

γ Chain (cont'd.)

PCR9γ and PCR11γ amplify a 304 bp fragment to sequence exon IX

PCR9γ. CTTCATAGACTTGCAGAG	forward from γ 9276
PCR11γ. GTGGGTCAATAGAAGTTAGCAGTTA	reverse from γ 9580

PCR9γ and PCR12γ amplify a 402 bp fragment to sequence exon IX

PCR9γ. CTTCATAGACTTGCAGAG	forward from γ 9276
PCR12γ. TCCATTGAAGGCTAAATGTCCTTA	reverse from γ 9677

Anti-Fibrinogen Antibodies

CONTRIBUTED BY

John Owen, M.D., M.B.A., FRCP(C), FIBMS
Department of Medicine
Section on Hematology/Oncology
The Bowman Gray School of Medicine
Wake Forest University
Winston-Salem, North Carolina 27157 USA
Telefax: 910-716-5687

The information in this section was assembled under the auspices of the Fibrinogen Subcommittee of the Scientific and Standardization Committee of the International Society on Thrombosis and Haemostasis. The intent of this endeavor was to compile a database of available monoclonal and polyclonal antibodies against fibrinogen. The present listing is by no means exhaustive, and investigators with antibodies to share are encouraged to contact me so that their contributions might be included in future editions of this book.

Individuals wishing to obtain access to these antibodies will need to contact the appropriate investigator to determine availability and cost.

***PLEASE NOTE:** This compilation is intended to promote the study of fibrinogen. However, the listing of an antibody does not represent an unrestricted offering and does not obligate the investigator to provide it to any individual.*

Anti-Fibrinogen Antibodies

List of Investigators

Jean Amiral, PhD
SERBIO P.A.E. Parispace 3
125 Avenue Louis Roche
92230 Gennevilliers France

David L. Amrani, PhD
Dept. of Health Sciences
Univ. of Wisconsin-Milwaukee
PO Box 413
Milwaukee, WI 53201 USA

Frank Brosstad, MD
Research Inst. for Internal Med.
Rikshospitalet Pilestredet 32
0027 Oslo Norway

James P. Chen, PhD
Dept of Medical Biology
Univ. of Tennessee Medical Center
1924 Alcoa Highway
Knoxville, TN 37920 USA

Paul Declerck, PhD
Center Thromb Vasc Res
Univ. of Leuven
Herestraat 49
B-3000 Leuven Belgium

Patrick J. Gaffney, PhD
NIBSC, Blanche Lane
South Mimms, Potters Bar
Hertfordshire, EN6 3QG UK

Patricia J. Haidaris, PhD
Hematology; P.O. Box 610
Univ. of Rochester S.M.D.
601 Elmwood Avenue
Rochester, NY 14642 USA

Stephen J. Kennel, PhD
Biology Division
Oak Ridge National Laboratory
PO Box 2009
Oak Ridge, TN 37831-8077 USA

Bohdan Kudryk, PhD
Blood Coag. & Biochem. Lab
Kimball Research Institute, NYBC
310 East 67th St
New York, NY 10021 USA

Michio Matsuda, MD
Div. Hematol. & Thrombosis Research
Jichi Medical School
Tochigi-Ken 329-04 Japan

Robert R. Montgomery, MD
Coag. Res. Lab.
Blood Center of SE Wisconsin
1701 W. Wisconsin Ave.
Milwaukee, WI 53233 USA

Willem Nieuwenhuizen, PhD
TNO Institute of Ageing and Vascular Research
Zemikedreef 9 P.O. Box 430
2300 AK Leiden
The Netherlands

John Owen, MD
Department of Medicine
Bowman Gray School of Medicine
Medical Center Boulevard
Winston-Salem, NC 27157 USA

John R. Shainoff, PhD
Research Division FF4
Cleveland Clinic
Cleveland, Ohio 44195 USA

Joan Sobel, PhD
Columbia University
College of Physicians & Surgeons
ICCR; PH 10
622 West 168th Street
New York, NY 10032 USA

Jeffrey Weitz, MD
Henderson General Hospital
711 Concession Street
Hamilton, Ontario L8V 1C3
Canada

Anti-Fibrinogen Antibodies

Investigator	Antibody I.D.	Specificity	Immunizing Antigen	Origin	Species/ Isotype	Known Applications	Remarks
J. Amiral	Assera E	FDP-E and fibrinogen	FDP-E	Polyclonal	---	Serum FDP-E	No reaction with FDP-D.
	Assera D	FDP-D and fibrinogen	FDP-D	Polyclonal	---		No reaction with FDP-E.
	Assera Fi	Fibrinogen, FgDP & FbDP	Fibrinogen	Polyclonal	---		
	13F3	Early FDP; not fibrinogen	Fibrin Degradation Products	Monoclonal	---	Plasma FDP	No reaction with D, D-dimer.
	Cx1-F2	D-dimer; not fibrinogen; low avidity for D	D dimer	Monoclonal	---	Plasma D-dimer	
	gC3	FDP neoantigen; not fibrinogen	Fibrinogen degradation products	Monoclonal	---		
D.L. Amrani	MAb 65.1	Bovine D-dimer; not fibrinogen (ELISA)	Bovine D-dimer	Monoclonal	Mouse IgG	ELISA; Western blot	
	MAb 65.2	Bovine D-dimer; not fibrinogen (ELISA)	Bovine D-dimer	Monoclonal	Mouse IgG	ELISA; Western blot	
	MSb 65.5	Bovine D-dimer and fibrinogen (ELISA)	Bovine D-dimer	Monoclonal	Mouse IgM	ELISA; Western blot	
	RAC-1	Fibrinogen	Chicken fibrinogen	Polyclonal	Rabbit	ELISA; Western blot immunoelectrophoresis	
F. Brosstad	S-4	D-dimer; X oligomers	D-dimer	Monoclonal	---	ELISA; Western blot; immunoaffinity purif.	Reacts 2:1 with D-dimer.
	D-2	D-dimer; X oligomers	D-dimer	Monoclonal	---	ELISA; Western blot; immunoaffinity purif.	Reacts 2:1 with D-dimer.
J.P. Chen	R46	D and E domains	fibrinogen	Polyclonal	Rabbit	TRCHI assays of FDP	
	R64	D and E domains of canine fibrinogen	Canine fibrinogen	Polyclonal	Rabbit	TRCHI assays of FDP	
	R23	D and E domains of bovine fibrinogen	Bovine fibrinogen	Polyclonal	Rabbit	TRCHI assays of FDP	
	R124	D and E domains of guinea pig fibrinogen	Guinea pig fibrinogen	Polyclonal	Rabbit	TRCHI assays of FDP	
	R132	D and E domains of porcine fibrinogen	Porcine fibrinogen	Polyclonal	Rabbit		
	R45	Fragment E neoantigen	Fragment E	Polyclonal	Rabbit	Serum & plasma fragment E RIA;	
	R42	Fragment D neoantigen	Fragment D	Polyclonal	Rabbit	Serum & plasma fragment E RIA	
	R119	D-dimer neoantigen	D-dimer	Polyclonal	Rabbit	Plasma D-dimer RIA	

Anti-Fibrinogen Antibodies

Investigator	Antibody I.D.	Specificity	Immunizing Antigen	Origin	Species/ Isotype	Known Applications	Remarks
P. Declerck	MA-15C5	D-dimer; γ-γ-crosslinked FDPs	D-dimer	Monoclonal	Mouse IgG_1	ELISA; imaging; drug targeting	
	MA-8D3	D-dimer; γ-γ-crosslinked FDPs	D-dimer	Monoclonal	Mouse IgG_1	ELISA; imaging	
P.J. Gaffney	NIBn 12B3.B10	Crosslinked fibrin	Denatured human fibrinogen	Monoclonal	Mouse IgG	Imaging	
	NIBn 54-5-8	X-oligomer	X-oligomer	Monoclonal	Mouse IgG	ELISA	
	NIBn 91-11	X-oligomer	D-dimer	Monoclonal	Mouse IgG	ELISA	
	NIBn 123	X-oligomer	X-oligomer	Monoclonal	Mouse IgM	ELISA; imaging	
	NIBn 52	X-oligomer	X-oligomer	Monoclonal	Mouse IgM	ELISA	
	NIBn 54-7-4	X-oligomer	X-oligomer	Monoclonal	Mouse IgG	ELISA	
P.J. Haidaris	L2B	γ(408-416)	CVREHPAET-BSA	Monoclonal	Mouse IgG_1	ELISA; Western blot; immunohistochemistry	
	H9B7	γ-Val411; γ-Leu427	GQQHHLGGAKQAGDV	Monoclonal	Mouse IgM		
	J88B	γ chain & γ chain dimers	FDPs	Monoclonal	Mouse IgG_1	ELISA; Western blot; immunohistochemistry	
	IF10	γ-Leu427(417-427)	YEYDSLYPEDDL	Monoclonal	Mouse IgG_1	ELISA; Western blot	
	D73H	fibrinogen β chain	fibrinogen	Monoclonal	Mouse IgM	ELISA; Western blot	
	D77H	fibrinogen β chain	fibrinogen	Monoclonal	Mouse IgM	ELISA; Western blot	
S.J. Kennel	104-14B	Fibrinogen; fibrin; fragment D	Fragment D	Monoclonal	Rat IgG_{2a}	ELISA; immunoprecipitation	$K_a = 4 \times 10^9$ L/mol
	231-12B	Fragment D, no binding to fibrinogen	Fragment D	Monoclonal	Rat IgG	ELISA	$K_a = 9 \times 10^6$ L/mol
	280-4A	D domain	Fragment D	Monoclonal	Mouse	ELISA; RIA	$K_a = 1.1 \times 10^{10}$ L/mol

Anti-Fibrinogen Antibodies

Investigator	Antibody I.D.	Specificity	Immunizing Antigen	Origin	Species/ Isotype	Known Applications	Remarks
B. Kudryk	T2G1	Bß15-42, ß chain of fibrin, No reaction with Fibrinogen	Thrombin digested NDSK, Mr 52,000	Monoclonal	Mouse IgG_1	Imaging; immuno-histochemistry	
	GC4	Fg-Ds, D-dimer, NO reaction with fibrinogen	Human Fg-Ds, Mr 93,000	Monoclonal	Mouse IgG_1	Imaging; immuno-histochemistry	
	1-8C6	Bß1-42, fibrinogen, Bß chain of fibrinogen	Human NDSK	Monoclonal	Mouse IgG_2	Immunohistochemistry	
	8C2-5	Free FPA, no reactivity with fibrinogen	Synthetic Aα7-16	Monoclonal	Mouse IgG_1	ELISA	
	D21-7	Free FPA, no reactivity with fibrinogen	Tyr-FPA (human)	Monoclonal	Mouse IgG_1	ELISA	
	1D4 xl-f	Fibrinogen, Hi2-DSK (Aα241-476)	Mixture of chains from cross linked fibrin	Monoclonal	Mouse IgG_1		
	4-2 xl-f	COOH end of fibrinogen gamma chain, gamma-gamma dimer, gamma chain of fragment D	Mixture of chains from cross linked fibrin	Monoclonal	Mouse IgG_1		
	2G10	Gamma 15-35, no reactivity with fibrinogen	gamma dimer	Monoclonal	Mouse IgG_2	Western blot; immuno-histochemistry	
	44-3	Fibrinogen gamma chain, cross linked fibrin, fragment D, D dimer, NOT fibrinogen	Mixture of chains from crosslinked fibrin	Monoclonal	Mouse IgG_1	Western blot; immuno-histochemistry	
	Fd4	Fibrinogen, most if not all D fragments, D dimer	Fg-Ds, Mr 93,000	Monoclonal	Mouse IgG_1	Western blot	
	1C2-2 xl-f	Fibrinogen and Aα chain of fibrinogen	Mixture of chains from cross linked fibrin	Monoclonal	Mouse IgG_1	Western blot	
	Ea3	Fibrinogen, Bß and ß chains, most if not all D fragments and D dimer	Fg-Ds, Mr 93,000	Monoclonal	Mouse IgG_1	Western blot	
M. Matsuda	JIF-25	γ(86-302); plasmin-resistant core	Fragment D_1	Monoclonal	Mouse IgG		
	JIF-23	N-termini of D_1,D_2, & D_3	Fragment D_1	Monoclonal	Mouse IgG	D & D-dimer ELISA	Available from IATRON (Japan) in a D-dimer assay.
R.R. Montgomery	A-γ'	γLeu427	γLeu427	Monoclonal	Mouse		Other MAbs with similar specificity are available.

Anti-Fibrinogen Antibodies

Investigator	Antibody I.D.	Specificity	Immunizing Antigen	Origin	Species/ Isotype	Known Applications	Remarks
W. Nieuwenhuizen	FDP-14	Plasmin degradation products; not fibrinogen or fibrin	Fibrin degradation products	Monoclonal	Mouse IgG_1	ELISA	Available in ELISA kit from Organon Teknika.
	Y22	Fibrin, Fg-Y, Fg-D of different species. Weak reaction with fibrinogen	Fragment Y	Monoclonal	Mouse IgG_1	Imaging	
	Y-18	Fibrinogen; FPA-containing fragments	Fragment Y	Monoclonal	Mouse IgM	ELISA	
	Anti-Fb-1/2	Soluble fibrin; D_{EGTA}; D-dimer; not with fibrinogen, D_{CATE}, or Fg-E	Peptide Aα(148-160)	Monoclonal	Mouse IgM	ELISA	
J. Owen	R2..R35	FpA or FpB; variable reactivity with fibrinogen	FpA; FpB	Polyclonal	Rabbit		Only small volumes are available.
J.R. Shainoff	anti-β15-2	Fibrin >> fibrinogen	Peptide β(15-22)	Monoclonal	Mouse IgG		
	anti-h-FP	Mid-region of FpA, both as free peptide and in fibrinogen	FpA-hemocyanin	Monoclonal	Mouse IgG	Immunoaffinity purif. of fibrinogen	
J. Sobel	F-102	Aα(540-554)	CNBr derivative of crosslinked fibrin	Monoclonal	Mouse	ELISA; Western blot	
	F-103	Aα(259-576)	CNBr derivative of crosslinked fibrin	Monoclonal	Mouse	ELISA; Western blot	
J. Weitz	S-847	Aα1-21, no reactivity with FPA, Aα1-19 or Aα1-20	Synthetic Aα14-21	Polyclonal	Sheep	Assay for Aα(1-21)	
	R20-3	Aα1-19, Aα1-20 and Aα1-21, No reaction with FPA	Aα1-20	Polyclonal	Rabbit	Assay for Aα(1-21)	
	R142	Bβ1-42, Bβ1-21. No reactivity with FPB or with Bβ15-42	Bβ1-42	Polyclonal	Rabbit	Assay for Bβ(1-42)	

Detailed Description of Fields

The *Index* is generated from a medium-sized computer database. Each table or Dysfibrinogen Report represents a "merge" of this database with a "template" that instructs the computer to select and print some of the information. Thus, the *Index* differs from a review article in that it can be revised almost instantaneously as new information becomes available.

This important advantage is accompanied by an equally important requirement that the information contained in the database be in a specific format, and that certain rules be followed during data entry. Thus, each "record" [Dysfibrinogen Report] contains 39 "fields" [related information elements that may be as short as a single word (Yes/No) or as long as a list of references].

In this section, those fields will be described. To avoid misinterpretation of the results, the user is advised to browse this list before using the *Index.*

Name: As proposed by Beck et al. [*Blood* **24**:853, **1964** and *Nature* (London) **203**:143, **1965**], variant human fibrinogens are named for the hometown of the index patient or the city in which they were discovered or studied. Customarily, the first report from a city is not assigned a numeric qualifier until a second variant from the same city has been discovered. However, *to simplify updating and retrieval, all dysfibrinogens in this Index have been assigned a numeric qualifier, regardless of whether multiple reports from the same city have been published.* When a city name has two possible spellings, the English version is used. If the variant has been described *only* in a published abstract, the superscript "Abs" (*Abstract*) is placed after the numeric qualifier. If the variant has not been described in a publication, the superscript "Unp" (*Unpublished*) is placed after the numeric qualifier, and the contributing investigator's name(s) will be found under "**Remarks.**" For unpublished variants, only the **name, structural defect, functional defect(s), clinical manifestation(s)** and **thrombin time** will be reported.

Last update: Refers to the date a Dysfibrinogen Report or Table was generated. The date is changed *only* when new information has been entered. For the 1991 edition, all dates were set at 1 December 1990. Additions or corrections have been made to 87 of these entries (including 21 new variants). For these variants this field has been revised to 10 January 1994.

Alphacode: This is an unique sequence of letters and numbers assigned to each variant. The alphacode functions mainly for database management. It contains a maximum of eight characters, with the first six taken from the city name [e.g., Baltimore → BALTIM]. If the city name contains fewer than six letters, all letters in the city name are used [e.g., Paris → PARIS]. If the city name begins with "Saint," the first two letters in the alphacode are "ST," and the remaining four letters are taken from the second word in the city name [e.g., Saint Louis → STLOUI]. The last two elements in the alphacode always contain the numeric qualifier converted from Roman to Arabic numerals. Thus, Roman numeral "I" → "01;" Roman numeral "II" → "02," etc. [e.g., BALTIM02 or PARIS04].

Reference type: Refers to the nature of the information from which a dysfibrinogen report was compiled. Possible entries are: *Article* [At least one publication was from a refereed journal or book chapter]; *Abstract* [The information was published in the abstracts or proceedings of a scientific meeting or congress]; and *Unpublished* [The information was communicated by the individual(s) listed under "**Remarks**"]. As noted earlier, for unpublished variants, only the **name, structural defect, functional defect(s), clinical manifestation(s)** and **thrombin time** will be reported.

Structural defect: Refers to the amino acid substitution presumed to be responsible for the functional defect. For example, "Aα(16) Arg → His" means that at position 16 of the Aα-chain, arginine has been replaced by histidine. If the information required by this field is "not available," the abbreviation "n.a." will be printed between the brackets.

Mutation: Refers to the genetic alteration as determined by DNA sequencing. Typically these data are from polymerase chain reaction (PCR)-based analyses. Often the mutation may be deduced by reference to the relevant genetic sequence. However, only *published* sequencing results are reported in this field. If the information is "not available," the abbreviation "n.a." will be printed between the brackets.

Family studies

Homozygote?: Refers to whether homozygous patients exist among the affected kindreds. Direct evidence must be published. Possible entries are *Yes, No,* or *n.a.* (information is *not available*).

Pedigree published?: Refers to whether a family tree or a paragraph describing affected individuals has been reported. Possible entries are *Yes, No,* or *n.a.* (information is *not available*).

Functional defect

Functional defect determination requires an investigation of the three phases of coagulation. In the *proteolytic* phase, fibrinopeptides A and B are released by thrombin. Most of the pre-1980 literature contains estimates of "Total" (fibrinopeptide A + B) release. In this case, the results usually will be qualified in a footnote. The more recent development of RIA and HPLC methods has made possible the routine measurement of individual fibrinopeptide release. In the *polymerization* phase, fibrin monomers assemble to form the fibrin gel. When compiling this information no distinction was made between polymerization-rate measurements from pre-formed fibrin monomers or from fibrinogen clotted by an excess of thrombin. In the *stabilization* phase, factor XIII catalyzes the formation of amide bonds between lysine (ε-NH_2) and glutamine (γ-$CONH_2$). When compiling this information, no distinction was made between stabilization determinations from clot solubility in denaturants (e.g., in acid or urea), or from direct measurements of γ-γ dimer formation (e.g., by gel electrophoresis).

FpA (fibrinopeptide A) release: Refers to the *rate* of fibrinopeptide A release by thrombin (not to the total amount released, which will be specified in a footnote if abnormal). Possible entries are *Normal, Abnormal,* or *n.a.* (information is *not available*).

FpB (fibrinopeptide B) release: Refers to the *rate* of fibrinopeptide B release by thrombin (not to the total amount released, which will be specified in a footnote if abnormal). Possible entries are *Normal, Abnormal,* or *n.a.* (information is *not available*).

Polymerization: Refers to the rate of fibrin monomer polymerization. No distinction is made between polymerization-rate measurements from pre-formed fibrin monomers or from fibrinogen clotted at high thrombin concentrations. Possible entries are *Normal, Abnormal,* or *n.a.* (information is *not available*).

Stabilization: Refers to the factor XIII-catalyzed formation of intermolecular crosslinks in the fibrin polymer. No distinction is made between stabilization determinations from clot solubility in denaturants such as acid or urea, or from direct measurements of γ-γ dimer formation (e.g., by gel electrophoresis). Possible entries are *Normal, Abnormal,* or *n.a.* (information is *not available*).

Clinical manifestation(s)

Bleeding?: Refers to whether abnormal bleeding has been reported for the index patient or affected kindred. More specific information (e.g., postpartum bleeding, post-trauma bleeding, etc.) usually will be found in a footnote. Possible entries are *Yes*, *No*, or *n.a.* (information is *not available*).

Thrombosis?: Refers to whether a thrombotic event has been reported for the index patient or affected kindred. More specific information (e.g., deep vein thrombosis, myocardial infarction, etc.) usually will be found in a footnote. Possible entries are *Yes*, *No*, or *n.a.* (information is *not available*).

Clinical laboratory results

Unless otherwise noted, clinical laboratory results were obtained from the index patient. **Normal (control) values or ranges are placed in parentheses.** Results may be expressed in seconds (s), minutes (m), hours (h), or percent (%).

Plasma fibrinogen concentration (mg/dL):

Chronometric: Refers to the plasma fibrinogen concentration as determined with an assay that depends on the rate of coagulation [e.g., the method of von Clauss, *Acta Haematol.* **17**:237, **1957**]. A subnormal value has been reported for >99% of the variants described to date.

Rate-indep'nt (-independent): Refers to the plasma fibrinogen concentration as determined with a non-immunologic assay that is independent of the coagulation rate (e.g., the method of Ratnoff and Menzie *J. Lab. Clin. Med.* **37**:316, **1951**; heat precipitation, etc.). Except in cases of hypodysfibrinogenemia, this value typically is within normal limits.

Immunologic: Refers to the plasma fibrinogen concentration as determined with a method using an anti-fibrinogen antibody. This method also is independent of the coagulation rate, and the result typically is within normal limits.

Hypodysfibrinogen?: Refers to whether dysfibrinogenemia is accompanied by subnormal plasma fibrinogen concentration, as determined with a coagulation rate-independent technique. Possible entries are *Yes*, *No*, or *n.a.* (information is *not available*).

Thrombin time: Refers to a thrombin coagulation time determination on patient plasma. Only thrombin times determined without added calcium are reported. A prolonged thrombin time has been reported for >99% of the variants described to date.

Reptilase (batroxobin) time: Refers to a Reptilase (Batroxobin) coagulation time determination on patient plasma. This enzyme releases only fibrinopeptide A.

Prothrombin time: Self-explanatory. The results will be expressed in seconds or percent.

Partial thromboplastin time: Self-explanatory. When compiling this information for the database, no distinction was made between an activated and nonactivated partial thromboplastin time.

Euglobulin lysis time: Self-explanatory. Possible entries are *Normal*, *Abnormal*, *n.a.* (information is *not available*), or the actual results may be given.

Bleeding time: Refers to the bleeding time of the index patient using the Duke or Ivy methods. Possible entries are *Normal*, *Abnormal*, and *n.a.* (information is *not available*); occasionally the actual result will be given.

Immunoelectrophoresis: Refers to the mobility (relative to normal fibrinogen) of patient fibrinogen on an isoelectric focussing gel. Possible entries are *Normal* (same mobility as normal fibrinogen), *Anodal* (increased mobility toward the anode), *Cathodal* (increased mobility toward the cathode), or *n.a.* (information is *not available*).

Platelet aggregation: Refers to the platelet aggregation results for the index patient. Abnormal platelet counts (if available) will be disclosed in a footnote. Possible entries are *Normal, Abnormal,* or *n.a.* (information is *not available*).

Other results with patient plasma

Ancrod (Arvin) time: Refers to an Ancrod (Arvin) coagulation time determination on patient plasma. This enzyme releases only fibrinopeptide A.

Recalcification time: Self-explanatory. Possible entries are *Normal, Abnormal, n.a.* (information is *not available*), or the actual results may be given.

Calcium corrects c.t. (clotting time)?: Refers to whether addition of calcium shortens the thrombin coagulation time to *normal* or *near-normal* values. Calcium always reduces the thrombin time to some extent, but the proportionate reduction is usually greater for variants with abnormal fibrin monomer polymerization. Possible entries are *Yes, No,* or *n.a.* (information is *not available*).

Inhib. (Inhibits) normal plasma?: Refers to whether mixing of normal and patient plasma prolongs the thrombin time of the former. Possible entries are *Yes, No,* or *n.a.* (information is *not available*).

In vivo synthesis: Refers to the results of a study to determine the fibrinogen synthetic rate in a patient with hypodysfibrinogenemia. Possible entries are *Normal, Abnormal,* or *n.a.* (information is *not available*).

In vivo catabolism: Refers to the results of a study to determine the fibrinogen catabolic rate in a patient with hypodysfibrinogenemia. Possible entries are *Normal, Abnormal,* or *n.a.* (information is *not available*).

Evaluation of isolated patient fibrinogen

Thrombin time: Refers to a thrombin coagulation time determination on fibrinogen isolated from patient plasma. Only thrombin times determined without added calcium are reported. If reduced or defective thrombin binding to fibrin has been reported, this will be indicated in a footnote.

Reptilase time: Refers to a Reptilase (Batroxobin) coagulation time determination on fibrinogen isolated from patient plasma. This enzyme releases only fibrinopeptide A.

Ancrod time: Refers to an Ancrod (Arvin) coagulation time determination on fibrinogen isolated from patient plasma. This enzyme releases only fibrinopeptide A.

Abnormal subunit?: Refers to whether a physicochemical abnormality has been detected in one of the dysfibrinogen subunits. More specific information usually will be found in a footnote. Possible entries are *Yes, No,* or *n.a.* (information is *not available*).

Abnormal FDPs [fibrin(ogen) degradation products]?: Refers to whether a physicochemical abnormality has been detected in a fibrin(ogen) degradation product generated by plasmin from the variant. More specific information, including whether the rate of FDP formation is abnormal, usually will be found in a footnote. Possible entries are *Yes*, *No*, or *n.a.* (information is *not available*).

Remarks: Footnotes, author acknowledgements and other comments will appear under this heading.

References: All known references, in reversed-chronological order, will appear under this heading. In general, abstracts are not included if a full article on the same subject has been published. Titles that have been translated into English are placed in square brackets.

Selected Database Information[1]

Last update: 10 January 1994

Number of variants indexed	263[2]	
Articles	225/261	(86%)[3]
Abstract(s) only	32/261	(12%)
Unpublished	4/261	(2%)
Variants with:		
Known structural defects	95/261	(36%)[3]
Abnormal fibrinopeptide release[4]	95/173	(55%)
Abnormal polymerization[4]	183/227	(81%)
Abnormal stabilization[4]	12/100	(12%)
Homozygotes	12/126	(10%)
Hypo(dys)fibrinogenemia	32/221	(14%)
Bleeding tendency	71/228	(31%)
Thrombotic tendency	47/228	(21%)
Bleeding and thrombotic tendency	5/228	(2%)
Bleeding *or* thrombotic tendency	113/228	(50%)
No clinical manifestations	115/228	(50%)

[1]The information on this page was obtained by inspection of the relevant tables (Section 2). Additional summaries will be found on the last page of Tables 3-9.

[2]Due to name duplication [Dusart I ↔ Paris V; Naples I ↔ Milan II] the actual number of variant fibrinogen kindreds listed in this book is 261.

[3]The numbers in this column are rounded to the nearest percent, and take into account the name duplication described in footnote 2.

[4]Note: Many variants exhibit more than one functional abnormality.

KNOWN MUTATIONS IN FIBRINOGEN

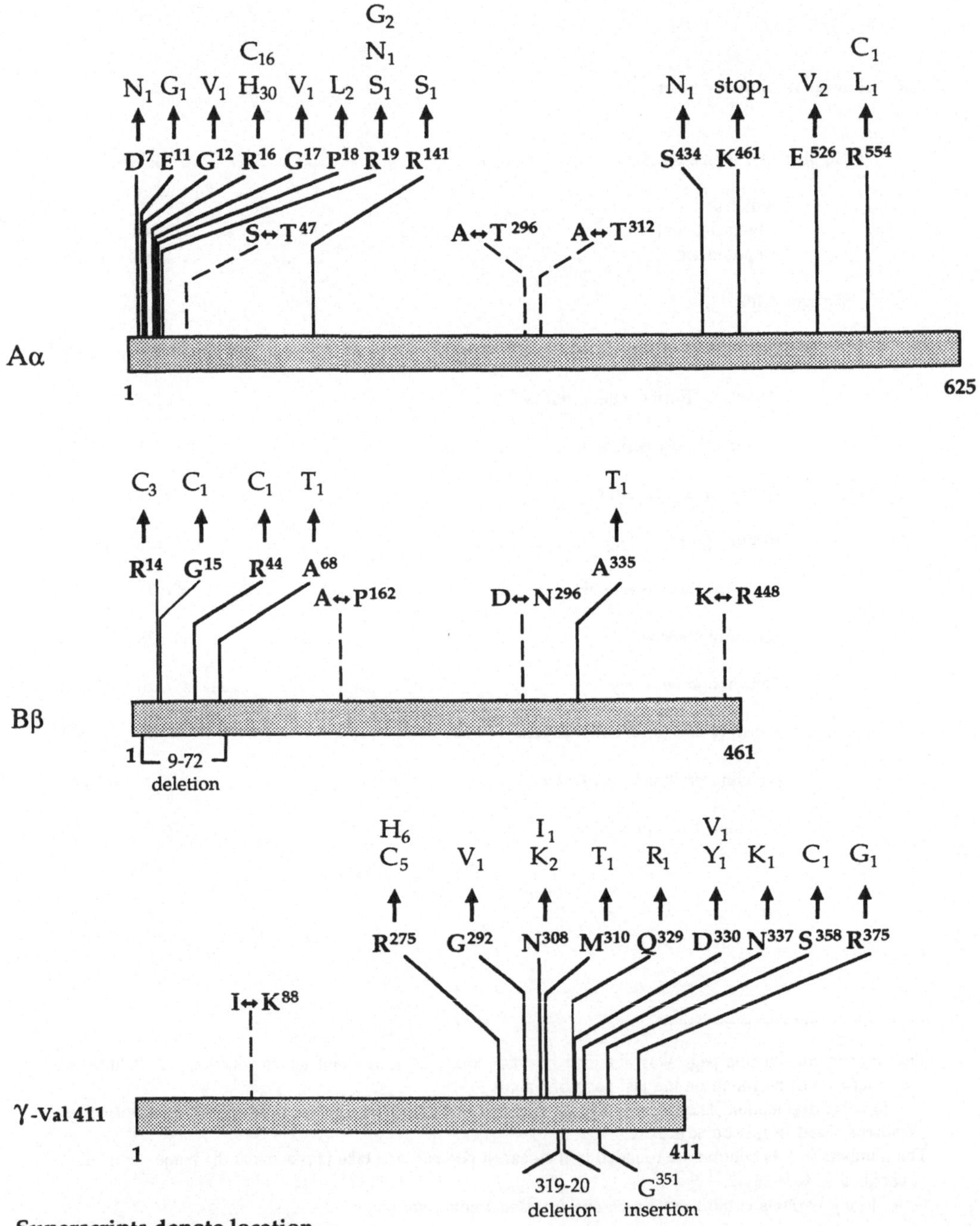

Superscripts denote location.
Subscripts denote frequency.
Dashed lines denote polymorphisms.

Last update: 10 January 1994

SECTION 2

TABULATED DATABASE INFORMATION

NOTES: *1. Additional summary information is located at the end of Tables 3 through 9.*

2. Results for fibrinogens Naples I and Paris V are italicized to emphasize that these are duplicate names (see Dusart I and Milan II, respectively).

Table 1: Alphabetical List of Variant Fibrinogens

Last Update: 10 January 1994 **Total: 261 (Corrected for name duplication)**

Fibrinogen	Last Update	Fibrinogen	Last Update
1. AARAU I[Abs]	10 January 1994	45. CARACAS III	10 January 1994
2. AARHUS I	1 December 1990	46. CARACAS IV	10 January 1994
3. ADELAIDE I	1 December 1990	47. CARACAS V	10 January 1994
4. ALBA/GENEVA I	1 December 1990	48. CARACAS VI	10 January 1994
5. ALÈS I	10 January 1994	49. CARACAS VII	10 January 1994
6. ALMÉRIA I	1 December 1990	50. CHAPEL HILL I	1 December 1990
7. AMIENS I	1 December 1990	51. CHAPEL HILL II	1 December 1990
8. AMIENS II	1 December 1990	52. CHAPEL HILL III	1 December 1990
9. AMSTERDAM I	1 December 1990	53. CHAPEL HILL IV	1 December 1990
10. AMSTERDAM II	1 December 1990	54. CHAPEL HILL V	10 January 1994
11. ARGENTEUIL I	1 December 1990	55. CHAPEL HILL VI	1 December 1990
12. ASAHI I	10 January 1994	56. CHAPEL HILL VII	1 December 1990
13. ASHFORD I	1 December 1990	57. CHARLOTTESVILLE I	1 December 1990
14. AWAJI I	1 December 1990	58. CHICAGO I[Abs]	1 December 1990
15. AWAJI II	1 December 1990	59. CHRISTCHURCH I	1 December 1990
16. BALTIMORE I	1 December 1990	60. CHRISTCHURCH II	1 December 1990
17. BALTIMORE II	1 December 1990	61. CLERMONT-FERRAND I	1 December 1990
18. BALTIMORE III	1 December 1990	62. CLEVELAND I	10 January 1994
19. BALTIMORE IV	1 December 1990	63. CLEVELAND II	10 January 1994
20. BARCELONA I	1 December 1990	64. COPENHAGEN I	1 December 1990
21. BARCELONA II	1 December 1990	65. COPENHAGEN II	1 December 1990
22. BERGAMO I	1 December 1990	66. DATE I	10 January 1994
23. BERGAMO II	1 December 1990	67. DETROIT I	1 December 1990
24. BERGAMO III	1 December 1990	68. DUSART I[1]	10 January 1994
25. BERLIN I	1 December 1990	69. ERFURT I	10 January 1994
26. BERLIN II[Abs]	10 January 1994	70. ERFURT II	1 December 1990
27. BERN I	10 January 1994	71. ESSEN I	1 December 1990
28. BERN II	1 December 1990	72. FRANKFURT I	1 December 1990
29. BERN III	10 January 1994	73. FRANKFURT II	1 December 1990
30. BETHESDA I	1 December 1990	74. FRANKFURT III	1 December 1990
31. BETHESDA II	1 December 1990	75. FRANKFURT IV[Unp]	1 December 1990
32. BETHESDA III	1 December 1990	76. FRANKFURT V[Unp]	1 December 1990
33. BICÊTRE I	1 December 1990	77. FRANKFURT XIII[1]	10 January 1994
34. BICÊTRE II	10 January 1994	78. FREIBURG I	1 December 1990
35. BIRMINGHAM I	1 December 1990	79. GENEVA I	1 December 1990
36. BODMIN I	1 December 1990	80. GENOVA I	1 December 1990
37. BONDY I	10 January 1994	81. GENOVA II	1 December 1990
38. BOULOGNE I[Abs]	10 January 1994	82. GENOVA III[Abs]	1 December 1990
39. BREMEN I	10 January 1994	83. GIESSEN I	1 December 1990
40. BRUSSELS I[Abs]	1 December 1990	84. GIESSEN II	1 December 1990
41. BUENOS AIRES I[Abs]	1 December 1990	85. GIESSEN III	1 December 1990
42. BUENOS AIRES II	1 December 1990	86. GRAND RAPIDS I	1 December 1990
43. CARACAS I	1 December 1990	87. GRENOBLE I	1 December 1990
44. CARACAS II	10 January 1994	88. GUADELOUPE I	1 December 1990

Superscripts refer to footnotes in Dysfibrinogen Reports (Section 3).

Table 1: Alphabetical List of Variant Fibrinogens (cont'd.)

Last Update: 10 January 1994 **Total: 261 (Corrected for name duplication)**

Fibrinogen	Last Update	Fibrinogen	Last Update
89. HAARLEM I	1 December 1990	133. LONDON III	1 December 1990
90. HAARLEM II	1 December 1990	134. LONDON IV	1 December 1990
91. HAIFA I	1 December 1990	135. LONDON V	1 December 1990
92. HANNOVER I	1 December 1990	136. LONDON VI	1 December 1990
93. HERSHEY I	1 December 1990	137. LONG BEACH I[Abs]	1 December 1990
94. HERSHEY II	1 December 1990	138. LOS ANGELES I[Abs]	1 December 1990
95. HOMBURG I	1 December 1990	139. LOUISVILLE I	1 December 1990
96. HOMBURG II	1 December 1990	140. MAASTRICHT I[Abs]	10 January 1994
97. HOMBURG III	1 December 1990	141. MADRID I	1 December 1990
98. HOMBURG IV	10 January 1994	142. MADRID II	1 December 1990
99. HOMBURG V	10 January 1994	143. MADRID III	1 December 1990
100. HOMBURG VI	1 December 1990	144. MAGDEBURG II[Abs]	10 January 1994
101. HOUSTON I	1 December 1990	145. MALAGA I	1 December 1990
102. HOUSTON II	1 December 1990	146. MALMÖE I	10 January 1994
103. IJMUIDEN I	10 January 1994	147. MANCHESTER I	1 December 1990
104. INDIANAPOLIS I	10 January 1994	148. MANNHEIM I	1 December 1990
105. INDIANAPOLIS II	10 January 1994	149. MANNHEIM II[Abs]	1 December 1990
106. INDIANAPOLIS III	10 January 1994	150. MARBURG I	10 January 1994
107. IOWA CITY I	1 December 1990	151. MARSEILLE I	1 December 1990
108. IRVINE I	1 December 1990	152. METZ I	10 January 1994
109. ISE I	10 January 1994	153. MÉXICO DF I[Abs]	10 January 1994
110. ISTANBUL I	1 December 1990	154. MILAN I[1]	1 December 1990
111. ISTANBUL II[Unp]	1 December 1990	155. MILAN II[1]	10 January 1994
112. JENA I	1 December 1990	156. MILAN III[Abs1]	10 January 1994
113. KANAZAWA I	10 January 1994	157. MILAN IV[1]	10 January 1994
114. KASSEL I	1 December 1990	158. MILAN VI[1]	1 December 1990
115. KAWAGUCHI I	1 December 1990	159. MILAN VII[Abs1]	10 January 1994
116. KENDAL I	1 December 1990	160. MITAKA I[Abs]	10 January 1994
117. KIEL I	10 January 1994	161. MITAKA II	10 January 1994
118. KYOTO I	10 January 1994	162. MONTEVIDEO I	10 January 1994
119. KYOTO II	10 January 1994	163. MONTREAL I	1 December 1990
120. KYOTO III	10 January 1994	164. MONTREAL II[Abs]	1 December 1990
121. LA CEVAINA I[Unp]	10 January 1994	165. MONTREAL III[Abs]	10 January 1994
122. LA GUAIRA I	10 January 1994	166. MORIOKA I[Abs]	1 December 1990
123. LA PLATA I	10 January 1994	167. MUNICH I[1]	1 December 1990
124. LEDYARD I	10 January 1994	168. MUNICH II[1]	10 January 1994
125. LEITCHFIELD I	1 December 1990	169. MÜNSTER I[Abs]	1 December 1990
126. LEOGAN I	1 December 1990	170. NAGOYA I	1 December 1990
127. LEUVEN I	1 December 1990	171. NANCY I	10 January 1994
128. LILLE I	10 January 1994	172. *NAPLES I*[1]	*10 January 1994*
129. LIMA I	10 January 1994	173. NEW ALBANY I	1 December 1990
130. LOGROÑO I	1 December 1990	174. NEWARK I[Abs]	1 December 1990
131. LONDON I	1 December 1990	175. NEW BRITAIN I[Abs]	10 January 1994
132. LONDON II	1 December 1990	176. NEW ORLEANS I	1 December 1990

Superscripts refer to footnotes in Dysfibrinogen Reports (Section 3).

Table 1: Alphabetical List of Variant Fibrinogens (cont'd.)

Last Update: 10 January 1994 **Total: 261 (Corrected for name duplication)**

Fibrinogen	Last Update
177. NEW ORLEANS II[Abs]	1 December 1990
178. NEW YORK I	1 December 1990
179. NEW YORK II	10 January 1994
180. NEW YORK III	10 January 1994
181. NEW YORK IV	10 January 1994
182. NIJMEGEN I	10 January 1994
183. NOTTINGHAM I	1 December 1990
184. OKLAHOMA I	10 January 1994
185. ORLEANS I	1 December 1990
186. ORSAY I	1 December 1990
187. OSAKA I	1 December 1990
188. OSAKA II	10 January 1994
189. OSAKA III	10 January 1994
190. OSAKA IV	10 January 1994
191. OSAKA V	10 January 1994
192. OSLO I	10 January 1994
193. OSLO II	1 December 1990
194. OSLO III	1 December 1990
195. OSLO IV	1 December 1990
196. OVIEDO I	1 December 1990
197. OVIEDO II[Abs]	1 December 1990
198. OVIEDO III[Abs]	1 December 1990
199. PAMPLONA I	1 December 1990
200. PAMPLONA II	1 December 1990
201. PARIS I	10 January 1994
202. PARIS II	1 December 1990
203. PARIS III	1 December 1990
204. PARIS IV	1 December 1990
205. *PARIS V*[A]	*10 January 1994*
206. PARIS VI	1 December 1990
207. PARMA I	10 January 1994
208. PERUGIA I	1 December 1990
209. PETOSKEY I	1 December 1990
210. PHILADELPHIA I	1 December 1990
211. PHILADELPHIA II	1 December 1990
212. POITIERS I	1 December 1990
213. PONTOISE I	10 January 1994
214. PRAHRAN I[1]	1 December 1990
215. QUEBEC I	10 January 1994
216. QUEBEC II	1 December 1990
217. RICHFIELD I[Abs]	1 December 1990
218. RIYADH I	10 January 1994
219. ROUEN I	1 December 1990
220. SAGA I	1 December 1990
221. SAINT LOUIS I	10 January 1994
222. SAINT MANDE I	10 January 1994
223. SAINT MANDE II	10 January 1994
224. SALAMANCA I[Abs]	1 December 1990
225. SAN FRANCISCO I[Abs1]	1 December 1990
226. SAN JUAN I	1 December 1990
227. SANTIAGO I	10 January 1994
228. SAPPORO I	1 December 1990
229. SCHWARZACH I	1 December 1990
230. SEATTLE I	1 December 1990
231. SEATTLE II	1 December 1990
232. SEVILLA I	1 December 1990
233. SHEFFIELD I	1 December 1990
234. STONY BROOK I	1 December 1990
235. STONY BROOK II	10 January 1994
236. STRASBOURG I[Abs]	10 January 1994
237. STRASBOURG II[Abs]	10 January 1994
238. SYDNEY I	1 December 1990
239. SYDNEY II	1 December 1990
240. TAMPERE I	10 January 1994
241. TEMPLE I	1 December 1990
242. TEMPLE II	1 December 1990
243. TOCHIGI I	1 December 1990
244. TOKUSHIMA I	1 December 1990
245. TOKYO I	1 December 1990
246. TOKYO II	1 December 1990
247. TORINO I	1 December 1990
248. TROYES I	1 December 1990
249. VALENCIA I	1 December 1990
250. VALHALLA I[Abs]	1 December 1990
251. VANCOUVER I	10 January 1994
252. VERSAILLES I	1 December 1990
253. VICENZA I	1 December 1990
254. VIENNA I[Abs]	1 December 1990
255. VILLEPARISIS I	1 December 1990
256. VILLIERS-SUR-MARNE I	10 January 1994
257. VITRY-SUR-SEINE I	10 January 1994
258. VLISSINGEN I	10 January 1994
259. WHITE MARSH I	10 January 1994
260. WIESBADEN I	1 December 1990
261. YERRES I	1 December 1990
262. ZÜRICH I	1 December 1990
263. ZÜRICH II	10 January 1994

Superscripts refer to footnotes in Dysfibrinogen Reports (Section 3).

Table 2A: Structural Defects Sorted Alphabetically

Last Update: 10 January 1994 Total: 95 (Corrected for name duplication)

Fibrinogen	Structural Defect	Mutation
AARHUS I	Aα(19) Arg → Gly	n.a.
AMIENS I	Aα(16) Arg → His	n.a.
AMIENS II	Aα(16) Arg → His	n.a.
ASAHI I	γ(310) Met → Thr[1]	ATG → ACG
BALTIMORE I	γ(292) Gly → Val[1]	GGC → GTC
BALTIMORE III	γ(308) Asn → Ile	n.a.
BALTIMORE IV	γ(275) Arg → Cys	n.a.
BARCELONA II	Aα(16) Arg → His	n.a.
BERGAMO I	Aα(16) Arg → Cys	n.a.
BERGAMO II	γ(275) Arg → His	n.a.
BERGAMO III	Aα(16) Arg → His	n.a.
BERN I	γ(337) Asn → Lys[1]	AAC → AAA
BERN II	Aα(16) Arg → His	n.a.
BERN III	Aα(16) Arg → Cys	n.a.
BICÊTRE I	Aα(16) Arg → His	n.a.
BICÊTRE II	γ(308) Asn → Lys	AAT → AAG[1]
BIRMINGHAM I	Aα(16) Arg → His	n.a.
BREMEN I	Aα(17) Gly → Val	n.a.
CARACAS II	Aα(434) Ser → Asn	n.a.
CHAPEL HILL II	Aα(16) Arg → His	n.a.
CHRISTCHURCH II	Bβ(14) Arg → Cys	n.a.
CLERMONT-FERRAND I	Aα(16) Arg → His	n.a.
DETROIT I	Aα(19) Arg → Ser	n.a.
DUSART I[1]	Aα(554) Arg → Cys[2]	CGT → TGT
ESSEN I	γ(275) Arg → His	n.a.
FRANKFURT XIII[1]	Aα(16) Arg → Cys[2]	n.a.[3]
GENEVA I	Aα(16) Arg → Cys	n.a.
GIESSEN I	Aα(16) Arg → His	n.a.
HAIFA I	γ(275) Arg → His	n.a.
HERSHEY II	Aα(16) Arg → Cys[1]	CGT → TGT
HOMBURG II	Aα(16) Arg → Cys	n.a.
HOMBURG III	Aα(16) Arg → Cys	n.a.
IJMUIDEN I	Bβ(14) Arg → Cys[1]	CGT →TGT
INDIANAPOLIS I	Aα(554) Arg → Leu[1]	CGT → CTT
INDIANAPOLIS II	Aα(526) Val → Glu	GAG → GTG
INDIANAPOLIS III	Aα(526) Val → Glu	GAG → GTG
ISE I	Bβ(15) Gly → Cys	n.a.
KANAZAWA I	Aα(18) Pro → Leu	n.a.
KAWAGUCHI I	Aα(16) Arg → Cys	n.a.
KENDAL I	Aα(16) Arg → His	n.a.

Superscripts refer to footnotes in Dysfibrinogen Reports (Section 3).

Table 2A: Structural Defects Sorted Alphabetically (cont'd.)

Last Update: 10 January 1994 Total: 95 (Corrected for name duplication)

Fibrinogen	Structural Defect	Mutation
KIEL I	Aα(16) Arg → His	n.a.
KYOTO I	γ(308) Asn → Lys[1]	AAT → AAG
KYOTO II	Aα(18) Pro → Leu	n.a.
KYOTO III	γ(330) Asp → Tyr[1]	GAT → TAT
LEDYARD I	Aα(16) Arg → Cys	n.a.
LEITCHFIELD I	Aα(16) Arg → His	n.a.
LEOGAN I	Aα(16) Arg → Cys[1]	CGT → TGT
LILLE I	Aα(7) Asp → Asn	n.a.
LIMA I	Aα(141) Arg → Ser[1]	n.a.
LONG BEACH I[Abs]	Aα(16) Arg → His	n.a.
LOUISVILLE I	Aα(16) Arg → His	n.a.
MANCHESTER I	Aα(16) Arg → His[1]	CGT → CAT
MANNHEIM I	Aα(19) Arg → Gly	n.a.
MARBURG I	Aα(461) Lys → stop[1]	AAA → TAA
METZ I	Aα(16) Arg → Cys	n.a.
MILAN I[1]	γ(330) Asp → Val	n.a.
MILAN II[1]	Bβ(68) Ala → Thr[2]	GCT → ACT
MILAN IV[1]	Aα(16) Arg → His	n.a.
MILAN VI[1]	Aα(16) Arg → His	n.a.
MILAN VII[Abs1]	γ(358) Ser → Cys[2]	TCT → TGT
MITAKA II	Aα(11) Glu → Gly	n.a.
MORIOKA I[Abs]	γ(275) Arg → Cys	n.a.
MUNICH I[1]	Aα(19) Arg → Asn	n.a.
NAGOYA I	γ(329) Gln → Arg	n.a.
NAPLES I[1]	*Bβ(68) Ala → Thr[2]*	*GCT → ACT*
NEW ALBANY I	Aα(16) Arg → His	n.a.
NEW BRITAIN I[Abs]	Aα(16) Arg → His	n.a.
NEW YORK I	Bβ(9-72) deletion[1]	Exon 2 deletion
NIJMEGEN I	Bβ(44) Arg → Cys[1]	CGT → TGT
OSAKA I	Aα(16) Arg → Cys	n.a.
OSAKA II	γ(275) Arg → Cys[1]	CGC → TGC
OSAKA III	γ(275) Arg → His	n.a.
OSAKA IV	Aα(16) Arg → His	n.a.
OSAKA V	γ(375) Arg → Gly	n.a.
PARIS I	γ(351) Gly → Insertion[1]	GGT → GTT...[1]
PARIS V[1]	*Aα(554) Arg → Cys[2]*	*CGT → TGT*
PARIS VI	Aα(16) Arg → His[1]	n.a.
PERUGIA I	γ(275) Arg → His	n.a.
PETOSKEY I	Aα(16) Arg → His[1]	n.a.
PONTOISE I	Bβ(335) Ala → Thr[1]	n.a.

Superscripts refer to footnotes in Dysfibrinogen Reports (Section 3).

Table 2A: Structural Defects Sorted Alphabetically (cont'd.)

Last Update: 10 January 1994 Total: 95 (Corrected for name duplication)

Fibrinogen	Structural Defect	Mutation
ROUEN I	Aα(12) Gly → Val	n.a.
SAGA I	γ(275) Arg → His	n.a.
SAPPORO I	Aα(16) Arg → His[1]	n.a.
SCHWARZACH I	Aα(16) Arg → Cys	n.a.
SEATTLE I	Bβ(14) Arg → Cys	n.a.
SEATTLE II	Aα(16) Arg → His	n.a.
SHEFFIELD I	Aα(16) Arg → His	n.a.
STONY BROOK I	Aα(16) Arg → Cys	n.a.
STONY BROOK II	Aα(16) Arg → His[1]	n.a.
SYDNEY I	Aα(16) Arg → His	n.a.
SYDNEY II	Aα(16) Arg → His	n.a.
TOCHIGI I	γ(275) Arg → Cys	n.a.
TOKYO II	γ(275) Arg → Cys[1]	n.a.
TORINO I	Aα(16) Arg → Cys	n.a.
VLISSINGEN I	γ(319-320) deletion[1]	AATGAT deletion[1]
WHITE MARSH I	Aα(16) Arg → His	n.a.
ZÜRICH I	Aα(16) Arg → Cys	n.a.

Superscripts refer to footnotes in Dysfibrinogen Reports (Section 3).

Table 2B: Structural Defects Sorted by Location

Last Update: 10 January 1994 Total: 95 (Corrected for name duplication)

Fibrinogen	Structural Defect	Mutation
LILLE I	Aα(7) Asp → Asn	n.a.
MITAKA II	Aα(11) Glu → Gly	n.a.
ROUEN I	Aα(12) Gly → Val	n.a.
BERGAMO I	Aα(16) Arg → Cys	n.a.
BERN III	Aα(16) Arg → Cys	n.a.
FRANKFURT XIII[1]	Aα(16) Arg → Cys[2]	n.a.[3]
GENEVA I	Aα(16) Arg → Cys	n.a.
KAWAGUCHI I	Aα(16) Arg → Cys	n.a.
LEDYARD I	Aα(16) Arg → Cys	n.a.
LEOGAN I	Aα(16) Arg → Cys[1]	CGT → TGT
METZ I	Aα(16) Arg → Cys	n.a.
OSAKA I	Aα(16) Arg → Cys	n.a.
SCHWARZACH I	Aα(16) Arg → Cys	n.a.
STONY BROOK I	Aα(16) Arg → Cys	n.a.
TORINO I	Aα(16) Arg → Cys	n.a.
ZÜRICH I	Aα(16) Arg → Cys	n.a.
HERSHEY II	Aα(16) Arg → Cys[1]	CGT → TGT
HOMBURG II	Aα(16) Arg → Cys	n.a.
HOMBURG III	Aα(16) Arg → Cys	n.a.
AMIENS I	Aα(16) Arg → His	n.a.
AMIENS II	Aα(16) Arg → His	n.a.
BARCELONA II	Aα(16) Arg → His	n.a.
BERGAMO III	Aα(16) Arg → His	n.a.
BERN II	Aα(16) Arg → His	n.a.
BICÊTRE I	Aα(16) Arg → His	n.a.
BIRMINGHAM I	Aα(16) Arg → His	n.a.
CHAPEL HILL II	Aα(16) Arg → His	n.a.
CLERMONT-FERRAND I	Aα(16) Arg → His	n.a.
GIESSEN I	Aα(16) Arg → His	n.a.
KENDAL I	Aα(16) Arg → His	n.a.
KIEL I	Aα(16) Arg → His	n.a.
LEITCHFIELD I	Aα(16) Arg → His	n.a.
LONG BEACH I[Abs]	Aα(16) Arg → His	n.a.
LOUISVILLE I	Aα(16) Arg → His	n.a.
MANCHESTER I	Aα(16) Arg → His[1]	CGT → CAT
MILAN IV[1]	Aα(16) Arg → His	n.a.
MILAN VI[1]	Aα(16) Arg → His	n.a.
NEW ALBANY I	Aα(16) Arg → His	n.a.
NEW BRITAIN I[Abs]	Aα(16) Arg → His	n.a.
OSAKA IV	Aα(16) Arg → His	n.a.
PARIS VI	Aα(16) Arg → His[1]	n.a.

Superscripts refer to footnotes in Dysfibrinogen Reports (Section 3).

Table 2B: Structural Defects Sorted by Location (cont'd.)

Last Update: 10 January 1994 Total: 95 (Corrected for name duplication)

Fibrinogen	Structural Defect	Mutation
PETOSKEY I	Aα(16) Arg → His[1]	n.a.
SAPPORO I	Aα(16) Arg → His[1]	n.a.
SEATTLE II	Aα(16) Arg → His	n.a.
SHEFFIELD I	Aα(16) Arg → His	n.a.
STONY BROOK II	Aα(16) Arg → His[1]	n.a.
SYDNEY I	Aα(16) Arg → His	n.a.
SYDNEY II	Aα(16) Arg → His	n.a.
WHITE MARSH I	Aα(16) Arg → His	n.a.
BREMEN I	Aα(17) Gly → Val	n.a.
KANAZAWA I	Aα(18) Pro → Leu	n.a.
KYOTO II	Aα(18) Pro → Leu	n.a.
MUNICH I[1]	Aα(19) Arg → Asn	n.a.
AARHUS I	Aα(19) Arg → Gly	n.a.
MANNHEIM I	Aα(19) Arg → Gly	n.a.
DETROIT I	Aα(19) Arg → Ser	n.a.
LIMA I	Aα(141) Arg → Ser[1]	n.a.
CARACAS II	Aα(434) Ser → Asn	n.a.
MARBURG I	Aα(461) Lys → stop[1]	AAA → TAA
INDIANAPOLIS II	Aα(526) Val → Glu	GAG → GTG
INDIANAPOLIS III	Aα(526) Val → Glu	GAG → GTG
DUSART I[1]	Aα(554) Arg → Cys[2]	CGT → TGT
PARIS V[1]	*Aα(554) Arg → Cys*[2]	*CGT → TGT*
INDIANAPOLIS I	Aα(554) Arg → Leu[1]	CGT → CTT
NEW YORK I	Bβ(9-72) deletion[1]	Exon 2 deletion
CHRISTCHURCH II	Bβ(14) Arg → Cys	n.a.
IJMUIDEN I	Bβ(14) Arg → Cys[1]	CGT →TGT
SEATTLE I	Bβ(14) Arg → Cys	n.a.
ISE I	Bβ(15) Gly → Cys	n.a.
NIJMEGEN I	Bβ(44) Arg → Cys[1]	CGT → TGT
MILAN II[1]	Bβ(68) Ala → Thr[2]	GCT → ACT
NAPLES I[1]	*Bβ(68) Ala → Thr*[2]	*GCT → ACT*
PONTOISE I	Bβ(335) Ala → Thr[1]	n.a.
BALTIMORE IV	γ(275) Arg → Cys	n.a.
MORIOKA I[Abs]	γ(275) Arg → Cys	n.a.
OSAKA II	γ(275) Arg → Cys[1]	CGC → TGC
TOCHIGI I	γ(275) Arg → Cys	n.a.
TOKYO II	γ(275) Arg → Cys[1]	n.a.
BERGAMO II	γ(275) Arg → His	n.a.
ESSEN I	γ(275) Arg → His	n.a.
HAIFA I	γ(275) Arg → His	n.a.
OSAKA III	γ(275) Arg → His	n.a.
PERUGIA I	γ(275) Arg → His	n.a.
SAGA I	γ(275) Arg → His	n.a.

Superscripts refer to footnotes in Dysfibrinogen Reports (Section 3).

Table 2B: Structural Defects Sorted by Location (cont'd.)

Last Update: 10 January 1994 Total: 95 (Corrected for name duplication)

Fibrinogen	Structural Defect	Mutation
BALTIMORE I	γ(292) Gly → Val[1]	GGC → GTC
BALTIMORE III	γ(308) Asn → Ile	n.a.
BICÊTRE II	γ(308) Asn → Lys	AAT → AAG[1]
KYOTO I	γ(308) Asn → Lys[1]	AAT → AAG
ASAHI I	γ(310) Met → Thr[1]	ATG → ACG
VLISSINGEN I	γ(319-320) deletion[1]	AATGAT deletion[1]
NAGOYA I	γ(329) Gln → Arg	n.a.
KYOTO III	γ(330) Asp → Tyr[1]	GAT → TAT
MILAN I[1]	γ(330) Asp → Val	n.a.
BERN I	γ(337) Asn → Lys[1]	AAC → AAA
PARIS I	γ(351) Gly → Insertion[1]	GGT → GTT...[1]
MILAN VII[Abs1]	γ(358) Ser → Cys[2]	TCT → TGT
OSAKA V	γ(375) Arg → Gly	n.a.

Superscripts refer to footnotes in Dysfibrinogen Reports (Section 3).

Table 3: Summary of Functional Defects

Last Update: 10 January 1994

Fibrinogen	Fibrinopeptide Release			Polymer-ization	Stabili-zation
	Total*	FpA	FpB		
AARAU I[Abs]		n.a.	n.a.	n.a.	n.a.
AARHUS I		Abnormal	Abnormal	Abnormal	Normal
ADELAIDE I		n.a.	n.a.	Normal	n.a.
ALBA/GENEVA I	Abnormal	n.a.[1]	n.a.[1]	Abnormal	Normal
ALÈS I		Normal	Normal	Abnormal	Normal
ALMÉRIA I		n.a.	n.a.	Abnormal	Normal
AMIENS I		Abnormal	Abnormal	Abnormal	n.a.
AMIENS II		Abnormal	Abnormal	Abnormal	n.a.
AMSTERDAM I		Abnormal	Normal	Abnormal	n.a.
AMSTERDAM II		Normal	Normal	n.a.	n.a.
ARGENTEUIL I		Abnormal[1]	n.a.	n.a.	n.a.
ASAHI I		Normal	Normal	Abnormal	Abnormal
ASHFORD I		Normal	Abnormal[1]	Abnormal	n.a.
AWAJI I		Normal	n.a.	Abnormal	n.a.
AWAJI II		Normal	Normal	Abnormal	Normal
BALTIMORE I		Normal	Normal	Abnormal	Abnormal
BALTIMORE II		Normal	Abnormal	Normal	Normal
BALTIMORE III		Normal	Normal	Abnormal	Normal
BALTIMORE IV		Normal	Normal	Abnormal	Normal
BARCELONA I		Abnormal	n.a.	Abnormal	Normal
BARCELONA II		Abnormal[1]	Abnormal	Abnormal	n.a.
BERGAMO I		Abnormal	Normal	Abnormal	n.a.
BERGAMO II		Normal	Normal	Abnormal	n.a.
BERGAMO III		Abnormal[1]	Abnormal[1]	Abnormal	n.a.
BERLIN I		Normal	Abnormal	n.a.	n.a.
BERLIN II[Abs]		n.a.	n.a.	n.a.	n.a.
BERN I		Normal	Normal	Abnormal	n.a.
BERN II		Abnormal	Abnormal[1]	Abnormal	n.a.
BERN III		Abnormal[1]	Normal	Abnormal	n.a.
BETHESDA I		Abnormal	Abnormal	Normal	n.a.
BETHESDA II	Abnormal	n.a.[1]	n.a.[1]	Abnormal	n.a.
BETHESDA III		Normal	Normal	Abnormal	Normal
BICÊTRE I		Abnormal	Abnormal	n.a.[2]	n.a.
BICÊTRE II		n.a.	n.a.	n.a.	n.a.
BIRMINGHAM I		Abnormal	Abnormal	Normal[1]	n.a.
BODMIN I		n.a.	n.a.	n.a.	n.a.
BONDY I		Abnormal	n.a.	Abnormal	n.a.
BOULOGNE I[Abs]		Normal	Normal	Abnormal	Normal
BREMEN I		Abnormal	Abnormal	Abnormal	Normal
BRUSSELS I[Abs]		Normal	Normal	Abnormal	n.a.

Superscripts refer to footnotes in Dysfibrinogen Reports (Section 3).

*An entry will appear in this column if release of individual fibrinopeptides was not determined.

Table 3: Summary of Functional Defects (cont'd.)

Last Update: 10 January 1994

Fibrinogen	Fibrinopeptide Release			Polymer-ization	Stabili-zation
	Total*	FpA	FpB		
BUENOS AIRES I[Abs]		n.a.	n.a.	Abnormal[1]	n.a.
BUENOS AIRES II		Normal[1]	Normal[1]	Abnormal	Normal
CARACAS I		Normal[1]	Normal[1]	Abnormal	Abnormal
CARACAS II		Normal	Normal	Abnormal	Normal
CARACAS III		n.a.	n.a.	Abnormal	Normal
CARACAS IV		Normal	Normal	Abnormal	n.a.
CARACAS V		Normal	Normal	Abnormal	Normal
CARACAS VI		Normal	Normal	Abnormal	n.a.
CARACAS VII		n.a.	n.a.	Abnormal	Normal
CHAPEL HILL I	Normal	Normal[1]	Normal[1]	Abnormal	n.a.
CHAPEL HILL II	Abnormal	n.a.[1]	n.a.[1]	Abnormal	Abnormal[2]
CHAPEL HILL III	Abnormal	n.a.[1]	n.a.[1]	Abnormal	Normal
CHAPEL HILL IV		n.a.	n.a.	Abnormal	Normal
CHAPEL HILL V		n.a.	n.a.	Abnormal	Normal
CHAPEL HILL VI		n.a.	n.a.	Abnormal[1]	Normal
CHAPEL HILL VII		n.a.	n.a.	n.a.	Normal
CHARLOTTESVILLE I	Abnormal	n.a.[1]	n.a.[1]	Normal[2]	Normal[2]
CHICAGO I[Abs]		n.a.	n.a.	n.a.	n.a.
CHRISTCHURCH I		Normal	Normal	n.a.	n.a.
CHRISTCHURCH II		Normal	Abnormal	n.a.	n.a.
CLERMONT-FERRAND I		n.a.	n.a.	Abnormal	Abnormal
CLEVELAND I		Normal	Normal	Abnormal	Normal
CLEVELAND II		Abnormal	Normal	Abnormal	Abnormal
COPENHAGEN I		Abnormal	n.a.	Abnormal	n.a.
COPENHAGEN II		n.a.	n.a.	Abnormal	n.a.
DATE I		Normal	Normal	Abnormal	n.a.
DETROIT I		Normal[1]	Abnormal[1]	Abnormal	Normal
DUSART I[1]	Normal	Normal[3]	Normal[3]	Abnormal	Normal
ERFURT I		Normal	Normal	n.a.	n.a.
ERFURT II		Abnormal[1]	Normal	n.a.	n.a.
ESSEN I		Normal	Normal	Abnormal	n.a.
FRANKFURT I		Normal	Normal	Abnormal	n.a.
FRANKFURT II		Abnormal[1]	n.a.	Abnormal[2]	n.a.
FRANKFURT III		Abnormal[2]	n.a.	Abnormal[3]	n.a.
FRANKFURT IV[Unp]		n.a.	n.a.	Abnormal	n.a.
FRANKFURT V[Unp]		n.a.	n.a.	Abnormal	n.a.
FRANKFURT XIII[1]		Abnormal	Normal	Abnormal	n.a.
FREIBURG I		Abnormal	n.a.	Abnormal	n.a.
GENEVA I		Abnormal[1]	Normal	Abnormal	n.a.
GENOVA I		Normal[1]	Normal[1]	Abnormal	n.a.

Superscripts refer to footnotes in Dysfibrinogen Reports (Section 3).

*An entry will appear in this column if release of individual fibrinopeptides was not determined.

Table 3: Summary of Functional Defects (cont'd.)

Last Update: 10 January 1994

Fibrinogen	Fibrinopeptide Release			Polymer-ization	Stabili-zation
	Total*	FpA	FpB		
GENOVA II		Normal	Normal	Abnormal	Abnormal[1]
GENOVA III[Abs]		Normal	Normal	Abnormal	Normal
GIESSEN I		Abnormal	Normal[1]	Abnormal	n.a.
GIESSEN II		Abnormal	n.a.	Abnormal	n.a.
GIESSEN III		n.a.	n.a.	Abnormal	n.a.
GRAND RAPIDS I		Abnormal	Abnormal	Abnormal	Abnormal[1]
GRENOBLE I		n.a.	n.a.	Abnormal	n.a.
GUADELOUPE I		n.a.	n.a.	n.a.	n.a.
HAARLEM I		Normal	n.a.	Abnormal	n.a.
HAARLEM II		Abnormal	n.a.	Normal	n.a.
HAIFA I	Normal	Normal[1]	Normal[1]	Abnormal	Normal
HANNOVER I		n.a.	n.a.	n.a.	n.a.
HERSHEY I		Normal	Normal	Abnormal	Normal
HERSHEY II		Abnormal[2]	n.a.	Abnormal	Normal
HOMBURG I		Abnormal	n.a.	Abnormal	Normal
HOMBURG II		Abnormal[1]	n.a.	Abnormal[1]	Normal
HOMBURG III		Abnormal[1]	Abnormal[1]	Abnormal[1]	Normal
HOMBURG IV		Normal	Normal[1]	Abnormal	Normal[1]
HOMBURG V		Abnormal	Abnormal[1]	Abnormal	Normal[1]
HOMBURG VI		n.a.	n.a.	n.a.	n.a.
HOUSTON I	Normal	Normal[1]	Normal[1]	Abnormal[2]	Normal
HOUSTON II		n.a.	n.a.	n.a.	n.a.
IJMUIDEN I		n.a.	Abnormal[2]	Abnormal	n.a.
INDIANAPOLIS I		n.a.	n.a.	n.a.	n.a.
INDIANAPOLIS II		n.a.	n.a.	n.a.	n.a.
INDIANAPOLIS III		n.a.	n.a.	n.a.	n.a.
IOWA CITY I		n.a.	n.a.	n.a.	Normal
IRVINE I		Abnormal	n.a.	n.a.	Normal
ISE I		Normal	Abnormal[1]	Abnormal[2]	n.a.
ISTANBUL I		n.a.	n.a.	n.a.	n.a.
ISTANBUL II[Unp]		Abnormal	Abnormal	Normal	n.a.
JENA I		Abnormal[1]	n.a.	n.a.	n.a.
KANAZAWA I		n.a.[1]	n.a.[1]	Abnormal	n.a.
KASSEL I		Normal	Normal	n.a.	n.a.
KAWAGUCHI I		Abnormal[1]	n.a.	Abnormal	n.a.
KENDAL I		n.a.	n.a.	n.a.	n.a.
KIEL I		Abnormal[1]	n.a.	n.a.	n.a.
KYOTO I		Normal	Normal	Abnormal	Normal
KYOTO II		Normal	Normal	Abnormal	n.a.
KYOTO III		Normal	Normal	Abnormal	Normal

Superscripts refer to footnotes in Dysfibrinogen Reports (Section 3).

*An entry will appear in this column if release of individual fibrinopeptides was not determined.

Table 3: Summary of Functional Defects (cont'd.)

Last Update: 10 January 1994

Fibrinogen	Fibrinopeptide Release			Polymer-ization	Stabili-zation
	Total*	FpA	FpB		
LA CEVAINA I[Unp]		Normal	Normal	Abnormal	Normal
LA GUAIRA I		Normal	Normal	Abnormal	Normal
LA PLATA I		Normal	Normal	Abnormal	Normal[1]
LEDYARD I		Abnormal[1]	Abnormal	Abnormal	n.a.
LEITCHFIELD I		n.a.	n.a.	n.a.	n.a.
LEOGAN I		Abnormal[2]	n.a.	Abnormal	Normal
LEUVEN I		n.a.	n.a.	Abnormal	Normal
LILLE I	Abnormal	n.a.[1]	n.a.[1]	Abnormal	Normal
LIMA I		n.a.	n.a.	Abnormal[3]	n.a.
LOGROÑO I		n.a.	n.a.	Abnormal	n.a.
LONDON I		Normal	Normal	Abnormal	n.a.
LONDON II		Normal	n.a.	Abnormal	n.a.
LONDON III		Abnormal[1]	Abnormal	Abnormal	n.a.
LONDON IV		Abnormal	Abnormal	Abnormal	n.a.
LONDON V		Normal	Normal	Abnormal	n.a.
LONDON VI		Abnormal[1]	n.a.	n.a.	n.a.
LONG BEACH I[Abs]		n.a.	n.a.	n.a.	n.a.
LOS ANGELES I[Abs]		n.a.	n.a.	Abnormal	Normal
LOUISVILLE I		Abnormal[1]	n.a.	Normal	n.a.
MAASTRICHT I[Abs]		n.a.	n.a.	n.a.	n.a.
MADRID I		Normal	Abnormal	Normal	n.a.
MADRID II		Abnormal[1]	Abnormal	Normal	n.a.
MADRID III		Abnormal[1]	n.a.	Normal	Normal
MAGDEBURG II[Abs]		n.a.	n.a.	n.a.	n.a.
MALAGA I		Abnormal[1]	n.a.	Abnormal	Normal
MALMÖE I		Normal	Normal	Abnormal	Normal
MANCHESTER I		Abnormal	Abnormal	Abnormal	Normal
MANNHEIM I		Abnormal	n.a.	Abnormal	Normal
MANNHEIM II[Abs]		Normal	n.a.	Abnormal	Normal
MARBURG I		Normal	Normal	Abnormal	Normal
MARSEILLE I		Abnormal[1]	Normal	Abnormal	Normal
METZ I		Abnormal[1]	Normal	Abnormal	Normal
MÉXICO DF I[Abs]		Abnormal	Abnormal	Abnormal	n.a.
MILAN I[1]		Normal	Normal	Abnormal	n.a.
MILAN II[1]		Abnormal	Abnormal	Normal	Normal
MILAN III[Abs1]		n.a.	n.a.	Abnormal	n.a.
MILAN IV[1]		Abnormal[2]	n.a.	Abnormal	n.a.
MILAN VI[1]		n.a.	n.a.	Abnormal	n.a.
MILAN VII[Abs1]		Normal	Normal	Abnormal[3]	n.a.
MITAKA I[Abs]		Normal	Normal	Abnormal	Normal

Superscripts refer to footnotes in Dysfibrinogen Reports (Section 3).

*An entry will appear in this column if release of individual fibrinopeptides was not determined.

Table 3: Summary of Functional Defects (cont'd.)

Last Update: 10 January 1994

Fibrinogen	Fibrinopeptide Release			Polymer-ization	Stabili-zation
	Total*	FpA	FpB		
MITAKA II		Abnormal	Abnormal	Normal	n.a.
MONTEVIDEO I		Normal	Normal	Abnormal	Normal
MONTREAL I	Normal	Normal[1]	Normal[1]	Abnormal	n.a.
MONTREAL II[Abs]		n.a.	n.a.	Abnormal	n.a.
MONTREAL III[Abs]		n.a.	n.a.	n.a.	n.a.
MORIOKA I[Abs]		n.a.	n.a.	Abnormal	Normal
MUNICH I[1]		Abnormal	n.a.	Abnormal	n.a.
MUNICH II[1]		Abnormal	n.a.	Abnormal	n.a.
MÜNSTER I[Abs]		n.a.	n.a.	n.a.	n.a.
NAGOYA I		Normal	Normal	Abnormal	Normal
NANCY I		n.a.[1]	n.a.[1]	Abnormal	n.a.
NAPLES I[1]		*Abnormal*	*Abnormal*	*Normal*	*Normal*
NEW ALBANY I		n.a.	n.a.	n.a.	n.a.
NEWARK I[Abs]		n.a.	n.a.	n.a.	n.a.
NEW BRITAIN I[Abs]		Abnormal	n.a.	Abnormal	n.a.
NEW ORLEANS I		Abnormal[1]	Abnormal[1]	Normal	Normal
NEW ORLEANS II[Abs]		n.a.	n.a.	Normal	n.a.
NEW YORK I		Abnormal	Abnormal	Abnormal	Normal
NEW YORK II		Abnormal	Abnormal	Abnormal	n.a.
NEW YORK III		Normal	Normal	Abnormal	n.a.
NEW YORK IV		Normal	Normal	Abnormal	n.a.
NIJMEGEN I		Normal	Normal	Abnormal	n.a.
NOTTINGHAM I		n.a.	n.a.	n.a.	n.a.
OKLAHOMA I	Normal	Normal[1]	Normal[1]	Normal	Normal
ORLEANS I	Abnormal	n.a.[1]	n.a.[1]	Abnormal	n.a.
ORSAY I		n.a.	n.a.	n.a.	n.a.
OSAKA I		Abnormal[1]	n.a.	Abnormal[1]	n.a.
OSAKA II		Normal	Normal	Abnormal	Normal
OSAKA III		Normal	Normal	Abnormal	Normal
OSAKA IV		Abnormal[1]	Normal	Abnormal	n.a.
OSAKA V		n.a.	n.a.	Abnormal[1]	n.a.
OSLO I		n.a.[1]	n.a.[1]	n.a.	n.a.
OSLO II		Normal	Normal	Abnormal	n.a.
OSLO III		n.a.[1]	n.a.[1]	n.a.	Normal
OSLO IV		n.a.[1]	n.a.[1]	Abnormal	n.a.
OVIEDO I		Normal	Normal	Abnormal	Normal
OVIEDO II[Abs]		Normal	Normal	Abnormal	Normal
OVIEDO III[Abs]		Normal	Normal	Abnormal	Normal
PAMPLONA I		n.a.	n.a.	Abnormal	Normal
PAMPLONA II		Normal	Abnormal[1]	Abnormal	Normal

Superscripts refer to footnotes in Dysfibrinogen Reports (Section 3).

*An entry will appear in this column if release of individual fibrinopeptides was not determined.

Table 3: Summary of Functional Defects (cont'd.)

Last Update: 10 January 1994

Fibrinogen	Fibrinopeptide Release			Polymer-ization	Stabili-zation
	Total*	FpA	FpB		
PARIS I	Normal	Normal[2]	Normal[2]	Abnormal	Abnormal
PARIS II	Normal	Normal[1]	Normal[1]	Abnormal	n.a.
PARIS III	Normal	Normal[1]	Normal[1]	Abnormal	Normal
PARIS IV		n.a.	n.a.	Abnormal	n.a.
PARIS V[1]		*Normal*[3]	*Normal*[3]	*Abnormal*	*Normal*
PARIS VI		n.a.[2]	n.a.[2]	n.a.[2]	n.a.
PARMA I		n.a.	n.a.	n.a.	n.a.
PERUGIA I		Normal	Normal	Abnormal	n.a.
PETOSKEY I		Abnormal	Abnormal	Abnormal	Normal
PHILADELPHIA I	Normal	Normal[1]	Normal[1]	Abnormal	n.a.
PHILADELPHIA II		n.a.[1]	n.a.[1]	n.a.	n.a.
POITIERS I		Abnormal	n.a.	n.a.	n.a.
PONTOISE I		Normal	Normal	Abnormal	Normal
PRAHRAN I[1]		n.a.	n.a.	n.a.	n.a.
QUEBEC I	Normal	Normal[1]	Normal[1]	Abnormal	n.a.
QUEBEC II	Abnormal	n.a.[1]	n.a.[1]	Abnormal	n.a.
RICHFIELD I[Abs]		Normal	n.a.	Abnormal	n.a.
RIYADH I		n.a.	n.a.	Abnormal	Normal
ROUEN I		Abnormal	Normal	Normal	n.a.
SAGA I		Normal	Normal	Abnormal	Normal
SAINT LOUIS I	Normal	Normal[1]	Normal[1]	Abnormal	n.a.
SAINT MANDE I		n.a.	n.a.	Abnormal	n.a.
SAINT MANDE II		n.a.	n.a.	Abnormal	n.a.
SALAMANCA I[Abs]		Normal	Normal	Abnormal	Normal
SAN FRANCISCO I[Abs1]		n.a.	n.a.	Abnormal	n.a.
SAN JUAN I		n.a.	n.a.	n.a.	n.a.
SANTIAGO I		Abnormal	Abnormal	Abnormal	n.a.
SAPPORO I		Abnormal	Abnormal	Normal	Normal
SCHWARZACH I		Abnormal[1]	n.a.	Abnormal	n.a.
SEATTLE I		Normal	Abnormal[1]	Abnormal	Normal
SEATTLE II		Abnormal[1]	Abnormal	Abnormal	Normal
SEVILLA I	Normal	Normal[1]	Normal[1]	Abnormal	Normal
SHEFFIELD I		n.a.[1]	n.a.[1]	n.a.[1]	n.a.
STONY BROOK I		Abnormal	n.a.	Abnormal	n.a.
STONY BROOK II		Abnormal	n.a.	Abnormal	n.a.
STRASBOURG I[Abs]		n.a.	n.a.	Abnormal[1]	n.a.
STRASBOURG II[Abs]		n.a.	n.a.	n.a.	n.a.
SYDNEY I		Abnormal	Abnormal[1]	Abnormal	n.a.
SYDNEY II		Abnormal	Abnormal	n.a.[1]	n.a.
TAMPERE I		n.a.	n.a.	n.a.	n.a.

Superscripts refer to footnotes in Dysfibrinogen Reports (Section 3).

*An entry will appear in this column if release of individual fibrinopeptides was not determined.

Table 3: Summary of Functional Defects (cont'd.)

Last Update: 10 January 1994

Fibrinogen	Fibrinopeptide Release			Polymer-ization	Stabili-zation
	Total*	FpA	FpB		
TEMPLE I		n.a.[1]	n.a.[1]	n.a.	n.a.
TEMPLE II		n.a.[1]	n.a.[1]	n.a.	n.a.
TOCHIGI I		Normal	Normal	Abnormal	Normal
TOKUSHIMA I		Normal[1]	Normal[1]	Abnormal	Normal
TOKYO I		n.a.	n.a.	n.a.	Abnormal
TOKYO II	Normal	Normal[2]	Normal[2]	Abnormal	Normal
TORINO I		n.a.[1]	n.a.[1]	Abnormal	n.a.
TROYES I		Normal	Normal	Abnormal	n.a.
VALENCIA I		n.a.	n.a.	Normal	Abnormal[6]
VALHALLA I^{Abs}		Normal	Abnormal[1]	Abnormal	n.a.
VANCOUVER I		n.a.	n.a.	n.a.	n.a.
VERSAILLES I		n.a.	n.a.	Abnormal	n.a.
VICENZA I	Normal	Normal[1]	Normal[1]	Abnormal	Normal
VIENNA I^{Abs}		n.a.	n.a.	Abnormal	n.a.
VILLEPARISIS I		n.a.	n.a.	n.a.	n.a.
VILLIERS-SUR-MARNE I		n.a.	n.a.	n.a.	n.a.
VITRY-SUR-SEINE I		n.a.	n.a.	n.a.	n.a.
VLISSINGEN I		Normal	Normal	Abnormal	n.a.
WHITE MARSH I		Abnormal	Abnormal	Abnormal	n.a.[1]
WIESBADEN I		n.a.	n.a.	n.a.	Abnormal[1]
YERRES I		n.a.	n.a.	n.a.	n.a.
ZÜRICH I		Abnormal[1]	n.a.	Abnormal	Normal
ZÜRICH II		Normal[1]	Normal[1]	Abnormal	Normal

Superscripts refer to footnotes in Dysfibrinogen Reports (Section 3).

*An entry will appear in this column if release of individual fibrinopeptides was not determined.

Summary of Functional Defect Data

Variants with abnormal fibrinopeptide release:	95/173	55%
Variants with abnormal fibrin monomer polymerization:	183/227	81%
Variants with abnormal fibrin stabilization:	12/100	12%

NOTE: Many variants are defective in more than one phase of coagulation.

Table 4: Family Studies

Last Update: 10 January 1994

Fibrinogen	Homozygote? [Yes/No/n.a.]	Pedigree Published? [Yes/No)]
AARAU I[Abs]	n.a.	No
AARHUS I	Yes	Yes[1]
ADELAIDE I	No	Yes
ALBA/GENEVA I	n.a.	No
ALÈS I	Yes	No
ALMÉRIA I	n.a.	No
AMIENS I	No	No
AMIENS II	No	No
AMSTERDAM I	No	Yes
AMSTERDAM II	n.a.	No
ARGENTEUIL I	n.a.	Yes
ASAHI I	No	No
ASHFORD I	n.a.	No
AWAJI I	No	Yes
AWAJI II	n.a.	Yes
BALTIMORE I	No	Yes
BALTIMORE II	No	Yes
BALTIMORE III	No	No
BALTIMORE IV	No	Yes
BARCELONA I	n.a.	No
BARCELONA II	No	Yes
BERGAMO I	No	No
BERGAMO II	No	No
BERGAMO III	No	No
BERLIN I	No	No
BERLIN II[Abs]	No	No
BERN I	No	Yes
BERN II	No	No
BERN III	No	Yes
BETHESDA I	No	Yes
BETHESDA II	n.a.	No
BETHESDA III	No	Yes
BICÊTRE I	Yes[1]	No
BICÊTRE II	No	Yes
BIRMINGHAM I	No	No
BODMIN I	n.a.	No
BONDY I	No	No
BOULOGNE I[Abs]	n.a.	No
BREMEN I	No	No
BRUSSELS I[Abs]	n.a.	No

Superscripts refer to footnotes in Dysfibrinogen Reports (Section 3).

Table 4: Family Studies (cont'd.)

Last Update: 10 January 1994

Fibrinogen	Homozygote? [Yes/No/n.a.]	Pedigree Published? [Yes/No)]
BUENOS AIRES I[Abs]	n.a.	No
BUENOS AIRES II	n.a.	No
CARACAS I	No[1]	Yes
CARACAS II	n.a.	No
CARACAS III	n.a.	No
CARACAS IV	n.a.	No
CARACAS V	n.a.	No
CARACAS VI	n.a.	No
CARACAS VII	n.a.	No
CHAPEL HILL I	n.a.	No
CHAPEL HILL II	No	No
CHAPEL HILL III	n.a.	Yes
CHAPEL HILL IV	n.a.	No
CHAPEL HILL V	n.a.	No
CHAPEL HILL VI	n.a.	No
CHAPEL HILL VII	n.a.	No
CHARLOTTESVILLE I	Yes	Yes
CHICAGO I[Abs]	No	No
CHRISTCHURCH I	n.a.	No
CHRISTCHURCH II	No	No
CLERMONT-FERRAND I	n.a.	No
CLEVELAND I	n.a.	Yes
CLEVELAND II	n.a.	Yes
COPENHAGEN I	n.a.	Yes
COPENHAGEN II	n.a.	No
DATE I	n.a.	Yes
DETROIT I	Yes	Yes
DUSART I[1]	No	Yes
ERFURT I	No	Yes
ERFURT II	No	No
ESSEN I	No	No
FRANKFURT I	n.a.	No
FRANKFURT II	n.a.	No
FRANKFURT III	n.a.	No
FRANKFURT IV[Unp]	n.a.	No
FRANKFURT V[Unp]	n.a.	No
FRANKFURT XIII[1]	No	Yes
FREIBURG I	n.a.	No
GENEVA I	No	Yes
GENOVA I	n.a.	Yes

Superscripts refer to footnotes in Dysfibrinogen Reports (Section 3).

Table 4: Family Studies (cont'd.)

Last Update: 10 January 1994

Fibrinogen	Homozygote? [Yes/No/n.a.]	Pedigree Published? [Yes/No)]
GENOVA II	n.a.	No
GENOVA III[Abs]	n.a.	No
GIESSEN I	Yes	No[2]
GIESSEN II	n.a.	No
GIESSEN III	n.a.	No
GRAND RAPIDS I	No	No
GRENOBLE I	No	No
GUADELOUPE I	n.a.	No
HAARLEM I	No	Yes
HAARLEM II	No	No
HAIFA I	n.a.	No
HANNOVER I	n.a.	No
HERSHEY I	n.a.	Yes
HERSHEY II	No	No
HOMBURG I	No	Yes
HOMBURG II	No	Yes
HOMBURG III	No	Yes
HOMBURG IV	No[1]	No
HOMBURG V	No[1]	No
HOMBURG VI	n.a.	No
HOUSTON I	n.a.	No
HOUSTON II	n.a.	No
IJMUIDEN I	No	No
INDIANAPOLIS I	No	Yes
INDIANAPOLIS II	No	Yes
INDIANAPOLIS III	No	Yes
IOWA CITY I	n.a.	No
IRVINE I	n.a.	Yes
ISE I	No	Yes
ISTANBUL I	n.a.	No
ISTANBUL II[Unp]	n.a.	No
JENA I	No	Yes
KANAZAWA I	No	Yes
KASSEL I	n.a.	No
KAWAGUCHI I	No	Yes
KENDAL I	n.a.	No
KIEL I	No	Yes
KYOTO I	No	Yes
KYOTO II	n.a.	No
KYOTO III	No	No

Superscripts refer to footnotes in Dysfibrinogen Reports (Section 3).

Table 4: Family Studies (cont'd.)

Last Update: 10 January 1994

Fibrinogen	Homozygote? [Yes/No/n.a.]	Pedigree Published? [Yes/No)]
LA CEVAINA I[Unp]	n.a.	No
LA GUAIRA I	n.a.	No
LA PLATA I	n.a.	No
LEDYARD I	No	No
LEITCHFIELD I	No	n.a.
LEOGAN I	No	No
LEUVEN I	n.a.	Yes[1]
LILLE I	No	No[2]
LIMA I	Yes	No[2]
LOGROÑO I	No	Yes
LONDON I	n.a.	Yes
LONDON II	n.a.	No
LONDON III	Yes	No
LONDON IV	n.a.	No
LONDON V	n.a.	No
LONDON VI	No	No
LONG BEACH I[Abs]	n.a.	No
LOS ANGELES I[Abs]	n.a.	No
LOUISVILLE I	No	Yes
MAASTRICHT I[Abs]	n.a.	No
MADRID I	n.a.	No
MADRID II	No	No
MADRID III	No	No
MAGDEBURG II[Abs]	n.a.	No
MALAGA I	No	No
MALMÖE I	n.a.	No
MANCHESTER I	No	Yes
MANNHEIM I	No	Yes
MANNHEIM II[Abs]	n.a.	No
MARBURG I	Yes	Yes
MARSEILLE I	n.a.	No
METZ I	Yes	Yes[2]
MÉXICO DF I[Abs]	n.a.	No
MILAN I[1]	No	No
MILAN II[1]	Yes[3]	Yes[3]
MILAN III[Abs1]	Yes	No
MILAN IV[1]	No	No
MILAN VI[1]	No	Yes
MILAN VII[Abs1]	No	No
MITAKA I[Abs]	n.a.	No

Superscripts refer to footnotes in Dysfibrinogen Reports (Section 3).

Table 4: Family Studies (cont'd.)

Last Update: 10 January 1994

Fibrinogen	Homozygote? [Yes/No/n.a.]	Pedigree Published? [Yes/No)]
MITAKA II	No	No
MONTEVIDEO I	n.a.	No
MONTREAL I	n.a.	No
MONTREAL II[Abs]	n.a.	No
MONTREAL III[Abs]	n.a.	No
MORIOKA I[Abs]	No	No
MUNICH I[1]	n.a.	No
MUNICH II[1]	n.a.	No
MÜNSTER I[Abs]	n.a.	No
NAGOYA I	No	No
NANCY I	n.a.	No
NAPLES I[1]	*Yes*[3]	*Yes*[3]
NEW ALBANY I	No	No
NEWARK I[Abs]	n.a.	No
NEW BRITAIN I[Abs]	n.a.	No
NEW ORLEANS I	No	Yes
NEW ORLEANS II[Abs]	n.a.	No
NEW YORK I	No	Yes
NEW YORK II	n.a.	No
NEW YORK III	n.a.	No
NEW YORK IV	n.a.	No
NIJMEGEN I	No	Yes
NOTTINGHAM I	n.a.	No
OKLAHOMA I	n.a.	Yes
ORLEANS I	n.a.	No
ORSAY I	n.a.	No
OSAKA I	No	No
OSAKA II	No	No
OSAKA III	No	No
OSAKA IV	No	Yes
OSAKA V	No	No
OSLO I	No	Yes
OSLO II	n.a.	Yes
OSLO III	No	No
OSLO IV	n.a.	Yes
OVIEDO I	n.a.	No[1]
OVIEDO II[Abs]	n.a.	No
OVIEDO III[Abs]	n.a.	No
PAMPLONA I	No	Yes
PAMPLONA II	No[1]	No

Superscripts refer to footnotes in Dysfibrinogen Reports (Section 3).

Table 4: Family Studies (cont'd.)

Last Update: 10 January 1994

Fibrinogen	Homozygote? [Yes/No/n.a.]	Pedigree Published? [Yes/No)]
PARIS I	No	No
PARIS II	n.a.	Yes
PARIS III	n.a.	No
PARIS IV	n.a.	No
PARIS V[A]	*No*	*Yes*
PARIS VI	No	No
PARMA I	n.a.	Yes
PERUGIA I	No	No
PETOSKEY I	No	Yes
PHILADELPHIA I	n.a.	Yes
PHILADELPHIA II	n.a.	No
POITIERS I	n.a.	Yes
PONTOISE I	No	No
PRAHRAN I[1]	n.a.	No
QUEBEC I	n.a.	No
QUEBEC II	n.a.	No
RICHFIELD I[Abs]	n.a.	No
RIYADH I	n.a.	No[1]
ROUEN I	No	No
SAGA I	No	No
SAINT LOUIS I	n.a.	Yes
SAINT MANDE I	n.a.	No
SAINT MANDE II	n.a.	No
SALAMANCA I[Abs]	n.a.	No
SAN FRANCISCO I[Abs1]	No	No
SAN JUAN I	n.a.	Yes
SANTIAGO I	n.a.	No
SAPPORO I	No	Yes
SCHWARZACH I	No	No
SEATTLE I	No	Yes
SEATTLE II	No	No
SEVILLA I	No[2]	No
SHEFFIELD I	No	No
STONY BROOK I	No	No
STONY BROOK II	No	No[2]
STRASBOURG I[Abs]	n.a.	n.a.
STRASBOURG II[Abs]	n.a.	n.a.
SYDNEY I	No	No
SYDNEY II	No	No
TAMPERE I	n.a.	No

Superscripts refer to footnotes in Dysfibrinogen Reports (Section 3).

Table 4: Family Studies (cont'd.)

Last Update: 10 January 1994

Fibrinogen	Homozygote? [Yes/No/n.a.]	Pedigree Published? [Yes/No)]
TEMPLE I	n.a.	No
TEMPLE II	n.a.	No
TOCHIGI I	No	No
TOKUSHIMA I	n.a.	Yes
TOKYO I	n.a.	No[1]
TOKYO II	No	Yes
TORINO I	No	No
TROYES I	n.a.	Yes
VALENCIA I	n.a.	Yes[1]
VALHALLA I[Abs]	No	No
VANCOUVER I	n.a.	Yes
VERSAILLES I	n.a.	Yes
VICENZA I	No	No
VIENNA I[Abs]	n.a.	No
VILLEPARISIS I	n.a.	No
VILLIERS-SUR-MARNE I	n.a.	No
VITRY-SUR-SEINE I	n.a.	No
VLISSINGEN I	No	No
WHITE MARSH I	No	No
WIESBADEN I	n.a.	No
YERRES I	n.a.	No
ZÜRICH I	No	No
ZÜRICH II	n.a.	No

Superscripts refer to footnotes in Dysfibrinogen Reports (Section 3).

Summary of Family Study Data

Variants with homozygotic patients:	12/126	10%
Variants with published pedigrees:	77/261	30%

Table 5: Clinical Manifestations

Last Update: 10 January 1994

Fibrinogen	Bleeding?	Thrombosis?
AARAU I[Abs]	No	No
AARHUS I	No	Yes[2]
ADELAIDE I	Yes[1]	No
ALBA/GENEVA I	No[2]	No[2]
ALÈS I	No	Yes[1]
ALMÉRIA I	No	No
AMIENS I	n.a.	n.a.
AMIENS II	n.a.	n.a.
AMSTERDAM I	No	No
AMSTERDAM II	n.a.	n.a.
ARGENTEUIL I	No	Yes[2]
ASAHI I	Yes[2]	No
ASHFORD I	n.a.	n.a.
AWAJI I	No	No
AWAJI II	No	Yes[1]
BALTIMORE I	Yes[2]	Yes[2]
BALTIMORE II	Yes[2]	No
BALTIMORE III	No	No
BALTIMORE IV	No	No
BARCELONA I	Yes[1]	No
BARCELONA II	Yes[2]	No
BERGAMO I	No	No
BERGAMO II	No	Yes[1]
BERGAMO III	No	No
BERLIN I	No	No
BERLIN II[Abs]	n.a.	n.a.
BERN I	No	No
BERN II	No	No
BERN III	No	No
BETHESDA I	Yes[1]	No
BETHESDA II	No	No
BETHESDA III	Yes[1]	Yes[1]
BICÊTRE I	n.a.	n.a.
BICÊTRE II	No	Yes[2]
BIRMINGHAM I	Yes[2]	No
BODMIN I	n.a.	n.a.
BONDY I	No	No
BOULOGNE I[Abs]	No	No
BREMEN I	Yes[1]	No
BRUSSELS I[Abs]	No	No

Superscripts refer to footnotes in Dysfibrinogen Reports (Section 3).

Table 5: Clinical Manifestations (cont'd.)

Last Update: 10 January 1994

Fibrinogen	Bleeding?	Thrombosis?
BUENOS AIRES I[Abs]	Yes[2]	No
BUENOS AIRES II	No	No
CARACAS I	Yes[2]	No
CARACAS II	No	No
CARACAS III	No	No
CARACAS IV	Yes[1]	No
CARACAS V	No	Yes[1]
CARACAS VI	Yes[1]	No
CARACAS VII	No	No
CHAPEL HILL I	Yes[2]	No
CHAPEL HILL II	Yes[3]	No
CHAPEL HILL III	No	Yes[2]
CHAPEL HILL IV	No[1]	No[1]
CHAPEL HILL V	n.a.	n.a.
CHAPEL HILL VI	n.a.	n.a.
CHAPEL HILL VII	n.a.[1]	n.a.[1]
CHARLOTTESVILLE I	No	Yes[3]
CHICAGO I[Abs]	No	Yes[1]
CHRISTCHURCH I	n.a.	n.a.
CHRISTCHURCH II	Yes[1]	No
CLERMONT-FERRAND I	n.a.	n.a.
CLEVELAND I	No[1]	No[1]
CLEVELAND II	No	No
COPENHAGEN I	No	Yes[1]
COPENHAGEN II	No	Yes[1]
DATE I	No	Yes[1]
DETROIT I	Yes[2]	No
DUSART I[1]	No	Yes[4]
ERFURT I	No	No
ERFURT II	Yes[2]	No
ESSEN I	No[1]	No[1]
FRANKFURT I	No	Yes[1]
FRANKFURT II	Yes	No
FRANKFURT III	Yes[3]	No[3]
FRANKFURT IV[Unp]	No	Yes
FRANKFURT V[Unp]	No	Yes
FRANKFURT XIII[1]	No	No
FREIBURG I	Yes[1]	No
GENEVA I	No[2]	No[2]
GENOVA I	No	No

Superscripts refer to footnotes in Dysfibrinogen Reports (Section 3).

Table 5: Clinical Manifestations (cont'd.)

Last Update: 10 January 1994

Fibrinogen	Bleeding?	Thrombosis?
GENOVA II	No	No
GENOVA III[Abs]	Yes	No
GIESSEN I	Yes[3]	No
GIESSEN II	Yes[1]	No
GIESSEN III	No	No
GRAND RAPIDS I	No	No
GRENOBLE I	No[1]	No[1]
GUADELOUPE I	n.a.	n.a.
HAARLEM I	No	No
HAARLEM II	No	No
HAIFA I	No	Yes[2]
HANNOVER I	Yes[1]	No
HERSHEY I	No[1]	Yes[1]
HERSHEY II	No	Yes[3]
HOMBURG I	No	No
HOMBURG II	No	No
HOMBURG III	Yes[2]	No
HOMBURG IV	No	No
HOMBURG V	No	No
HOMBURG VI	No	No
HOUSTON I	Yes[3]	No
HOUSTON II	Yes[1]	No
IJMUIDEN I	No	Yes
INDIANAPOLIS I	No[2]	No[2]
INDIANAPOLIS II	No[1]	No[1]
INDIANAPOLIS III	No[1]	No[1]
IOWA CITY I	No[1]	No[1]
IRVINE I	No	Yes[1]
ISE I	No	No
ISTANBUL I	No	Yes[1]
ISTANBUL II[Unp]	Yes	No
JENA I	No	No
KANAZAWA I	No	No
KASSEL I	n.a.	n.a.
KAWAGUCHI I	No	No
KENDAL I	n.a.	n.a.
KIEL I	No	No
KYOTO I	No[2]	No[2]
KYOTO II	Yes[1]	No
KYOTO III	No	No

Superscripts refer to footnotes in Dysfibrinogen Reports (Section 3).

Table 5: Clinical Manifestations (cont'd.)

Last Update: 10 January 1994

Fibrinogen	Bleeding?	Thrombosis?
LA CEVAINA I[Unp]	No	No
LA GUAIRA I	No	No
LA PLATA I	No	No
LEDYARD I	Yes[2]	No
LEITCHFIELD I	n.a.	n.a.
LEOGAN I	No[3]	No[3]
LEUVEN I	No	No
LILLE I	No	No
LIMA I	Yes[4]	No
LOGROÑO I	No	No
LONDON I	No	Yes[1]
LONDON II	No	Yes
LONDON III	No	No
LONDON IV	No	No
LONDON V	No	Yes[1]
LONDON VI	n.a.	n.a.
LONG BEACH I[Abs]	n.a.	n.a.
LOS ANGELES I[Abs]	No	No
LOUISVILLE I	Yes[2]	No
MAASTRICHT I[Abs]	Yes[1]	No
MADRID I	No	No
MADRID II	No	No
MADRID III	No	No
MAGDEBURG II[Abs]	Yes[1]	No
MALAGA I	No	No
MALMÖE I	No	Yes[1]
MANCHESTER I	No	No
MANNHEIM I	Yes[1]	No
MANNHEIM II[Abs]	Yes[1]	Yes[2]
MARBURG I	Yes[2]	Yes[3]
MARSEILLE I	No	No
METZ I	Yes[3]	No
MÉXICO DF I[Abs]	No	No
MILAN I[1]	No	No
MILAN II[1]	No	Yes[4]
MILAN III[Abs1]	No	Yes[2]
MILAN IV[1]	No[3]	No[3]
MILAN VI[1]	Yes[2]	No
MILAN VII[Abs1]	No	No
MITAKA I[Abs]	No	No

Superscripts refer to footnotes in Dysfibrinogen Reports (Section 3).

Table 5: Clinical Manifestations (cont'd.)

Last Update: 10 January 1994

Fibrinogen	Bleeding?	Thrombosis?
MITAKA II	Yes[1]	No
MONTEVIDEO I	Yes[1]	No
MONTREAL I	No	No
MONTREAL II[Abs]	Yes[1]	No
MONTREAL III[Abs]	No	No
MORIOKA I[Abs]	No	No
MUNICH I[1]	Yes[2]	No
MUNICH II[1]	Yes	No
MÜNSTER I[Abs]	n.a.	n.a.
NAGOYA I	No	No
NANCY I	No	Yes[2]
NAPLES I[1]	*No*	*Yes*[4]
NEW ALBANY I	No	No
NEWARK I[Abs]	Yes[1]	No
NEW BRITAIN I[Abs]	No	No
NEW ORLEANS I	Yes[2]	No
NEW ORLEANS II[Abs]	No	Yes
NEW YORK I	No	Yes[2]
NEW YORK II	Yes[1]	No
NEW YORK III	Yes[1]	No
NEW YORK IV	Yes[1]	No
NIJMEGEN I	No	Yes[2]
NOTTINGHAM I	n.a.	n.a.
OKLAHOMA I	Yes[2]	No
ORLEANS I	No	No
ORSAY I	No	No
OSAKA I	No	No
OSAKA II	No	No
OSAKA III	No	No
OSAKA IV	No[2]	No[2]
OSAKA V	No	No
OSLO I	No	Yes[2]
OSLO II	No	No
OSLO III	No	No
OSLO IV	No	No
OVIEDO I	No	No
OVIEDO II[Abs]	No	No
OVIEDO III[Abs]	No	No
PAMPLONA I	No	No
PAMPLONA II	No	Yes[2]

Superscripts refer to footnotes in Dysfibrinogen Reports (Section 3).

Table 5: Clinical Manifestations (cont'd.)

Last Update: 10 January 1994

Fibrinogen	Bleeding?	Thrombosis?
PARIS I	No	No
PARIS II	No	Yes[2]
PARIS III	No	No
PARIS IV	No	No
PARIS V[4]	*No*	*Yes*[4]
PARIS VI	n.a.	n.a.
PARMA I	Yes	No
PERUGIA I	No	No
PETOSKEY I	No	No
PHILADELPHIA I	Yes[2]	No
PHILADELPHIA II	n.a.	n.a.
POITIERS I	No	Yes[1]
PONTOISE I	n.a.	n.a.
PRAHRAN I[1]	Yes[2]	No[2]
QUEBEC I	No	No
QUEBEC II	Yes[2]	No
RICHFIELD I[Abs]	No	Yes[1]
RIYADH I	Yes[2]	No
ROUEN I	n.a.	n.a.
SAGA I	Yes[1]	No
SAINT LOUIS I	Yes[2]	No
SAINT MANDE I	Yes	No
SAINT MANDE II	No	No
SALAMANCA I[Abs]	n.a.	n.a.
SAN FRANCISCO I[Abs1]	No	No
SAN JUAN I	Yes[1]	No
SANTIAGO I	Yes[1]	No
SAPPORO I	No	No
SCHWARZACH I	No	No
SEATTLE I	No[2]	No[2]
SEATTLE II	No	No
SEVILLA I	No	No
SHEFFIELD I	Yes[2]	No
STONY BROOK I	No	No
STONY BROOK II	Yes[3]	No
STRASBOURG I[Abs]	No	Yes[2]
STRASBOURG II[Abs]	n.a.	Yes[1]
SYDNEY I	No	No
SYDNEY II	n.a.	n.a.
TAMPERE I	No	Yes[1]

Superscripts refer to footnotes in Dysfibrinogen Reports (Section 3).

Table 5: Clinical Manifestations (cont'd.)

Last Update: 10 January 1994

Fibrinogen	Bleeding?	Thrombosis?
TEMPLE I	n.a.	n.a.
TEMPLE II	n.a.	n.a.
TOCHIGI I	No	No
TOKUSHIMA I	No	No
TOKYO I	Yes[2]	No
TOKYO II	No	No
TORINO I	No	No
TROYES I	No	No
VALENCIA I	Yes[2]	No
VALHALLA I[Abs]	Yes[2]	No
VANCOUVER I	Yes[1]	No
VERSAILLES I	No	No
VICENZA I	Yes[2]	No
VIENNA I[Abs]	Yes[1]	No
VILLEPARISIS I	n.a.	n.a.
VILLIERS-SUR-MARNE I	n.a.	n.a.
VITRY-SUR-SEINE I	n.a.	n.a.
VLISSINGEN I	No	Yes[2]
WHITE MARSH I	n.a.	n.a.
WIESBADEN I	Yes	Yes
YERRES I	n.a.	n.a.
ZÜRICH I	No	No
ZÜRICH II	No[2]	No[2]

Superscripts refer to footnotes in Dysfibrinogen Reports (Section 3).

Summary of Clinical Manifestations

Variants with abnormal bleeding:	**71/228**	**31%**
Variants with thrombotic episodes:	**47/228**	**21%**
Variants with abnormal bleeding and thrombosis:	**5/228**	**2%**
Variants with bleeding or thrombotic complications:	**113/228**	**50%**
Asymptomatic variants	**115/228**	**50%**

Table 6: Plasma Fibrinogen Determinations

Last Update: 10 January 1994

Fibrinogen	Plasma Fibrinogen Concentration (mg/dL)			
	Chronometric	**Rate Independent**	**Immunologic**	***Hypo*dysfibrinogen?**
AARAU I[Abs]	n.a.	n.a.	Normal[1]	No
AARHUS I	No clot	Normal[3]	Normal[3]	No
ADELAIDE I	55/(150-400)	110/(150-400)	120/(150-400)	Yes
ALBA/GENEVA I	20/(250)	95/(250)	15-60[3]	Yes
ALÈS I	n.a.	n.a.	n.a.	n.a.
ALMÉRIA I	97/(250)	250/(250)	n.a.	No
AMIENS I	n.a.	n.a.	n.a.	n.a.
AMIENS II	n.a.	n.a.	n.a.	n.a.
AMSTERDAM I	152/(>200)	200/(>200)	1:80/(1:80)[1]	No
AMSTERDAM II	n.a.	n.a.	n.a.	n.a.
ARGENTEUIL I	23/(150-300)	120/(150-300)	n.a.	Yes
ASAHI I	<50/(200-400)	565[3,4]	525[4]	No
ASHFORD I	n.a.	n.a.	140[2]	No
AWAJI I	73[1]	296[1]	n.a.	No
AWAJI II	86/(200-350)	230/(200-350)	248/(200-400)	No
BALTIMORE I	35/(175)	104/(180)	180/(180)	No
BALTIMORE II	36/(150-400)	82/(150-400)	62-96/(150-400)	Yes
BALTIMORE III	107/(150-400)	170/(150-400)	180/(150-400)	No
BALTIMORE IV	32/(>150)	192/(>150)	n.a.	No
BARCELONA I	0/(250)	350/(250)	n.a.	No
BARCELONA II	57[3]	416[4]	450[4]	No
BERGAMO I	40/(240)	200/(245)	220/(240)	No
BERGAMO II	22/(200)	240/(200)	230/(200)	No
BERGAMO III	30/(200)	250/(200)	250/(200)	No
BERLIN I	n.a.	n.a.	n.a.	n.a.
BERLIN II[Abs]	Subnormal[1]	Normal[1]	n.a.	No
BERN I	25/(150-300)	180/(150-300)	140/(150-300)	Yes
BERN II	30/(150-300)	260/(150-300)	200/(150-300)	No
BERN III	20/(150-300)	240/(150-300)	260/(150-300)	No
BETHESDA I	36/(186-380)	330/(200-400)	300/(250)	No
BETHESDA II	94/(190-380)	179/(200-400)	180/(300)	No
BETHESDA III	30-41/(190-380)	90-117/(186-360)	100-120/(200-390)	Yes
BICÊTRE I	n.a.	n.a.	n.a.	n.a.
BICÊTRE II	130/(200-400)	350/(200-400)	370/(200-400)	No
BIRMINGHAM I	50/(200-400)	n.a.	342/(200-400)	No
BODMIN I	n.a.	n.a.	n.a.	n.a.
BONDY I	30/(410)	70/(375)	750/(420)	No
BOULOGNE I[Abs]	Abnormal	n.a.	Normal	No
BREMEN I	80/(180-400)	n.a.	234/(200-430)	No
BRUSSELS I[Abs]	Subnormal[1]	Normal[1]	Normal[1]	No

Superscripts refer to footnotes in Dysfibrinogen Reports (Section 3).

Table 6: Plasma Fibrinogen Determinations (cont'd.)

Last Update: 10 January 1994

Fibrinogen	Plasma Fibrinogen Concentration (mg/dL)			
	Chronometric	**Rate Independent**	**Immunologic**	***Hypo*dysfibrinogen?**
BUENOS AIRES I[Abs]	Normal[1]	Normal[1]	n.a.	No
BUENOS AIRES II	50/(200-450)	365/(200-450)	n.a.	No
CARACAS I	n.a.	280/(200-350)	286/(200-350)	No
CARACAS II	39/(180-400)	420/(200-400)	500/(210-450)	No
CARACAS III	80[1]	330[1]	250[1]	No
CARACAS IV	45[2]	300[2]	300[2]	No
CARACAS V	80/(180-400)[2]	530/(200-400)[2]	540/(210-450)[2]	No
CARACAS VI	75[2]	120[2]	120[2]	Yes
CARACAS VII	50[1]	305[1]	300[1]	No
CHAPEL HILL I	119/(280)	94/(270)	131/(355)	Yes
CHAPEL HILL II	116/(263)	427/(272)	408/(235)	No
CHAPEL HILL III	258/(216)	249/(256)	332/(235)	No
CHAPEL HILL IV	131/(219)	352/(299)	372/(300)	No
CHAPEL HILL V	99/(225)	n.a.	398/(252)	No
CHAPEL HILL VI	n.a.	n.a.	155/(252)	n.a.
CHAPEL HILL VII	16/(250)	n.a.	11/(300)	Yes
CHARLOTTESVILLE I	13/(200-400)	390/(200-390)	300/(200-400)	No
CHICAGO I[Abs]	135[2]	150[2]	320[2]	No
CHRISTCHURCH I	n.a.	n.a.	n.a.	n.a.
CHRISTCHURCH II	n.a.	n.a.	n.a.	n.a.
CLERMONT-FERRAND I	n.a.	n.a.	n.a.	n.a.
CLEVELAND I	n.a.	332/(177-415)	n.a.	No
CLEVELAND II	n.a.	289/(177-415)	n.a.	No
COPENHAGEN I	n.a.	Normal[2]	Normal[2]	No
COPENHAGEN II	n.a.	n.a.	1071/(204-442)	No
DATE I	45/(200-400)	n.a.	106/(180-460)	Yes
DETROIT I	0/(200-300)	300/(200-350)	960/(397-641)	No
DUSART I[1]	165/(200-400)	n.a.	190/(200-400)	No
ERFURT I	193[1]	198[1]	n.a.	No
ERFURT II	n.a.	n.a.	n.a.	n.a.
ESSEN I	10/(200)	240/(200)	200/(200)	No
FRANKFURT I	27.5/(200-400)[2]	180/(160-320)[2]	162/(160-300)[2]	No
FRANKFURT II	44/(200-400)	240/(160-320)	286/(160-300)	No
FRANKFURT III	36/(200-400)[3]	180/(160-320)[3]	308/(160-300)[3]	No[3]
FRANKFURT IV[Unp]	n.a.	n.a.	n.a.	n.a.
FRANKFURT V[Unp]	n.a.	n.a.	n.a.	n.a.
FRANKFURT XIII[1]	35[4]	n.a.	n.a.	No
FREIBURG I	10-20[2]	n.a.	Subnormal[3]	Yes
GENEVA I	14/(150-400)	180/(150-400)	180/(150-400)	No
GENOVA I	140/(200-400)	n.a.	350/(200-450)	No

Superscripts refer to footnotes in Dysfibrinogen Reports (Section 3).

Table 6: Plasma Fibrinogen Determinations (cont'd.)

Last Update: 10 January 1994

Fibrinogen	Plasma Fibrinogen Concentration (mg/dL)			
	Chronometric	**Rate Independent**	**Immunologic**	***Hypo*dysfibrinogen?**
GENOVA II	59/(200-400)	370/(180-400)	350/(200-450)	No
GENOVA III[Abs]	Subnormal[1]	Normal[1]	Normal[1]	No
GIESSEN I	45/(200)	160/(200)	215/(240)	No
GIESSEN II	0/(250)	33/(260)	50/(300)	Yes
GIESSEN III	180/(345)	160/(262)	304/(345)	No
GRAND RAPIDS I	48/(280)	93/(280)	120/(280)	Yes
GRENOBLE I	50/(200-400)	120/(200-400)	210/(200-400)	No
GUADELOUPE I	80[1]	265[1]	220[1]	No
HAARLEM I	50/(200-400)	n.a.	240/(200-400)	No
HAARLEM II	85/(200-400)	n.a.	260/(200-400)	No
HAIFA I	n.a.	260/(150-500)	n.a.	No
HANNOVER I	57/(200-280)	124/(180-280)	240/(210-320)	No
HERSHEY I	275/(176-377)	480/(200-450)[2]	630/(215-400)[2]	No
HERSHEY II	38-112/(200-399)[4]	n.a.	664/(200-399)[4]	No
HOMBURG I	58/(150-430)	250/(180-360)	270/(190-450)	No
HOMBURG II	88/(150-430)[1]	282/(180-360)[1]	210/(190-450)[1]	No
HOMBURG III	55/(150-430)[1]	275/(180-360)[1]	240/(190-450)[1]	No
HOMBURG IV	64/(150-430)[1]	230/(180-360)[1]	180/(190-450)[1]	No
HOMBURG V	29/(150-430)[1]	180/(180-360)[1]	388/(190-450)[1]	No
HOMBURG VI	48/(150-430)[1]	120/(180-360)[1]	543/(190-450)[1]	n.a.
HOUSTON I	n.a.	n.a.	640/(150-350)	No
HOUSTON II	n.a.	n.a.	n.a.	n.a.
IJMUIDEN I	90/(180-490)	n.a.	270/(160-500)	No
INDIANAPOLIS I	n.a.	n.a.	n.a.	n.a.
INDIANAPOLIS II	Normal	n.a.	Normal	No
INDIANAPOLIS III	Normal	n.a.	Normal	No
IOWA CITY I	71[2]	141[2]	238[2]	No
IRVINE I	170/(200-370)	290/(200-370)	300/(200-370)	No
ISE I	129/(150-350)	277/(150-350)	256/(150-350)	No
ISTANBUL I	0/(200-300)	260/(200-300)[1]	320/(240)	No
ISTANBUL II[Unp]	n.a.	n.a.	n.a.	n.a.
JENA I	n.a.	186[2]	436[2]	No
KANAZAWA I	65/(150-350)	337/(150-350)	371/(150-350)	No
KASSEL I	n.a.	n.a.	n.a.	n.a.
KAWAGUCHI I	<40/(200-400)	230/(200-400)	262/(200-400)	No
KENDAL I	n.a.	n.a.	n.a.	Yes
KIEL I	87/(200-450)	177/(200-450)	258/(200-450)	No
KYOTO I	77/(150-350)	150/(150-350)	210/(150-350)	No
KYOTO II	64/(150-350)	201/(150-350)	216/(150-350)	No
KYOTO III	68/(200-400)	n.a.	290/(200-400)	No

Superscripts refer to footnotes in Dysfibrinogen Reports (Section 3).

Table 6: Plasma Fibrinogen Determinations (cont'd.)

Last Update: 10 January 1994

Fibrinogen	Plasma Fibrinogen Concentration (mg/dL)			
	Chronometric	**Rate Independent**	**Immunologic**	***Hypo*dysfibrinogen?**
LA CEVAINA I[Unp]	n.a.	n.a.	n.a.	No
LA GUAIRA I	85[1]	340[1]	350[1]	No
LA PLATA I	n.a.	230[2]	230[2]	No
LEDYARD I	40/(150-350)	n.a.	315/(150-350)	No
LEITCHFIELD I	n.a.	n.a.	n.a.	n.a.
LEOGAN I	55[4]	n.a.	525[4]	No
LEUVEN I	78/(200-400)	159/(200-400)	128/(200-400)	Yes
LILLE I	<20/(410)	340/(375)	505/(420)	No
LIMA I	50[5]	240[5]	n.a.	No
LOGROÑO I	n.a.	40/(200-400)	170/(150-350)	No
LONDON I	n.a.	239/(230)	400/(400)	No
LONDON II	100/(220)	n.a.	130/(220-550)	Yes
LONDON III	n.a.	110/(200-400)	420/(200-400)	No
LONDON IV	n.a.	260/(200-400)	n.a.	No
LONDON V	n.a.	n.a.	n.a.[2]	Yes
LONDON VI	n.a.	90[2]	n.a.	Yes
LONG BEACH I[Abs]	n.a.	n.a.	n.a.	No
LOS ANGELES I[Abs]	Subnormal[1]	Normal[1]	Normal[1]	No
LOUISVILLE I	60-80[3]	n.a.	Normal[4]	No
MAASTRICHT I[Abs]	20[2]	n.a.	n.a.	n.a.[2]
MADRID I	59[1]	248[1]	300[1]	No
MADRID II	45[2]	266[2]	260[2]	No
MADRID III	70/(200-400)	n.a.	248/(200-400)	No
MAGDEBURG II[Abs]	Subnormal[2]	Normal[2]	n.a.	No
MALAGA I	55/(200-400)	n.a.	164/(200-400)	No
MALMÖE I	n.a.	70[2]	n.a.	Yes
MANCHESTER I	n.a.	562[2]	n.a.	No
MANNHEIM I	55-80[2]	n.a.	370-380[2]	No
MANNHEIM II[Abs]	50-80[3]	n.a.	150-180[3]	Yes
MARBURG I	<25/(250)	190/(280)	60/(250)[4]	Yes[4]
MARSEILLE I	25/(240)	n.a.	220/(240)	No
METZ I	0/(300-450)	250/(300-450)	300/(200-400)	No
MÉXICO DF I[Abs]	n.a.	n.a.	n.a.	n.a.
MILAN I[1]	40/(150-300)	300/(150-300)	240/(150-300)	No
MILAN II[1]	170/(200-400)	320[5]	300/(200-400)	No
MILAN III[Abs1]	<20[3]	Normal[4]	Normal[4]	No
MILAN IV[1]	35/(150-400)	180/(150-400)	187/(150-400)	No
MILAN VI[1]	30/(230)	n.a.	190/(230)	No
MILAN VII[Abs1]	n.a.	n.a.	n.a.	n.a.
MITAKA I[Abs]	67-156[1]	n.a.	125-174[1]	Yes

Superscripts refer to footnotes in Dysfibrinogen Reports (Section 3).

Table 6: Plasma Fibrinogen Determinations (cont'd.)

Last Update: 10 January 1994

Fibrinogen	Plasma Fibrinogen Concentration (mg/dL)			
	Chronometric	**Rate Independent**	**Immunologic**	***Hypo*dysfibrinogen?**
MITAKA II	91/(350)	308/(350)	n.a.	No
MONTEVIDEO I	60[2]	144[2]	109[2].	Yes
MONTREAL I	170/(250-450)	110/(200-400)	360/(350-700)	No
MONTREAL II[Abs]	n.a.	Normal[2]	Normal[2]	No
MONTREAL III[Abs]	40-80[1]	n.a.	360[1]	No
MORIOKA I[Abs]	n.a.	n.a.	n.a.	n.a.
MUNICH I[1]	n.a.	210/(150-400)	n.a.	No
MUNICH II[1]	37[2]	180[2]	n.a.	No
MÜNSTER I[Abs]	n.a.	n.a.	n.a.	n.a.
NAGOYA I	80/(180-360)	228/(200-400)	220/(200-400)	No
NANCY I	270[3]	380/(300-450)	290[3]	No
NAPLES I[1]	*170/(200-400)*	*320*[5]	*300/(200-400)*	*No*
NEW ALBANY I	n.a.	n.a.	n.a.	n.a.
NEWARK I[Abs]	230[2]	n.a.	140[2]	No
NEW BRITAIN I[Abs]	120[1]	225[1]	n.a.	No
NEW ORLEANS I	50-73/(200-400)	445/(180-290)	640/(200-450)	No[3]
NEW ORLEANS II[Abs]	95[1]	n.a.	262[1]	No
NEW YORK I	n.a.	64/(200-450)	156/(200-450)	No
NEW YORK II	n.a.	200/(200-400)	n.a.	No
NEW YORK III	n.a.	195/(200-400)	n.a.	No
NEW YORK IV	n.a.	100/(200-400)	n.a.	Yes
NIJMEGEN I	120/(180-490)	n.a.	350/(160-500)	No
NOTTINGHAM I	n.a.	n.a.	n.a.	Yes
OKLAHOMA I	n.a.	237[3]	n.a.	No
ORLEANS I	50[2]	n.a.	370[2]	No
ORSAY I	275[1]	330[1]	350[1]	No
OSAKA I	n.a.	n.a.	n.a.	n.a.
OSAKA II	40/(200-400)	Normal[2]	n.a.	No
OSAKA III	93/(150-350)	181/(150-350)	270/(150-350)	No
OSAKA IV	54/(150-350)	n.a.	335/(180-350)	No
OSAKA V	90/(150-350)	218/(150-350)	250/(150-350)	No
OSLO I	n.a.	270/(195-330)	n.a.	No
OSLO II	70/(200-400)	240/(200-400)	270/(200-400)	No
OSLO III	n.a.	n.a.	n.a.	n.a.
OSLO IV	48/(170-374)	150/(170-374)	n.a.	Yes
OVIEDO I	74/(200-400)	n.a.	370/(200-400)	No
OVIEDO II[Abs]	Subnormal[1]	n.a.	Normal[1]	No
OVIEDO III[Abs]	Subnormal[1]	n.a.	Normal[1]	No
PAMPLONA I	n.a.	124/(200-400)	200/(200-400)	No
PAMPLONA II	145/(200-400)	340/(200-400)	310/(200-400)	No

Superscripts refer to footnotes in Dysfibrinogen Reports (Section 3).

Table 6: Plasma Fibrinogen Determinations (cont'd.)

Last Update: 10 January 1994

Fibrinogen	Plasma Fibrinogen Concentration (mg/dL)			
	Chronometric	**Rate Independent**	**Immunologic**	***Hypo*dysfibrinogen?**
PARIS I	n.a.	n.a.	n.a.	n.a.
PARIS II	90[3]	270[3]	300[3]	No
PARIS III	240/(250-400)	300/(250-400)	300/(250-400)	No
PARIS IV	55/(200-450)	315/(200-450)	300/(200-450)	No
PARIS V[4]	*165/(200-400)*	*n.a.*	*190/(200-400)*	*No*
PARIS VI	n.a.	250[3]	n.a.	No
PARMA I	n.a.	60[1]	n.a.	Yes
PERUGIA I	28/(200)	150/(200)	150/(200)	No
PETOSKEY I	96/(>200)	298/(>200)	n.a.	No
PHILADELPHIA I	73/(232-444)	78/(160-380)	78[3]	Yes
PHILADELPHIA II	n.a.	n.a.	n.a.	n.a.
POITIERS I	100/(150-300)	500/(150-300)	n.a.	No
PONTOISE I	n.a.	n.a.	n.a.	n.a.
PRAHRAN I[1]	n.a.	85/(246-550)	n.a.	Yes
QUEBEC I	174/(175-375)	265/(200-400)	254/(200-400)	No
QUEBEC II	130/(175-375)	280/(200-400)	311/(200-400)	No
RICHFIELD I[Abs]	32/(190-440)	n.a.	189/(200-450)	No
RIYADH I	<50[3]	n.a.	n.a.	No[4]
ROUEN I	n.a.	n.a.	n.a.	n.a.
SAGA I	<40/(150-350)	345[2]	245[2]	No
SAINT LOUIS I	n.a.	177/(200-400)[3]	n.a.	No[3]
SAINT MANDE I	334/(>150)[1]	320/(>150)	n.a.	No
SAINT MANDE II	35/(>150)	180/(>150)	n.a.	No
SALAMANCA I[Abs]	Subnormal[1]	n.a.	Normal[1]	No
SAN FRANCISCO I[Abs1]	n.a.	n.a.	n.a.	n.a.
SAN JUAN I	50/(190-365)[2]	n.a.	n.a.	n.a.[2]
SANTIAGO I	80[2]	185[2]	200[2]	No
SAPPORO I	64/(243)	186/(176)	n.a.	No
SCHWARZACH I	57/(200-400)	n.a.	404/(200-400)	No
SEATTLE I	57/(200-300)	215/(200-300)	n.a.	No
SEATTLE II	57/(200-400)	297/(200-400)	n.a.	No
SEVILLA I	49/(200-400)	123/(200-400)	280/(200-400)	No
SHEFFIELD I	n.a.	210[3]	n.a.	No
STONY BROOK I	56[1]	160[1]	210[1]	No
STONY BROOK II	77[4]	n.a.	408[4]	No
STRASBOURG I[Abs]	n.a.	n.a.	n.a.	n.a.
STRASBOURG II[Abs]	n.a.	n.a.	n.a.	n.a.
SYDNEY I	n.a.	n.a.	Normal[2]	No
SYDNEY II	n.a.	n.a.	n.a.	n.a.
TAMPERE I	140-180/(170-360)	n.a.	250/(200-450)	No

Superscripts refer to footnotes in Dysfibrinogen Reports (Section 3).

Table 6: Plasma Fibrinogen Determinations (cont'd.)

Last Update: 10 January 1994

Fibrinogen	Plasma Fibrinogen Concentration (mg/dL)			
	Chronometric	**Rate Independent**	**Immunologic**	***Hypo*dysfibrinogen?**
TEMPLE I	n.a.	n.a.	n.a.	n.a.
TEMPLE II	n.a.	n.a.	n.a.	n.a.
TOCHIGI I	44/(150-350)	142/(150-350)	210/(150-350)	No
TOKUSHIMA I	105[2]	627[2]	581[2]	No
TOKYO I	n.a.	163-320/(150-350)	182-263/(200-400)	No
TOKYO II	27/(200-400)	197/(200-350)	378/(200-400)	No
TORINO I	20/(200)	270/(200)	230/(200)	No
TROYES I	55/(300-450)	250/(300-450)	360/(240-480)	No
VALENCIA I	n.a.	76-80/(250)[3]	n.a.	Yes
VALHALLA I[Abs]	n.a.	n.a.	n.a.	n.a.
VANCOUVER I	n.a.	76[2]	n.a.	Yes[3]
VERSAILLES I	40/(200-400)	240[1]	180[1]	No
VICENZA I	84/(200-400)	240/(180-400)	280/(200-450)	No
VIENNA I[Abs]	Subnormal[2]	n.a.	Normal[2]	No
VILLEPARISIS I	55[1]	90[1]	90[1]	Yes[2]
VILLIERS-SUR-MARNE I	45[1]	215[1]	350[1]	No
VITRY-SUR-SEINE I	170[1]	500[1]	550[1]	No
VLISSINGEN I	40/(200-400)	180/(200-400)	310/(200-400)	No
WHITE MARSH I	79[2]	n.a.	384[2]	No
WIESBADEN I	38/(280)	91/(334)	440/(240)	No
YERRES I	45[1]	175[1]	200[1]	No
ZÜRICH I	20-50/(150-500)	400/(200-400)	n.a.	No
ZÜRICH II	Subnormal[1]	Normal[1]	Normal[1]	No

Superscripts refer to footnotes in Dysfibrinogen Reports (Section 3).

Summary of Plasma Fibrinogen Data

Variants evaluated for plasma fibrinogen:	221/261	85%
Variants with subnormal plasma fibrinogen:		
by chronometric method	171/182	94%
by rate-independent or immunologic method	32/216	15%
Variants with hypodysfibrinogenemia:	32/221	14%

Table 7: Clinical Laboratory Results

Last Update: 10 January 1994

Fibrinogen	Thrombin Time	Reptilase (Batrox.) Time	Prothrombin Time	Partial T'plastin Time	Euglobulin Lysis Time	Bleeding Time	Immuno-electro-phoresis	Platelet Aggrega-tion
AARAU I^{Abs}	Abnormal[1]	n.a.	n.a.	n.a.	n.a.	n.a.	Anodal	n.a.
AARHUS I	>600s/(<30s)	n.a.	245s/(16s)	473s/(32s)	n.a.	n.a.	Normal	Normal
ADELAIDE I	19s/(7-12s)	25s/(15-20s)	1.54/(0.95-1.2)[2]	45s/(35-45s)	1.75h/(>2h)	Normal	Normal[3]	Normal[3]
ALBA/GENEVA I	60s/(11s)	n.a.	n.a.	n.a.	>5h/(>5h)	n.a.	Normal	n.a.
ALÈS I	165s/(14s)	No Clot	n.a.	n.a.	n.a.	n.a.	n.a.	n.a.
ALMÉRIA I	23s/(10s)	55s/(18s)	Normal[1]	Normal[1]	Normal	n.a.	n.a.	n.a.
AMIENS I	n.a.	n.a.	n.a.	n.a.	n.a.	n.a.	n.a.	n.a.
AMIENS II	n.a.	n.a.	n.a.	n.a.	n.a.	n.a.	n.a.	n.a.
AMSTERDAM I	32s/(16s)	14m/(2m)	16s/(11.5s)	n.a.	n.a.	n.a.	Cathodal	n.a.
AMSTERDAM II	n.a.	n.a.	n.a.	n.a.	n.a.	n.a.	n.a.	n.a.
ARGENTEUIL I	44s/(18-20s)	43s/(18-25s)	25.5s/(11-13s)	41s/(28-32s)	n.a.	n.a.	n.a.	n.a.
ASAHI I	>300s/(15.8s)	n.a.	14.9s/(10.9s)	41.7s/(33.5s)	n.a.	Normal	n.a.	Normal
ASHFORD I	160s/(18s)	45s/(17s)	n.a.	n.a.	n.a.	n.a.	n.a.	n.a.
AWAJI I	41.5s/(14s)	38.5s/(21s)	Normal[2]	Normal[2]	Abnormal	n.a.	Anodal	n.a.
AWAJI II	21.9s/(12.4s)	32.3s/(21s)	79%/(100%)	23.2s/(40s)	n.a.	n.a.	n.a.	n.a.
BALTIMORE I	>120s/(11.7s)	84s/(27s)	45%/(60-100%)	n.a.	Normal	n.a.	Anodal	Normal
BALTIMORE II	n.a.	n.a.	14.5s/(13-17s)	73s/(<100s)	Normal	n.a.	n.a.	Normal
BALTIMORE III	n.a.	n.a.	Normal	Normal	Normal	n.a.	n.a.	Normal
BALTIMORE IV	n.a.	n.a.	22s/(13-17s)	88s/(<100s)	2h/(>2h)	n.a.	n.a.	n.a.
BARCELONA I	600s/(19s)	1000s/(31s)	430s/(15s)	254s/(30s)	n.a.	n.a.	n.a.	Normal
BARCELONA II	35s[3]	35s[3]	45%[3]	29s[4]	n.a.	n.a.	n.a.	n.a.
BERGAMO I	120s/(17.4s)	n.a.	16.9s/(14.7s)	30.1s/(28.7s)	n.a.	n.a.	n.a.	n.a.
BERGAMO II	37.0s/(12.5s)	37.8s/(17.6)	n.a.	n.a.	n.a.	n.a.	n.a.	n.a.
BERGAMO III	37s/(18s)	74s/(20s)	n.a.	n.a.	n.a.	n.a.	n.a.	n.a.
BERLIN I	Abnormal[1]	n.a.	n.a.	n.a.	n.a.	n.a.	n.a.	n.a.
BERLIN II^{Abs}	n.a.	n.a.	Abnormal[1]	n.a.	n.a.	n.a.	n.a.	n.a.
BERN I	21.8s/(12-15s)	32.1s/(13-14s)	70%/(>70%)[2]	45s/(40-60s)[2]	n.a.	n.a.	n.a.	Normal
BERN II	41s/(14.5s)	77s/(17s)	n.a.	n.a.	n.a.	n.a.	n.a.	Normal
BERN III	46.7s/(12-15s)	>120s/(14-17s)[2]	70%/(70-130%)	61s/(40-60s)	n.a.	n.a.	n.a.	n.a.
BETHESDA I	148s/(<35s)	106s/(24s)	16.2s/(11-14s)	45.4s/(30-35s)	>180m/(>180m)	Normal	Anodal	n.a.
BETHESDA II	48s/(<30s)	49s/(<22s)	12.9s/(12.3s)	32.6s/(31s)	>180m/(>180m)	n.a.	Anodal	n.a.
BETHESDA III	65-300s/(<30s)	31-67s/(19-24s)	15s/(11-13.5s)	31.8s/(27-35s)	143m/(>180m)	n.a.	Normal	Normal
BICÊTRE I	n.a.	n.a.	n.a.	n.a.	n.a.	n.a.	n.a.	n.a.
BICÊTRE II	40s/(<20s)	29s/(<23s)	70%/(>60%)[3]	39s/(<48s)[3]	Normal[3]	n.a.	Normal[3]	n.a.
BIRMINGHAM I	52.1s/(22.6s)	25.8s/(9.7s)	n.a.	n.a.	n.a.	Abnormal	n.a.	Normal
BODMIN I	n.a.	n.a.	n.a.	n.a.	n.a.	n.a.	n.a.	n.a.
BONDY I	>120s/(21s)	>120s/(21s)	19s/(13s)	n.a.	n.a.	Normal	Normal	n.a.
BOULOGNE I^{Abs}	Abnormal	n.a.	n.a.	n.a.	n.a.	n.a.	Normal	n.a.
BREMEN I	61s/(24s)	n.a.	62%/(>70%)	57s/(27s)	n.a.	Abnormal	n.a.	n.a.
BRUSSELS I^{Abs}	n.a.	n.a.	Normal[1]	Normal[1]	n.a.	n.a.	n.a.	n.a.

Superscripts refer to footnotes in Dysfibrinogen Reports (Section 3).

Table 7: Clinical Laboratory Results (cont'd.) **Last Update: 10 January 1994**

Fibrinogen	Thrombin Time	Reptilase (Batrox.) Time	Prothrombin Time	Partial T'plastin Time	Euglobulin Lysis Time	Bleeding Time	Immuno-electro-phoresis	Platelet Aggrega-tion
BUENOS AIRES I[Abs]	Abnormal[1]	n.a.	n.a.	n.a.	n.a.	Abnormal	Anodal	n.a.
BUENOS AIRES II	60s/(18-29s)	45s/(18-22s)	65%/(>70%)	39s/(36s)	n.a.	Normal	n.a.	n.a.
CARACAS I	23s/(15-18s)	25s/(15-18s)	18.3s/(11-13s)	40.2s/(42-48s)	n.a.	Normal	Anodal	Normal
CARACAS II	85.2s/(14s)	Abnormal[1]	n.a.	n.a.	n.a.	n.a.	Anodal	n.a.
CARACAS III	24s/(15-18s)[2]	Abnormal[3]	n.a.	n.a.	n.a.	n.a.	Normal	n.a.
CARACAS IV	36s/(15-18s)[3]	Abnormal[4]	n.a.	n.a.	n.a.	n.a.	Normal	n.a.
CARACAS V	25s/(15-18s)[2]	n.a.	29.5s/(11-13s)[2]	65s/(42-48s)[2]	n.a.	n.a.	n.a.	n.a.
CARACAS VI	31s/(15-18s)[3]	Abnormal[4]	n.a.	n.a.	n.a.	n.a.	Normal	n.a.
CARACAS VII	30s/(13-15s)[2]	Abnormal[3]	n.a.	n.a.	n.a.	n.a.	Normal	n.a.
CHAPEL HILL I	13.3s/(10.5s)	26.6s/(20.0s)	Normal[3]	Normal[3]	Normal	Normal	n.a.	n.a.
CHAPEL HILL II	29.2s/(12.4s)	38.2s/(14.8s)	14.3s/(12.2s)	51.3s/(51.2s)	n.a.	n.a.	n.a.	n.a.
CHAPEL HILL III	12.6s/(11.5s)	31.0s/(16.3s)	Normal[3]	Normal[3]	>3h/(>3h)	n.a.	Anodal	n.a.
CHAPEL HILL IV	20.3s/(11.4s)	90s/(14s)	n.a.	n.a.	n.a.	n.a.	n.a.	n.a.
CHAPEL HILL V	24.1s/(11.4s)	78s/(16.3s)	n.a.	n.a.	n.a.	n.a.	n.a.	n.a.
CHAPEL HILL VI	14.1s/(11.5s)	13.8s/(16.3s)	n.a.	n.a.	n.a.	n.a.	n.a.	n.a.
CHAPEL HILL VII	34.5s/(11.6s)	52s/(14s)	n.a.	n.a.	n.a.	n.a.	n.a.	n.a.
CHARLOTTESVILLE I	>200s/(13-19s)	>700s/(20-25s)	29s/(11-15s)	47s/(25-41s)	n.a.	n.a.	n.a.	n.a.
CHICAGO I[Abs]	Abnormal[3]	Abnormal[3]	n.a.	n.a.	n.a.	n.a.	Normal[4]	n.a.
CHRISTCHURCH I	n.a.	n.a.	n.a.	n.a.	n.a.	n.a.	n.a.	n.a.
CHRISTCHURCH II	38s/(20s)	26s/(18s)	n.a.	n.a.	n.a.	n.a.	n.a.	n.a.
CLERMONT-FERRAND I	n.a.	n.a.	n.a.	n.a.	n.a.	n.a.	n.a.	n.a.
CLEVELAND I	80s/(26-34s)	165s/(70-80s)	16.5s/(12-14s)	119s/(60-100s)	>180m/(>180m)	Normal	Abnormal	Normal
CLEVELAND II	68s/(30s)	50s/(21s)	16.8s/(13.4s)	53.6s/(52.7s)	n.a.	Normal	Normal	Normal
COPENHAGEN I	30s/(13-17s)	n.a.	n.a.	n.a.	Normal	n.a.	Normal	n.a.
COPENHAGEN II	22s/(13-17s)	31s/(16s)	n.a.	Normal[2]	5.3h/(2-4h)	n.a.	Normal[3]	n.a.
DATE I	48.5s/(13.5-20.4s)	n.a.	16.8/(10.3-11.5)	n.a.	n.a.	n.a.	n.a.	n.a.
DETROIT I	>60s/(14.5s)	n.a.[3]	>30s/(12.6s)	>600s/(50-70s)	>180m/(>180m)	Normal	Anodal	n.a.
DUSART I[1]	35s/(20s)	29.5s/(20s)	17.5s/(12s)	n.a.	n.a.	n.a.	n.a.	Normal
ERFURT I	Normal[2]	Normal[2]	Normal[2]	Normal[2]	n.a.	n.a.	n.a.	n.a.
ERFURT II	Abnormal[3]	n.a.	n.a.	n.a.	n.a.	n.a.	n.a.	n.a.
ESSEN I	46.4s/(12.5s)	53.8s/(17.6s)	n.a.	n.a.	n.a.	n.a.	n.a.	n.a.
FRANKFURT I	60s/(<22s)	>85s/(<20s)[2]	22s/(16s)[2]	37.5s/(20-40s)[2]	n.a.	Normal	n.a.[3]	Normal
FRANKFURT II	52s/(<22s)[2]	>55s/(<20s)[2]	19s/(16s)[2]	38s/(20-40s)	n.a.	Normal	n.a.[3]	Normal
FRANKFURT III	48s/(<22s)[3]	71s/(<20s)[3]	21s/(16s)[3]	39s/(20-40s)[3]	n.a.	Normal[3]	n.a.	Normal[3]
FRANKFURT IV[Unp]	40s/<22s)	n.a.	n.a.	n.a.	n.a.	n.a.	n.a.	n.a.
FRANKFURT V[Unp]	>120s/(22s)	n.a.	n.a.	n.a.	n.a.	n.a.	n.a.	n.a.
FRANKFURT XIII[1]	n.a.	n.a.	Abnormal	Abnormal	n.a.	n.a.	n.a.	n.a.
FREIBURG I	Abnormal[3]	Abnormal[3]	n.a.	n.a.	n.a.	n.a.	n.a.	n.a.
GENEVA I	38.9s/(12-15s)	60s/(16-18s)	66%/(100%)	27.6s/(25-30s)	n.a.	n.a.	n.a.	n.a.
GENOVA I	58s/(18s)	61.5s/(17s)	18.5s/(14s)	Normal[2]	n.a.	n.a.	n.a.	n.a.

Superscripts refer to footnotes in Dysfibrinogen Reports (Section 3).

Table 7: Clinical Laboratory Results (cont'd.)

Last Update: 10 January 1994

Fibrinogen	Thrombin Time	Reptilase (Batrox.) Time	Prothrombin Time	Partial T'plastin Time	Euglobulin Lysis Time	Bleeding Time	Immuno-electro-phoresis	Platelet Aggrega-tion
GENOVA II	43s/(13-17s)	61s/(15-20s)	16.8s/(12-14s)	35s/(27-33s)	n.a.	Normal	Normal	n.a.
GENOVA III[Abs]	Abnormal[1]	Abnormal[1]	n.a.	n.a.	n.a.	n.a.	n.a.	n.a.
GIESSEN I	>120s/(11-14s)	>120s/(11-14s)	28.4s/(11-14s)	37.7s/(22-34s)	Normal	Normal	Normal	Normal
GIESSEN II	222s/(18s)	277s/(20s)	15%/(80%)	67s/(45s)	n.a.	Normal	Normal	n.a.
GIESSEN III	40.4s/(19-24s)	54.2s/(20-25s)	100%/(70-120%)	48s/(37-50s)	n.a.	Normal	Normal	Abnormal
GRAND RAPIDS I	16.8s/(7.6s)	n.a.	14.5s/(10.5s)	32.2s/(27.5s)	n.a.	n.a.	n.a.	n.a.
GRENOBLE I	n.a.	n.a.	n.a.	n.a.	n.a.	n.a.	n.a.	n.a.
GUADELOUPE I	40s/(20s)	36s/(23s)	64%/(>70%)	40s/(38s)	n.a.	n.a.	n.a.	Normal
HAARLEM I	11s/(<8s)	24s/(<20s)	14s/(<13s)	45s/(<40s)	n.a.	Normal	n.a.	n.a.
HAARLEM II	12s/(12s)	n.a.	13s/(13s)	43s/(43s)	n.a.	Normal	n.a.	n.a.
HAIFA I	33s/(11s)	28s/(14s)	15.5s/(14s)	28.5s/(26s)	Normal	Normal	n.a.	Normal
HANNOVER I	34s/(17-23s)	87s/(13-20s)	76%/(90-112%)	44s/(35-45s)	n.a.	Normal	n.a.	n.a.
HERSHEY I	26s/(20s)	60s/(49s)	16s/(12s)	66s/(42s)	Normal	n.a.	Normal	Normal
HERSHEY II	70s/(20s)[4]	n.a.	12.8s/(12s)[4]	31s/(42s)[4]	Normal	n.a.	Normal[4]	Normal[4]
HOMBURG I	44s/(<23s)	58s/(<18s)	47%/(>75%)	43s/(<39s)	n.a.	Normal	Normal[2]	Abnormal[2]
HOMBURG II	42s/(<23s)[1]	54s/(<18s)[1]	48%/(>75%)[1]	44s/(<39s)[1]	n.a.	Normal	Normal	Normal
HOMBURG III	42s/(<23s)[1]	80s/(<18s)[1]	50%/(>75%)[1]	35s/(<39s)	n.a.	Normal	Normal	Abnormal
HOMBURG IV	29s/(<23s)[1]	40.5s/(<18s)[1]	46%/(>75%)[1]	42s/(<39s)[1]	n.a.	Normal[1]	n.a.	n.a.
HOMBURG V	40s/(<23s)[1]	49s/(<18s)[1]	54%/(>75%)[1]	41s/(<39s)[1]	n.a.	Normal[1]	n.a.	n.a.
HOMBURG VI	38s/(<23s)[1]	42s/(<18s)[1]	59%/(>75%)[1]	39s/(<39s)[1]	n.a.	Normal[1]	n.a.	Abnormal[1]
HOUSTON I	32s/(18-22s)	21s/(21-22s)	27s/(11-13s)	87s/(<35s)	n.a.	Normal	Normal	Normal
HOUSTON II	27s/(<19s)	n.a.	13s/(11-12s)	42s/(24-36s)	n.a.	Normal	n.a.	n.a.
IJMUIDEN I	25.0s/(18.5s)	26.0s/(20s)	n.a.	n.a.	n.a.	n.a.	n.a.	n.a.
INDIANAPOLIS I	n.a.	n.a.	n.a.	n.a.	n.a.	n.a.	n.a.	n.a.
INDIANAPOLIS II	Normal	Normal	n.a.	n.a.	n.a.	n.a.	n.a.	n.a.
INDIANAPOLIS III	Normal	Normal	n.a.	n.a.	n.a.	n.a.	n.a.	n.a.
IOWA CITY I	278s/(34-38s)	173s/(18s)	n.a.	n.a.	n.a.	Normal	Normal	Normal
IRVINE I	Abnormal[2]	n.a.	Normal[2]	Normal[2]	n.a.	n.a.	Cathodal	n.a.
ISE I	22.4s/(12-13.8s)	n.a.	Normal[3]	Normal[3]	n.a.	Normal	n.a.	Normal
ISTANBUL I	120s/(10s)	80s/(14s)	>120s/(12s)	300s/(45s)	No clot	n.a.	Normal	Abnormal
ISTANBUL II[Unp]	35s/(11s)	n.a.	n.a.	n.a.	n.a.	n.a.	n.a.	n.a.
JENA I	26s[2]	60s[3]	34%[3]	40s[2]	n.a.	n.a.	n.a.	n.a.
KANAZAWA I	18.4s/(10.5s)	187s/(31.3s)	Normal	Normal	Normal	Normal	n.a.	Normal
KASSEL I	n.a.	n.a.	n.a.	n.a.	n.a.	n.a.	n.a.	n.a.
KAWAGUCHI I	55.1s/(13s)	114s/(23.6s)	19.1s/(11.4s)	29.9s/(24.8s)	n.a.	Normal	n.a.	Normal
KENDAL I	n.a.	n.a.	n.a.	n.a.	n.a.	n.a.	n.a.	n.a.
KIEL I	18s/(9-10.5s)	n.a.	89%/(70-100%)	31.7s/(<42s)	n.a.	n.a.	n.a.	n.a.
KYOTO I	47.6s/(16-18s)	>200/(13-18s)	Normal[3]	Normal[3]	n.a.	n.a.	n.a.	n.a.
KYOTO II	22.3s/(11.7-12.7)	>100s/(11.2-14.3s)	Abnormal[2]	Abnormal[2]	n.a.	n.a.	n.a.	n.a.
KYOTO III	20.4s(10.1s)	n.a.	13.9s/(10.9s)	Normal[2]	n.a.	n.a.	n.a.	n.a.

Superscripts refer to footnotes in Dysfibrinogen Reports (Section 3).

Table 7: Clinical Laboratory Results (cont'd.)

Last Update: 10 January 1994

Fibrinogen	Thrombin Time	Reptilase (Batrox.) Time	Prothrombin Time	Partial T'plastin Time	Euglobulin Lysis Time	Bleeding Time	Immuno-electro-phoresis	Platelet Aggrega-tion
LA CEVAINA I[Unp]	60s/(15-18s)	n.a.	n.a.	n.a.	n.a.	n.a.	n.a.	n.a.
LA GUAIRA I	Abnormal[2]	Abnormal[2]	n.a.	n.a.	n.a.	n.a.	Normal	n.a.
LA PLATA I	28s/(15-18s)[1]	Abnormal[3]	n.a.	n.a.	n.a.	n.a.	Normal	n.a.
LEDYARD I	62.3s/(16-20s)	30.2s/(13-16.9s)	13.2s/(9.6-12s)	28.8s/(25.6-35.2s)	n.a.	n.a.	n.a.	n.a.[3]
LEITCHFIELD I	n.a.	n.a.	n.a.	n.a.	n.a.	n.a.	n.a.	n.a.
LEOGAN I	48s/(20s)	n.a.	n.a.	n.a.	Normal	n.a.	n.a.	n.a.
LEUVEN I	29.2s/(19s)[2]	47.2s/(20s)	n.a.	Normal[3]	Normal[3]	Normal	n.a.	n.a.
LILLE I	No clot	No clot	55s/(15s)	88s/(50s)	n.a.	Normal	Normal	n.a.
LIMA I	38.4s/(12.2)	Abnormal[6]	n.a.	n.a.	n.a.	n.a.	Anodal	n.a.
LOGROÑO I	54s/(18-20s)	127s/(15-18s)	18s/(11-13s)	43s/(35-40s)	210m/(>180m)	Normal	Normal	Normal
LONDON I	91s/(10.6s)[2]	45s/(15.6s)	n.a.	80.8s/(50.6s)	n.a.	n.a.	Normal	n.a.
LONDON II	30-180s/(15s)	45s/(11s)	14s/(12s)	44s/(33s)	n.a.	n.a.	n.a.	n.a.
LONDON III	25s/(9-12s)	n.a.	Normal[2]	43s/(38-41s)	n.a.	n.a.	n.a.	n.a.
LONDON IV	19s/(9-12s)	38s/(18s)	Normal[1]	57s/(38-41s)	n.a.	Normal	n.a.	n.a.
LONDON V	n.a.	n.a.	44s/(14s)	n.a.	n.a.	n.a.	n.a.	n.a.
LONDON VI	25s/(11s)	n.a.	n.a.	n.a.	n.a.	n.a.	n.a.	n.a.
LONG BEACH I[Abs]	n.a.	n.a.	n.a.	n.a.	n.a.	n.a.	n.a.	n.a.
LOS ANGELES I[Abs]	Abnormal[1]	n.a.	Abnormal[1]	Normal[1]	n.a.	n.a.	Abnormal	n.a.
LOUISVILLE I	Abnormal[4]	n.a.	n.a.	n.a.	n.a.	n.a.	n.a.	n.a.[5]
MAASTRICHT I[Abs]	n.a.	n.a.	n.a.	n.a.	n.a.	n.a.	n.a.	n.a.
MADRID I	60s/(17s)	42s/(16s)	85%[2]	39s/(45s)	n.a.	n.a.	Normal	n.a.
MADRID II	Abnormal[3]	58s/(16s)	43%[2]	n.a.	n.a.	n.a.	Normal	n.a.
MADRID III	32s/(18-20s)	35s/(15-18s)	16s/(12-14s)	40s/(35-45s)	>180m/(>180m)[2]	Normal[2]	n.a.	Normal[2]
MAGDEBURG II[Abs]	n.a.	n.a.	Abnormal[2]	n.a.	n.a.	n.a.	n.a.	n.a.
MALAGA I	31s/(18-20s)	23s/(15-18s)	16s/(12-14s)	46s/(35-45s)	>180/(>180)[2]	Normal[2]	n.a.	Normal[2]
MALMÖE I	25-30s/(<20s)	22-24s/(19s)	n.a.	n.a.	n.a.	n.a.	n.a.	Normal
MANCHESTER I	110s/(24s)	n.a.	21s/(14s)	36.5s/(34.5s)	n.a.	n.a.	Normal	n.a.
MANNHEIM I	34.5s[3]	57.5s[3]	n.a.	n.a.	n.a.	Normal	n.a.	Normal
MANNHEIM II[Abs]	27.5s[4]	22s[4]	n.a.	n.a.	85-110m[5]	Normal	n.a.	n.a.
MARBURG I	240s/(20s)[5]	>1 hr/(20s)	31s/(15s)	78s/(40s)	>120m/(>120m)	Normal	Normal	n.a.
MARSEILLE I	73s/(25s)	>60s/(19s)	16.5s/(12s)	Normal[2]	Normal	Normal	Normal	Abnormal[3]
METZ I	No clot	No clot	No clot	No clot	120m/(240m)[4]	Normal	Cathodal[5]	Abnormal[6]
MÉXICO DF I[Abs]	n.a.	n.a.	n.a.	n.a.	n.a.	n.a.	Normal	n.a.
MILAN I[1]	21s/(11-14s)	24.7s/(14-15s)	n.a.	n.a.	n.a.	Normal	n.a.	n.a.
MILAN II[1]	>180s/(19.8s)	21.8s/(22.1s)	21s/(13s)	28s/(28-43s)[6]	167m/(281m)	Normal[6]	n.a.	Normal
MILAN III[Abs1]	Abnormal[4]	Abnormal[4]	n.a.	n.a.	n.a.	n.a.	n.a.	n.a.
MILAN IV[1]	25s/(12-15s)	>180s/(16-18s)	n.a.	n.a.	n.a.	n.a.	n.a.	n.a.
MILAN VI[1]	51s/(17s)	51s/(20s)	n.a.	n.a.	n.a.	Normal	n.a.	Abnormal
MILAN VII[Abs1]	Abnormal	n.a.	n.a.	n.a.	n.a.	n.a.	n.a.	n.a.
MITAKA I[Abs]	Abnormal	Abnormal	Abnormal	Normal	n.a.	n.a.	Anodal	n.a.

Superscripts refer to footnotes in Dysfibrinogen Reports (Section 3).

Table 7: Clinical Laboratory Results (cont'd.)

Last Update: 10 January 1994

Fibrinogen	Thrombin Time	Reptilase (Batrox.) Time	Prothrombin Time	Partial T'plastin Time	Euglobulin Lysis Time	Bleeding Time	Immuno-electro-phoresis	Platelet Aggrega-tion
MITAKA II	28.3s/(13.2s)	n.a.	77%[2]	42.6s/(27-40s)	n.a.	n.a.	n.a.	n.a.
MONTEVIDEO I	Abnormal[3]	n.a.	n.a.	n.a.	n.a.	n.a.	Normal	n.a.
MONTREAL I	46s/(10s)[2]	80s/(18s)	18s/(12s)	n.a.	240m/(240m)	Abnormal	Normal	n.a.
MONTREAL II[Abs]	Abnormal[2]	Abnormal[2]	Abnormal[2]	Abnormal[2]	n.a.	n.a.	n.a.	n.a.
MONTREAL III[Abs]	>3m/(15s)	Abnormal	Abnormal	n.a.	n.a.	n.a.	n.a.	n.a.
MORIOKA I[Abs]	n.a.	n.a.	n.a.	n.a.	n.a.	n.a.	n.a.	n.a.
MUNICH I[1]	29s/(12-14s)	>300s/(18-20s)	51%/(>70%)	n.a.	n.a.	Normal	n.a.	Normal
MUNICH II[1]	31s[3]	104s[3]	45s[3]	47.5s[3]	Normal	Abnormal	n.a.	n.a.
MÜNSTER I[Abs]	n.a.	n.a.	n.a.	n.a.	n.a.	n.a.	n.a.	n.a.
NAGOYA I	20.8s/(10.2s)	n.a.	16.8s/(12.3s)	58s/(47-57s)	n.a.	Normal	n.a.	Normal
NANCY I	75s/(23s)	67s/(32s)	77%[3]	n.a.	n.a.	Normal	Anodal	n.a.
NAPLES I[1]	*>180s/(19.8s)*	*21.8s/(22.1s)*	*21s/(13s)*	*28s/(28-43s)*[6]	*167m/(281m)*	*Normal*[6]	*n.a.*	*Normal*
NEW ALBANY I	n.a.	n.a.	n.a.	n.a.	n.a.	n.a.	n.a.	n.a.
NEWARK I[Abs]	n.a.	n.a.	n.a.	n.a.	Normal[3]	Normal	Normal	Normal
NEW BRITAIN I[Abs]	Abnormal	Abnormal	n.a.	n.a.	n.a.	n.a.	n.a.	n.a.
NEW ORLEANS I	43.5s/(15s)	1320s/(55s)	15s/(11.5s)	58.5s/(30-39s)	n.a.	n.a.	Anodal	n.a.
NEW ORLEANS II[Abs]	34s/(19s)	Normal[2]	15.4s/(12s)	Normal[2]	n.a.	n.a.	Normal	n.a.
NEW YORK I	72s/(7.5s)[3]	73.5s/(33s)	Abnormal[4]	n.a.[5]	>120m/(>120m)	n.a.	Anodal	Normal
NEW YORK II	45.2s/(12-15s)	80s/(17-23s)	13s/(11-12.5s)	40.9s/(31-36s)	n.a.	n.a.	n.a.	n.a.
NEW YORK III	32.9s/(12-15s)	47.8s/(17-23s)	13.1s/(11-12.5s)	56.3s/(31-36s)	n.a.	n.a.	n.a.	n.a.
NEW YORK IV	20.7s/(12-15s)	180s/(17-23s)	17.6s/(11-12.5s)	39.4s/(31-36s)	n.a.	n.a.	n.a.	n.a.
NIJMEGEN I	20.2s/(18.5s)	22.7s/(<20s)	n.a.	n.a.	n.a.	n.a.	n.a.	n.a.
NOTTINGHAM I	n.a.	n.a.	n.a.	n.a.	n.a.	n.a.	n.a.	n.a.
OKLAHOMA I	n.a.	n.a.	15s/(15-17s)	n.a.	2.5-7h/(21-30h)	Normal	Normal	n.a.
ORLEANS I	58s/(20s)	n.a.	64%[3]	n.a.	n.a.	Normal	Normal	n.a.
ORSAY I	50s/(19s)	36s/(16s)	48%/(>70%)	30s/(30s)	n.a.	n.a.	n.a.	n.a.
OSAKA I	n.a.	n.a.	n.a.	n.a.	n.a.	n.a.	n.a.	n.a.
OSAKA II	107.9s/(14.3s)	n.a.	n.a.	n.a.	n.a.	n.a.	n.a.	n.a.
OSAKA III	43.8s/(14.8-16.4s)	>100s/(12.1-13.7s)	15.2s/(11.3-12.1s)	n.a.	n.a.	Normal	n.a.	n.a.
OSAKA IV	80.9s/(14.4s)	106s/(20.9s)	57%/(80-120%)	28s/(20-35s)	n.a.	n.a.	n.a.	n.a.
OSAKA V	14.3s/(9.7s)	n.a.	n.a.	n.a.	n.a.	n.a.	n.a.	n.a.
OSLO I	24.5/(25-36)[3]	n.a.	15.3s/(12.6-17s)	56.9s/(54-60s)	n.a.	n.a.	n.a.	n.a.
OSLO II	41s/(18-23s)	n.a.	18s/(13-17s)	33s/(25-35s)	n.a.	n.a.	n.a.	n.a.[4]
OSLO III	n.a.	n.a.	n.a.	n.a.	n.a.	n.a.	n.a.	n.a.
OSLO IV	40.7s/(16-19s)	38.5s/(15-18s)	17.5s/(15-18s)	31s/(25-35s)	6h/(>2.5h)	Normal	n.a.	n.a.
OVIEDO I	43s/(17-20s)	50s/(15-18s)	13s/(11-13s)	45s/(40-45s)	180m/(180m)	n.a.	Normal	Normal
OVIEDO II[Abs]	Abnormal[1]	Abnormal[1]	n.a.	n.a.	n.a.	n.a.	Normal	n.a.
OVIEDO III[Abs]	Abnormal[1]	Abnormal[1]	n.a.	n.a.	n.a.	n.a.	Normal	n.a.
PAMPLONA I	75s/(18-20s)	72s/(15-18s)	17s/(11-13s)	58s/(35-45s)	>180m/(>180m)	Normal	Cathodal	Normal
PAMPLONA II	63s/(18-20s)	13s/(15-18s)	15s/(11-13s)	40s/(35-40s)	200m/(>180m)	Normal[1]	Normal[1]	Normal[1]

Superscripts refer to footnotes in Dysfibrinogen Reports (Section 3).

Table 7: Clinical Laboratory Results (cont'd.)

Last Update: 10 January 1994

Fibrinogen	Thrombin Time	Reptilase (Batrox.) Time	Prothrombin Time	Partial T'plastin Time	Euglobulin Lysis Time	Bleeding Time	Immuno-electro-phoresis	Platelet Aggrega-tion
PARIS I	No clot	40s/(18s)	No clot	n.a.	n.a.	Normal	Normal	n.a.
PARIS II	85s/(20s)[4]	60s/(18s)	18s/(12s)	n.a.	n.a.	Normal	Normal	n.a.
PARIS III	50s/(20s)	45s/(18s)	15s/(12s)	n.a.	>3h/(>3h)	Normal	Normal	Normal
PARIS IV	72s/(18-29s)	45s/(18-22s)	50%	n.a.	n.a.	Normal	n.a.	n.a.
PARIS V[1]	*35s/(20s)*	*29.5s/(20s)*	*17.5s/(12s)*	*n.a.*	*n.a.*	*n.a.*	*n.a.*	*Normal*
PARIS VI	54s/(20s)	60s/(22s)	n.a.	n.a.	n.a.	n.a.	n.a.	n.a.
PARMA I	n.a.	n.a.	28s/(16s)	n.a.	n.a.	Normal	n.a.	Normal
PERUGIA I	26.1s/(12.5s)	31.6s/(17.6s)	n.a.	n.a.	n.a.	n.a.	n.a.	n.a.
PETOSKEY I	13.6s/(8-9s)	n.a.	11s/(13s)	30.1s/(35s)	n.a.	n.a.	n.a.	n.a.
PHILADELPHIA I	83.6s/(18-22s)	300s/(38.5s)	16s/(11.5-13.5s)	76s/(45-90s)	120m/(>120m)	Normal	Normal	n.a.
PHILADELPHIA II	n.a.	n.a.	n.a.	n.a.	n.a.	n.a.	n.a.	n.a.
POITIERS I	105s/(18-20s)	60s/(18-25s)	13.9s/(11-13s)	60s/(28-32s)	n.a.	n.a.	n.a.	Normal
PONTOISE I	88s/(20s)	n.a.	n.a.	n.a.	n.a.	n.a.	n.a.	n.a.
PRAHRAN I[1]	114s/(4s)	n.a.	Normal[3]	Normal[3]	Abnormal[4]	n.a.	Cathodal	n.a.
QUEBEC I	25s/(15-19s)	21.5s/(14-16s)	10.5s/(9.5-11.5s)	36s/(32-45s)	Normal[2]	Normal[2]	Normal	Normal[2]
QUEBEC II	24s/(15-19s)	23s/(14-16s)	14s/(9.5-11.5s)	47s/(32-45s)	Normal[2]	Normal[2]	Normal	Normal[2]
RICHFIELD I[Abs]	28.6s/(11.5-16.5s)	35s/(13-17s)	n.a.	n.a.	Abnormal	Normal	n.a.	n.a.
RIYADH I	49.7s/(13.8s)	>50.5s/(15s)	41.4s/(11.4s)	90s/(53.1s)	n.a.	n.a.	n.a.	n.a.
ROUEN I	n.a.	n.a.	n.a.	n.a.	n.a.	n.a.	n.a.	n.a.
SAGA I	23.4s/(9.4s)	n.a.	n.a.	n.a.	n.a.	n.a.	n.a.	n.a.
SAINT LOUIS I	34.7s/(12-18s)[4]	n.a.	25.6s/(14-16s)	114s/(35-53s)	n.a.	Abnormal	Normal	Normal
SAINT MANDE I	Abnormal	Abnormal[2]	Normal	Normal	n.a.	Normal	n.a.	n.a.
SAINT MANDE II	Abnormal	Abnormal	Abnormal	Abnormal	n.a.	Normal	n.a.	n.a.
SALAMANCA I[Abs]	Abnormal[1]	Abnormal[1]	n.a.	n.a.	n.a.	n.a.	Normal	n.a.
SAN FRANCISCO I[Abs1]	45s/(7s)	n.a.	n.a.	n.a.	n.a.	n.a.	Normal	n.a.
SAN JUAN I	n.a.[3]	n.a.[4]	n.a.	n.a.	n.a.	Abnormal	n.a.	n.a.
SANTIAGO I	24s/(12-15s)[3]	Abnormal[4]	n.a.	n.a.	n.a.	n.a.	Normal	n.a.
SAPPORO I	57.3s/(11.3s)	47.4s/(11.1s)	14.3s/(11s)	25.4s/(25s)	n.a.	n.a.	n.a.	n.a.
SCHWARZACH I	30s/(12-18s)	71s/(12-16s)	48%/(75-110%)	39s/(35-45s)	n.a.	n.a.	Normal	n.a.
SEATTLE I	50s/(17s)	n.a.	13.3s/(12s)	35s/(39s)	n.a.	9.5m/(4-8m)	Normal	n.a.
SEATTLE II	37s/(20-25s)	47s/(18-22s)	Normal[2]	Normal[2]	n.a.	n.a.	n.a.	n.a.
SEVILLA I	38s/(18-20s)	41s/(15-18s)	12s/(11-13s)	56s/(35-40s)	180m/(>180m)	n.a.	Normal	n.a.
SHEFFIELD I	36s/(10s)	32s/(15s)	n.a.	n.a.	n.a.	n.a.	n.a.	n.a.
STONY BROOK I	65s/(18s)	88s/(21s)	18s/(9-11s)	56s/(26-37s)	Normal[2]	Normal	n.a.	Normal[3]
STONY BROOK II	n.a.	n.a.	n.a.	n.a.	Normal	n.a.	n.a.	n.a.
STRASBOURG I[Abs]	n.a.	n.a.	n.a.	n.a.	n.a.	n.a.	n.a.	n.a.
STRASBOURG II[Abs]	n.a.	n.a.	n.a.	n.a.	n.a.	n.a.	n.a.	n.a.
SYDNEY I	85s/(20s)	n.a.	n.a.	n.a.	n.a.	n.a.	n.a.	n.a.
SYDNEY II	n.a.	n.a.	n.a.	n.a.	n.a.	n.a.	n.a.	n.a.
TAMPERE I	>90s/(<18s)	64s/(<11.5s)	98%/(70-120%)	41.4s/(32-42s)	n.a.	n.a.	n.a.	n.a.

Superscripts refer to footnotes in Dysfibrinogen Reports (Section 3).

Table 7: Clinical Laboratory Results (cont'd.)

Last Update: 10 January 1994

Fibrinogen	Thrombin Time	Reptilase (Batrox.) Time	Prothrombin Time	Partial T'plastin Time	Euglobulin Lysis Time	Bleeding Time	Immuno-electro-phoresis	Platelet Aggrega-tion
TEMPLE I	n.a.	n.a.	n.a.	n.a.	n.a.	n.a.	n.a.	n.a.
TEMPLE II	n.a.	n.a.	n.a.	n.a.	n.a.	n.a.	n.a.	n.a.
TOCHIGI I	>150s/(8-12s)	>150s/(13-18s)	Normal[1]	Normal	n.a.	n.a.	Normal	n.a.
TOKUSHIMA I	58s/(11s)	86.2s/(19.5s)	15.2s/(11.4s)	51.4s/(40.2s)	10h/(9.5h)	Normal	n.a.	Normal
TOKYO I	11s/(10-11s)	Normal[3]	12.5s/(11-13s)	64s/(55-75s)	Normal[3]	Normal	Anodal	Normal
TOKYO II	155s/(11.8s)	172s/(18.7s)	15.8s/(11.3s)	37.9s/(21.3s)	n.a.	Normal	Normal	Normal
TORINO I	40s/(18s)	53s/(20s)	n.a.	n.a.	n.a.	n.a.	n.a.	n.a.
TROYES I	60s/(19s)	98s/(22s)	18s/(12s)	n.a.	240m/(240m)	Normal	Normal	Abnormal
VALENCIA I	No clot	No clot	n.a.	<5%[4]	n.a.[5]	Abnormal	n.a.	n.a.
VALHALLA I[Abs]	Normal[3]	n.a.	Normal[3]	Normal[3]	Normal	Abnormal	n.a.	n.a.
VANCOUVER I	Abnormal[4]	n.a.	63%[2]	n.a.	n.a.	Normal	n.a.	n.a.
VERSAILLES I	62s/(23.5s)	36.5s/(19s)	50%[1]	38s/(34s)	>3h/(>3h)	Normal	Normal	n.a.
VICENZA I	58s/(13-17s)	67s/(15-20s)	17.4s/(12-14s)	34s/(27-33s)	Normal	Normal	Normal	Normal
VIENNA I[Abs]	Abnormal[2]	Abnormal[2]	Abnormal[2]	n.a.	n.a.	n.a.	Normal	Normal
VILLEPARISIS I	33s/(20s)	23s/(15s)	39%/(>70%)	41s/(37s)	n.a.	n.a.	n.a.	n.a.
VILLIERS-SUR-MARNE I	>60s/(21s)	>60s/(21s)	44%/(>70%)	39s/(32s)	n.a.	n.a.	n.a.	n.a.
VITRY-SUR-SEINE I	>60s/(20s)	38s/(18s)	44%/(>70%)	38s/(35s)	n.a.	n.a.	n.a.	n.a.
VLISSINGEN I	57.5s/(18.6s)	41.3s/(20.1s)	n.a.	n.a.	n.a.	n.a.	n.a.	n.a.
WHITE MARSH I	44s/(19s)	34s/(13s)	14s/(12s)	26s/(25s)	n.a.	n.a.	n.a.	n.a.
WIESBADEN I	No clot	No clot	23.5s/(11.6s)	40.6s/(34.5s)	n.a.	n.a.	Normal	n.a.
YERRES I	43s/(20s)	55s/(22s)	64%/(>70%)	48s/(42s)	n.a.	n.a.	n.a.	n.a.
ZÜRICH I	38s/(15s)	n.a.	17s/(12s)	n.a.	n.a.	Normal	Normal	n.a.
ZÜRICH II	Abnormal[1]	n.a.	Abnormal[1]	n.a.	n.a.	n.a.	Anodal[3]	n.a.

Superscripts refer to footnotes in Dysfibrinogen Reports (Section 3).

Summary of Clinical Laboratory Data

Variants with abnormal thrombin time:	214/220	97%
Variants with abnormal Reptilase (batroxobin) time:	159/167	95%
Variants with abnormal prothrombin time:	121/158	77%
Variants with abnormal partial thromboplastin time:	70/134	52%
Variants with abnormal euglobulin lysis time:	9/57	16%
Variants with abnormal bleeding time:	10/87	12%
Variants with abnormal immunoelectrophoresis:	23/92	25%
Variants with abnormal platelet aggregation:	9/63	14%

Table 8: Other Results with Patient Plasma

Last Update: 10 January 1994

Fibrinogen	Ancrod (Arvin) Time	Recalcification Time	Calcium Corrects C.T.?	Inhib. Normal Plasma?	In vivo Synthesis	In vivo Catabolism
AARAU I[Abs]	n.a.	n.a.	n.a.	n.a.	n.a.	n.a.
AARHUS I	n.a.	n.a.	n.a.	Yes	n.a.	n.a.
ADELAIDE I	n.a.	n.a.	n.a.	No	n.a.	n.a.
ALBA/GENEVA I	n.a.	n.a.	No	n.a.	n.a.	n.a.
ALÈS I	n.a.	n.a.	n.a.	n.a.	n.a.	n.a.
ALMÉRIA I	n.a.	n.a.	n.a.	n.a.	n.a.	n.a.
AMIENS I	n.a.	n.a.	n.a.	n.a.	n.a.	n.a.
AMIENS II	n.a.	n.a.	n.a.	n.a.	n.a.	n.a.
AMSTERDAM I	70s/(6.5s)	Normal	n.a.	Yes	n.a.	n.a.
AMSTERDAM II	n.a.	n.a.	n.a.	n.a.	n.a.	n.a.
ARGENTEUIL I	n.a.	n.a.	No	n.a.	n.a.	n.a.
ASAHI I	>300s/(9.8s)	n.a.	No	n.a.	n.a.	n.a.
ASHFORD I	n.a.	n.a.	n.a.	n.a.	n.a.	n.a.
AWAJI I	n.a.	n.a.	No	No	n.a.	n.a.
AWAJI II	n.a.	n.a.	No	n.a.	n.a.	n.a.
BALTIMORE I	n.a.	Abnormal	Yes	No	n.a.	Normal
BALTIMORE II	n.a.	n.a.	No	No	Decreased	Normal
BALTIMORE III	n.a.	n.a.	Yes	No	n.a.	n.a.
BALTIMORE IV	n.a.	n.a.	Yes	Yes	n.a.	n.a.
BARCELONA I	n.a.	n.a.	n.a.	Yes	n.a.	n.a.
BARCELONA II	n.a.	n.a.	n.a.	n.a.	n.a.	n.a.
BERGAMO I	n.a.	n.a.	No	n.a.	n.a.	n.a.
BERGAMO II	n.a.	n.a.	No	n.a.	n.a.	n.a.
BERGAMO III	n.a.	n.a.	No	n.a.	n.a.	n.a.
BERLIN I	n.a.	n.a.	n.a.	n.a.	n.a.	n.a.
BERLIN II[Abs]	n.a.	n.a.	n.a.	n.a.	n.a.	n.a.
BERN I	n.a.	n.a.	Yes	n.a.	n.a.	n.a.
BERN II	n.a.	n.a.	No	n.a.	n.a.	n.a.
BERN III	n.a.	n.a.	n.a.	n.a.	n.a.	n.a.
BETHESDA I	n.a.	n.a.	n.a.	Yes	Normal	Normal
BETHESDA II	n.a.	n.a.	No	Yes	n.a.	Increased
BETHESDA III	n.a.	n.a.	n.a.	Yes	n.a.	Increased
BICÊTRE I	n.a.	n.a.	n.a.	n.a.	n.a.	n.a.
BICÊTRE II	n.a.	n.a.	n.a.	n.a.	n.a.	n.a.
BIRMINGHAM I	n.a.	n.a.	n.a.	n.a.	n.a.	n.a.
BODMIN I	n.a.	n.a.	n.a.	n.a.	n.a.	n.a.
BONDY I	n.a.	n.a.	n.a.	n.a.	n.a.	n.a.
BOULOGNE I[Abs]	n.a.	n.a.	n.a.	n.a.	n.a.	n.a.
BREMEN I	n.a.	n.a.	No	n.a.	n.a.	n.a.
BRUSSELS I[Abs]	n.a.	n.a.	Yes	Yes	n.a.	n.a.

Superscripts refer to footnotes in Dysfibrinogen Reports (Section 3).

Table 8: Other Results with Patient Plasma (cont'd.)

Last Update: 10 January 1994

Fibrinogen	Ancrod (Arvin) Time	Recalci-fication Time	Calcium Corrects C.T.?	Inhib. Normal Plasma?	In vivo Synthesis	In vivo Catabolism
BUENOS AIRES I[Abs]	n.a.	n.a.	n.a.	n.a.	n.a.	n.a.
BUENOS AIRES II	n.a.	n.a.	n.a.	No	n.a.	n.a.
CARACAS I	n.a.	n.a.	No	Yes	n.a.	n.a.
CARACAS II	>300s/(15.7s)	n.a.	No	No	n.a.	n.a.
CARACAS III	n.a.	n.a.	Yes	No	n.a.	n.a.
CARACAS IV	n.a.	n.a.	Yes	No	n.a.	n.a.
CARACAS V	n.a.	n.a.	n.a.	n.a.	n.a.	n.a.
CARACAS VI	n.a.	n.a.	No	No	n.a.	n.a.
CARACAS VII	n.a.	n.a.	Yes	No	n.a.	n.a.
CHAPEL HILL I	n.a.	n.a.	n.a.	n.a.	Normal	Normal
CHAPEL HILL II	n.a.	n.a.	No	No	n.a.	n.a.
CHAPEL HILL III	43.0s/(21.2s)	n.a.	n.a.	n.a.	n.a.	n.a.
CHAPEL HILL IV	n.a.	n.a.	n.a.	n.a.	n.a.	n.a.
CHAPEL HILL V	No clot	n.a.	n.a.	No	n.a.	n.a.
CHAPEL HILL VI	n.a.	n.a.	n.a.	n.a.	n.a.	n.a.
CHAPEL HILL VII	n.a.	n.a.	n.a.	No	n.a.	n.a.
CHARLOTTESVILLE I	n.a.	n.a.	n.a.	Yes	n.a.	n.a.
CHICAGO I[Abs]	n.a.	n.a.	No	n.a.	n.a.	n.a.
CHRISTCHURCH I	n.a.	n.a.	n.a.	n.a.	n.a.	n.a.
CHRISTCHURCH II	n.a.	n.a.	n.a.	n.a.	n.a.	n.a.
CLERMONT-FERRAND I	n.a.	n.a.	n.a.	n.a.	n.a.	n.a.
CLEVELAND I	n.a.	n.a.	No	Yes	n.a.	n.a.
CLEVELAND II	n.a.	n.a.	Yes	Yes	n.a.	n.a.
COPENHAGEN I	63s/(18-33s)	n.a.	No	No	n.a.	n.a.
COPENHAGEN II	n.a.	n.a.	n.a.	n.a.	n.a.	n.a.
DATE I	n.a.	n.a.	No	n.a.	n.a.	n.a.
DETROIT I	n.a.	>600s/(80-120s)	No	Yes	n.a.	n.a.
DUSART I[1]	n.a.	n.a.	n.a.	n.a.	n.a.	n.a.
ERFURT I	n.a.	n.a.	n.a.	n.a.	n.a.	n.a.
ERFURT II	n.a.	n.a.	n.a.	n.a.	n.a.	n.a.
ESSEN I	n.a.	n.a.	n.a.	n.a.	n.a.	n.a.
FRANKFURT I	n.a.	n.a.	n.a.	No	n.a.	n.a.
FRANKFURT II	n.a.	n.a.	n.a.	No	n.a.	n.a.
FRANKFURT III	n.a.	n.a.	n.a.	No[3]	n.a.	n.a.
FRANKFURT IV[Unp]	n.a.	n.a.	n.a.	n.a.	n.a.	n.a.
FRANKFURT V[Unp]	n.a.	n.a.	n.a.	n.a.	n.a.	n.a.
FRANKFURT XIII[1]	n.a.	n.a.	n.a.	n.a.	n.a.	n.a.
FREIBURG I	n.a.	n.a.	Yes	Yes	n.a.	n.a.
GENEVA I	n.a.	n.a.	n.a.	n.a.	n.a.	n.a.
GENOVA I	n.a.	n.a.	Yes	n.a.	n.a.	n.a.

Superscripts refer to footnotes in Dysfibrinogen Reports (Section 3).

Table 8: Other Results with Patient Plasma (cont'd.)

Last Update: 10 January 1994

Fibrinogen	Ancrod (Arvin) Time	Recalcification Time	Calcium Corrects C.T.?	Inhib. Normal Plasma?	In vivo Synthesis	In vivo Catabolism
GENOVA II	87s/(12-18s)	n.a.	No	Yes	n.a.	n.a.
GENOVA III[Abs]	n.a.	n.a.	n.a.	Yes	n.a.	n.a.
GIESSEN I	n.a.	n.a.	No	n.a.	n.a.	n.a.
GIESSEN II	298s/(20s)	n.a.	n.a.	Yes	n.a.	Increased
GIESSEN III	n.a.	n.a.	Yes	n.a.	n.a.	n.a.
GRAND RAPIDS I	n.a.	n.a.	n.a.	n.a.	n.a.	n.a.
GRENOBLE I	n.a.	n.a.	n.a.	n.a.	n.a.	n.a.
GUADELOUPE I	n.a.	n.a.	n.a.	n.a.	n.a.	n.a.
HAARLEM I	n.a.	n.a.	Yes	n.a.	n.a.	n.a.
HAARLEM II	n.a.	n.a.	Yes	n.a.	n.a.	n.a.
HAIFA I	n.a.	n.a.	Yes	n.a.	n.a.	n.a.
HANNOVER I	n.a.	n.a.	Yes	Yes	n.a.	n.a.
HERSHEY I	n.a.	n.a.	Yes	Yes	n.a.	n.a.
HERSHEY II	n.a.	n.a.	n.a.	Yes[4]	n.a.	n.a.
HOMBURG I	n.a.	n.a.	No[2]	No	n.a.	n.a.
HOMBURG II	n.a.	n.a.	No[1]	No[1]	n.a.	n.a.
HOMBURG III	n.a.	n.a.	No[1]	No	n.a.	n.a.
HOMBURG IV	n.a.	n.a.	No[1]	No[1]	n.a.	n.a.
HOMBURG V	n.a.	n.a.	n.a.	n.a.	n.a.	n.a.
HOMBURG VI	n.a.	n.a.	No[1]	No[1]	n.a.	n.a.
HOUSTON I	n.a.	>1800s/(<135s)	No	Yes[3]	n.a.	n.a.
HOUSTON II	n.a.	n.a.	n.a.	n.a.	n.a.	n.a.
IJMUIDEN I	n.a.	n.a.	n.a.	n.a.	n.a.	n.a.
INDIANAPOLIS I	n.a.	n.a.	n.a.	n.a.	n.a.	n.a.
INDIANAPOLIS II	n.a.	n.a.	n.a.	n.a.	n.a.	n.a.
INDIANAPOLIS III	n.a.	n.a.	n.a.	n.a.	n.a.	n.a.
IOWA CITY I	8-10h/(10s)	n.a.	No	n.a.	n.a.	n.a.
IRVINE I	n.a.	n.a.	n.a.	n.a.	n.a.	n.a.
ISE I	n.a.	n.a.	n.a.	n.a.	n.a.	n.a.
ISTANBUL I	n.a.	360s/(90s)	No	No	n.a.	n.a.
ISTANBUL II[Unp]	n.a.	n.a.	n.a.	n.a.	n.a.	n.a.
JENA I	n.a.	n.a.	n.a.	n.a.	n.a.	n.a.
KANAZAWA I	n.a.	n.a.	No	n.a.	n.a.	n.a.
KASSEL I	n.a.	n.a.	n.a.	n.a.	n.a.	n.a.
KAWAGUCHI I	n.a.	n.a.	n.a.	Yes	n.a.	n.a.
KENDAL I	n.a.	n.a.	n.a.	n.a.	n.a.	n.a.
KIEL I	n.a.	n.a.	n.a.	n.a.	n.a.	n.a.
KYOTO I	n.a.	n.a.	Yes	n.a.	n.a.	n.a.
KYOTO II	n.a.	n.a.	n.a.	n.a.	n.a.	n.a.
KYOTO III	34.1s/(17s)	n.a.	Yes	n.a.	n.a.	n.a.

Superscripts refer to footnotes in Dysfibrinogen Reports (Section 3).

Table 8: Other Results with Patient Plasma (cont'd.)

Last Update: 10 January 1994

Fibrinogen	Ancrod (Arvin) Time	Recalcification Time	Calcium Corrects C.T.?	Inhib. Normal Plasma?	In vivo Synthesis	In vivo Catabolism
LA CEVAINA I[Unp]	n.a.	n.a.	n.a.	n.a.	n.a.	n.a.
LA GUAIRA I	n.a.	n.a.	Yes	No	n.a.	n.a.
LA PLATA I	n.a.	n.a.	No	No	n.a.	n.a.
LEDYARD I	n.a.	n.a.	n.a.	n.a.	n.a.	n.a.
LEITCHFIELD I	n.a.	n.a.	n.a.	n.a.	n.a.	n.a.
LEOGAN I	n.a.	n.a.	n.a.	n.a.	n.a.	n.a.
LEUVEN I	110s/(27s)	Normal[3]	No	Yes	n.a.	n.a.
LILLE I	n.a.	190s/(130s)	n.a.	No	n.a.	n.a.
LIMA I	28.4s/(11.5)	n.a.	Yes	n.a.	n.a.	n.a.
LOGROÑO I	n.a.	n.a.	n.a.	Yes	n.a.	n.a.
LONDON I	n.a.	n.a.	No	Yes	n.a.	n.a.
LONDON II	n.a.	n.a.	n.a.	n.a.	n.a.	Normal
LONDON III	n.a.	n.a.	n.a.	No	n.a.	n.a.
LONDON IV	n.a.	n.a.	n.a.	No	n.a.	n.a.
LONDON V	n.a.	n.a.	n.a.	n.a.	n.a.	n.a.
LONDON VI	n.a.	n.a.	n.a.	n.a.	n.a.	n.a.
LONG BEACH I[Abs]	n.a.	n.a.	n.a.	n.a.	n.a.	n.a.
LOS ANGELES I[Abs]	n.a.	n.a.	Yes	Yes	n.a.	n.a.
LOUISVILLE I	n.a.	n.a.	n.a.	Yes	n.a.	n.a.
MAASTRICHT I[Abs]	n.a.	n.a.	n.a.	n.a.	n.a.	n.a.
MADRID I	n.a.	n.a.	n.a.	n.a.	n.a.	n.a.
MADRID II	n.a.	n.a.	n.a.	n.a.	n.a.	n.a.
MADRID III	n.a.	n.a.	No	Yes	n.a.	n.a.
MAGDEBURG II[Abs]	n.a.	n.a.	n.a.	n.a.	n.a.	n.a.
MALAGA I	n.a.	n.a.	No	Yes	n.a.	n.a.
MALMÖE I	n.a.	n.a.	n.a.	n.a.	n.a.	Normal
MANCHESTER I	Abnormal[3]	30s/(15s)	No	No	n.a.	n.a.
MANNHEIM I	n.a.	n.a.	n.a.	n.a.	n.a.	n.a.
MANNHEIM II[Abs]	n.a.	n.a.	n.a.	n.a.	n.a.	n.a.
MARBURG I	n.a.	n.a.	No	Yes	n.a.	n.a.
MARSEILLE I	n.a.	n.a.	No	n.a.	n.a.	n.a.
METZ I	No clot	n.a.	No	n.a.	n.a.	n.a.
MÉXICO DF I[Abs]	n.a.	n.a.	n.a.	n.a.	n.a.	n.a.
MILAN I[1]	n.a.	n.a.	n.a.	n.a.	n.a.	n.a.
MILAN II[1]	23s/(23s)	n.a.	No	Yes[6]	n.a.	n.a.
MILAN III[Abs1]	n.a.	n.a.	n.a.	Yes	n.a.	n.a.
MILAN IV[1]	n.a.	n.a.	n.a.	n.a.	n.a.	n.a.
MILAN VI[1]	n.a.	n.a.	n.a.	n.a.	n.a.	n.a.
MILAN VII[Abs1]	n.a.	n.a.	n.a.	n.a.	n.a.	n.a.
MITAKA I[Abs]	Abnormal	n.a.	n.a.	n.a.	n.a.	n.a.

Superscripts refer to footnotes in Dysfibrinogen Reports (Section 3).

Table 8: Other Results with Patient Plasma (cont'd.)

Last Update: 10 January 1994

Fibrinogen	Ancrod (Arvin) Time	Recalci-fication Time	Calcium Corrects C.T.?	Inhib. Normal Plasma?	In vivo Synthesis	In vivo Catabolism
MITAKA II	18.7s/(20.1s)	n.a.	No	n.a.	n.a.	n.a.
MONTEVIDEO I	n.a.	n.a.	No	No	n.a.	n.a.
MONTREAL I	n.a.	n.a.	No	n.a.	n.a.	n.a.
MONTREAL II[Abs]	n.a.	n.a.	n.a.	No	n.a.	n.a.
MONTREAL III[Abs]	n.a.	n.a.	n.a.	n.a.	n.a.	n.a.
MORIOKA I[Abs]	n.a.	n.a.	n.a.	n.a.	n.a.	n.a.
MUNICH I[1]	>300s/(11-12s)	n.a.	n.a.	n.a.	n.a.	n.a.
MUNICH II[1]	n.a.	n.a.	n.a.	n.a.	n.a.	n.a.
MÜNSTER I[Abs]	n.a.	n.a.	n.a.	n.a.	n.a.	n.a.
NAGOYA I	n.a.	n.a.	No	Yes	n.a.	n.a.
NANCY I	n.a.	n.a.	Yes	No	n.a.	n.a.
NAPLES I[1]	*23s/(23s)*	*n.a.*	*No*	*Yes*[6]	*n.a.*	*n.a.*
NEW ALBANY I	n.a.	n.a.	n.a.	n.a.	n.a.	n.a.
NEWARK I[Abs]	n.a.	n.a.	n.a.	No	n.a.	n.a.
NEW BRITAIN I[Abs]	n.a.	n.a.	n.a.	n.a.	n.a.	n.a.
NEW ORLEANS I	50s/(31.5s)	n.a.	n.a.	Yes[4]	n.a.	n.a.
NEW ORLEANS II[Abs]	Normal[2]	n.a.	n.a.	No[3]	n.a.	n.a.
NEW YORK I	n.a.	n.a.	No	No	n.a.	n.a.
NEW YORK II	n.a.	n.a.	No	n.a.	n.a.	n.a.
NEW YORK III	n.a.	n.a.	No	n.a.	n.a.	n.a.
NEW YORK IV	n.a.	n.a.	Yes	n.a.	n.a.	n.a.
NIJMEGEN I	n.a.	n.a.	n.a.	n.a.	n.a.	n.a.
NOTTINGHAM I	n.a.	n.a.	n.a.	n.a.	n.a.	n.a.
OKLAHOMA I	n.a.	200s/(100-200s)	n.a.	No	n.a.	Normal
ORLEANS I	n.a.	n.a.	n.a.	No	n.a.	n.a.
ORSAY I	n.a.	n.a.	n.a.	n.a.	n.a.	n.a.
OSAKA I	n.a.	n.a.	n.a.	n.a.	n.a.	n.a.
OSAKA II	n.a.	n.a.	n.a.	n.a.	n.a.	n.a.
OSAKA III	n.a.	n.a.	No	n.a.	n.a.	n.a.
OSAKA IV	n.a.	n.a.	No	n.a.	n.a.	n.a.
OSAKA V	n.a.	n.a.	Yes[2]	n.a.	n.a.	n.a.
OSLO I	n.a.	n.a.	n.a.	n.a.	n.a.	n.a.
OSLO II	n.a.	n.a.	No	n.a.	n.a.	n.a.
OSLO III	n.a.	n.a.	n.a.	n.a.	n.a.	n.a.
OSLO IV	n.a.	n.a.	n.a.	n.a.	n.a.	n.a.
OVIEDO I	n.a.	n.a.	Yes	Yes	n.a.	n.a.
OVIEDO II[Abs]	n.a.	n.a.	Yes	Yes	n.a.	n.a.
OVIEDO III[Abs]	n.a.	n.a.	Yes	Yes	n.a.	n.a.
PAMPLONA I	n.a.	n.a.	n.a.	Yes	n.a.	n.a.
PAMPLONA II	n.a.	n.a.	Yes[1]	No[1]	n.a.	n.a.

Superscripts refer to footnotes in Dysfibrinogen Reports (Section 3).

Table 8: Other Results with Patient Plasma (cont'd.)

Last Update: 10 January 1994

Fibrinogen	Ancrod (Arvin) Time	Recalcification Time	Calcium Corrects C.T.?	Inhib. Normal Plasma?	In vivo Synthesis	In vivo Catabolism
PARIS I	n.a.	150s/(150s)	No[3]	Yes	n.a.	n.a.
PARIS II	180s/(4s)	n.a.	No	No	n.a.	n.a.
PARIS III	n.a.	n.a.	n.a.	n.a.	n.a.	n.a.
PARIS IV	n.a.	n.a.	n.a.	No	n.a.	n.a.
PARIS V[A]	*n.a.*	*n.a.*	*n.a.*	*n.a.*	*n.a.*	*n.a.*
PARIS VI	n.a.	n.a.	n.a.	n.a.	n.a.	n.a.
PARMA I	n.a.	180s/(100-120s)	n.a.	n.a.	Decreased	Normal
PERUGIA I	n.a.	n.a.	n.a.	n.a.	n.a.	n.a.
PETOSKEY I	n.a.	n.a.	n.a.	No	n.a.	n.a.
PHILADELPHIA I	n.a.	n.a.	No	Yes	Normal[4]	Increased
PHILADELPHIA II	n.a.	n.a.	n.a.	n.a.	n.a.	n.a.
POITIERS I	n.a.	n.a.	No	n.a.	n.a.	n.a.
PONTOISE I	n.a.	n.a.	n.a.	n.a.	n.a.	n.a.
PRAHRAN I[1]	n.a.	Normal	n.a.	No	n.a.	n.a.
QUEBEC I	n.a.	n.a.	Yes[2]	No	n.a.	n.a.
QUEBEC II	n.a.	n.a.	Yes[2]	No	n.a.	n.a.
RICHFIELD I[Abs]	n.a.	n.a.	n.a.	n.a.	n.a.	n.a.
RIYADH I	n.a.	n.a.	n.a.	No	n.a.	n.a.
ROUEN I	n.a.	n.a.	n.a.	n.a.	n.a.	n.a.
SAGA I	82.4s/(11.3s)	n.a.	Yes	n.a.	n.a.	n.a.
SAINT LOUIS I	n.a.	n.a.	No	No	n.a.	n.a.
SAINT MANDE I	n.a.	n.a.	n.a.	Yes	n.a.	n.a.
SAINT MANDE II	n.a.	n.a.	n.a.	Yes	n.a.	n.a.
SALAMANCA I[Abs]	n.a.	n.a.	Yes	Yes	n.a.	n.a.
SAN FRANCISCO I[Abs1]	n.a.	n.a.	n.a.	Yes	n.a.	n.a.
SAN JUAN I	n.a.	n.a.	n.a.	n.a.	n.a.	n.a.
SANTIAGO I	n.a.	n.a.	n.a.	No	n.a.	n.a.
SAPPORO I	n.a.	n.a.	No	Yes	n.a.	n.a.
SCHWARZACH I	n.a.	n.a.	No	No	n.a.	n.a.
SEATTLE I	n.a.	n.a.	No	No	n.a.	n.a.
SEATTLE II	n.a.	n.a.	n.a.	n.a.	n.a.	n.a.
SEVILLA I	n.a.	n.a.	Yes	No	n.a.	n.a.
SHEFFIELD I	n.a.	n.a.	n.a.	n.a.	n.a.	n.a.
STONY BROOK I	n.a.	n.a.	n.a.	Yes	n.a.	n.a.
STONY BROOK II	n.a.	n.a.	n.a.	Yes	n.a.	n.a.
STRASBOURG I[Abs]	n.a.	n.a.	n.a.	n.a.	n.a.	n.a.
STRASBOURG II[Abs]	n.a.	n.a.	n.a.	n.a.	n.a.	n.a.
SYDNEY I	n.a.	n.a.	n.a.	n.a.	n.a.	n.a.
SYDNEY II	n.a.	n.a.	n.a.	n.a.	n.a.	n.a.
TAMPERE I	n.a.	112s/(<113s)	n.a.	n.a.	n.a.	n.a.

Superscripts refer to footnotes in Dysfibrinogen Reports (Section 3).

Table 8: Other Results with Patient Plasma (cont'd.)

Last Update: 10 January 1994

Fibrinogen	Ancrod (Arvin) Time	Recalcification Time	Calcium Corrects C.T.?	Inhib. Normal Plasma?	In vivo Synthesis	In vivo Catabolism
TEMPLE I	n.a.	n.a.	n.a.	n.a.	n.a.	n.a.
TEMPLE II	n.a.	n.a.	n.a.	n.a.	n.a.	n.a.
TOCHIGI I	n.a.	n.a.	Yes	n.a.	n.a.	n.a.
TOKUSHIMA I	n.a.	n.a.	n.a.	n.a.	n.a.	n.a.
TOKYO I	n.a.	Normal[3]	n.a.	No	n.a.	n.a.
TOKYO II	n.a.	n.a.	Yes	n.a.	n.a.	n.a.
TORINO I	n.a.	n.a.	n.a.	n.a.	n.a.	n.a.
TROYES I	n.a.	n.a.	No	n.a.	n.a.	n.a.
VALENCIA I	n.a.	n.a.	No	No	n.a.	n.a.
VALHALLA I[Abs]	n.a.	n.a.	n.a.	n.a.	n.a.	n.a.
VANCOUVER I	n.a.	n.a.	n.a.	n.a.	n.a.	n.a.
VERSAILLES I	n.a.	n.a.	No	n.a.	n.a.	n.a.
VICENZA I	41s/(12-18s)	n.a.	No	Yes	n.a.	n.a.
VIENNA I[Abs]	n.a.	n.a.	n.a.	n.a.	n.a.	n.a.
VILLEPARISIS I	n.a.	n.a.	n.a.	No	n.a.	n.a.
VILLIERS-SUR-MARNE I	n.a.	n.a.	n.a.	n.a.	n.a.	n.a.
VITRY-SUR-SEINE I	n.a.	n.a.	n.a.	n.a.	n.a.	n.a.
VLISSINGEN I	n.a.	n.a.	n.a.	n.a.	n.a.	n.a.
WHITE MARSH I	n.a.	n.a.	n.a.	n.a.	n.a.	n.a.
WIESBADEN I	n.a.	n.a.	n.a.	Yes	n.a.	n.a.
YERRES I	n.a.	n.a.	n.a.	No	n.a.	n.a.
ZÜRICH I	n.a.	105s/(<120s)	Yes	Yes	n.a.	n.a.
ZÜRICH II	n.a.	n.a.	n.a.	Yes	n.a.	n.a.

Superscripts refer to footnotes in Dysfibrinogen Reports (Section 3).

Summary of Other Results with Patient Plasma

Variants with abnormal Ancrod (Arvin) time:	**20/23**	**87%**
Variants with abnormal recalcification time:	**5/13**	**39%**
Variants with clotting times corrected by calcium:	**37/101**	**37%**
Variants that inhibit normal plasma:	**51/106**	**48%**
Variants with abnormal in vivo synthesis:	**3/6**	**50%**
Variants with abnormal in vivo catabolism:	**4/12**	**33%**

NOTE: Regarding in vivo studies of fibrinogen synthesis and catabolism, of the 12 variants that were evaluated, 8 presented with hypodysfibrinogenemia (Table 6). Of these 8, 2 had normal fibrinogen synthesis, 2 had decreased fibrinogen synthesis, 5 had normal fibrinogen catabolism, and 3 had increased fibrinogen catabolism. Of the remaining 4 variants with normal plasma fibrinogen concentrations, 1 (fibrinogen Bethesda II) exhibited increased fibrinogen catabolism.

Table 9: Results with Isolated Patient Fibrinogen

Last Update: 10 January 1994

Fibrinogen	Thrombin Time	Reptilase (Batroxobin) Time	Ancrod (Arvin) Time	Abnormal Subunit?	Abnormal FDPs?
AARAU I[Abs]	n.a.	n.a.	n.a.	n.a.	n.a.
AARHUS I	n.a.	Abnormal[3]	n.a.	No	n.a.
ADELAIDE I	Abnormal[3]	Abnormal[3]	Abnormal[3]	No[4]	n.a.
ALBA/GENEVA I	n.a.	n.a.	n.a.	No	n.a.
ALÈS I	n.a.	n.a.	n.a.	n.a.	Yes[2]
ALMÉRIA I	n.a.	n.a.	n.a.	No	n.a.
AMIENS I	n.a.	n.a.	n.a.	n.a.	n.a.
AMIENS II	n.a.	n.a.	n.a.	n.a.	n.a.
AMSTERDAM I	n.a.	n.a.	n.a.	n.a.	No
AMSTERDAM II	n.a.	n.a.	n.a.	n.a.	n.a.
ARGENTEUIL I	>500s/(45s)[3]	>500s/(58s)	n.a.	n.a.	Yes[4]
ASAHI I	>180s/(12.8s)	n.a.	>180s/(5.5s)	Yes[5]	Yes[6]
ASHFORD I	27s/(17s)	n.a.	n.a.	n.a.	n.a.
AWAJI I	n.a.	n.a.	n.a.	Yes[3]	n.a.
AWAJI II	n.a.	n.a.	n.a.	n.a.	n.a.
BALTIMORE I	>120s/(14.2s)	n.a.	n.a.	No	n.a.
BALTIMORE II	n.a.	n.a.	n.a.	No	n.a.
BALTIMORE III	n.a.	n.a.	n.a.	Yes[1]	n.a.
BALTIMORE IV	n.a.	n.a.	n.a.	Yes	n.a.
BARCELONA I	n.a.	n.a.	n.a.	No	No[2]
BARCELONA II	n.a.	n.a.	n.a.	n.a.	n.a.
BERGAMO I	37s/(10.4s)	51.2s/(10.6s)	n.a.	No	n.a.
BERGAMO II	n.a.	n.a.	n.a.	No	n.a.
BERGAMO III	n.a.	n.a.	n.a.	n.a.	n.a.
BERLIN I	n.a.	n.a.	n.a.	No	n.a.
BERLIN II[Abs]	n.a.	n.a.	n.a.	Yes[2]	n.a.
BERN I	n.a.	n.a.	n.a.	Yes[3]	Yes[4]
BERN II	n.a.	n.a.	n.a.	No	n.a.
BERN III	n.a.	n.a.	n.a.	n.a.	n.a.
BETHESDA I	Abnormal[2]	n.a.	n.a.	No	n.a.
BETHESDA II	n.a.	n.a.	n.a.	n.a.	n.a.
BETHESDA III	n.a.	n.a.	n.a.	No	No[2]
BICÊTRE I	n.a.	Abnormal[3]	n.a.	n.a.	n.a.
BICÊTRE II	n.a.	n.a.	n.a.	Yes[4]	No[5]
BIRMINGHAM I	164s/(22s)	n.a.	n.a.	n.a.	n.a.
BODMIN I	n.a.	n.a.	n.a.	n.a.	n.a.
BONDY I	n.a.	n.a.	n.a.	No	No[1]
BOULOGNE I[Abs]	n.a.	n.a.	n.a.	No	n.a.
BREMEN I	61.7s/(13.2s)	n.a.	167s/(12.7s)	No	n.a.
BRUSSELS I[Abs]	n.a.	n.a.	n.a.	n.a.	n.a.

Superscripts refer to footnotes in Dysfibrinogen Reports (Section 3).

Table 9: Results with Isolated Patient Fibrinogen (cont'd.)

Last Update: 10 January 1994

Fibrinogen	Thrombin Time	Reptilase (Batroxobin) Time	Ancrod (Arvin) Time	Abnormal Subunit?	Abnormal FDPs?
BUENOS AIRES I[Abs]	n.a.	n.a.	n.a.	n.a.	n.a.
BUENOS AIRES II	n.a.	n.a.	n.a.	No	No
CARACAS I	22s/(12-13s)[1]	n.a.	n.a.	Yes	No[1]
CARACAS II	n.a.	n.a.	n.a.	Yes[2]	Yes[3]
CARACAS III	n.a.	n.a.	n.a.	No	n.a.
CARACAS IV	n.a.	n.a.	n.a.	n.a.	No[5]
CARACAS V	n.a.	n.a.	n.a.	n.a.	n.a.
CARACAS VI	n.a.	n.a.	n.a.	No	No[5]
CARACAS VII	n.a.	n.a.	n.a.	n.a.	No[4]
CHAPEL HILL I	18.1s/(16.3s)	n.a.	n.a.	No	No[4]
CHAPEL HILL II	n.a.	n.a.	n.a.	No	No[4]
CHAPEL HILL III	n.a.	n.a.	n.a.	No	No[4]
CHAPEL HILL IV	n.a.	n.a.	n.a.	n.a.	n.a.
CHAPEL HILL V	n.a.	n.a.	n.a.	n.a.	n.a.
CHAPEL HILL VI	n.a.	n.a.	n.a.	n.a.	n.a.
CHAPEL HILL VII	n.a.	n.a.	n.a.	n.a.	n.a.
CHARLOTTESVILLE I	n.a.	n.a.	n.a.	n.a.	n.a.
CHICAGO I[Abs]	n.a.	n.a.	n.a.	n.a.	n.a.
CHRISTCHURCH I	n.a.	n.a.	n.a.	n.a.	n.a.
CHRISTCHURCH II	n.a.	n.a.	n.a.	No	n.a.
CLERMONT-FERRAND I	n.a.	n.a.	n.a.	n.a.	No
CLEVELAND I	n.a.	n.a.	n.a.	Yes[2]	n.a.
CLEVELAND II	77s/(27.4s)	196s/(84s)	>1200s/(33.3s)	No	n.a.
COPENHAGEN I	n.a.	n.a.	n.a.	No	n.a.
COPENHAGEN II	33s/(18s)	n.a.	n.a.	n.a.	n.a.
DATE I	32.3s/(<20.5s)	n.a.	n.a.	No	No[2]
DETROIT I	n.a.	n.a.[3]	n.a.	No	n.a.
DUSART I[1]	22s/(12s)	27s/(18s)	n.a.	No	No[5]
ERFURT I	n.a.	n.a.	n.a.	Yes[3]	n.a.
ERFURT II	n.a.	n.a.	n.a.	No	n.a.
ESSEN I	n.a.	n.a.	n.a.	n.a.	n.a.
FRANKFURT I	n.a.	n.a.	n.a.	n.a.	n.a.
FRANKFURT II	n.a.	n.a.	n.a.	n.a.	n.a.
FRANKFURT III	n.a.	n.a.	n.a.	n.a.	n.a.
FRANKFURT IV[Unp]	n.a.	n.a.	n.a.	n.a.	n.a.
FRANKFURT V[Unp]	n.a.	n.a.	n.a.	n.a.	n.a.
FRANKFURT XIII[1]	n.a.	n.a.	n.a.	No	n.a.
FREIBURG I	n.a.	n.a.	n.a.	No	n.a.
GENEVA I	n.a.	n.a.	n.a.	No	n.a.
GENOVA I	116s/(17s)	90s/(20s)	n.a.	No	No

Superscripts refer to footnotes in Dysfibrinogen Reports (Section 3).

Table 9: Results with Isolated Patient Fibrinogen (cont'd.)

Last Update: 10 January 1994

Fibrinogen	Thrombin Time	Reptilase (Batroxobin) Time	Ancrod (Arvin) Time	Abnormal Subunit?	Abnormal FDPs?
GENOVA II	36s/(15-20s)	n.a.	n.a.	No	No
GENOVA III[Abs]	n.a.	n.a.	n.a.	No	Yes
GIESSEN I	n.a.	n.a.	n.a.	No	No
GIESSEN II	n.a.	n.a.	n.a.	n.a.	No[2]
GIESSEN III	n.a.	n.a.	n.a.	n.a.	n.a.
GRAND RAPIDS I	n.a.	n.a.	n.a.	No	No
GRENOBLE I	n.a.	n.a.	n.a.	Yes[2]	n.a.
GUADELOUPE I	n.a.	n.a.	n.a.	n.a.	n.a.
HAARLEM I	21s/(18s)	>180s/(30s)	n.a.	No	No
HAARLEM II	29s/(18s)	43s/(30s)	n.a.	No	No
HAIFA I	36s/(16s)	30s/(16s)	n.a.	No	Yes[3]
HANNOVER I	n.a.	n.a.	n.a.	n.a.	n.a.
HERSHEY I	n.a.	60s/(49s)	n.a.	No	n.a.
HERSHEY II	n.a.	62s/(25s)[4]	n.a.	No	n.a.
HOMBURG I	n.a.	n.a.	n.a.	n.a.	n.a.
HOMBURG II	n.a.	n.a.	n.a.	n.a.	n.a.
HOMBURG III	n.a.	n.a.	n.a.	n.a.	n.a.
HOMBURG IV	n.a.	n.a.	n.a.	n.a.	n.a.
HOMBURG V	n.a.	n.a.	n.a.	n.a.	n.a.
HOMBURG VI	n.a.	n.a.	n.a.	n.a.	n.a.
HOUSTON I	21s/(20-22s)	n.a.	n.a.	No	Yes
HOUSTON II	n.a.	n.a.	n.a.	n.a.	n.a.
IJMUIDEN I	n.a.	n.a.	n.a.	n.a.	n.a.[3]
INDIANAPOLIS I	n.a.	n.a.	n.a.	n.a.	n.a.
INDIANAPOLIS II	n.a.	n.a.	n.a.	n.a.	n.a.
INDIANAPOLIS III	n.a.	n.a.	n.a.	n.a.	n.a.
IOWA CITY I	n.a.	n.a.	n.a.	n.a.	n.a.
IRVINE I	n.a.	n.a.	n.a.	n.a.	n.a.
ISE I	12.5s/(5.2-7.2s)	16.3s/(14.8-19.9s)	n.a.	No	No
ISTANBUL I	n.a.	n.a.	n.a.	Yes	n.a.
ISTANBUL II[Unp]	n.a.	n.a.	n.a.	n.a.	n.a.
JENA I	n.a.	n.a.	n.a.	n.a.	n.a.
KANAZAWA I	n.a.	n.a.	n.a.	No	n.a.
KASSEL I	n.a.	n.a.	n.a.	n.a.	n.a.
KAWAGUCHI I	n.a.	n.a.	n.a.	No	n.a.
KENDAL I	n.a.	n.a.	n.a.	n.a.	n.a.
KIEL I	n.a.	n.a.	n.a.	n.a.	n.a.
KYOTO I	179s/(17-18s)	n.a.	n.a.	Yes[4]	Yes[5]
KYOTO II	>100s/(10.2s)	>100s/(11.7s)	n.a.	No	No
KYOTO III	135s/(11.1s)	n.a.	>300s/(15.3s)	Yes[3]	Yes

Superscripts refer to footnotes in Dysfibrinogen Reports (Section 3).

Table 9: Results with Isolated Patient Fibrinogen (cont'd.)

Last Update: 10 January 1994

Fibrinogen	Thrombin Time	Reptilase (Batroxobin) Time	Ancrod (Arvin) Time	Abnormal Subunit?	Abnormal FDPs?
LA CEVAINA I[Unp]	n.a.	n.a.	n.a.	n.a.	n.a.
LA GUAIRA I	n.a.	n.a.	n.a.	n.a.	No[3]
LA PLATA I	n.a.	n.a.	n.a.	n.a.	No
LEDYARD I	n.a.	n.a.	n.a.	n.a.	n.a.
LEITCHFIELD I	n.a.	n.a.	n.a.	n.a.	n.a.
LEOGAN I	n.a.	n.a.	n.a.	No	n.a.
LEUVEN I	n.a.	n.a.	n.a.	No	n.a.
LILLE I	19m/(24s)	No clot	n.a.	No	Yes[3]
LIMA I	n.a.	n.a.	n.a.	Yes[7]	No[8]
LOGROÑO I	n.a.	n.a.	n.a.	No	No
LONDON I	65s/(5.2s)[2]	n.a.	n.a.	No	n.a.
LONDON II	30-180s/(12.6s)	n.a.	n.a.	n.a.	n.a.
LONDON III	95s/(20s)	n.a.	n.a.	No	n.a.
LONDON IV	30s/(20s)	n.a.	n.a.	No	No
LONDON V	n.a.	n.a.	n.a.	n.a.	n.a.
LONDON VI	n.a.	n.a.	n.a.	n.a.	n.a.
LONG BEACH I[Abs]	n.a.	n.a.	n.a.	n.a.	n.a.
LOS ANGELES I[Abs]	n.a.	n.a.	n.a.	n.a.	n.a.
LOUISVILLE I	Abnormal[4]	n.a.	n.a.	No	n.a.
MAASTRICHT I[Abs]	n.a.	n.a.	n.a.	n.a.	n.a.
MADRID I	n.a.	n.a.	n.a.	n.a.	n.a.
MADRID II	65s/(18s)	n.a.	n.a.	n.a.	n.a.
MADRID III	n.a.	n.a.	n.a.	No[2]	No[2]
MAGDEBURG II[Abs]	n.a.	n.a.	n.a.	n.a.	n.a.
MALAGA I	n.a.	n.a.	n.a.	No[2]	No[2]
MALMÖE I	20.5s/(15s)	30s/(21s)	n.a.	No	No
MANCHESTER I	147s/(12.4s)	n.a.	n.a.	No	No
MANNHEIM I	n.a.	n.a.	n.a.	No	n.a.[4]
MANNHEIM II[Abs]	n.a.	n.a.	n.a.	No	n.a.[6]
MARBURG I	640s/(20s)[5]	n.a.	n.a.	Yes[6]	n.a.
MARSEILLE I	46s/(20s)	46s/(15s)	n.a.	No	No
METZ I	n.a.	n.a.	n.a.	Yes[5]	No
MÉXICO DF I[Abs]	n.a.	n.a.	n.a.	n.a.	No
MILAN I[1]	n.a.	n.a.	n.a.	Yes[2]	Yes
MILAN II[1]	90s/(23s)[7]	38s/(65s)[8]	16s/(23s)[8]	n.a.	n.a.
MILAN III[Abs1]	n.a.	n.a.	n.a.	Yes[5]	n.a.
MILAN IV[1]	n.a.	n.a.	n.a.	n.a.	n.a.
MILAN VI[1]	n.a.	n.a.	n.a.	No	n.a.
MILAN VII[Abs1]	n.a.	n.a.	n.a.	n.a.	n.a.
MITAKA I[Abs]	n.a.	n.a.	n.a.	No	n.a.

Superscripts refer to footnotes in Dysfibrinogen Reports (Section 3).

Table 9: Results with Isolated Patient Fibrinogen (cont'd.)

Last Update: 10 January 1994

Fibrinogen	Thrombin Time	Reptilase (Batroxobin) Time	Ancrod (Arvin) Time	Abnormal Subunit?	Abnormal FDPs?
MITAKA II	41.2s/(16.7s)[3]	n.a.	21.2s/(19.7s)	No	n.a.
MONTEVIDEO I	n.a.	n.a.	n.a.	No	n.a.
MONTREAL I	n.a.	n.a.	n.a.	Yes	n.a.
MONTREAL II[Abs]	n.a.	n.a.	n.a.	n.a.	n.a.
MONTREAL III[Abs]	n.a.	n.a.	n.a.	n.a.	n.a.
MORIOKA I[Abs]	n.a.	n.a.	n.a.	Yes[1]	Yes
MUNICH I[1]	n.a.	n.a.	n.a.	n.a.	n.a.
MUNICH II[1]	n.a.	n.a.	n.a.	n.a.	n.a.
MÜNSTER I[Abs]	n.a.	n.a.	n.a.	n.a.	n.a.
NAGOYA I	n.a.	n.a.	n.a.	Yes[1]	No
NANCY I	n.a.	n.a.	n.a.	No[4]	n.a.
NAPLES I[1]	*90s/(23s)*[7]	*38s/(65s)*[8]	*16s/(23s)*[8]	*n.a.*	*n.a.*
NEW ALBANY I	n.a.	n.a.	n.a.	n.a.	n.a.
NEWARK I[Abs]	n.a.	n.a.	n.a.	n.a.	Yes[4]
NEW BRITAIN I[Abs]	n.a.	n.a.	n.a.	n.a.	n.a.
NEW ORLEANS I	125s/(26s)	n.a.	n.a.	No	n.a.
NEW ORLEANS II[Abs]	Abnormal[3]	n.a.	n.a.	n.a.	n.a.
NEW YORK I	Abnormal	n.a.	n.a.	Yes	n.a.
NEW YORK II	48.4s/(16s)	n.a.	n.a.	No	n.a.
NEW YORK III	n.a.	n.a.	n.a.	No	n.a.
NEW YORK IV	28.4s/(16s)	n.a.	n.a.	No	n.a.
NIJMEGEN I	22.7s/(20s)	30s/(25s)	n.a.	No	n.a.[2]
NOTTINGHAM I	n.a.	n.a.	n.a.	n.a.	n.a.
OKLAHOMA I	n.a.	n.a.	n.a.	No	n.a.
ORLEANS I	n.a.	n.a.	n.a.	n.a.	n.a.
ORSAY I	n.a.	n.a.	n.a.	n.a.	n.a.
OSAKA I	n.a.	n.a.	n.a.	n.a.	n.a.
OSAKA II	>300s/(15.3s)	n.a.	>300s/(17.6s)	Yes[3]	Yes[4]
OSAKA III	>100s/(10.2-12s)	n.a.	n.a.	Yes[1]	Yes[2]
OSAKA IV	n.a.	n.a.	n.a.	No	No[3]
OSAKA V	23.7s/(8.7s)	37.3s/(10s)	n.a.	Yes[3]	Yes[4]
OSLO I	n.a.	n.a.	n.a.	Yes[5]	n.a.
OSLO II	n.a.	n.a.	n.a.	No	n.a.
OSLO III	n.a.	n.a.	n.a.	Yes[2]	n.a.
OSLO IV	n.a.	n.a.	n.a.	n.a.	n.a.
OVIEDO I	Abnormal[2]	n.a.	n.a.	No	No
OVIEDO II[Abs]	Abnormal[1]	n.a.	n.a.	No	n.a.
OVIEDO III[Abs]	Abnormal[1]	n.a.	n.a.	No	n.a.
PAMPLONA I	180s/(15-20s)	n.a.	n.a.	No	No[1]
PAMPLONA II	n.a.[3]	n.a.	n.a.	No	No

Superscripts refer to footnotes in Dysfibrinogen Reports (Section 3).

Table 9: Results with Isolated Patient Fibrinogen (cont'd.)

Last Update: 10 January 1994

Fibrinogen	Thrombin Time	Reptilase (Batroxobin) Time	Ancrod (Arvin) Time	Abnormal Subunit?	Abnormal FDPs?
PARIS I	150s/(15s)[3]	n.a.	n.a.	Yes[4]	Yes[5]
PARIS II	n.a.[4]	n.a.	n.a.	n.a.	n.a.
PARIS III	n.a.	n.a.	n.a.	No	No
PARIS IV	n.a.	n.a.	n.a.	n.a.	No
PARIS V[A]	*22s/(12s)*	*27s/(18s)*	*n.a.*	*No*	*No*[5]
PARIS VI	n.a.	n.a.	n.a.	n.a.	n.a.
PARMA I	n.a.	n.a.	n.a.	n.a.	n.a.
PERUGIA I	n.a.	n.a.	n.a.	n.a.	n.a.
PETOSKEY I	n.a.	Abnormal[2]	n.a.	No	No
PHILADELPHIA I	n.a.	n.a.	n.a.	No	n.a.
PHILADELPHIA II	n.a.	n.a.	n.a.	n.a.	n.a.
POITIERS I	>500s/(45s)[3]	>500s/(58s)	n.a.	n.a.	Yes[2]
PONTOISE I	n.a.	n.a.	n.a.	Yes[2]	Yes[3]
PRAHRAN I[1]	n.a.	n.a.	n.a.	n.a.	n.a.
QUEBEC I	n.a.	n.a.	n.a.	n.a.	n.a.
QUEBEC II	n.a.	n.a.	n.a.	n.a.	n.a.
RICHFIELD I[Abs]	n.a.	n.a.	n.a.	Yes[2]	Yes[3]
RIYADH I	n.a.	n.a.	n.a.	n.a.	n.a.
ROUEN I	n.a.	n.a.	n.a.	n.a.	n.a.
SAGA I	114s/(14.7s)	n.a.	>180s/(11.3s)	No	Yes[3]
SAINT LOUIS I	n.a.[4]	n.a.	n.a.	n.a.	n.a.
SAINT MANDE I	n.a.	n.a.	n.a.	n.a.	n.a.
SAINT MANDE II	n.a.	n.a.	n.a.	n.a.	n.a.
SALAMANCA I[Abs]	Abnormal[1]	n.a.	n.a.	No	n.a.
SAN FRANCISCO I[Abs1]	n.a.	n.a.	n.a.	n.a.	n.a.
SAN JUAN I	21s/(16s)	n.a.	n.a.	n.a.	n.a.
SANTIAGO I	n.a.	n.a.	n.a.	No	No[5]
SAPPORO I	101s/(20.1s)	n.a.	>200s/(28.3s)	No	n.a.
SCHWARZACH I	n.a.	n.a.	n.a.	No	n.a.
SEATTLE I	n.a.	n.a.	n.a.	No	n.a.
SEATTLE II	n.a.	n.a.	n.a.	No	n.a.
SEVILLA I	n.a.	n.a.	n.a.	No	No[3]
SHEFFIELD I	n.a.	n.a.	n.a.	n.a.	n.a.
STONY BROOK I	n.a.	n.a.	n.a.	Yes[4]	n.a.
STONY BROOK II	Abnormal	Abnormal	n.a.	No	n.a.
STRASBOURG I[Abs]	n.a.	n.a.	n.a.	n.a.	n.a.
STRASBOURG II[Abs]	n.a.	n.a.	n.a.	n.a.	n.a.
SYDNEY I	n.a.	n.a.	n.a.	No	n.a.
SYDNEY II	n.a.	n.a.	n.a.	n.a.	n.a.
TAMPERE I	n.a.	n.a.	n.a.	n.a.	n.a.

Superscripts refer to footnotes in Dysfibrinogen Reports (Section 3).

Table 9: Results with Isolated Patient Fibrinogen (cont'd.)

Last Update: 10 January 1994

Fibrinogen	Thrombin Time	Reptilase (Batroxobin) Time	Ancrod (Arvin) Time	Abnormal Subunit?	Abnormal FDPs?
TEMPLE I	n.a.	n.a.	n.a.	n.a.	n.a.
TEMPLE II	n.a.	n.a.	n.a.	n.a.	n.a.
TOCHIGI I	>150s/(15-17s)	>150s/(12-14s)	n.a.	Yes[2]	Yes[3]
TOKUSHIMA I	188s/(30.8s)	>1800s/(78.6s)	n.a.	No	n.a.
TOKYO I	n.a.	n.a.	n.a.	Yes	Yes[4]
TOKYO II	n.a.	n.a.	n.a.	No	n.a.
TORINO I	n.a.	n.a.	n.a.	n.a.	n.a.
TROYES I	n.a.	n.a.	n.a.	No	n.a.
VALENCIA I	n.a.	n.a.	n.a.	No	n.a.[5]
VALHALLA I[Abs]	73s/(45s)	n.a.	n.a.	No	n.a.
VANCOUVER I	n.a.	n.a.	n.a.	n.a.	n.a.
VERSAILLES I	n.a.	n.a.	n.a.	n.a.	n.a.
VICENZA I	48s/(15-20s)	n.a.	n.a.	No	No
VIENNA I[Abs]	n.a.	n.a.	n.a.	No	n.a.
VILLEPARISIS I	n.a.	n.a.	n.a.	n.a.	n.a.
VILLIERS-SUR-MARNE I	n.a.	n.a.	n.a.	n.a.	n.a.
VITRY-SUR-SEINE I	n.a.	n.a.	n.a.	n.a.	n.a.
VLISSINGEN I	n.a.	n.a.	n.a.	Yes[3]	Yes[4]
WHITE MARSH I	n.a.	n.a.	n.a.	No	n.a.
WIESBADEN I	n.a.	n.a.	n.a.	n.a.	n.a.
YERRES I	n.a.	n.a.	n.a.	n.a.	n.a.
ZÜRICH I	n.a.	n.a.	n.a.	No	n.a.
ZÜRICH II	n.a.	n.a.	n.a.	No[3]	n.a.

Superscripts refer to footnotes in Dysfibrinogen Reports (Section 3).

Summary of Results with Isolated Patient Fibrinogen

Variants with abnormal thrombin time:	61/62	98%
Variants with abnormal Reptilase (batroxobin) time:	23/25	92%
Variants with abnormal ancrod (Arvin) time:	9/10	90%
Variants with abnormal subunits:	28/129	22%
Variants with abnormal FDPs:	19/67	28%

SECTION 3

DYSFIBRINOGEN REPORTS

Variant fibrinogens are listed in alphabetical order.

FIBRINOGEN AARAU I[Abs]

Last update	[10 January 1994]	**Structural defect**	[n.a.]
Alphacode	[AARAU01]	**Mutation**	[n.a.]
Ref. type	[Abstract]		

Functional defect(s)

FpA release:	[n.a.]
FpB release:	[n.a.]
Polymerization:	[n.a.]
Stabilization:	[n.a.]

Family studies

Homozygote? [n.a.]

Pedigree published? [No]

Clinical manifestation(s) Bleeding? [No] Thrombosis? [No]

Clinical laboratory results

Plasma fibrinogen concentration (mg/dL)

Chronometric: [n.a.]

Rate-indep'nt: [n.a.]

Immunologic: [Normal[1]]

*Hypo*dysfibrinogen? [No]

Thrombin time:	[Abnormal[1]]
Reptilase (batroxobin) time:	[n.a.]
Prothrombin time:	[n.a.]
Partial thromboplastin time:	[n.a.]
Euglobulin lysis time:	[n.a.]
Bleeding time:	[n.a.]
Immunoelectrophoresis:	[Anodal]
Platelet aggregation:	[n.a.]

Other results with patient plasma

Ancrod (Arvin) time:	[n.a.]	Inhib. normal plasma?	[n.a.]
Recalcification time:	[n.a.]	In vivo synthesis:	[n.a.]
Calcium corrects c.t.?	[n.a.]	In vivo catabolism:	[n.a.]

Evaluation of isolated patient fibrinogen

Thrombin time:	[n.a.]	Abnormal subunit?	[n.a.]
Reptilase time:	[n.a.]	Abnormal FDPs?	[n.a.]
Ancrod (Arvin) time:	[n.a.]		

Remarks

[1]Data not reported.

Results are from review articles; Beck & Duckert (1973) is not on file.

References

1. Beck, E.A. and Duckert, F. Congenital dysfibrinogenemia: fibrinogen Aarau. *Proc. II Congr. Europ. Afr. Div. Int. Soc. Haematol.* 253, **1973**. ABSTRACT

FIBRINOGEN AARHUS I

Last update [1 December 1990]
Alphacode [AARHUS01]
Ref. type [Article]

Family studies
Homozygote? [Yes]
Pedigree published? [Yes[1]]

Structural defect [Aα(19) Arg → Gly]
Mutation [n.a.]

Functional defect(s)
FpA release: [Abnormal]
FpB release: [Abnormal]
Polymerization: [Abnormal]
Stabilization: [Normal]

Clinical manifestation(s) Bleeding? [No] Thrombosis? [Yes[2]]

Clinical laboratory results
Plasma fibrinogen concentration (mg/dL)
Chronometric: [No clot]
Rate-indep'nt: [Normal[3]]
Immunologic: [Normal[3]]

*Hypo*dysfibrinogen? [No]

Thrombin time:	[>600s/(<30s)]
Reptilase (batroxobin) time:	[n.a.]
Prothrombin time:	[245s/(16s)]
Partial thromboplastin time:	[473s/(32s)]
Euglobulin lysis time:	[n.a.]
Bleeding time:	[n.a.]
Immunoelectrophoresis:	[Normal]
Platelet aggregation:	[Normal]

Other results with patient plasma
Ancrod (Arvin) time: [n.a.]
Recalcification time: [n.a.]
Calcium corrects c.t.? [n.a.]

Inhib. normal plasma? [Yes]
In vivo synthesis: [n.a.]
In vivo catabolism: [n.a.]

Evaluation of isolated patient fibrinogen
Thrombin time: [n.a.]
Reptilase time: [Abnormal[3]]
Ancrod (Arvin) time: [n.a.]

Abnormal subunit? [No]
Abnormal FDPs? [n.a.]

Remarks
[1]There is evidence of consanguinity.
[2]Thrombotic tendency is based on finding of transient ischemic attacks after surgery. These symptoms were *not* observed in Mannheim I.

Parents of proposita are cousins, and exhibit prolonged PTT and thrombin time; proposita was more severely affected than either parent, and no clots were detected during chronometric fibrinogen determinations or incubation with batroxobin.

References

1. Blombäck, B., Hessel, B., Fields, R. and Procyk, R. Fibrinogen Aarhus: An abnormal fibrinogen with Aα19 Arg → Gly substitution. In: *Fibrinogen 3. Biochemistry, Biological Functions, Gene Regulation and Expression*, M.W. Mosesson, D.L. Amrani, K.R. Siebenlist and J.P. DiOrio (eds.), Elsevier, Amsterdam. pp. 263-266, **1988**.
2. Hessel, B., Stenbjerg, S., Dyr, J., Kudryk, B., Therkildsen, L. and Blombäck, B. Fibrinogen Aarhus -- a new case of dysfibrinogenemia. *Thromb. Res.* **42**:21-37, **1986**.

FIBRINOGEN ADELAIDE I

Last update [1 December 1990]
Alphacode [ADELAI01]
Ref. type [Article]

Structural defect [n.a.]
Mutation [n.a.]

Family studies
Homozygote? [No]
Pedigree published? [Yes]

Functional defect(s)
FpA release: [n.a.]
FpB release: [n.a.]
Polymerization: [Normal]
Stabilization: [n.a.]

Clinical manifestation(s) Bleeding? [Yes[1]] Thrombosis? [No]

Clinical laboratory results
Plasma fibrinogen concentration (mg/dL)
Chronometric: [55/(150-400)]
Rate-indep'nt: [110/(150-400)]
Immunologic: [120/(150-400)]

*Hypo*dysfibrinogen? [Yes]

Thrombin time:	[19s/(7-12s)]
Reptilase (batroxobin) time:	[25s/(15-20s)]
Prothrombin time:	[1.54/(0.95-1.2)[2]]
Partial thromboplastin time:	[45s/(35-45s)]
Euglobulin lysis time:	[1.75h/(>2h)]
Bleeding time:	[Normal]
Immunoelectrophoresis:	[Normal[3]]
Platelet aggregation:	[Normal[3]]

Other results with patient plasma
Ancrod (Arvin) time: [n.a.]
Recalcification time: [n.a.]
Calcium corrects c.t.? [n.a.]

Inhib. normal plasma? [No]
In vivo synthesis: [n.a.]
In vivo catabolism: [n.a.]

Evaluation of isolated patient fibrinogen
Thrombin time: [Abnormal[3]]
Reptilase time: [Abnormal[3]]
Ancrod (Arvin) time: [Abnormal[3]]

Abnormal subunit? [No[4]]
Abnormal FDPs? [n.a.]

Remarks
[1]Excessive postpartum and post-surgical bleeding was controlled in the 32 year-old proposita with fibrinogen infusion; similar symptoms in her 24 year-old sister were refractory to this treatment.
[2]Prothrombin time ratio.
[3]T. Exner, personal communication.
[4]Increased anodal mobility of the α-chain on isoelectric focusing implicates this subunit as the site of the molecular defect.

References

1. Exner, T., Barber, S., Sage, R.E. and Kronenberg, H. Fibrinogen Adelaide: a familial hypodysfibrinogenaemia associated with abnormal α-chains. *Br. J. Haematol.* **56**:95-106, **1984**.

FIBRINOGEN ALBA/GENEVA I

Last update [1 December 1990]
Alphacode [ALBAGE01]
Ref. type [Article]

Family studies
Homozygote? [n.a.]
Pedigree published? [No]

Structural defect [n.a.]
Mutation [n.a.]

Functional defect(s)
FpA release: [n.a.[1]]
FpB release: [n.a.[1]]
Polymerization: [Abnormal]
Stabilization: [Normal]

Clinical manifestation(s) Bleeding? [No[2]] Thrombosis? [No[2]]

Clinical laboratory results
Plasma fibrinogen concentration (mg/dL)
Chronometric: [20/(250)]
Rate-indep'nt: [95/(250)]
Immunologic: [15-60[3]]

*Hypo*dysfibrinogen? [Yes]

Thrombin time:	[60s/(11s)]
Reptilase (batroxobin) time:	[n.a.]
Prothrombin time:	[n.a.]
Partial thromboplastin time:	[n.a.]
Euglobulin lysis time:	[>5h/(>5h)]
Bleeding time:	[n.a.]
Immunoelectrophoresis:	[Normal]
Platelet aggregation:	[n.a.]

Other results with patient plasma
Ancrod (Arvin) time: [n.a.]
Recalcification time: [n.a.]
Calcium corrects c.t.? [No]

Inhib. normal plasma? [n.a.]
In vivo synthesis: [n.a.]
In vivo catabolism: [n.a.]

Evaluation of isolated patient fibrinogen
Thrombin time: [n.a.]
Reptilase time: [n.a.]
Ancrod (Arvin) time: [n.a.]

Abnormal subunit? [No]
Abnormal FDPs? [n.a.]

Remarks
[1]The rate of *total* fibrinopeptide release was reduced; individual fibrinopeptide release was not reported.
[2]Two spontaneous abortions and an episode of retinal detachment were reported.
[3]Normal range not reported.

Results are a composite of data from the proposita (deceased) and affected relatives.

References

1. Aguercif, M., Soria, J., Soria, C., Ritschard, J., Samama, M. and Bouvier, C. A new family with dysfibrinogenaemia, fibrinogen Alba/Geneva. *Proc. IV Int. Congr. Thrombos. Haemostas.* p. 38, **1973**. ABSTRACT

2. Aguercif, M., Anner, R., Ritschard, J., Nydegger, U., Soria, J. and Bouvier, C.A. [Syndromes of congenital and familial disfibrinogenemia. Apropos of 2 additional families]. *Pediatrie* **27**:317-323, **1972**.

FIBRINOGEN ALÈS I

Last update	[10 January 1994]	**Structural defect**	[n.a.]
Alphacode	[ALES01]	**Mutation**	[n.a.]
Ref. type	[Article]		

Family studies
Homozygote? [Yes]
Pedigree published? [No]

Functional defect(s)
FpA release: [Normal]
FpB release: [Normal]
Polymerization: [Abnormal]
Stabilization: [Normal]

Clinical manifestation(s) Bleeding? [No] Thrombosis? [Yes[1]]

Clinical laboratory results
Plasma fibrinogen concentration (mg/dL)
Chronometric: [n.a.]
Rate-indep'nt: [n.a.]
Immunologic: [n.a.]

*Hypo*dysfibrinogen? [n.a.]

Thrombin time:	[165s/(14s)]
Reptilase (batroxobin) time:	[No Clot]
Prothrombin time:	[n.a.]
Partial thromboplastin time:	[n.a.]
Euglobulin lysis time:	[n.a.]
Bleeding time:	[n.a.]
Immunoelectrophoresis:	[n.a.]
Platelet aggregation:	[n.a.]

Other results with patient plasma

Ancrod (Arvin) time:	[n.a.]	Inhib. normal plasma?	[n.a.]
Recalcification time:	[n.a.]	In vivo synthesis:	[n.a.]
Calcium corrects c.t.?	[n.a.]	In vivo catabolism:	[n.a.]

Evaluation of isolated patient fibrinogen

Thrombin time:	[n.a.]	Abnormal subunit?	[n.a.]
Reptilase time:	[n.a.]	Abnormal FDPs?	[Yes[2]]
Ancrod (Arvin) time:	[n.a.]		

Remarks

[1]Arterial thrombosis (stroke) "at a young age" was reported. Defective thrombin binding to fibrinogen was postulated to be responsible for the clinical manifestations.

[2]Isoelectric focusing disclosed an abnormal γ-chain. Defective binding of fragment D_1 to immobilized des-FpA-fibrin monomers and decreased ability to accelerate t-PA-catalyzed plasmin generation were reported.

FIBRINOGEN ALÈS I

References

1. Soria, J., Lu, H., Mirshahi, M., Vasse, M., Mirshahi, S.S., Woimant, F., Favier, J.P., Desvignes, P., Bonnet, P., Schved, J.F. and Soria, C. Defective fibrin polymerization: a risk for stroke at young age. The case of fibrinogen Alès. *Blood Coag. & Fibrinol.* **4**:820-821, **1993**. ABSTRACT

2. Soria, C., Soria, J., Mirshahi, M., Desvignes, P., Bonnet, P. and Caen, J.P. [Importance of the structure of the clot in thrombolysis]. *Ann. Biol. Clin. (Paris)* **45**:207-211, **1987**.

3. Soria, J., Soria, C., Samama, M. and Caen, J. Study of ten cases of congenital dysfibrinogenemia. Clinical and molecular biological aspects. In: *Fibrinogen - Structural Variants and Interactions*, A. Henschen, B. Hessel, J. McDonagh and T. Saldeen (eds.), Walter de Gruyter, Berlin. pp. 165-183, **1985**.

4. Soria, J., Soria, C., Mirshahi, M., Desvignes, P., Dunn, F. and Bonnet, P. Homozygous dysfibrinogen variant characterized by an absence of reactivity of the polymerizing site 'a' located in the γ-chain: fibrinogen Alès. *Proc. VIII Int. Congr. Thrombos.* p. 81, **1984**. ABSTRACT

FIBRINOGEN ALMÉRIA I

Last update	[1 December 1990]	**Structural defect**	[n.a.]
Alphacode	[ALMERI01]	**Mutation**	[n.a.]
Ref. type	[Article]		

Family studies
Homozygote? [n.a.]
Pedigree published? [No]

Functional defect(s)
FpA release: [n.a.]
FpB release: [n.a.]
Polymerization: [Abnormal]
Stabilization: [Normal]

Clinical manifestation(s) Bleeding? [No] Thrombosis? [No]

Clinical laboratory results

Plasma fibrinogen concentration (mg/dL)
Chronometric: [97/(250)]
Rate-indep'nt: [250/(250)]
Immunologic: [n.a.]

*Hypo*dysfibrinogen? [No]

Thrombin time:	[23s/(10s)]
Reptilase (batroxobin) time:	[55s/(18s)]
Prothrombin time:	[Normal[1]]
Partial thromboplastin time:	[Normal[1]]
Euglobulin lysis time:	[Normal]
Bleeding time:	[n.a.]
Immunoelectrophoresis:	[n.a.]
Platelet aggregation:	[n.a.]

Other results with patient plasma

Ancrod (Arvin) time:	[n.a.]	Inhib. normal plasma?	[n.a.]
Recalcification time:	[n.a.]	In vivo synthesis:	[n.a.]
Calcium corrects c.t.?	[n.a.]	In vivo catabolism:	[n.a.]

Evaluation of isolated patient fibrinogen

Thrombin time:	[n.a.]	Abnormal subunit?	[No]
Reptilase time:	[n.a.]	Abnormal FDPs?	[n.a.]
Ancrod (Arvin) time:	[n.a.]		

Remarks

[1]Data not reported.

References

1. Vila, V., Regañon, E., Fernández-Pavon, A. and Aznar, J. Dysfibrinogenemaemia associated with a defect in the aggregation of the fibrin monomers (Alméria I fibrinogen). A preliminary study. *Scand. J. Haematol.* **33**:460-465, **1984**.

FIBRINOGEN AMIENS I

Last update [1 December 1990]
Alphacode [AMIENS01]
Ref. type [Article]

Family studies
Homozygote? [No]
Pedigree published? [No]

Structural defect [Aα(16) Arg → His]
Mutation [n.a.]

Functional defect(s)
FpA release: [Abnormal]
FpB release: [Abnormal]
Polymerization: [Abnormal]
Stabilization: [n.a.]

Clinical manifestation(s) Bleeding? [n.a.] Thrombosis? [n.a.]

Clinical laboratory results
Plasma fibrinogen concentration (mg/dL)
Chronometric: [n.a.]
Rate-indep'nt: [n.a.]
Immunologic: [n.a.]

*Hypo*dysfibrinogen? [n.a.]

Thrombin time:	[n.a.]
Reptilase (batroxobin) time:	[n.a.]
Prothrombin time:	[n.a.]
Partial thromboplastin time:	[n.a.]
Euglobulin lysis time:	[n.a.]
Bleeding time:	[n.a.]
Immunoelectrophoresis:	[n.a.]
Platelet aggregation:	[n.a.]

Other results with patient plasma
Ancrod (Arvin) time: [n.a.]
Recalcification time: [n.a.]
Calcium corrects c.t.? [n.a.]

Inhib. normal plasma? [n.a.]
In vivo synthesis: [n.a.]
In vivo catabolism: [n.a.]

Evaluation of isolated patient fibrinogen
Thrombin time: [n.a.]
Reptilase time: [n.a.]
Ancrod (Arvin) time: [n.a.]

Abnormal subunit? [n.a.]
Abnormal FDPs? [n.a.]

Remarks

References

1. Soria, J., Soria, C., Bertrand, O., Roussel, B., Dieval, J., Vendrely, C. and Delobel, J. Molecular basis for the Aα-chain substitutions in dysfibrinogenemia with a description of two new cases of the disorder: Fibrinogen Amiens I and fibrinogen Amiens II. In: *Fibrinogen 2. Biochemistry, Physiology and Clinical Relevance*, G.D.O. Lowe, J.T. Douglas, C.D. Forbes and A. Henschen (eds.), Elsevier, Amsterdam. pp. 57-62, **1987**.

2. Soria, J., Soria, C., Samama, M. and Caen, J. Study of ten cases of congenital dysfibrinogenemia. Clinical and molecular biological aspects. In: *Fibrinogen - Structural Variants and Interactions*, A. Henschen, B. Hessel, J. McDonagh and T. Saldeen (eds.), Walter de Gruyter, Berlin. pp. 165-183, **1985**.

FIBRINOGEN AMIENS II

Last update [1 December 1990]
Alphacode [AMIENS02]
Ref. type [Article]

Family studies
Homozygote? [No]
Pedigree published? [No]

Structural defect [Aα(16) Arg → His]
Mutation [n.a.]

Functional defect(s)
FpA release: [Abnormal]
FpB release: [Abnormal]
Polymerization: [Abnormal]
Stabilization: [n.a.]

Clinical manifestation(s) Bleeding? [n.a.] Thrombosis? [n.a.]

Clinical laboratory results
Plasma fibrinogen concentration (mg/dL)
Chronometric: [n.a.]
Rate-indep'nt: [n.a.]
Immunologic: [n.a.]

*Hypo*dysfibrinogen? [n.a.]

Thrombin time:	[n.a.]
Reptilase (batroxobin) time:	[n.a.]
Prothrombin time:	[n.a.]
Partial thromboplastin time:	[n.a.]
Euglobulin lysis time:	[n.a.]
Bleeding time:	[n.a.]
Immunoelectrophoresis:	[n.a.]
Platelet aggregation:	[n.a.]

Other results with patient plasma
Ancrod (Arvin) time: [n.a.]
Recalcification time: [n.a.]
Calcium corrects c.t.? [n.a.]

Inhib. normal plasma? [n.a.]
In vivo synthesis: [n.a.]
In vivo catabolism: [n.a.]

Evaluation of isolated patient fibrinogen
Thrombin time: [n.a.]
Reptilase time: [n.a.]
Ancrod (Arvin) time: [n.a.]

Abnormal subunit? [n.a.]
Abnormal FDPs? [n.a.]

Remarks
The single published report for fibrinogen Amiens II summarizes conclusions but does not provide data related to determination of the structural and functional defect.

References

1. Soria, J., Soria, C., Bertrand, O., Roussel, B., Dieval, J., Vendrely, C. and Delobel, J. Molecular basis for the Aα-chain substitutions in dysfibrinogenemia with a description of two new cases of the disorder: Fibrinogen Amiens I and fibrinogen Amiens II. In: *Fibrinogen 2. Biochemistry, Physiology and Clinical Relevance*, G.D.O. Lowe, J.T. Douglas, C.D. Forbes and A. Henschen (eds.), Elsevier, Amsterdam. pp. 57-62, **1987**.

FIBRINOGEN AMSTERDAM I

Last update [1 December 1990]
Alphacode [AMSTER01]
Ref. type [Article]

Family studies
Homozygote? [No]
Pedigree published? [Yes]

Structural defect [n.a.]
Mutation [n.a.]

Functional defect(s)
FpA release: [Abnormal]
FpB release: [Normal]
Polymerization: [Abnormal]
Stabilization: [n.a.]

Clinical manifestation(s) Bleeding? [No] Thrombosis? [No]

Clinical laboratory results
Plasma fibrinogen concentration (mg/dL)
Chronometric: [152/(>200)]
Rate-indep'nt: [200/(>200)]
Immunologic: [1:80/(1:80)[1]]

*Hypo*dysfibrinogen? [No]

Thrombin time:	[32s/(16s)]
Reptilase (batroxobin) time:	[14m/(2m)]
Prothrombin time:	[16s/(11.5s)]
Partial thromboplastin time:	[n.a.]
Euglobulin lysis time:	[n.a.]
Bleeding time:	[n.a.]
Immunoelectrophoresis:	[Cathodal]
Platelet aggregation:	[n.a.]

Other results with patient plasma
Ancrod (Arvin) time: [70s/(6.5s)]
Recalcification time: [Normal]
Calcium corrects c.t.? [n.a.]

Inhib. normal plasma? [Yes]
In vivo synthesis: [n.a.]
In vivo catabolism: [n.a.]

Evaluation of isolated patient fibrinogen
Thrombin time: [n.a.]
Reptilase time: [n.a.]
Ancrod (Arvin) time: [n.a.]

Abnormal subunit? [n.a.]
Abnormal FDPs? [No]

Remarks
[1]This is a plasma titration; mg/dL not reported.

References

1. Henschen, A., Kehl, M., Southan, C., Lottspeich, F. and Georgopoulos, D. Genetically abnormal fibrinogens — some current characterisation strategies. In: *Fibrinogen —Structure, Functional Aspects, Metabolism*, F. Haverkate, A. Henschen, W. Nieuwenhuizen and P.W. Straub (eds.), Walter de Gruyter, Berlin. pp. 125-144, **1983**.

2. Janssen, C.L. and Vreeken, J. Fibrinogen Amsterdam, another hereditary abnormality of fibrinogen. *Br. J. Haematol.* **20**:287-298, **1971**.

FIBRINOGEN AMSTERDAM II

Last update [1 December 1990]
Alphacode [AMSTER02]
Ref. type [Article[1]]

Family studies
Homozygote? [n.a.]
Pedigree published? [No]

Structural defect [n.a.]
Mutation [n.a.]

Functional defect(s)
FpA release: [Normal]
FpB release: [Normal]
Polymerization: [n.a.]
Stabilization: [n.a.]

Clinical manifestation(s) Bleeding? [n.a.] Thrombosis? [n.a.]

Clinical laboratory results
Plasma fibrinogen concentration (mg/dL)
Chronometric: [n.a.]
Rate-indep'nt: [n.a.]
Immunologic: [n.a.]

*Hypo*dysfibrinogen? [n.a.]

Thrombin time:	[n.a.]
Reptilase (batroxobin) time:	[n.a.]
Prothrombin time:	[n.a.]
Partial thromboplastin time:	[n.a.]
Euglobulin lysis time:	[n.a.]
Bleeding time:	[n.a.]
Immunoelectrophoresis:	[n.a.]
Platelet aggregation:	[n.a.]

Other results with patient plasma
Ancrod (Arvin) time: [n.a.]
Recalcification time: [n.a.]
Calcium corrects c.t.? [n.a.]

Inhib. normal plasma? [n.a.]
In vivo synthesis: [n.a.]
In vivo catabolism: [n.a.]

Evaluation of isolated patient fibrinogen
Thrombin time: [n.a.]
Reptilase time: [n.a.]
Ancrod (Arvin) time: [n.a.]

Abnormal subunit? [n.a.]
Abnormal FDPs? [n.a.]

Remarks
[1]Review article only; F. Haverkate, personal communication.

References

1. Henschen, A., Kehl, M. and Southan, C. Genetically abnormal fibrinogens — strategies for structure elucidation, including fibrinopeptide analysis. In: *Variants of Human Fibrinogen*, E.A. Beck and M. Furlan (eds.), Hans Huber Publ., Berne, pp. 273-320, **1984**.

FIBRINOGEN ARGENTEUIL I

Last update [1 December 1990]
Alphacode [ARGENT01]
Ref. type [Article]

Structural defect [n.a.]
Mutation [n.a.]

Family studies
Homozygote? [n.a.]
Pedigree published? [Yes]

Functional defect(s)
FpA release: [Abnormal[1]]
FpB release: [n.a.]
Polymerization: [n.a.]
Stabilization: [n.a.]

Clinical manifestation(s) Bleeding? [No] Thrombosis? [Yes[2]]

Clinical laboratory results
Plasma fibrinogen concentration (mg/dL)
Chronometric: [23/(150-300)]
Rate-indep'nt: [120/(150-300)]
Immunologic: [n.a.]

*Hypo*dysfibrinogen? [Yes]

Thrombin time:	[44s/(18-20s)]
Reptilase (batroxobin) time:	[43s/(18-25s)]
Prothrombin time:	[25.5s/(11-13s)]
Partial thromboplastin time:	[41s/(28-32s)]
Euglobulin lysis time:	[n.a.]
Bleeding time:	[n.a.]
Immunoelectrophoresis:	[n.a.]
Platelet aggregation:	[n.a.]

Other results with patient plasma
Ancrod (Arvin) time: [n.a.]
Recalcification time: [n.a.]
Calcium corrects c.t.? [No]

Inhib. normal plasma? [n.a.]
In vivo synthesis: [n.a.]
In vivo catabolism: [n.a.]

Evaluation of isolated patient fibrinogen
Thrombin time: [>500s/(45s)[3]]
Reptilase time: [>500s/(58s)]
Ancrod (Arvin) time: [n.a.]

Abnormal subunit? [n.a.]
Abnormal FDPs? [Yes[4]]

Remarks
[1]Approximately 50% of fibrinopeptide A was not released.
[2]The propositus presented with deep vein thrombosis.
[3]Reduced binding of thrombin to fibrin was reported.
[4]The *rate* of FDP formation was reduced.

This is the first report of combined dysfibrinogenemia and protein C deficiency (See also POITIERS I).

References

1. Gandrille, S., Priollet, P., Capron, L., Roncato, M., Fiessinger, J.N. and Aiach, M. Association of inherited dysfibrinogenaemia and protein C deficiency in two unrelated families. *Brit. J. Haematol.* **68**:329-337, **1988**.

FIBRINOGEN ASAHI I

Last update	[10 January 1994]	**Structural defect**	[γ(310) Met → Thr[1]]
Alphacode	[ASAHI01]	**Mutation**	[ATG → ACG]
Ref. type	[Article]		

Family studies
Homozygote? [No]
Pedigree published? [No]

Functional defect(s)
FpA release: [Normal]
FpB release: [Normal]
Polymerization: [Abnormal]
Stabilization: [Abnormal]

Clinical manifestation(s) Bleeding? [Yes[2]] Thrombosis? [No]

Clinical laboratory results

Plasma fibrinogen concentration (mg/dL)

Chronometric: [<50/(200-400)]
Rate-indep'nt: [565[3,4]]
Immunologic: [525[4]]

*Hypo*dysfibrinogen? [No]

Thrombin time:	[>300s/(15.8s)]
Reptilase (batroxobin) time:	[n.a.]
Prothrombin time:	[14.9s/(10.9s)]
Partial thromboplastin time:	[41.7s/(33.5s)]
Euglobulin lysis time:	[n.a.]
Bleeding time:	[Normal]
Immunoelectrophoresis:	[n.a.]
Platelet aggregation:	[Normal]

Other results with patient plasma

Ancrod (Arvin) time:	[>300s/(9.8s)]	Inhib. normal plasma?	[n.a.]
Recalcification time:	[n.a.]	In vivo synthesis:	[n.a.]
Calcium corrects c.t.?	[No]	In vivo catabolism:	[n.a.]

Evaluation of isolated patient fibrinogen

Thrombin time:	[>180s/(12.8s)]	Abnormal subunit?	[Yes[5]]
Reptilase time:	[n.a.]	Abnormal FDPs?	[Yes[6]]
Ancrod (Arvin) time:	[>180s/(5.5s)]		

Remarks

[1]Fibrinogen Asahi has dual structural abnormalities: The amino acid substitution noted above plus *N*-glycosylation at γ(308) Asn — the first variant to be so identified. See also CARACAS II, LIMA I and PONTOISE I. Also noteworthy are the dual functional defects of fibrin polymerization and stabilization. The structural defect was confirmed with the PCR method (Mimuro et al., 1990; 1992).

[2]Post-traumatic bleeding and delayed wound healing were reported.

[3]Determined turbidimetrically per Matsuda et al. [*J. Clin. Invest.* **72**:1034-1041, **1983**].

[4]Normal range not reported.

[5]SDS-PAGE disclosed an oversized γ-chain.

[6]About half of fragments D_1 and D_2 were larger than normal; fragment D_3 was the normal size.

FIBRINOGEN ASAHI I

References

1. Mimuro, J., Muramatsu, S., Maekawa, H., Sakata, Y., Kaneko, M., Yoshitake, S., Okuma, M., Ito, Y., Takeda, Y. and Matsuda, M. Gene analyses of abnormal fibrinogens with a mutation in the γ chain. *Intl. J. Hematol.* **56**:129-134, **1992**.

2. Muramatsu, S., Mimuro, J., Maekawa, H., Sakata, Y., Matsuda, M., Yoshitake, S. and Okuma, M. Gene analysis of abnormal fibrinogens characterized by a mutation in the γ chain. *Thromb. Haemostas.* **65**:821, **1991**. ABSTRACT

3. Matsuda, M., Terukina, S., Yoshida, N., Yamazumi, K. and Maekawa, H. Abnormal fibrinogens with two structural defects. *Adv. Exp. Med. Biol.* **281**:63-72, **1990**.

4. Yamazumi, K., Shimura, K., Maekawa, H., Muramatsu, S., Terukina, S., and Matsuda, M. Delayed intermolecular γ-chain cross-linking by factor XIIIa in fibrinogen Asahi characterized by a γ-Met-310 to Thr substitution with an *N*-glycosylated γ-Asn-308. *Blood Coag. & Fibrinol.* **1**:557-559, **1990**.

5. Mimuro, J., Yamazumi, K., Terukina, S., and Matsuda, M. A T→C exchange in exon VIII of the fibrinogen γ chain gene defined by the polymerase chain reaction for fibrinogen Asahi with a γ Met-310 to Thr substitution and *N*-glycosylated Asn-308. *Proc. X Intl. Fgen. Wkshp.*, **1990** ABSTRACT.

6. Yamazumi, K., Shimura, K., Terukina, S., Takahashi, N. and Matsuda, M. A γ methionine-310 to threonine substitution and consequent *N*-glycosylation at γ asparagine-308 identified in a congenital dysfibrinogenemia associated with posttraumatic bleeding, fibrinogen Asahi. *J. Clin. Invest.* **83**:1590-1597, **1989**.

7. Yamazumi, K., Terukina, S., Shimura, K., Matsuda, M. and Takahashi, N. A substitution of γ Met-310 to Thr and an extra glycosylation at γ Asn-308 in an abnormal fibrinogen "Asahi." In: *Fibrinogen 3. Biochemistry, Biological Functions, Gene Regulation and Expression*, M.W. Mosesson, D.L. Amrani, K.R. Siebenlist and J.P. DiOrio (eds.), Elsevier Science Publ., B.V., Amsterdam. pp. 269-269, **1988**.

FIBRINOGEN ASHFORD I

Last update	[1 December 1990]	**Structural defect**	[n.a.]
Alphacode	[ASHFOR01]	**Mutation**	[n.a.]
Ref. type	[Article]		

Family studies
Homozygote? [n.a.]
Pedigree published? [No]

Functional defect(s)
FpA release: [Normal]
FpB release: [Abnormal[1]]
Polymerization: [Abnormal]
Stabilization: [n.a.]

Clinical manifestation(s) Bleeding? [n.a.] Thrombosis? [n.a.]

Clinical laboratory results

Plasma fibrinogen concentration (mg/dL)
Chronometric: [n.a.]
Rate-indep'nt: [n.a.]
Immunologic: [140[2]]

*Hypo*dysfibrinogen? [No]

Thrombin time:	[160s/(18s)]
Reptilase (batroxobin) time:	[45s/(17s)]
Prothrombin time:	[n.a.]
Partial thromboplastin time:	[n.a.]
Euglobulin lysis time:	[n.a.]
Bleeding time:	[n.a.]
Immunoelectrophoresis:	[n.a.]
Platelet aggregation:	[n.a.]

Other results with patient plasma

Ancrod (Arvin) time:	[n.a.]	Inhib. normal plasma?	[n.a.]
Recalcification time:	[n.a.]	In vivo synthesis:	[n.a.]
Calcium corrects c.t.?	[n.a.]	In vivo catabolism:	[n.a.]

Evaluation of isolated patient fibrinogen

Thrombin time:	[27s/(17s)]	Abnormal subunit?	[n.a.]
Reptilase time:	[n.a.]	Abnormal FDPs?	[n.a.]
Ancrod (Arvin) time:	[n.a.]		

Remarks

[1]A reduced rate of fibrinopeptide B release was detected only at low thrombin concentrations.
[2]This value was characterized as "slightly low." The normal range was not reported.

References

1. Ruf, W., Bender, A., Lane, D.A., Preissner, K.T., Selmayr, E. and Muller-Berghaus, G. Thrombin-induced fibrinopeptide B release from normal and variant fibrinogens: influence of inhibitors of fibrin polymerization. *Biochim. Biophys. Acta* **965**:169-175, **1988**.

2. Southan, C., Thompson, E. and Lane, D.A. Direct analysis of plasma fibrinogen-derived fibrinopeptides by high-performance liquid chromatography: investigation of nine congenital fibrinogen abnormalities. *Br. J. Haematol.* **65**:469-473, **1987**.

FIBRINOGEN AWAJI I

Last update [1 December 1990]
Alphacode [AWAJI01]
Ref. type [Article]

Family studies
Homozygote? [No]
Pedigree published? [Yes]

Structural defect [n.a.]
Mutation [n.a.]

Functional defect(s)
FpA release: [Normal]
FpB release: [n.a.]
Polymerization: [Abnormal]
Stabilization: [n.a.]

Clinical manifestation(s) Bleeding? [No] Thrombosis? [No]

Clinical laboratory results
Plasma fibrinogen concentration (mg/dL)
Chronometric: [73[1]]
Rate-indep'nt: [296[1]]
Immunologic: [n.a.]

*Hypo*dysfibrinogen? [No]

Thrombin time:	[41.5s/(14s)]
Reptilase (batroxobin) time:	[38.5s/(21s)]
Prothrombin time:	[Normal[2]]
Partial thromboplastin time:	[Normal[2]]
Euglobulin lysis time:	[Abnormal]
Bleeding time:	[n.a.]
Immunoelectrophoresis:	[Anodal]
Platelet aggregation:	[n.a.]

Other results with patient plasma
Ancrod (Arvin) time: [n.a.]
Recalcification time: [n.a.]
Calcium corrects c.t.? [No]

Inhib. normal plasma? [No]
In vivo synthesis: [n.a.]
In vivo catabolism: [n.a.]

Evaluation of isolated patient fibrinogen
Thrombin time: [n.a.]
Reptilase time: [n.a.]
Ancrod (Arvin) time: [n.a.]

Abnormal subunit? [Yes[3]]
Abnormal FDPs? [n.a.]

Remarks
[1]Normal range not reported.
[2]Data not reported.
[3]Two-dimensional electrophoresis disclosed a charge abnormality (increased anodal mobility) in the γ-chain.

References

1. Matsuo, T., Okuno, S., Mukaida, T., Ueshima, S., Okada, K. and Matsuo, O. A hereditary dysfibrinogenemia: fibrinogen Awaji. *Haemostas.* **17**:89-97, **1987**.

2. Matsuo, T., Okuno, S., Mukaida, T. and Matsuo, O. [Fibrinogen Awaji: a congenital dysfibrinogenemia characterized by abnormal fibrin monomer polymerization]. *Nippon Ketsueki Gakkai Zasshi* **48**:1594-1597, **1985**.

FIBRINOGEN AWAJI II

Last update [1 December 1990]
Alphacode [AWAJI02]
Ref. type [Article]

Structural defect [n.a.]
Mutation [n.a.]

Family studies
Homozygote? [n.a.]
Pedigree published? [Yes]

Functional defect(s)
FpA release: [Normal]
FpB release: [Normal]
Polymerization: [Abnormal]
Stabilization: [Normal]

Clinical manifestation(s) Bleeding? [No] Thrombosis? [Yes[1]]

Clinical laboratory results
Plasma fibrinogen concentration (mg/dL)
Chronometric: [86/(200-350)]
Rate-indep'nt: [230/(200-350)]
Immunologic: [248/(200-400)]

*Hypo*dysfibrinogen? [No]

Thrombin time:	[21.9s/(12.4s)]
Reptilase (batroxobin) time:	[32.3s/(21s)]
Prothrombin time:	[79%/(100%)]
Partial thromboplastin time:	[23.2s/(40s)]
Euglobulin lysis time:	[n.a.]
Bleeding time:	[n.a.]
Immunoelectrophoresis:	[n.a.]
Platelet aggregation:	[n.a.]

Other results with patient plasma
Ancrod (Arvin) time: [n.a.]
Recalcification time: [n.a.]
Calcium corrects c.t.? [No]

Inhib. normal plasma? [n.a.]
In vivo synthesis: [n.a.]
In vivo catabolism: [n.a.]

Evaluation of isolated patient fibrinogen
Thrombin time: [n.a.]
Reptilase time: [n.a.]
Ancrod (Arvin) time: [n.a.]

Abnormal subunit? [n.a.]
Abnormal FDPs? [n.a.]

Remarks
[1]Left internal carotid artery occlusion in the 55 year-old propositus was treated successfully with urokinase.

References

1. Matsuo, T., Mukaida, T., Mori, E. and Matsuo, O. [Congenital dysfibrinogenemia in a patient with left internal carotid artery occlusion]. *Nippon Naika Gakkai Zasshi* **75**:51-56, **1986**.

FIBRINOGEN BALTIMORE I

Last update [1 December 1990]
Alphacode [BALTIM01]
Ref. type [Article]

Structural defect [γ(292) Gly → Val[1]]
Mutation [GGC → GTC]

Family studies
Homozygote? [No]
Pedigree published? [Yes]

Functional defect(s)
FpA release: [Normal]
FpB release: [Normal]
Polymerization: [Abnormal]
Stabilization: [Abnormal]

Clinical manifestation(s) Bleeding? [Yes[2]] Thrombosis? [Yes[2]]

Clinical laboratory results
Plasma fibrinogen concentration (mg/dL)
Chronometric: [35/(175)]
Rate-indep'nt: [104/(180)]
Immunologic: [180/(180)]

*Hypo*dysfibrinogen? [No]

Thrombin time:	[>120s/(11.7s)]
Reptilase (batroxobin) time:	[84s/(27s)]
Prothrombin time:	[45%/(60-100%)]
Partial thromboplastin time:	[n.a.]
Euglobulin lysis time:	[Normal]
Bleeding time:	[n.a.]
Immunoelectrophoresis:	[Anodal]
Platelet aggregation:	[Normal]

Other results with patient plasma
Ancrod (Arvin) time: [n.a.]
Recalcification time: [Abnormal]
Calcium corrects c.t.? [Yes]

Inhib. normal plasma? [No]
In vivo synthesis: [n.a.]
In vivo catabolism: [Normal]

Evaluation of isolated patient fibrinogen
Thrombin time: [>120s/(14.2s)]
Reptilase time: [n.a.]
Ancrod (Arvin) time: [n.a.]

Abnormal subunit? [No]
Abnormal FDPs? [n.a.]

Remarks
[1]The structural defect was determined by peptide mapping and with the PCR method.
[2]Proposita presented with femoral vein thrombosis following minor trauma. Her history included frequent bruising, epistaxis, menorrhagia, and a "severe thrombotic episode" lasting several months. A 25-year follow-up disclosed no thrombotic or hemorrhagic events (Bantia et al., 1990); 8 affected offspring also were asymptomatic.

FIBRINOGEN BALTIMORE I

References

1. Bantia, S., Mane, S.M., Bell, W.R., and Dang, C.V. Fibrinogen Baltimore I: Polymerization defect associated with a γ^{292}Gly → Val (GGC→GTC) mutation. *Blood* **76**:2279-2283, **1990**

2. Brown, C.H. and Crowe, M.F. Defective α-polymerization in the conversion of fibrinogen Baltimore to fibrin. *J. Clin. Invest.* **55**:1190-1194, **1975**.

3. Beck, E.A., Shainoff, J.R., Vogel, A. and Jackson, D.P. Functional evaluation of an inherited abnormal fibrinogen: fibrinogen "Baltimore." *J. Clin. Invest.* **50**:1874-1884, **1971**.

4. Smith, E.B. and Holder, W.R. Stasis ulcer and "fibrinogen Baltimore." *Arch. Dermatol.* **104**:221-222, **1971**.

5. Mosesson, M.W. Fibrinogen Baltimore: physiochemical characterization. In: *Hemophilia and New Hemorrhagic States*, K.M. Brinkhous (ed.), University of North Carolina Press, Chapel Hill. pp. 247-253, **1970**.

6. Mosesson, M.W. and Beck, E.A. Chromatographic, ultracentrifugal, and related studies of fibrinogen "Baltimore." *J. Clin. Invest.* **48**:1656-1662, **1969**.

7. Vogel, A. and Beck, E.A. [Qualitative electromicroscopic study on the fibrin structure originating from Baltimore fibrinogen]. *Schweiz. Med. Wochenschr.* **98**:1651-1653, **1968**.

8. Beck, E.A., Mosesson, M.W., Charache, P. and Jackson, D.P. [Hemorrhagic diathesis with dominant heredity, caused by an abnormal fibrinogen (fibrinogen Baltimore)]. *Schweiz. Med. Wochenschr.* **96**:1196-1199, **1966**.

9. Beck, E.A., Charache, P. and Jackson, D.P. A new inherited coagulation disorder caused by an abnormal fibrinogen ('fibrinogen Baltimore'). *Nature* **208**:143-145, **1965**.

10. Beck, E. Abnormal fibrinogen (fibrinogen 'Baltimore') as a cause of a familial hemorrhagic disorder. *Blood* **24**:853-854, **1964**.

FIBRINOGEN BALTIMORE II

Last update [1 December 1990]
Alphacode [BALTIM02]
Ref. type [Article]

Family studies
Homozygote? [No]
Pedigree published? [Yes]

Structural defect [n.a.[1]]
Mutation [n.a.]

Functional defect(s)
FpA release: [Normal]
FpB release: [Abnormal]
Polymerization: [Normal]
Stabilization: [Normal]

Clinical manifestation(s) Bleeding? [Yes[2]] Thrombosis? [No]

Clinical laboratory results

Plasma fibrinogen concentration (mg/dL)
Chronometric: [36/(150-400)]
Rate-indep'nt: [82/(150-400)]
Immunologic: [62-96/(150-400)]

*Hypo*dysfibrinogen? [Yes]

Thrombin time:	[n.a.]
Reptilase (batroxobin) time:	[n.a.]
Prothrombin time:	[14.5s/(13-17s)]
Partial thromboplastin time:	[73s/(<100s)]
Euglobulin lysis time:	[Normal]
Bleeding time:	[n.a.]
Immunoelectrophoresis:	[n.a.]
Platelet aggregation:	[Normal]

Other results with patient plasma
Ancrod (Arvin) time: [n.a.]
Recalcification time: [n.a.]
Calcium corrects c.t.? [No]

Inhib. normal plasma? [No]
In vivo synthesis: [Decreased]
In vivo catabolism: [Normal]

Evaluation of isolated patient fibrinogen
Thrombin time: [n.a.]
Reptilase time: [n.a.]
Ancrod (Arvin) time: [n.a.]

Abnormal subunit? [No]
Abnormal FDPs? [n.a.]

Remarks

[1]A polymorphism [Bβ(448) Arg → Lys], presumably not responsible for the functional defect, has been detected in this variant (Schmelzer et al., 1988).

[2]Excessive postpartum bleeding not requiring transfusion was reported.

References

1. Ebert, R.F. and Schmelzer, C.H. Isolation and comparative peptide mapping of fibrinogen subunits by reversed-phase high-performance liquid chromatography. *J. Chromatogr.* **443**:309-316, **1988**.

2. Schmelzer, C.H., Ebert, R.F. and Bell, W.R. A polymorphism at $B\beta_{448}$ of fibrinogen identified during structural studies of fibrinogen Baltimore II. *Thromb. Res.* **52**:173-177, **1988**.

3. Ebert, R.F. and Bell, W.R. Fibrinogen Baltimore II: congenital hypo-dysfibrinogenemia with delayed release of fibrinopeptide B and decreased rate of fibrinogen synthesis. *Proc. Natl. Acad. Sci. U.S.A.* **80**:7318-7322, **1983**.

FIBRINOGEN BALTIMORE III

Last update [1 December 1990]
Alphacode [BALTIM03]
Ref. type [Article]

Structural defect [γ(308) Asn → Ile]
Mutation [n.a.]

Family studies
Homozygote? [No]
Pedigree published? [No]

Functional defect(s)
FpA release: [Normal]
FpB release: [Normal]
Polymerization: [Abnormal]
Stabilization: [Normal]

Clinical manifestation(s) Bleeding? [No] Thrombosis? [No]

Clinical laboratory results
Plasma fibrinogen concentration (mg/dL)
Chronometric: [107/(150-400)]
Rate-indep'nt: [170/(150-400)]
Immunologic: [180/(150-400)]

*Hypo*dysfibrinogen? [No]

Thrombin time:	[n.a.]
Reptilase (batroxobin) time:	[n.a.]
Prothrombin time:	[Normal]
Partial thromboplastin time:	[Normal]
Euglobulin lysis time:	[Normal]
Bleeding time:	[n.a.]
Immunoelectrophoresis:	[n.a.]
Platelet aggregation:	[Normal]

Other results with patient plasma
Ancrod (Arvin) time: [n.a.]
Recalcification time: [n.a.]
Calcium corrects c.t.? [Yes]

Inhib. normal plasma? [No]
In vivo synthesis: [n.a.]
In vivo catabolism: [n.a.]

Evaluation of isolated patient fibrinogen
Thrombin time: [n.a.]
Reptilase time: [n.a.]
Ancrod (Arvin) time: [n.a.]

Abnormal subunit? [Yes[1]]
Abnormal FDPs? [n.a.]

Remarks
[1]About 50% of the γ-chains migrate on SDS-PAGE with an apparent M_r of 45,500 (approx. 1,500 kDa smaller than normal).

In their discussion, Bantia et al. (1990) suggest that the entire γ275-405 region is "important for fibrin monomer polymerization."

References

1. Bantia, S., Bell, W.R. and Dang, C.V. Polymerization defect of fibrinogen Baltimore III due to a γAsn^{308}→Ile mutation. *Blood* **75**:1659-1663, **1990**.

2. Bantia, S., Dang, C.V. and Bell, W.R. γAsn^{308} → Ile substitution in fibrinogen Baltimore III with impaired fibrin monomer polymerization. In: *Fibrinogen 4. Current Basic and Clinical Aspects*, M. Matsuda, S. Iwanaga, A. Takada and A. Henschen (eds.), Elsevier Science Publ. B.V., Amsterdam. pp. 167-170, **1990**.

3. Ebert, R.F. and Bell, W.R. Fibrinogen Baltimore III: congenital dysfibrinogenemia with a shortened γ-subunit. *Thromb. Res.* **51**:251-258, **1988**.

FIBRINOGEN BALTIMORE IV

Last update [1 December 1990]
Alphacode [BALTIM04]
Ref. type [Article]

Structural defect [γ(275) Arg → Cys]
Mutation [n.a.]

Family studies
Homozygote? [No]
Pedigree published? [Yes]

Functional defect(s)
FpA release: [Normal]
FpB release: [Normal]
Polymerization: [Abnormal]
Stabilization: [Normal]

Clinical manifestation(s) Bleeding? [No] Thrombosis? [No]

Clinical laboratory results
Plasma fibrinogen concentration (mg/dL)
Chronometric: [32/(>150)]
Rate-indep'nt: [192/(>150)]
Immunologic: [n.a.]

*Hypo*dysfibrinogen? [No]

Thrombin time: [n.a.]
Reptilase (batroxobin) time: [n.a.]
Prothrombin time: [22s/(13-17s)]
Partial thromboplastin time: [88s/(<100s)]
Euglobulin lysis time: [2h/(>2h)]
Bleeding time: [n.a.]
Immunoelectrophoresis: [n.a.]
Platelet aggregation: [n.a.]

Other results with patient plasma
Ancrod (Arvin) time: [n.a.]
Recalcification time: [n.a.]
Calcium corrects c.t.? [Yes]

Inhib. normal plasma? [Yes]
In vivo synthesis: [n.a.]
In vivo catabolism: [n.a.]

Evaluation of isolated patient fibrinogen
Thrombin time: [n.a.]
Reptilase time: [n.a.]
Ancrod (Arvin) time: [n.a.]

Abnormal subunit? [Yes]
Abnormal FDPs? [n.a.]

Remarks

References

1. Schmelzer, C.H., Ebert, R.F. and Bell, W.R. Fibrinogen Baltimore IV: Congenital dysfibrinogenemia with a γ(275) (Arg → Cys) substitution. *Thromb. Res.* **56**:307-316, **1989**.

2. Ebert, R.F. and Schmelzer, C.H. Isolation and comparative peptide mapping of fibrinogen subunits by reversed-phase high-performance liquid chromatography. *J. Chromatogr.* **443**:309-316, **1988**.

3. Ebert, R.F. and Bell, W.R. Fibrinogen Baltimore IV: congenital dysfibrinogenemia with delayed fibrin monomer polymerization. *Thromb. Res.* **38**:121-128, **1985**.

FIBRINOGEN BARCELONA I

Last update [1 December 1990]
Alphacode [BARCEL01]
Ref. type [Article]

Structural defect [n.a.]
Mutation [n.a.]

Family studies
Homozygote? [n.a.]
Pedigree published? [No]

Functional defect(s)
FpA release: [Abnormal]
FpB release: [n.a.]
Polymerization: [Abnormal]
Stabilization: [Normal]

Clinical manifestation(s) Bleeding? [Yes[1]] Thrombosis? [No]

Clinical laboratory results

Plasma fibrinogen concentration (mg/dL)
Chronometric: [0/(250)]
Rate-indep'nt: [350/(250)]
Immunologic: [n.a.]

*Hypo*dysfibrinogen? [No]

Thrombin time:	[600s/(19s)]
Reptilase (batroxobin) time:	[1000s/(31s)]
Prothrombin time:	[430s/(15s)]
Partial thromboplastin time:	[254s/(30s)]
Euglobulin lysis time:	[n.a.]
Bleeding time:	[n.a.]
Immunoelectrophoresis:	[n.a.]
Platelet aggregation:	[Normal]

Other results with patient plasma
Ancrod (Arvin) time: [n.a.]
Recalcification time: [n.a.]
Calcium corrects c.t.? [n.a.]

Inhib. normal plasma? [Yes]
In vivo synthesis: [n.a.]
In vivo catabolism: [n.a.]

Evaluation of isolated patient fibrinogen
Thrombin time: [n.a.]
Reptilase time: [n.a.]
Ancrod (Arvin) time: [n.a.]

Abnormal subunit? [No]
Abnormal FDPs? [No[2]]

Remarks

[1]Severe postpartum bleeding in the 28 year-old proposita was reported.
[2]The *rate* of FDP formation was reduced.

The sialic acid content of this variant was about 25% of normal.

References

1. Vila, V., Regañon, E., Aznar, J., Navarro, G. and Salas, M. Fibrinogen Barcelona I. Congenital dysfibrinogenemia characterized by defective release of fibrinopeptide A and fibrinogen degradation products. *Thromb. Res.* **45**:437-449, **1987**.

FIBRINOGEN BARCELONA II

Last update [1 December 1990]
Alphacode [BARCEL02]
Ref. type [Article]

Structural defect [Aα(16) Arg → His]
Mutation [n.a.]

Family studies
Homozygote? [No]
Pedigree published? [Yes]

Functional defect(s)
FpA release: [Abnormal[1]]
FpB release: [Abnormal]
Polymerization: [Abnormal]
Stabilization: [n.a.]

Clinical manifestation(s) Bleeding? [Yes[2]] Thrombosis? [No]

Clinical laboratory results
Plasma fibrinogen concentration (mg/dL)
Chronometric: [57[3]]
Rate-indep'nt: [416[4]]
Immunologic: [450[4]]

*Hypo*dysfibrinogen? [No]

Thrombin time:	[35s[3]]
Reptilase (batroxobin) time:	[35s[3]]
Prothrombin time:	[45%[3]]
Partial thromboplastin time:	[29s[4]]
Euglobulin lysis time:	[n.a.]
Bleeding time:	[n.a.]
Immunoelectrophoresis:	[n.a.]
Platelet aggregation:	[n.a.]

Other results with patient plasma
Ancrod (Arvin) time: [n.a.]
Recalcification time: [n.a.]
Calcium corrects c.t.? [n.a.]

Inhib. normal plasma? [n.a.]
In vivo synthesis: [n.a.]
In vivo catabolism: [n.a.]

Evaluation of isolated patient fibrinogen
Thrombin time: [n.a.]
Reptilase time: [n.a.]
Ancrod (Arvin) time: [n.a.]

Abnormal subunit? [n.a.]
Abnormal FDPs? [n.a.]

Remarks
[1]Only half the normal amount of fibrinopeptide A was released.
[2]Excessive bleeding after tooth extraction was reported. Excessive bleeding was *not* observed in two other surgical procedures for bursitis of the left knee and repair of an anal fissure. Surgery for intervertebral disk herniation also was uneventful, but in this case the patient was pre-treated with cryoprecipitate and calcium heparin.
[3]This value is abnormal; the normal range was not reported.
[4]This value is normal; the normal range was not reported.

References

1. Borrell, M. Vila, L., Solá, J., Coll, I., and Fontcuberta, J. Fibrinogen Barcelona II: A new case of Aα 16 Arg → His substitution. *Haemostas.* **20**:1-7, **1990**

FIBRINOGEN BERGAMO I

Last update	[1 December 1990]	**Structural defect**	[Aα(16) Arg → Cys]
Alphacode	[BERGAM01]	**Mutation**	[n.a.]
Ref. type	[Article]		

Family studies
Homozygote? [No]
Pedigree published? [No]

Functional defect(s)
FpA release: [Abnormal]
FpB release: [Normal]
Polymerization: [Abnormal]
Stabilization: [n.a.]

Clinical manifestation(s) Bleeding? [No] Thrombosis? [No]

Clinical laboratory results

Plasma fibrinogen concentration (mg/dL)
Chronometric: [40/(240)]
Rate-indep'nt: [200/(245)]
Immunologic: [220/(240)]

*Hypo*dysfibrinogen? [No]

Thrombin time:	[120s/(17.4s)]
Reptilase (batroxobin) time:	[n.a.]
Prothrombin time:	[16.9s/(14.7s)]
Partial thromboplastin time:	[30.1s/(28.7s)]
Euglobulin lysis time:	[n.a.]
Bleeding time:	[n.a.]
Immunoelectrophoresis:	[n.a.]
Platelet aggregation:	[n.a.]

Other results with patient plasma

Ancrod (Arvin) time:	[n.a.]	Inhib. normal plasma?	[n.a.]
Recalcification time:	[n.a.]	In vivo synthesis:	[n.a.]
Calcium corrects c.t.?	[No]	In vivo catabolism:	[n.a.]

Evaluation of isolated patient fibrinogen

Thrombin time:	[37s/(10.4s)]	Abnormal subunit?	[No]
Reptilase time:	[51.2s/(10.6s)]	Abnormal FDPs?	[n.a.]
Ancrod (Arvin) time:	[n.a.]		

Remarks

Both father and son were affected. Clinical laboratory results are those of the father.

References

1. Reber, P., Furlan, M. and Beck, E.A. Fibrinogen "Bergamo I" (Aα-16 Arg → Cys): Alternative methods for structure elucidation. In: *Fibrinogen, Fibrin Formation and Fibrinolysis*, D.A. Lane, A. Henschen and M.K. Jasani (eds.), W. de Gruyter, Berlin. pp. 103-110, **1986**.

2. Reber, P., Furlan, M., Beck, E.A., Finazzi, G., Buelli, M. and Barbui, T. Fibrinogen Bergamo I (Aα 16Arg → Cys): susceptibility towards thrombin following aminoethylation, methylation or carboxamidomethylation of cysteine residues. *Thromb. Haemostas.* **54**:390-393, **1985**.

FIBRINOGEN BERGAMO II

Last update [1 December 1990]
Alphacode [BERGAM02]
Ref. type [Article]

Family studies
Homozygote? [No]
Pedigree published? [No]

Structural defect [γ(275) Arg → His]
Mutation [n.a.]

Functional defect(s)
FpA release: [Normal]
FpB release: [Normal]
Polymerization: [Abnormal]
Stabilization: [n.a.]

Clinical manifestation(s) Bleeding? [No] Thrombosis? [Yes[1]]

Clinical laboratory results
Plasma fibrinogen concentration (mg/dL)
Chronometric: [22/(200)]
Rate-indep'nt: [240/(200)]
Immunologic: [230/(200)]

*Hypo*dysfibrinogen? [No]

Thrombin time:	[37.0s/(12.5s)]
Reptilase (batroxobin) time:	[37.8s/(17.6)]
Prothrombin time:	[n.a.]
Partial thromboplastin time:	[n.a.]
Euglobulin lysis time:	[n.a.]
Bleeding time:	[n.a.]
Immunoelectrophoresis:	[n.a.]
Platelet aggregation:	[n.a.]

Other results with patient plasma
Ancrod (Arvin) time: [n.a.]
Recalcification time: [n.a.]
Calcium corrects c.t.? [No]

Inhib. normal plasma? [n.a.]
In vivo synthesis: [n.a.]
In vivo catabolism: [n.a.]

Evaluation of isolated patient fibrinogen
Thrombin time: [n.a.]
Reptilase time: [n.a.]
Ancrod (Arvin) time: [n.a.]

Abnormal subunit? [No]
Abnormal FDPs? [n.a.]

Remarks
[1]Deep vein thrombosis and two episodes of pulmonary embolism followed interruption of proposita's first pregnancy. Patients from two other families (Essen I and Perugia I) with the same amino acid substitution were asymptomatic.

References

1. Reber, P., Furlan, M., Henschen, A., Kaudewitz, H., Barbui, T., Hilgard, P., Nenci, G.G., Berrettini, M. and Beck, E.A. Three abnormal fibrinogen variants with the same amino acid substitution (γ-275 Arg → His): fibrinogens Bergamo II, Essen and Perugia. *Thromb. Haemostas.* **56**:401-406, **1986**.

2. Reber, P., Furlan, M., Henschen, A. and Beck, E.A. Three new fibrinogen variants with defective polymerization site in the γ-chain. In: *Fibrinogen and Its Derivatives. Biochemistry, Physiology and Pathophysiology*, G. Muller-Berghaus, U. Scheefers-Borchel, E. Selmayr and A. Henschen (eds.), Excerpta Medica, Amsterdam. pp. 41-42, **1986**.

FIBRINOGEN BERGAMO III

Last update [1 December 1990]
Alphacode [BERGAM03]
Ref. type [Article]

Family studies
Homozygote? [No]
Pedigree published? [No]

Structural defect [Aα(16) Arg → His]
Mutation [n.a.]

Functional defect(s)
FpA release: [Abnormal[1]]
FpB release: [Abnormal[1]]
Polymerization: [Abnormal]
Stabilization: [n.a.]

Clinical manifestation(s) Bleeding? [No] Thrombosis? [No]

Clinical laboratory results

Plasma fibrinogen concentration (mg/dL)
Chronometric: [30/(200)]
Rate-indep'nt: [250/(200)]
Immunologic: [250/(200)]

*Hypo*dysfibrinogen? [No]

Thrombin time:	[37s/(18s)]
Reptilase (batroxobin) time:	[74s/(20s)]
Prothrombin time:	[n.a.]
Partial thromboplastin time:	[n.a.]
Euglobulin lysis time:	[n.a.]
Bleeding time:	[n.a.]
Immunoelectrophoresis:	[n.a.]
Platelet aggregation:	[n.a.]

Other results with patient plasma
Ancrod (Arvin) time: [n.a.]
Recalcification time: [n.a.]
Calcium corrects c.t.? [No]

Inhib. normal plasma? [n.a.]
In vivo synthesis: [n.a.]
In vivo catabolism: [n.a.]

Evaluation of isolated patient fibrinogen
Thrombin time: [n.a.]
Reptilase time: [n.a.]
Ancrod (Arvin) time: [n.a.]

Abnormal subunit? [n.a.]
Abnormal FDPs? [n.a.]

Remarks

[1]Rates of fibrinopeptide release were not reported. Other variants with this molecular defect exhibit delayed fibrinopeptide A and B release plus delayed polymerization of fibrin monomers.

References

1. Reber, P., Furlan, M., Beck, E.A. and Barbui, T. Fibrinogen Bergamo III and fibrinogen Torino: two further variants with hereditary molecular defects in fibrinopeptide A. *Thromb. Res.* **46**:163-167, **1987**.

FIBRINOGEN BERLIN I

Last update [1 December 1990]
Alphacode [BERLIN01]
Ref. type [Article]

Family studies
Homozygote? [No]
Pedigree published? [No]

Structural defect [n.a.]
Mutation [n.a.]

Functional defect(s)
FpA release: [Normal]
FpB release: [Abnormal]
Polymerization: [n.a.]
Stabilization: [n.a.]

Clinical manifestation(s) Bleeding? [No] Thrombosis? [No]

Clinical laboratory results

Plasma fibrinogen concentration (mg/dL)
Chronometric: [n.a.]
Rate-indep'nt: [n.a.]
Immunologic: [n.a.]

*Hypo*dysfibrinogen? [n.a.]

Thrombin time:	[Abnormal[1]]
Reptilase (batroxobin) time:	[n.a.]
Prothrombin time:	[n.a.]
Partial thromboplastin time:	[n.a.]
Euglobulin lysis time:	[n.a.]
Bleeding time:	[n.a.]
Immunoelectrophoresis:	[n.a.]
Platelet aggregation:	[n.a.]

Other results with patient plasma
Ancrod (Arvin) time: [n.a.]
Recalcification time: [n.a.]
Calcium corrects c.t.? [n.a.]

Inhib. normal plasma? [n.a.]
In vivo synthesis: [n.a.]
In vivo catabolism: [n.a.]

Evaluation of isolated patient fibrinogen
Thrombin time: [n.a.]
Reptilase time: [n.a.]
Ancrod (Arvin) time: [n.a.]

Abnormal subunit? [No]
Abnormal FDPs? [n.a.]

Remarks

References

1. Meyer, M., Vogel, G., Gromnica-Ihle, E., Schellenberg, I. and Ostermann, G. Hereditary dysfibrinogenaemia: structural and functional studies on three fibrinogen variants. *Folia Haematol. (Leipz.)* **115**:499-502, **1988**.

FIBRINOGEN BERLIN II[Abs]

Last update [10 January 1994]
Alphacode [BERLIN02]
Ref. type [Abstract]

Family studies
Homozygote? [No]
Pedigree published? [No]

Structural defect [n.a.]
Mutation [n.a.]

Functional defect(s)
FpA release: [n.a.]
FpB release: [n.a.]
Polymerization: [n.a.]
Stabilization: [n.a.]

Clinical manifestation(s) Bleeding? [n.a.] Thrombosis? [n.a.]

Clinical laboratory results
Plasma fibrinogen concentration (mg/dL)
Chronometric: [Subnormal[1]]
Rate-indep'nt: [Normal[1]]
Immunologic: [n.a.]

*Hypo*dysfibrinogen? [No]

Thrombin time:	[n.a.]
Reptilase (batroxobin) time:	[n.a.]
Prothrombin time:	[Abnormal[1]]
Partial thromboplastin time:	[n.a.]
Euglobulin lysis time:	[n.a.]
Bleeding time:	[n.a.]
Immunoelectrophoresis:	[n.a.]
Platelet aggregation:	[n.a.]

Other results with patient plasma
Ancrod (Arvin) time: [n.a.]
Recalcification time: [n.a.]
Calcium corrects c.t.? [n.a.]

Inhib. normal plasma? [n.a.]
In vivo synthesis: [n.a.]
In vivo catabolism: [n.a.]

Evaluation of isolated patient fibrinogen
Thrombin time: [n.a.]
Reptilase time: [n.a.]
Ancrod (Arvin) time: [n.a.]

Abnormal subunit? [Yes[2]]
Abnormal FDPs? [n.a.]

Remarks
[1]Data not reported.
[2]SDS-PAGE disclosed an oversized Bβ-chain. Increased glycosylation of this subunit also was reported.

References

1. Meyer, M., Lutze, G. and Gromnica-Ilhe, E. Dysfibrinogenemia: Abnormalities in the Bβ chains of fibrinogens Berlin II and Magdeburg II. *Thromb. Haemostas.* **65**:903, **1991**. ABSTRACT

FIBRINOGEN BERN I

Last update [10 January 1994]
Alphacode [BERN01]
Ref. type [Article]

Structural defect [γ(337) Asn → Lys[1]]
Mutation [AAC → AAA]

Family studies
Homozygote? [No]
Pedigree published? [Yes]

Functional defect(s)
FpA release: [Normal]
FpB release: [Normal]
Polymerization: [Abnormal]
Stabilization: [n.a.]

Clinical manifestation(s) Bleeding? [No] Thrombosis? [No]

Clinical laboratory results
Plasma fibrinogen concentration (mg/dL)
Chronometric: [25/(150-300)]
Rate-indep'nt: [180/(150-300)]
Immunologic: [140/(150-300)]

*Hypo*dysfibrinogen? [Yes]

Thrombin time:	[21.8s/(12-15s)]
Reptilase (batroxobin) time:	[32.1s/(13-14s)]
Prothrombin time:	[70%/(>70%)[2]]
Partial thromboplastin time:	[45s/(40-60s)[2]]
Euglobulin lysis time:	[n.a.]
Bleeding time:	[n.a.]
Immunoelectrophoresis:	[n.a.]
Platelet aggregation:	[Normal]

Other results with patient plasma
Ancrod (Arvin) time: [n.a.]
Recalcification time: [n.a.]
Calcium corrects c.t.? [Yes]

Inhib. normal plasma? [n.a.]
In vivo synthesis: [n.a.]
In vivo catabolism: [n.a.]

Evaluation of isolated patient fibrinogen
Thrombin time: [n.a.]
Reptilase time: [n.a.]
Ancrod (Arvin) time: [n.a.]

Abnormal subunit? [Yes[3]]
Abnormal FDPs? [Yes[4]]

Remarks
[1]The structural defect was determined with the PCR method.
[2]This value is within normal limits.
[3]2D electrophoresis disclosed an abnormal γ-chain.
[4]2D electrophoresis disclosed an abnormal γ-chain remnant (γ_2).

Sialic acid content was higher than normal.

FIBRINOGEN BERN I

References

1. Steinmann, C., Reber, P., Jungo, M., Lämmle, B., Heinemann, G., Wermuth, B. and Furlan, M. Fibrinogen Bern I: Substitution γ 337 Asn → Lys is responsible for defective fibrin monomer polymerization. *Blood* **82**:2104-2108, **1993**.

2. Steinmann, C., Lämmle, B., Heinemann, G., Wermuth, B. and Furlan, M. Fibrinogen Bern I: Substitution γ 337 Asn → Lys is responsible for defective fibrin monomer polymerization and impaired interactions with calcium. *Proc. XI Int'l. F'gen. Wkshop.* p. 2, **1992**. ABSTRACT

3. Rupp, C., Kuyas, C., Häberli, A., Furlan, M., Perret, B.A. and Beck, E.A. Fibrinogen Bern I: A hereditary fibrinogen variant with defective conformational stabilization by calcium ions. In: *Fibrinogen —Recent Biochemical and Medical Aspects*, A. Henschen, H. Graeff and F. Lottspeich (eds.), W. de Gruyter, Berlin. pp. 167-182, **1982**.

4. Rupp, C., Kuyas, C., Häberli, A., Furlan, M., von Fliedner, V. and Beck, E.A. [Fibrinogen Bern I and fibrinogen Bern II: 2 hereditary fibrinogen variants with diverse biochemical properties]. *Schweiz. Med. Wochenschr.* **111**:1543-1545, **1981**.

5. Beck, E.A. Congenital abnormalities of fibrinogen. *Clin. Haematol.* **8**:169-181, **1979**.

FIBRINOGEN BERN II

Last update [1 December 1990]
Alphacode [BERN02]
Ref. type [Article]

Structural defect [Aα(16) Arg → His]
Mutation [n.a.]

Family studies
Homozygote? [No]
Pedigree published? [No]

Functional defect(s)
FpA release: [Abnormal]
FpB release: [Abnormal[1]]
Polymerization: [Abnormal]
Stabilization: [n.a.]

Clinical manifestation(s) Bleeding? [No] Thrombosis? [No]

Clinical laboratory results
Plasma fibrinogen concentration (mg/dL)
Chronometric: [30/(150-300)]
Rate-indep'nt: [260/(150-300)]
Immunologic: [200/(150-300)]

*Hypo*dysfibrinogen? [No]

Thrombin time:	[41s/(14.5s)]
Reptilase (batroxobin) time:	[77s/(17s)]
Prothrombin time:	[n.a.]
Partial thromboplastin time:	[n.a.]
Euglobulin lysis time:	[n.a.]
Bleeding time:	[n.a.]
Immunoelectrophoresis:	[n.a.]
Platelet aggregation:	[Normal]

Other results with patient plasma
Ancrod (Arvin) time: [n.a.]
Recalcification time: [n.a.]
Calcium corrects c.t.? [No]

Inhib. normal plasma? [n.a.]
In vivo synthesis: [n.a.]
In vivo catabolism: [n.a.]

Evaluation of isolated patient fibrinogen
Thrombin time: [n.a.]
Reptilase time: [n.a.]
Ancrod (Arvin) time: [n.a.]

Abnormal subunit? [No]
Abnormal FDPs? [n.a.]

Remarks
[1]The rate of fibrinopeptide B release was not reported. Other dysfibrinogens with this molecular defect exhibit delayed fibrinopeptide A and B release plus delayed polymerization of fibrin monomers.

References

1. Rupp, C., Sievi, R., Furlan, M. and Beck, E.A. [Fibrinogen Bern II: hereditary fibrinogen variant with amino acid substitution of arginine replaced by histidine in position 16 of the Aα-chain]. *Schweiz. Med. Wochenschr.* **113**:1460-1462, **1983**.

2. Rupp, C., Kuyas, C., Haeberli, A., Furlan, M., von Fliedner, V. and Beck, E.A. [Fibrinogen Bern I and fibrinogen Bern II: 2 hereditary fibrinogen variants with diverse biochemical properties]. *Schweiz. Med. Wochenschr.* **111**:1543-1545, **1981**.

FIBRINOGEN BERN III

Last update [10 January 1994]
Alphacode [BERN03]
Ref. type [Article]

Structural defect [Aα(16) Arg → Cys]
Mutation [n.a.]

Family studies
Homozygote? [No]
Pedigree published? [Yes]

Functional defect(s)
FpA release: [Abnormal[1]]
FpB release: [Normal]
Polymerization: [Abnormal]
Stabilization: [n.a.]

Clinical manifestation(s) Bleeding? [No] Thrombosis? [No]

Clinical laboratory results

Plasma fibrinogen concentration (mg/dL)
Chronometric: [20/(150-300)]
Rate-indep'nt: [240/(150-300)]
Immunologic: [260/(150-300)]

*Hypo*dysfibrinogen? [No]

Thrombin time:	[46.7s/(12-15s)]
Reptilase (batroxobin) time:	[>120s/(14-17s)[2]]
Prothrombin time:	[70%/(70-130%)]
Partial thromboplastin time:	[61s/(40-60s)]
Euglobulin lysis time:	[n.a.]
Bleeding time:	[n.a.]
Immunoelectrophoresis:	[n.a.]
Platelet aggregation:	[n.a.]

Other results with patient plasma
Ancrod (Arvin) time: [n.a.]
Recalcification time: [n.a.]
Calcium corrects c.t.? [n.a.]

Inhib. normal plasma? [n.a.]
In vivo synthesis: [n.a.]
In vivo catabolism: [n.a.]

Evaluation of isolated patient fibrinogen
Thrombin time: [n.a.]
Reptilase time: [n.a.]
Ancrod (Arvin) time: [n.a.]

Abnormal subunit? [n.a.]
Abnormal FDPs? [n.a.]

Remarks
[1]Only half the normal amount of Fibrinopeptide A was released.
[2]Clots failed to form when patient plasma was incubated with Reptilase.

References

1. Furlan, M., Leupin, L., Biasiutti, F.D. and Lämmle, B. Fibrinogen Bern III: A further case of the hereditary fibrinogen variant with substitution Aα 16 Arg → Cys. *Schweiz. Med. Wochenschr.* **121**:1068-1071, **1991**.

FIBRINOGEN BETHESDA I

Last update [1 December 1990]
Alphacode [BETHES01]
Ref. type [Article]

Structural defect [n.a.]
Mutation [n.a.]

Family studies
Homozygote? [No]
Pedigree published? [Yes]

Functional defect(s)
FpA release: [Abnormal]
FpB release: [Abnormal]
Polymerization: [Normal]
Stabilization: [n.a.]

Clinical manifestation(s) Bleeding? [Yes[1]] Thrombosis? [No]

Clinical laboratory results
Plasma fibrinogen concentration (mg/dL)
Chronometric: [36/(186-380)]
Rate-indep'nt: [330/(200-400)]
Immunologic: [300/(250)]

*Hypo*dysfibrinogen? [No]

Thrombin time:	[148s/(<35s)]
Reptilase (batroxobin) time:	[106s/(24s)]
Prothrombin time:	[16.2s/(11-14s)]
Partial thromboplastin time:	[45.4s/(30-35s)]
Euglobulin lysis time:	[>180m/(>180m)]
Bleeding time:	[Normal]
Immunoelectrophoresis:	[Anodal]
Platelet aggregation:	[n.a.]

Other results with patient plasma
Ancrod (Arvin) time: [n.a.]
Recalcification time: [n.a.]
Calcium corrects c.t.? [n.a.]

Inhib. normal plasma? [Yes]
In vivo synthesis: [Normal]
In vivo catabolism: [Normal]

Evaluation of isolated patient fibrinogen
Thrombin time: [Abnormal[2]]
Reptilase time: [n.a.]
Ancrod (Arvin) time: [n.a.]

Abnormal subunit? [No]
Abnormal FDPs? [n.a.]

Remarks
[1]The 9 year-old proposita exhibited a lifelong bleeding tendency and easy bruising.
[2]Data not reported.

Fibrinogen Bethesda I is the first in which the *rate* of fibrinopeptide release was included in the evaluation of the functional defect.

References

1. Gralnick, H.R., Givelber, H.M., Shainoff, J.R. and Finlayson, J.S. Fibrinogen Bethesda: a congenital dysfibrinogenemia with delayed fibrinopeptide release. *J. Clin. Invest.* **50**:1819-1830, **1971**.

FIBRINOGEN BETHESDA II

Last update [1 December 1990]
Alphacode [BETHES02]
Ref. type [Article]

Family studies
Homozygote? [n.a.]
Pedigree published? [No]

Structural defect [n.a.]
Mutation [n.a.]

Functional defect(s)
FpA release: [n.a.[1]]
FpB release: [n.a.[1]]
Polymerization: [Abnormal]
Stabilization: [n.a.]

Clinical manifestation(s) Bleeding? [No] Thrombosis? [No]

Clinical laboratory results
Plasma fibrinogen concentration (mg/dL)
Chronometric: [94/(190-380)]
Rate-indep'nt: [179/(200-400)]
Immunologic: [180/(300)]

*Hypo*dysfibrinogen? [No]

Thrombin time:	[48s/(<30s)]
Reptilase (batroxobin) time:	[49s/(<22s)]
Prothrombin time:	[12.9s/(12.3s)]
Partial thromboplastin time:	[32.6s/(31s)]
Euglobulin lysis time:	[>180m/(>180m)]
Bleeding time:	[n.a.]
Immunoelectrophoresis:	[Anodal]
Platelet aggregation:	[n.a.]

Other results with patient plasma
Ancrod (Arvin) time: [n.a.]
Recalcification time: [n.a.]
Calcium corrects c.t.? [No]

Inhib. normal plasma? [Yes]
In vivo synthesis: [n.a.]
In vivo catabolism: [Increased]

Evaluation of isolated patient fibrinogen
Thrombin time: [n.a.]
Reptilase time: [n.a.]
Ancrod (Arvin) time: [n.a.]

Abnormal subunit? [n.a.]
Abnormal FDPs? [n.a.]

Remarks
[1]The rate of *total* fibrinopeptide release was reduced slightly; individual fibrinopeptide release was not reported.

References

1. Gralnick, H.R., Givelber, H.M. and Finlayson, J.S. A new congenital abnormality of human fibrinogen. Fibrinogen Bethesda II. *Thromb. Diath. Haemorrh.* **29**:562-571, **1973**.

FIBRINOGEN BETHESDA III

Last update [1 December 1990]
Alphacode [BETHES03]
Ref. type [Article]

Family studies
Homozygote? [No]
Pedigree published? [Yes]

Structural defect [n.a.]
Mutation [n.a.]

Functional defect(s)
FpA release: [Normal]
FpB release: [Normal]
Polymerization: [Abnormal]
Stabilization: [Normal]

Clinical manifestation(s) Bleeding? [Yes[1]] Thrombosis? [Yes[1]]

Clinical laboratory results
Plasma fibrinogen concentration (mg/dL)
Chronometric: [30-41/(190-380)]
Rate-indep'nt: [90-117/(186-360)]
Immunologic: [100-120/(200-390)]

*Hypo*dysfibrinogen? [Yes]

Thrombin time:	[65-300s/(<30s)]
Reptilase (batroxobin) time:	[31-67s/(19-24s)]
Prothrombin time:	[15s/(11-13.5s)]
Partial thromboplastin time:	[31.8s/(27-35s)]
Euglobulin lysis time:	[143m/(>180m)]
Bleeding time:	[n.a.]
Immunoelectrophoresis:	[Normal]
Platelet aggregation:	[Normal]

Other results with patient plasma
Ancrod (Arvin) time: [n.a.]
Recalcification time: [n.a.]
Calcium corrects c.t.? [n.a.]

Inhib. normal plasma? [Yes]
In vivo synthesis: [n.a.]
In vivo catabolism: [Increased]

Evaluation of isolated patient fibrinogen
Thrombin time: [n.a.]
Reptilase time: [n.a.]
Ancrod (Arvin) time: [n.a.]

Abnormal subunit? [No]
Abnormal FDPs? [No[2]]

Remarks
[1]Three first-trimester abortions associated with excessive bleeding and two pregnancies associated with abnormal bleeding, excessive postpartum bleeding, and thrombophlebitis in the 27 year-old proposita were reported.
[2]A reduced *rate* of FDP formation was reported.

References

1. Gralnick, H.R., Coller, B.S., Fratantoni, J.C. and Martinez, J. Fibrinogen Bethesda III: A hypodysfibrinogenemia. *Blood* **53**:28-46, **1979**.

FIBRINOGEN BICÊTRE I

Last update [1 December 1990]
Alphacode [BICETR01]
Ref. type [Article]

Structural defect [Aα(16) Arg → His]
Mutation [n.a.]

Family studies
Homozygote? [Yes[1]]
Pedigree published? [No]

Functional defect(s)
FpA release: [Abnormal]
FpB release: [Abnormal]
Polymerization: [n.a.[2]]
Stabilization: [n.a.]

Clinical manifestation(s) Bleeding? [n.a.] Thrombosis? [n.a.]

Clinical laboratory results
Plasma fibrinogen concentration (mg/dL)
Chronometric: [n.a.]
Rate-indep'nt: [n.a.]
Immunologic: [n.a.]

*Hypo*dysfibrinogen? [n.a.]

Thrombin time:	[n.a.]
Reptilase (batroxobin) time:	[n.a.]
Prothrombin time:	[n.a.]
Partial thromboplastin time:	[n.a.]
Euglobulin lysis time:	[n.a.]
Bleeding time:	[n.a.]
Immunoelectrophoresis:	[n.a.]
Platelet aggregation:	[n.a.]

Other results with patient plasma
Ancrod (Arvin) time: [n.a.]
Recalcification time: [n.a.]
Calcium corrects c.t.? [n.a.]

Inhib. normal plasma? [n.a.]
In vivo synthesis: [n.a.]
In vivo catabolism: [n.a.]

Evaluation of isolated patient fibrinogen
Thrombin time: [n.a.]
Reptilase time: [Abnormal[3]]
Ancrod (Arvin) time: [n.a.]

Abnormal subunit? [n.a.]
Abnormal FDPs? [n.a.]

Remarks
[1]Fibrinogen Bicêtre I comprises both homo- and heterozygous patients. A case report has not been published.
[2]Polymerization of fibrin monomers was not reported. Other dysfibrinogens with this molecular defect exhibit delayed fibrinopeptide A and B release plus delayed polymerization of fibrin monomers.
[3]Data not reported.

References

1. Henschen, A., Kehl, M., Southan, C., Lottspeich, F. and Georgopoulos, D. Genetically abnormal fibrinogens — some current characterisation strategies. In: *Fibrinogen —Structure, Functional Aspects, Metabolism*, F. Haverkate, A. Henschen, W. Nieuwenhuizen and P.W. Straub (eds.), Walter de Gruyter, Berlin. pp. 125-144, **1983**.

FIBRINOGEN BICÊTRE II

Last update [10 January 1994]
Alphacode [BICETR02]
Ref. type [Article]

Family studies
Homozygote? [No]
Pedigree published? [Yes]

Structural defect [γ(308) Asn → Lys]
Mutation [AAT → AAG[1]]

Functional defect(s)
FpA release: [n.a.]
FpB release: [n.a.]
Polymerization: [n.a.]
Stabilization: [n.a.]

Clinical manifestation(s) Bleeding? [No] Thrombosis? [Yes[2]]

Clinical laboratory results

Plasma fibrinogen concentration (mg/dL)
Chronometric: [130/(200-400)]
Rate-indep'nt: [350/(200-400)]
Immunologic: [370/(200-400)]

*Hypo*dysfibrinogen? [No]

Thrombin time:	[40s/(<20s)]
Reptilase (batroxobin) time:	[29s/(<23s)]
Prothrombin time:	[70%/(>60%)[3]]
Partial thromboplastin time:	[39s/(<48s)[3]]
Euglobulin lysis time:	[Normal[3]]
Bleeding time:	[n.a.]
Immunoelectrophoresis:	[Normal[3]]
Platelet aggregation:	[n.a.]

Other results with patient plasma
Ancrod (Arvin) time: [n.a.]
Recalcification time: [n.a.]
Calcium corrects c.t.? [n.a.]

Inhib. normal plasma? [n.a.]
In vivo synthesis: [n.a.]
In vivo catabolism: [n.a.]

Evaluation of isolated patient fibrinogen
Thrombin time: [n.a.]
Reptilase time: [n.a.]
Ancrod (Arvin) time: [n.a.]

Abnormal subunit? [Yes[4]]
Abnormal FDPs? [No[5]]

Remarks

[1]Determined with the PCR method. See also fibrinogen Kyoto I.

[2]At age 40 the propositus presented with deep vein thrombosis and pulmonary embolism.

[3]P. Grailhe, personal communication.

[4]SDS-PAGE disclosed an abnormal γ-chain.

[5]Rates of t-PA and plasminogen activation, and plasminogen binding to the variant fibrin were within normal limits. This mutation generates a new plasmin cleavage site.

Affected family members were asymptomatic, and additional risk factors of smoking and obesity were associated with the index patient. The authors note that these findings, plus the observed normal fibrinolytic functionality indicate that the mutation may not be causally related to the thrombotic tendency in this patient.

References

1. Grailhe, P., Boyer-Neumann, C., Haverkate, F., Grimbergen, J., Larrieu, M.J. and Anglés-Cano, E. The mutation in fibrinogen Bicêtre II (γ Asn_{308} → Lys) does not affect the binding of t-PA and plasminogen to fibrin. *Blood Coag. & Fibrinol.* **4**:679-687, **1993**.

FIBRINOGEN BIRMINGHAM I

Last update [1 December 1990]
Alphacode [BIRMIN01]
Ref. type [Article]

Structural defect [Aα(16) Arg → His]
Mutation [n.a.]

Family studies
Homozygote? [No]
Pedigree published? [No]

Functional defect(s)
FpA release: [Abnormal]
FpB release: [Abnormal]
Polymerization: [Normal[1]]
Stabilization: [n.a.]

Clinical manifestation(s) Bleeding? [Yes[2]] Thrombosis? [No]

Clinical laboratory results

Plasma fibrinogen concentration (mg/dL)
Chronometric: [50/(200-400)]
Rate-indep'nt: [n.a.]
Immunologic: [342/(200-400)]

*Hypo*dysfibrinogen? [No]

Thrombin time:	[52.1s/(22.6s)]
Reptilase (batroxobin) time:	[25.8s/(9.7s)]
Prothrombin time:	[n.a.]
Partial thromboplastin time:	[n.a.]
Euglobulin lysis time:	[n.a.]
Bleeding time:	[Abnormal]
Immunoelectrophoresis:	[n.a.]
Platelet aggregation:	[Normal]

Other results with patient plasma
Ancrod (Arvin) time: [n.a.]
Recalcification time: [n.a.]
Calcium corrects c.t.? [n.a.]

Inhib. normal plasma? [n.a.]
In vivo synthesis: [n.a.]
In vivo catabolism: [n.a.]

Evaluation of isolated patient fibrinogen
Thrombin time: [164s/(22s)]
Reptilase time: [n.a.]
Ancrod (Arvin) time: [n.a.]

Abnormal subunit? [n.a.]
Abnormal FDPs? [n.a.]

Remarks
[1]Other variants with this molecular defect exhibit delayed polymerization of fibrin monomers.
[2]Epistaxis and occasional hematomas and hemarthroses in the 25 year-old proposita were reported.

References

1. Siebenlist, K.R., Prchal, J.T. and Mosesson, M.W. Fibrinogen Birmingham: a heterozygous dysfibrinogenemia (Aα-16 Arg → His) containing heterodimeric molecules. *Blood* 71:613-618, **1988**.

2. Siebenlist, K.R., Prchal, J.T. and Mosesson, M.W. Fibrinogen Birmingham: A new heterodimeric dysfibrinogenemia with defective fibrinopeptide A release (Aα-16 Arg → His). In: *Fibrinogen 2. Biochemistry, Physiology and Clinical Relevance*, G.D.O. Lowe, J.T. Douglas, C.D. Forbes and A. Henschen (eds.), Elsevier, Amsterdam. pp. 63-66, **1987**.

FIBRINOGEN BODMIN I

Last update [1 December 1990]
Alphacode [BODMIN01]
Ref. type [Article[2]]

Family studies
Homozygote? [n.a.]
Pedigree published? [No]

Structural defect [n.a.[1]]
Mutation [n.a.]

Functional defect(s)
FpA release: [n.a.]
FpB release: [n.a.]
Polymerization: [n.a.]
Stabilization: [n.a.]

Clinical manifestation(s) Bleeding? [n.a.] Thrombosis? [n.a.]

Clinical laboratory results
Plasma fibrinogen concentration (mg/dL)
Chronometric: [n.a.]
Rate-indep'nt: [n.a.]
Immunologic: [n.a.]

*Hypo*dysfibrinogen? [n.a.]

Thrombin time: [n.a.]
Reptilase (batroxobin) time: [n.a.]
Prothrombin time: [n.a.]
Partial thromboplastin time: [n.a.]
Euglobulin lysis time: [n.a.]
Bleeding time: [n.a.]
Immunoelectrophoresis: [n.a.]
Platelet aggregation: [n.a.]

Other results with patient plasma
Ancrod (Arvin) time: [n.a.]
Recalcification time: [n.a.]
Calcium corrects c.t.? [n.a.]

Inhib. normal plasma? [n.a.]
In vivo synthesis: [n.a.]
In vivo catabolism: [n.a.]

Evaluation of isolated patient fibrinogen
Thrombin time: [n.a.]
Reptilase time: [n.a.]
Ancrod (Arvin) time: [n.a.]

Abnormal subunit? [n.a.]
Abnormal FDPs? [n.a.]

Remarks
[1]A structural defect in the Bβ chain is suspected.
[2]Review article only; P. Gaffney, personal communication.

References

1. Lane, D.A., Thompson, E. and Southan, C. Rapid screening method of fibrinopeptide analysis applied to congenital dysfibrinogenaemia: Summary of 23 cases. In: *Fibrinogen 2. Biochemistry, Physiology and Clinical Relevance*, G.D.O. Lowe, J.T. Douglas, C.D. Forbes and A. Henschen (eds.), Elsevier, Amsterdam. pp. 71-74, **1987**.

FIBRINOGEN BONDY I

Last update [10 January 1994]
Alphacode [BONDY01]
Ref. type [Article]

Structural defect [n.a.]
Mutation [n.a.]

Family studies
Homozygote? [No]
Pedigree published? [No]

Functional defect(s)
FpA release: [Abnormal]
FpB release: [n.a.]
Polymerization: [Abnormal]
Stabilization: [n.a.]

Clinical manifestation(s) Bleeding? [No] Thrombosis? [No]

Clinical laboratory results
Plasma fibrinogen concentration (mg/dL)
Chronometric: [30/(410)]
Rate-indep'nt: [70/(375)]
Immunologic: [750/(420)]

*Hypo*dysfibrinogen? [No]

Thrombin time:	[>120s/(21s)]
Reptilase (batroxobin) time:	[>120s/(21s)]
Prothrombin time:	[19s/(13s)]
Partial thromboplastin time:	[n.a.]
Euglobulin lysis time:	[n.a.]
Bleeding time:	[Normal]
Immunoelectrophoresis:	[Normal]
Platelet aggregation:	[n.a.]

Other results with patient plasma
Ancrod (Arvin) time: [n.a.]
Recalcification time: [n.a.]
Calcium corrects c.t.? [n.a.]

Inhib. normal plasma? [n.a.]
In vivo synthesis: [n.a.]
In vivo catabolism: [n.a.]

Evaluation of isolated patient fibrinogen
Thrombin time: [n.a.]
Reptilase time: [n.a.]
Ancrod (Arvin) time: [n.a.]

Abnormal subunit? [No]
Abnormal FDPs? [No[1]]

Remarks
[1]A reduced *rate* of FDP formation was reported.

References

1. Jandrot-Perrus, M., Aurousseau, M.H., Rabiet, M.J. and Josso, F. Fibrinogen Bondy: a new case of dysfibrinogenemia. Isolation of the abnormal fibrinogen molecules. *Thromb. Res.* **27**:659-670, **1982**.

FIBRINOGEN BOULOGNE I[Abs]

Last update [10 January 1994]
Alphacode [BOULOG01]
Ref. type [Abstract]

Family studies
Homozygote? [n.a.]
Pedigree published? [No]

Structural defect [n.a.]
Mutation [n.a.]

Functional defect(s)
FpA release: [Normal]
FpB release: [Normal]
Polymerization: [Abnormal]
Stabilization: [Normal]

Clinical manifestation(s) Bleeding? [No] Thrombosis? [No]

Clinical laboratory results
Plasma fibrinogen concentration (mg/dL)
Chronometric: [Abnormal]
Rate-indep'nt: [n.a.]
Immunologic: [Normal]
*Hypo*dysfibrinogen? [No]

Thrombin time: [Abnormal]
Reptilase (batroxobin) time: [n.a.]
Prothrombin time: [n.a.]
Partial thromboplastin time: [n.a.]
Euglobulin lysis time: [n.a.]
Bleeding time: [n.a.]
Immunoelectrophoresis: [Normal]
Platelet aggregation: [n.a.]

Other results with patient plasma
Ancrod (Arvin) time: [n.a.]
Recalcification time: [n.a.]
Calcium corrects c.t.? [n.a.]
Inhib. normal plasma? [n.a.]
In vivo synthesis: [n.a.]
In vivo catabolism: [n.a.]

Evaluation of isolated patient fibrinogen
Thrombin time: [n.a.]
Reptilase time: [n.a.]
Ancrod (Arvin) time: [n.a.]
Abnormal subunit? [No]
Abnormal FDPs? [n.a.]

Remarks

References

1. Soria, J., Soria, C., Houbouyan, L. and Goguel, A. Fibrinogen Boulogne. A congenital abnormality in the aggregation of fibrin monomers. *Proc. III Congr. Europ. Afr. Div. Int. Soc. Haematol.* p. 23, **1975**. ABSTRACT

FIBRINOGEN BREMEN I

Last update [10 January 1994]
Alphacode [BREMEN01]
Ref. type [Article]

Structural defect [Aα(17) Gly → Val]
Mutation [n.a.]

Family studies
Homozygote? [No]
Pedigree published? [No]

Functional defect(s)
FpA release: [Abnormal]
FpB release: [Abnormal]
Polymerization: [Abnormal]
Stabilization: [Normal]

Clinical manifestation(s) Bleeding? [Yes[1]] Thrombosis? [No]

Clinical laboratory results
Plasma fibrinogen concentration (mg/dL)
Chronometric: [80/(180-400)]
Rate-indep'nt: [n.a.]
Immunologic: [234/(200-430)]

*Hypo*dysfibrinogen? [No]

Thrombin time:	[61s/(24s)]
Reptilase (batroxobin) time:	[n.a.]
Prothrombin time:	[62%/(>70%)]
Partial thromboplastin time:	[57s/(27s)]
Euglobulin lysis time:	[n.a.]
Bleeding time:	[Abnormal]
Immunoelectrophoresis:	[n.a.]
Platelet aggregation:	[n.a.]

Other results with patient plasma
Ancrod (Arvin) time: [n.a.]
Recalcification time: [n.a.]
Calcium corrects c.t.? [No]

Inhib. normal plasma? [n.a.]
In vivo synthesis: [n.a.]
In vivo catabolism: [n.a.]

Evaluation of isolated patient fibrinogen
Thrombin time: [61.7s/(13.2s)]
Reptilase time: [n.a.]
Ancrod (Arvin) time: [167s/(12.7s)]

Abnormal subunit? [No]
Abnormal FDPs? [n.a.]

Remarks
[1]Multiple skin hematomas (easy bruising) and impaired wound healing were reported. Fibrinogen concentrate was effective in preventing postoperative complications.

References

1. Wada, Y., Niwa, K., Maekawa, H., Asakura, S., Sugo, T., Nakanishi, M., Auerswald, G., Popp, M. and Matsuda, M. A new type of congenital dysfibrinogen, fibrinogen Bremen, with an Aα Gly-17 to Val substitution associated with hemorrhagic diathesis and delayed wound healing. *Thromb. Haemost.* **70**:397-403, **1993**.

2. Auerswald, G., Popp, M. and Matsuda, M. Clinical aspects combined with a new fibrinogen (fibrinogen Bremen) with an Aα Gly-17 to Val substitution. *Proc. XI Int'l. F'gen. Wkshop.* p. 9, **1992**. ABSTRACT

3. Wada, Y., Niwa, K., Maekawa, H., Nakanishi, M., Auerswald, G., Popp, M. and Matsuda, M. Fibrinogen Bremen with an Aα Gly-17 to Val substitution: Normal fibrin monomer polymerization despite the structural alteration in the "A" polymerization site. *Proc. XI Int'l. F'gen. Wkshop.* p. 10, **1992**. ABSTRACT

FIBRINOGEN BRUSSELS I^{Abs}

Last update [1 December 1990]
Alphacode [BRUSSE01]
Ref. type [Abstract]

Family studies
Homozygote? [n.a.]
Pedigree published? [No]

Structural defect [n.a.]
Mutation [n.a.]

Functional defect(s)
FpA release: [Normal]
FpB release: [Normal]
Polymerization: [Abnormal]
Stabilization: [n.a.]

Clinical manifestation(s) Bleeding? [No] Thrombosis? [No]

Clinical laboratory results
Plasma fibrinogen concentration (mg/dL)
Chronometric: [Subnormal[1]]
Rate-indep'nt: [Normal[1]]
Immunologic: [Normal[1]]

*Hypo*dysfibrinogen? [No]

Thrombin time:	[n.a.]
Reptilase (batroxobin) time:	[n.a.]
Prothrombin time:	[Normal[1]]
Partial thromboplastin time:	[Normal[1]]
Euglobulin lysis time:	[n.a.]
Bleeding time:	[n.a.]
Immunoelectrophoresis:	[n.a.]
Platelet aggregation:	[n.a.]

Other results with patient plasma
Ancrod (Arvin) time: [n.a.]
Recalcification time: [n.a.]
Calcium corrects c.t.? [Yes]

Inhib. normal plasma? [Yes]
In vivo synthesis: [n.a.]
In vivo catabolism: [n.a.]

Evaluation of isolated patient fibrinogen
Thrombin time: [n.a.]
Reptilase time: [n.a.]
Ancrod (Arvin) time: [n.a.]

Abnormal subunit? [n.a.]
Abnormal FDPs? [n.a.]

Remarks
[1]Data not reported.

References

1. Capel, P., Bosson, D., Heriga-Muller, Ch., Mandelbaum, I.M., Vertongen, F. and Fondu, P. Investigation of an inherited defect in fibrinogen polymerization, with special emphasis on ultrastructural disturbances (Fibrinogen Brussels). *Haemostas.* **12**:186, **1982**. ABSTRACT

FIBRINOGEN BUENOS AIRES I[Abs]

Last update [1 December 1990]
Alphacode [BUENOS01]
Ref. type [Article]

Structural defect [n.a.]
Mutation [n.a.]

Family studies
Homozygote? [n.a.]
Pedigree published? [No]

Functional defect(s)
FpA release: [n.a.]
FpB release: [n.a.]
Polymerization: [Abnormal[1]]
Stabilization: [n.a.]

Clinical manifestation(s) Bleeding? [Yes[2]] Thrombosis? [No]

Clinical laboratory results
Plasma fibrinogen concentration (mg/dL)
Chronometric: [Normal[1]]
Rate-indep'nt: [Normal[1]]
Immunologic: [n.a.]

*Hypo*dysfibrinogen? [No]

Thrombin time:	[Abnormal[1]]
Reptilase (batroxobin) time:	[n.a.]
Prothrombin time:	[n.a.]
Partial thromboplastin time:	[n.a.]
Euglobulin lysis time:	[n.a.]
Bleeding time:	[Abnormal]
Immunoelectrophoresis:	[Anodal]
Platelet aggregation:	[n.a.]

Other results with patient plasma
Ancrod (Arvin) time: [n.a.]
Recalcification time: [n.a.]
Calcium corrects c.t.? [n.a.]

Inhib. normal plasma? [n.a.]
In vivo synthesis: [n.a.]
In vivo catabolism: [n.a.]

Evaluation of isolated patient fibrinogen
Thrombin time: [n.a.]
Reptilase time: [n.a.]
Ancrod (Arvin) time: [n.a.]

Abnormal subunit? [n.a.]
Abnormal FDPs? [n.a.]

Remarks
[1]Data not reported.
[2]A lifelong bleeding tendency and defective wound healing in the 42 year-old proposita were reported. Antithrombin III levels were normal.

References

1. Buraschi, J.A., Sack, E.S., Quiroga, E. and Hendler, H. A new fibrinogen anomaly: Fibrinogen Buenos Aires *Thromb. Diath. Haemorrh.* **34**:570-571, **1975**. ABSTRACT

FIBRINOGEN BUENOS AIRES II

Last update [1 December 1990]
Alphacode [BUENOS02]
Ref. type [Article]

Structural defect [n.a.]
Mutation [n.a.]

Family studies
Homozygote? [n.a.]
Pedigree published? [No]

Functional defect(s)
FpA release: [Normal[1]]
FpB release: [Normal[1]]
Polymerization: [Abnormal]
Stabilization: [Normal]

Clinical manifestation(s) Bleeding? [No] Thrombosis? [No]

Clinical laboratory results
Plasma fibrinogen concentration (mg/dL)
Chronometric: [50/(200-450)]
Rate-indep'nt: [365/(200-450)]
Immunologic: [n.a.]

*Hypo*dysfibrinogen? [No]

Thrombin time:	[60s/(18-29s)]
Reptilase (batroxobin) time:	[45s/(18-22s)]
Prothrombin time:	[65%/(>70%)]
Partial thromboplastin time:	[39s/(36s)]
Euglobulin lysis time:	[n.a.]
Bleeding time:	[Normal]
Immunoelectrophoresis:	[n.a.]
Platelet aggregation:	[n.a.]

Other results with patient plasma
Ancrod (Arvin) time: [n.a.]
Recalcification time: [n.a.]
Calcium corrects c.t.? [n.a.]

Inhib. normal plasma? [No]
In vivo synthesis: [n.a.]
In vivo catabolism: [n.a.]

Evaluation of isolated patient fibrinogen
Thrombin time: [n.a.]
Reptilase time: [n.a.]
Ancrod (Arvin) time: [n.a.]

Abnormal subunit? [No]
Abnormal FDPs? [No]

Remarks
[1]Method not reported.

References

1. Amsellem, M., Samama, M., Conard, J., Levyne, S. and Ohlgiesser, C. [Congenital dysfibrinogenaemia. Two new cases]. *Nouv. Presse Med.* 7:3745-3748, **1978**.

FIBRINOGEN CARACAS I

Last update	[1 December 1990]	**Structural defect**	[n.a.]
Alphacode	[CARACA01]	**Mutation**	[n.a.]
Ref. type	[Article]		

Family studies
Homozygote? [No[1]]
Pedigree published? [Yes]

Functional defect(s)
FpA release: [Normal[1]]
FpB release: [Normal[1]]
Polymerization: [Abnormal]
Stabilization: [Abnormal]

Clinical manifestation(s) Bleeding? [Yes[2]] Thrombosis? [No]

Clinical laboratory results

Plasma fibrinogen concentration (mg/dL)
Chronometric: [n.a.]
Rate-indep'nt: [280/(200-350)]
Immunologic: [286/(200-350)]

*Hypo*dysfibrinogen? [No]

Thrombin time:	[23s/(15-18s)]
Reptilase (batroxobin) time:	[25s/(15-18s)]
Prothrombin time:	[18.3s/(11-13s)]
Partial thromboplastin time:	[40.2s/(42-48s)]
Euglobulin lysis time:	[n.a.]
Bleeding time:	[Normal]
Immunoelectrophoresis:	[Anodal]
Platelet aggregation:	[Normal]

Other results with patient plasma

Ancrod (Arvin) time:	[n.a.]	Inhib. normal plasma?	[Yes]
Recalcification time:	[n.a.]	In vivo synthesis:	[n.a.]
Calcium corrects c.t.?	[No]	In vivo catabolism:	[n.a.]

Evaluation of isolated patient fibrinogen

Thrombin time:	[22s/(12-13s)[1]]	Abnormal subunit?	[Yes]
Reptilase time:	[n.a.]	Abnormal FDPs?	[No[1]]
Ancrod (Arvin) time:	[n.a.]		

Remarks

[1]C.L. Arocha-Piñango, personal communication.

[2] Propositus was a 4 month-old male presenting with recurrent spontaneous rectal bleeding. Results are from his mother, who exhibited excessive bleeding after dental extraction and poor wound healing.

References

1. de Bosch, N.B., Arocha-Piñango, C.L., Soria, J., Soria, C., Rodríguez, A. and Rodríguez, S. An abnormal fibrinogen in a Venezuelan family. *Thromb. Res.* **10**:253-265, **1977**.

FIBRINOGEN CARACAS II

Last update [10 January 1994]
Alphacode [CARACA02]
Ref. type [Article]

Family studies
Homozygote? [n.a.]
Pedigree published? [No]

Structural defect [Aα(434) Ser → Asn]
Mutation [n.a.]

Functional defect(s)
FpA release: [Normal]
FpB release: [Normal]
Polymerization: [Abnormal]
Stabilization: [Normal]

Clinical manifestation(s) Bleeding? [No] Thrombosis? [No]

Clinical laboratory results
Plasma fibrinogen concentration (mg/dL)
Chronometric: [39/(180-400)]
Rate-indep'nt: [420/(200-400)]
Immunologic: [500/(210-450)]

*Hypo*dysfibrinogen? [No]

Thrombin time:	[85.2s/(14s)]
Reptilase (batroxobin) time:	[Abnormal[1]]
Prothrombin time:	[n.a.]
Partial thromboplastin time:	[n.a.]
Euglobulin lysis time:	[n.a.]
Bleeding time:	[n.a.]
Immunoelectrophoresis:	[Anodal]
Platelet aggregation:	[n.a.]

Other results with patient plasma
Ancrod (Arvin) time: [>300s/(15.7s)]
Recalcification time: [n.a.]
Calcium corrects c.t.? [No]

Inhib. normal plasma? [No]
In vivo synthesis: [n.a.]
In vivo catabolism: [n.a.]

Evaluation of isolated patient fibrinogen
Thrombin time: [n.a.]
Reptilase time: [n.a.]
Ancrod (Arvin) time: [n.a.]

Abnormal subunit? [Yes[2]]
Abnormal FDPs? [Yes[3]]

Remarks
[1]Reptilase time was reported as 50.2s longer than normal.
[2]SDS-PAGE disclosed an oversized γ-chain. See also ASAHI I, LIMA I, and PONTOISE I.
[3]Small glycoslyated FDPs were reported.

Electron microscopy of patient fibrinogen and fibrin (Marchi et al., 1990) disclosed no differences from normal.

FIBRINOGEN CARACAS II

References

1. Maekawa, H., Yamazumi, K., Muramatsu, S., Kaneko, M., Hirata, H., Takahashi, N., de Bosch, N.B., Carvajal, Z., Ojeda, A., Arocha-Piñango, C.L. and Matsuda, M. An Aα Ser-434 to *N*-glycosylated Asn substitution in a dysfibrinogen, fibrinogen Caracas II, characterized by impaired fibrin gel formation. *J. Biol. Chem.* **266**:11575-11581, **1991**.

2. Arocha-Piñango, C.L., Bosch, N., Torres, A., Caires-Tronchoni, D., Marchi, R., Vidal, H. and Rizzo, M.G. Dysfibrinogenemias in Latin America. A cooperative study group. *Rev. Iberoamer. Tromb. Hemostasia* **3**:110-122, **1990**.

3. Marchi, R., Arocha-Piñango, C.L. and Gil, F. Electron microscopy studies of 7 patients with dysfibrinogenemia and some of their relatives. *Rev. Iberoamer. Tromb. Hemostasia* **3**:185-190, **1990**.

4. Bosch, N.B., Arocha-Piñango, C.L., Rodríguez, A., Ojeda, A. and Carvajal, Z. Another inherited abnormality in plasma fibrinogen. *Thromb. Haemostas.* **38**:100, **1977**. ABSTRACT

FIBRINOGEN CARACAS III

Last update	[10 January 1994]	**Structural defect**	[n.a.]
Alphacode	[CARACA03]	**Mutation**	[n.a.]
Ref. type	[Article]		

Family studies

Homozygote?	[n.a.]
Pedigree published?	[No]

Functional defect(s)

FpA release:	[n.a.]
FpB release:	[n.a.]
Polymerization:	[Abnormal]
Stabilization:	[Normal]

Clinical manifestation(s) Bleeding? [No] Thrombosis? [No]

Clinical laboratory results

Plasma fibrinogen concentration (mg/dL)

Chronometric: [80[1]]
Rate-indep'nt: [330[1]]
Immunologic: [250[1]]

*Hypo*dysfibrinogen? [No]

Thrombin time:	[24s/(15-18s)[2]]
Reptilase (batroxobin) time:	[Abnormal[3]]
Prothrombin time:	[n.a.]
Partial thromboplastin time:	[n.a.]
Euglobulin lysis time:	[n.a.]
Bleeding time:	[n.a.]
Immunoelectrophoresis:	[Normal]
Platelet aggregation:	[n.a.]

Other results with patient plasma

Ancrod (Arvin) time:	[n.a.]	Inhib. normal plasma?	[No]
Recalcification time:	[n.a.]	In vivo synthesis:	[n.a.]
Calcium corrects c.t.?	[Yes]	In vivo catabolism:	[n.a.]

Evaluation of isolated patient fibrinogen

Thrombin time:	[n.a.]	Abnormal subunit?	[No]
Reptilase time:	[n.a.]	Abnormal FDPs?	[n.a.]
Ancrod (Arvin) time:	[n.a.]		

Remarks

[1]Normal range not reported.
[2]C.L. Arocha-Piñango, personal communication.
[3]Data not reported; Reptilase time was 75s longer than normal.

References

1. Arocha-Piñango, C.L., Bosch, N., Torres, A., Caires-Tronchoni, D., Marchi, R., Vidal, H. and Rizzo, M.G. Dysfibrinogenemias in Latin America. A cooperative study group. *Rev. Iberoamer. Tromb. Hemostasia* **3**:110-122, **1990**.

FIBRINOGEN CARACAS IV

Last update	[10 January 1994]	**Structural defect**	[n.a.]
Alphacode	[CARACA04]	**Mutation**	[n.a.]
Ref. type	[Article]		

Family studies

Homozygote? [n.a.]
Pedigree published? [No]

Functional defect(s)

FpA release: [Normal]
FpB release: [Normal]
Polymerization: [Abnormal]
Stabilization: [n.a.]

Clinical manifestation(s) Bleeding? [Yes[1]] Thrombosis? [No]

Clinical laboratory results

Plasma fibrinogen concentration (mg/dL)

Chronometric: [45[2]]
Rate-indep'nt: [300[2]]
Immunologic: [300[2]]

*Hypo*dysfibrinogen? [No]

Thrombin time:	[36s/(15-18s)[3]]
Reptilase (batroxobin) time:	[Abnormal[4]]
Prothrombin time:	[n.a.]
Partial thromboplastin time:	[n.a.]
Euglobulin lysis time:	[n.a.]
Bleeding time:	[n.a.]
Immunoelectrophoresis:	[Normal]
Platelet aggregation:	[n.a.]

Other results with patient plasma

Ancrod (Arvin) time:	[n.a.]	Inhib. normal plasma?	[No]
Recalcification time:	[n.a.]	In vivo synthesis:	[n.a.]
Calcium corrects c.t.?	[Yes]	In vivo catabolism:	[n.a.]

Evaluation of isolated patient fibrinogen

Thrombin time:	[n.a.]	Abnormal subunit?	[n.a.]
Reptilase time:	[n.a.]	Abnormal FDPs?	[No[5]]
Ancrod (Arvin) time:	[n.a.]		

Remarks

[1]"Moderate" bleeding was reported; details were not provided.
[2]Normal range not reported.
[3]C.L. Arocha-Piñango, personal communication.
[4]Data not reported; Reptilase time was 32s longer than normal.
[5]A decreased *rate* of FDP formation was reported.

Most of the studies were performed on fibrinogen from the proband's affected father.

References

1. Arocha-Piñango, C.L., Bosch, N., Torres, A., Caires-Tronchoni, D., Marchi, R., Vidal, H. and Rizzo, M.G. Dysfibrinogenemias in Latin America. A cooperative study group. *Rev. Iberoamer. Tromb. Hemostasia* **3**:110-122, **1990**.

FIBRINOGEN CARACAS V

Last update [10 January 1994]
Alphacode [CARACA05]
Ref. type [Abstract]

Family studies
Homozygote? [n.a.]
Pedigree published? [No]

Structural defect [n.a.]
Mutation [n.a.]

Functional defect(s)
FpA release: [Normal]
FpB release: [Normal]
Polymerization: [Abnormal]
Stabilization: [Normal]

Clinical manifestation(s) Bleeding? [No] Thrombosis? [Yes[1]]

Clinical laboratory results

Plasma fibrinogen concentration (mg/dL)
Chronometric: [80/(180-400)[2]]
Rate-indep'nt: [530/(200-400)[2]]
Immunologic: [540/(210-450)[2]]

*Hypo*dysfibrinogen? [No]

Thrombin time:	[25s/(15-18s)[2]]
Reptilase (batroxobin) time:	[n.a.]
Prothrombin time:	[29.5s/(11-13s)[2]]
Partial thromboplastin time:	[65s/(42-48s)[2]]
Euglobulin lysis time:	[n.a.]
Bleeding time:	[n.a.]
Immunoelectrophoresis:	[n.a.]
Platelet aggregation:	[n.a.]

Other results with patient plasma
Ancrod (Arvin) time: [n.a.]
Recalcification time: [n.a.]
Calcium corrects c.t.? [n.a.]

Inhib. normal plasma? [n.a.]
In vivo synthesis: [n.a.]
In vivo catabolism: [n.a.]

Evaluation of isolated patient fibrinogen
Thrombin time: [n.a.]
Reptilase time: [n.a.]
Ancrod (Arvin) time: [n.a.]

Abnormal subunit? [n.a.]
Abnormal FDPs? [n.a.]

Remarks

[1]Recurrent pulmonary embolism in mother and affected daughter were reported. Antithrombin III and protein C levels were normal.

[2]C.L. Arocha-Piñango, personal communication.

Electron microscopy of patient fibrinogen and fibrin (Marchi et al., 1990) disclosed no differences from normal.

References

1. Arocha-Piñango, C.L., Torres, A., Marchi, R., Rodríguez, S., Camarillo, H., Muller-Soyano, A. and Bosch, N.B. A new thrombotic dysfibrinogenemia present in several members of a venezuelan family. *Thromb. Haemostas.* **58**:149, **1987**. ABSTRACT

2. Marchi, R., Arocha-Piñango, C.L. and Gil, F. Electron microscopy studies of 7 patients with dysfibrinogenemia and some of their relatives. *Rev. Iberoamer. Tromb. Hemostasia* **3**:185-190, **1990**.

FIBRINOGEN CARACAS VI

Last update [10 January 1994]
Alphacode [CARACA06]
Ref. type [Article]

Family studies
Homozygote? [n.a.]
Pedigree published? [No]

Structural defect [n.a.]
Mutation [n.a.]

Functional defect(s)
FpA release: [Normal]
FpB release: [Normal]
Polymerization: [Abnormal]
Stabilization: [n.a.]

Clinical manifestation(s) Bleeding? [Yes[1]] Thrombosis? [No]

Clinical laboratory results

Plasma fibrinogen concentration (mg/dL)
Chronometric: [75[2]]
Rate-indep'nt: [120[2]]
Immunologic: [120[2]]

*Hypo*dysfibrinogen? [Yes]

Thrombin time:	[31s/(15-18s)[3]]
Reptilase (batroxobin) time:	[Abnormal[4]]
Prothrombin time:	[n.a.]
Partial thromboplastin time:	[n.a.]
Euglobulin lysis time:	[n.a.]
Bleeding time:	[n.a.]
Immunoelectrophoresis:	[Normal]
Platelet aggregation:	[n.a.]

Other results with patient plasma
Ancrod (Arvin) time: [n.a.]
Recalcification time: [n.a.]
Calcium corrects c.t.? [No]

Inhib. normal plasma? [No]
In vivo synthesis: [n.a.]
In vivo catabolism: [n.a.]

Evaluation of isolated patient fibrinogen
Thrombin time: [n.a.]
Reptilase time: [n.a.]
Ancrod (Arvin) time: [n.a.]

Abnormal subunit? [No]
Abnormal FDPs? [No[5]]

Remarks

[1]"Moderate" bleeding was reported; details were not provided.
[2]Normal range not reported.
[3]C.L. Arocha-Piñango, personal communication.
[4]Data not reported; Reptilase time was 45s longer than normal.
[5]An increased *rate* of FDP formation was reported.

Electron microscopy of patient fibrin (Marchi et al., 1990) disclosed a shortened fiber periodicity (18.4 ± 1 nm) compared to normal fibrin (22.2 ± 0.5 nm).

References

1. Arocha-Piñango, C.L., Bosch, N., Torres, A., Caires-Tronchoni, D., Marchi, R., Vidal, H. and Rizzo, M.G. Dysfibrinogenemias in Latin America. A cooperative study group. *Rev. Iberoamer. Tromb. Hemostasia* **3**:110-122, **1990**.

2. Marchi, R., Arocha-Piñango, C.L. and Gil, F. Electron microscopy studies of 7 patients with dysfibrinogenemia and some of their relatives. *Rev. Iberoamer. Tromb. Hemostasia* **3**:185-190, **1990**.

FIBRINOGEN CARACAS VII

Last update [10 January 1994]
Alphacode [CARACA07]
Ref. type [Article]

Family studies
Homozygote? [n.a.]
Pedigree published? [No]

Structural defect [n.a.]
Mutation [n.a.]

Functional defect(s)
FpA release: [n.a.]
FpB release: [n.a.]
Polymerization: [Abnormal]
Stabilization: [Normal]

Clinical manifestation(s) Bleeding? [No] Thrombosis? [No]

Clinical laboratory results
Plasma fibrinogen concentration (mg/dL)
Chronometric: [50[1]]
Rate-indep'nt: [305[1]]
Immunologic: [300[1]]

*Hypo*dysfibrinogen? [No]

Thrombin time:	[30s/(13-15s)[2]]
Reptilase (batroxobin) time:	[Abnormal[3]]
Prothrombin time:	[n.a.]
Partial thromboplastin time:	[n.a.]
Euglobulin lysis time:	[n.a.]
Bleeding time:	[n.a.]
Immunoelectrophoresis:	[Normal]
Platelet aggregation:	[n.a.]

Other results with patient plasma
Ancrod (Arvin) time: [n.a.]
Recalcification time: [n.a.]
Calcium corrects c.t.? [Yes]

Inhib. normal plasma? [No]
In vivo synthesis: [n.a.]
In vivo catabolism: [n.a.]

Evaluation of isolated patient fibrinogen
Thrombin time: [n.a.]
Reptilase time: [n.a.]
Ancrod (Arvin) time: [n.a.]

Abnormal subunit? [n.a.]
Abnormal FDPs? [No[4]]

Remarks
[1]Normal range not reported.
[2]C.L. Arocha-Piñango & N.B. Bosch, personal communication.
[3]Data not reported; Reptilase time was 45s longer than normal.
[4]A decreased *rate* of FDP formation was reported.

Electron microscopy of patient fibrinogen and fibrin (Marchi et al., 1990) disclosed no differences from normal.

References

1. Arocha-Piñango, C.L., Bosch, N., Torres, A., Caires-Tronchoni, D., Marchi, R., Vidal, H. and Rizzo, M.G. Dysfibrinogenemias in Latin America. A cooperative study group. *Rev. Iberoamer. Tromb. Hemostasia* **3**:110-122, **1990**.

2. Marchi, R., Arocha-Piñango, C.L. and Gil, F. Electron microscopy studies of 7 patients with dysfibrinogenemia and some of their relatives. *Rev. Iberoamer. Tromb. Hemostasia* **3**:185-190, **1990**.

FIBRINOGEN CHAPEL HILL I

Last update [1 December 1990]
Alphacode [CHAPEL01]
Ref. type [Article]

Family studies
Homozygote? [n.a.]
Pedigree published? [No]

Structural defect [n.a.]
Mutation [n.a.]

Functional defect(s)
FpA release: [Normal[1]]
FpB release: [Normal[1]]
Polymerization: [Abnormal]
Stabilization: [n.a.]

Clinical manifestation(s) Bleeding? [Yes[2]] Thrombosis? [No]

Clinical laboratory results
Plasma fibrinogen concentration (mg/dL)
Chronometric: [119/(280)]
Rate-indep'nt: [94/(270)]
Immunologic: [131/(355)]

*Hypo*dysfibrinogen? [Yes]

Thrombin time:	[13.3s/(10.5s)]
Reptilase (batroxobin) time:	[26.6s/(20.0s)]
Prothrombin time:	[Normal[3]]
Partial thromboplastin time:	[Normal[3]]
Euglobulin lysis time:	[Normal]
Bleeding time:	[Normal]
Immunoelectrophoresis:	[n.a.]
Platelet aggregation:	[n.a.]

Other results with patient plasma
Ancrod (Arvin) time: [n.a.]
Recalcification time: [n.a.]
Calcium corrects c.t.? [n.a.]

Inhib. normal plasma? [n.a.]
In vivo synthesis: [Normal]
In vivo catabolism: [Normal]

Evaluation of isolated patient fibrinogen
Thrombin time: [18.1s/(16.3s)]
Reptilase time: [n.a.]
Ancrod (Arvin) time: [n.a.]

Abnormal subunit? [No]
Abnormal FDPs? [No[4]]

Remarks
[1]The rate of *total* fibrinopeptide release was normal.
[2]Excessive bleeding after dental extraction was reported in the 20 year-old proposita.
[3]Data not reported.
[4]The *rate* of FDP formation was reduced.

Purified fibrinogen did not gel in the absence of calcium, and exhibited increased α-chain proteolysis when treated with Ancrod.

References

1. McDonagh, R.P., Carrell, N.A., Roberts, H.R., Blatt, P.M. and McDonagh, J. Fibrinogen Chapel Hill: Hypodysfibrinogenemia with a tertiary polymerization defect. *Am. J. Hematol.* **9**:23-38, **1980**.

FIBRINOGEN CHAPEL HILL II

Last update [1 December 1990]
Alphacode [CHAPEL02]
Ref. type [Article]

Structural defect [Aα(16) Arg → His]
Mutation [n.a.]

Family studies
Homozygote? [No]
Pedigree published? [No]

Functional defect(s)
FpA release: [n.a.[1]]
FpB release: [n.a.[1]]
Polymerization: [Abnormal]
Stabilization: [Abnormal[2]]

Clinical manifestation(s) Bleeding? [Yes[3]] Thrombosis? [No]

Clinical laboratory results
Plasma fibrinogen concentration (mg/dL)
Chronometric: [116/(263)]
Rate-indep'nt: [427/(272)]
Immunologic: [408/(235)]

*Hypo*dysfibrinogen? [No]

Thrombin time:	[29.2s/(12.4s)]
Reptilase (batroxobin) time:	[38.2s/(14.8s)]
Prothrombin time:	[14.3s/(12.2s)]
Partial thromboplastin time:	[51.3s/(51.2s)]
Euglobulin lysis time:	[n.a.]
Bleeding time:	[n.a.]
Immunoelectrophoresis:	[n.a.]
Platelet aggregation:	[n.a.]

Other results with patient plasma
Ancrod (Arvin) time: [n.a.]
Recalcification time: [n.a.]
Calcium corrects c.t.? [No]

Inhib. normal plasma? [No]
In vivo synthesis: [n.a.]
In vivo catabolism: [n.a.]

Evaluation of isolated patient fibrinogen
Thrombin time: [n.a.]
Reptilase time: [n.a.]
Ancrod (Arvin) time: [n.a.]

Abnormal subunit? [No]
Abnormal FDPs? [No[4]]

Remarks
[1]The rate of *total* fibrinopeptide release was reduced; individual fibrinopeptide release was not reported.
[2]The rate of factor XIII-catalyzed α-polymer formation was reduced.
[3]Unstable angina and mild bleeding in the 61 year-old propositus were reported.
[4]The *rate* of FDP formation was reduced.

Studies on purified fibrinogen were performed with plasma from the affected son of the propositus. Plasma treated with Ancrod or Reptilase failed to gel at room temperature. At 37 °C fragile clots formed.

References

1. Carrell, N. Functional defects in abnormal fibrinogens. In: *Fibrinogen — Structural Variants and Interactions*, A. Henschen, B. Hessel, J. McDonagh and T. Saldeen (eds.), Walter de Gruyter, Berlin. pp. 155-164, **1985**.

2. Carrell, N. and McDonagh, J. Fibrinogen Chapel Hill II: defective in reactions with thrombin, factor XIIIa and plasmin. *Br. J. Haematol.* **52**:35-47, **1982**.

FIBRINOGEN CHAPEL HILL III

Last update	[1 December 1990]	**Structural defect**	[n.a.]
Alphacode	[CHAPEL03]	**Mutation**	[n.a.]
Ref. type	[Article]		

Family studies
Homozygote? [n.a.]
Pedigree published? [Yes]

Functional defect(s)
FpA release: [n.a.[1]]
FpB release: [n.a.[1]]
Polymerization: [Abnormal]
Stabilization: [Normal]

Clinical manifestation(s) Bleeding? [No] Thrombosis? [Yes[2]]

Clinical laboratory results

Plasma fibrinogen concentration (mg/dL)
Chronometric: [258/(216)]
Rate-indep'nt: [249/(256)]
Immunologic: [332/(235)]

*Hypo*dysfibrinogen? [No]

Thrombin time:	[12.6s/(11.5s)]
Reptilase (batroxobin) time:	[31.0s/(16.3s)]
Prothrombin time:	[Normal[3]]
Partial thromboplastin time:	[Normal[3]]
Euglobulin lysis time:	[>3h/(>3h)]
Bleeding time:	[n.a.]
Immunoelectrophoresis:	[Anodal]
Platelet aggregation:	[n.a.]

Other results with patient plasma

Ancrod (Arvin) time:	[43.0s/(21.2s)]	Inhib. normal plasma?	[n.a.]
Recalcification time:	[n.a.]	In vivo synthesis:	[n.a.]
Calcium corrects c.t.?	[n.a.]	In vivo catabolism:	[n.a.]

Evaluation of isolated patient fibrinogen

Thrombin time:	[n.a.]	Abnormal subunit?	[No]
Reptilase time:	[n.a.]	Abnormal FDPs?	[No[4]]
Ancrod (Arvin) time:	[n.a.]		

Remarks

[1]The rate of *total* fibrinopeptide release was reduced; individual fibrinopeptide release was not reported.
[2]The thrombotic tendency apparently was related to impaired fibrinolysis. Factor XIII activity was 39%.
[3]Data not reported.
[4]The *rate* of FDP formation was reduced.

Fibrin gels were extremely rigid and resistant to lysis by plasmin.

References

1. Carrell, N. Functional defects in abnormal fibrinogens. In: *Fibrinogen — Structural Variants and Interactions*, A. Henschen, B. Hessel, J. McDonagh and T. Saldeen (eds.), Walter de Gruyter, Berlin. pp. 155-164, **1985**.

2. Carrell, N., Gabriel, D.A., Blatt, P.M., Carr, M.E. and McDonagh, J. Hereditary dysfibrinogenemia in a patient with thrombotic disease. *Blood* **62**:439-447, **1983**.

FIBRINOGEN CHAPEL HILL IV

Last update [1 December 1990]
Alphacode [CHAPEL04]
Ref. type [Article]

Family studies
Homozygote? [n.a.]
Pedigree published? [No]

Structural defect [n.a.]
Mutation [n.a.]

Functional defect(s)
FpA release: [n.a.]
FpB release: [n.a.]
Polymerization: [Abnormal]
Stabilization: [Normal]

Clinical manifestation(s) Bleeding? [No[1]] Thrombosis? [No[1]]

Clinical laboratory results
Plasma fibrinogen concentration (mg/dL)
Chronometric: [131/(219)]
Rate-indep'nt: [352/(299)]
Immunologic: [372/(300)]

*Hypo*dysfibrinogen? [No]

Thrombin time:	[20.3s/(11.4s)]
Reptilase (batroxobin) time:	[90s/(14s)]
Prothrombin time:	[n.a.]
Partial thromboplastin time:	[n.a.]
Euglobulin lysis time:	[n.a.]
Bleeding time:	[n.a.]
Immunoelectrophoresis:	[n.a.]
Platelet aggregation:	[n.a.]

Other results with patient plasma
Ancrod (Arvin) time: [n.a.]
Recalcification time: [n.a.]
Calcium corrects c.t.? [n.a.]

Inhib. normal plasma? [n.a.]
In vivo synthesis: [n.a.]
In vivo catabolism: [n.a.]

Evaluation of isolated patient fibrinogen
Thrombin time: [n.a.]
Reptilase time: [n.a.]
Ancrod (Arvin) time: [n.a.]

Abnormal subunit? [n.a.]
Abnormal FDPs? [n.a.]

Remarks
[1]The proposita presented with inflammatory bowel disease.

References

1. Carrell, N. Functional defects in abnormal fibrinogens. In: *Fibrinogen — Structural Variants and Interactions*, A. Henschen, B. Hessel, J. McDonagh and T. Saldeen (eds.), Walter de Gruyter, Berlin. pp. 155-164, **1985**.

FIBRINOGEN CHAPEL HILL V

Last update [10 January 1994]
Alphacode [CHAPEL05]
Ref. type [Article]

Family studies
Homozygote? [n.a.]
Pedigree published? [No]

Structural defect [n.a.]
Mutation [n.a.]

Functional defect(s)
FpA release: [n.a.]
FpB release: [n.a.]
Polymerization: [Abnormal]
Stabilization: [Normal]

Clinical manifestation(s) Bleeding? [n.a.] Thrombosis? [n.a.]

Clinical laboratory results
Plasma fibrinogen concentration (mg/dL)
Chronometric: [99/(225)]
Rate-indep'nt: [n.a.]
Immunologic: [398/(252)]

*Hypo*dysfibrinogen? [No]

Thrombin time: [24.1s/(11.4s)]
Reptilase (batroxobin) time: [78s/(16.3s)]
Prothrombin time: [n.a.]
Partial thromboplastin time: [n.a.]
Euglobulin lysis time: [n.a.]
Bleeding time: [n.a.]
Immunoelectrophoresis: [n.a.]
Platelet aggregation: [n.a.]

Other results with patient plasma
Ancrod (Arvin) time: [No clot]
Recalcification time: [n.a.]
Calcium corrects c.t.? [n.a.]

Inhib. normal plasma? [No]
In vivo synthesis: [n.a.]
In vivo catabolism: [n.a.]

Evaluation of isolated patient fibrinogen
Thrombin time: [n.a.]
Reptilase time: [n.a.]
Ancrod (Arvin) time: [n.a.]

Abnormal subunit? [n.a.]
Abnormal FDPs? [n.a.]

Remarks

References

1. Carrell, N. Functional defects in abnormal fibrinogens. In: *Fibrinogen —Structural Variants and Interactions*, A. Henschen, B. Hessel, J. McDonagh and T. Saldeen (eds.), Walter de Gruyter, Berlin. pp. 155-164, **1985**.

FIBRINOGEN CHAPEL HILL VI

Last update [1 December 1990]
Alphacode [CHAPEL06]
Ref. type [Article]

Family studies
Homozygote? [n.a.]
Pedigree published? [No]

Structural defect [n.a.]
Mutation [n.a.]

Functional defect(s)
FpA release: [n.a.]
FpB release: [n.a.]
Polymerization: [Abnormal[1]]
Stabilization: [Normal]

Clinical manifestation(s) Bleeding? [n.a.] Thrombosis? [n.a.]

Clinical laboratory results
Plasma fibrinogen concentration (mg/dL)
Chronometric: [n.a.]
Rate-indep'nt: [n.a.]
Immunologic: [155/(252)]

*Hypo*dysfibrinogen? [n.a.]

Thrombin time:	[14.1s/(11.5s)]
Reptilase (batroxobin) time:	[13.8s/(16.3s)]
Prothrombin time:	[n.a.]
Partial thromboplastin time:	[n.a.]
Euglobulin lysis time:	[n.a.]
Bleeding time:	[n.a.]
Immunoelectrophoresis:	[n.a.]
Platelet aggregation:	[n.a.]

Other results with patient plasma
Ancrod (Arvin) time: [n.a.]
Recalcification time: [n.a.]
Calcium corrects c.t.? [n.a.]

Inhib. normal plasma? [n.a.]
In vivo synthesis: [n.a.]
In vivo catabolism: [n.a.]

Evaluation of isolated patient fibrinogen
Thrombin time: [n.a.]
Reptilase time: [n.a.]
Ancrod (Arvin) time: [n.a.]

Abnormal subunit? [n.a.]
Abnormal FDPs? [n.a.]

Remarks
[1]An *increased* rate of fibrin monomer polymerization and α-chain crosslinking was observed (compare with fibrinogens Oslo I and Strasbourg I).

References

1. Carrell, N. Functional defects in abnormal fibrinogens. In: *Fibrinogen — Structural Variants and Interactions*, A. Henschen, B. Hessel, J. McDonagh and T. Saldeen (eds.), Walter de Gruyter, Berlin. pp. 155-164, **1985**.

FIBRINOGEN CHAPEL HILL VII

Last update [1 December 1990]
Alphacode [CHAPEL07]
Ref. type [Article]

Family studies
Homozygote? [n.a.]
Pedigree published? [No]

Structural defect [n.a.]
Mutation [n.a.]

Functional defect(s)
FpA release: [n.a.]
FpB release: [n.a.]
Polymerization: [n.a.]
Stabilization: [Normal]

Clinical manifestation(s) Bleeding? [n.a.[1]] Thrombosis? [n.a.[1]]

Clinical laboratory results
Plasma fibrinogen concentration (mg/dL)
Chronometric: [16/(250)]
Rate-indep'nt: [n.a.]
Immunologic: [11/(300)]

*Hypo*dysfibrinogen? [Yes]

Thrombin time:	[34.5s/(11.6s)]
Reptilase (batroxobin) time:	[52s/(14s)]
Prothrombin time:	[n.a.]
Partial thromboplastin time:	[n.a.]
Euglobulin lysis time:	[n.a.]
Bleeding time:	[n.a.]
Immunoelectrophoresis:	[n.a.]
Platelet aggregation:	[n.a.]

Other results with patient plasma
Ancrod (Arvin) time: [n.a.]
Recalcification time: [n.a.]
Calcium corrects c.t.? [n.a.]

Inhib. normal plasma? [No]
In vivo synthesis: [n.a.]
In vivo catabolism: [n.a.]

Evaluation of isolated patient fibrinogen
Thrombin time: [n.a.]
Reptilase time: [n.a.]
Ancrod (Arvin) time: [n.a.]

Abnormal subunit? [n.a.]
Abnormal FDPs? [n.a.]

Remarks
[1]Multiple spontaneous abortions in the first trimester of pregnancy were reported.

References

1. Carrell, N. Functional defects in abnormal fibrinogens. In: *Fibrinogen — Structural Variants and Interactions*, A. Henschen, B. Hessel, J. McDonagh and T. Saldeen (eds.), Walter de Gruyter, Berlin. pp. 155-164, **1985**.

FIBRINOGEN CHARLOTTESVILLE I

Last update [1 December 1990]
Alphacode [CHARLO01]
Ref. type [Article]

Family studies
Homozygote? [Yes]
Pedigree published? [Yes]

Structural defect [n.a.]
Mutation [n.a.]

Functional defect(s)
FpA release: [n.a.[1]]
FpB release: [n.a.[1]]
Polymerization: [Normal[2]]
Stabilization: [Normal[2]]

Clinical manifestation(s) Bleeding? [No] Thrombosis? [Yes[3]]

Clinical laboratory results
Plasma fibrinogen concentration (mg/dL)
Chronometric: [13/(200-400)]
Rate-indep'nt: [390/(200-390)]
Immunologic: [300/(200-400)]

*Hypo*dysfibrinogen? [No]

Thrombin time:	[>200s/(13-19s)]
Reptilase (batroxobin) time:	[>700s/(20-25s)]
Prothrombin time:	[29s/(11-15s)]
Partial thromboplastin time:	[47s/(25-41s)]
Euglobulin lysis time:	[n.a.]
Bleeding time:	[n.a.]
Immunoelectrophoresis:	[n.a.]
Platelet aggregation:	[n.a.]

Other results with patient plasma
Ancrod (Arvin) time: [n.a.]
Recalcification time: [n.a.]
Calcium corrects c.t.? [n.a.]

Inhib. normal plasma? [Yes]
In vivo synthesis: [n.a.]
In vivo catabolism: [n.a.]

Evaluation of isolated patient fibrinogen
Thrombin time: [n.a.]
Reptilase time: [n.a.]
Ancrod (Arvin) time: [n.a.]

Abnormal subunit? [n.a.]
Abnormal FDPs? [n.a.]

Remarks
[1]The rate of *total* fibrinopeptide release was reduced; individual fibrinopeptide release was not reported.
[2]Data not reported.
[3]Recurrent thrombophlebitis and pulmonary embolism in the 40 year-old proposita were reported.

References

1. Laugen, R.H. and Bithell, T.C. Hereditary dysfibrinogenemia characterized by slow fibrinopeptide release and competitive inhibition of thrombin. *Acta Haematol. (Basel)* **71**:150-157, **1984**.

FIBRINOGEN CHICAGO I^{Abs}

Last update [1 December 1990]
Alphacode [CHICAG01]
Ref. type [Abstract]

Structural defect [n.a.]
Mutation [n.a.]

Family studies
Homozygote? [No]
Pedigree published? [No]

Functional defect(s)
FpA release: [n.a.]
FpB release: [n.a.]
Polymerization: [n.a.]
Stabilization: [n.a.]

Clinical manifestation(s) Bleeding? [No] Thrombosis? [Yes[1]]

Clinical laboratory results
Plasma fibrinogen concentration (mg/dL)
Chronometric: [135[2]]
Rate-indep'nt: [150[2]]
Immunologic: [320[2]]

*Hypo*dysfibrinogen? [No]

Thrombin time:	[Abnormal[3]]
Reptilase (batroxobin) time:	[Abnormal[3]]
Prothrombin time:	[n.a.]
Partial thromboplastin time:	[n.a.]
Euglobulin lysis time:	[n.a.]
Bleeding time:	[n.a.]
Immunoelectrophoresis:	[Normal[4]]
Platelet aggregation:	[n.a.]

Other results with patient plasma
Ancrod (Arvin) time: [n.a.]
Recalcification time: [n.a.]
Calcium corrects c.t.? [No]

Inhib. normal plasma? [n.a.]
In vivo synthesis: [n.a.]
In vivo catabolism: [n.a.]

Evaluation of isolated patient fibrinogen
Thrombin time: [n.a.]
Reptilase time: [n.a.]
Ancrod (Arvin) time: [n.a.]

Abnormal subunit? [n.a.]
Abnormal FDPs? [n.a.]

Remarks
[1]Recurrent venous thrombosis in the 24 year-old propositus was reported.
[2]Normal range not reported.
[3]Data not reported.
[4]An abnormal pattern on crossed immunoelectrophoresis was reported.

References

1. Papp, A.C., Snopko, R.M., Cole, E.R., Sassetti, R.J. and Wu, K.K. Recurrent venous thrombosis related to a hereditary dysfibrinogen with abnormal crossed immunoelectrophoretic pattern. *Thromb. Haemostas.* **46**:360, **1981**. ABSTRACT

FIBRINOGEN CHRISTCHURCH I

Last update [1 December 1990]
Alphacode [CHRIST01]
Ref. type [Article[1]]

Family studies
Homozygote? [n.a.]
Pedigree published? [No]

Structural defect [n.a.]
Mutation [n.a.]

Functional defect(s)
FpA release: [Normal]
FpB release: [Normal]
Polymerization: [n.a.]
Stabilization: [n.a.]

Clinical manifestation(s) Bleeding? [n.a.] Thrombosis? [n.a.]

Clinical laboratory results
Plasma fibrinogen concentration (mg/dL)
Chronometric: [n.a.]
Rate-indep'nt: [n.a.]
Immunologic: [n.a.]

*Hypo*dysfibrinogen? [n.a.]

Thrombin time:	[n.a.]
Reptilase (batroxobin) time:	[n.a.]
Prothrombin time:	[n.a.]
Partial thromboplastin time:	[n.a.]
Euglobulin lysis time:	[n.a.]
Bleeding time:	[n.a.]
Immunoelectrophoresis:	[n.a.]
Platelet aggregation:	[n.a.]

Other results with patient plasma
Ancrod (Arvin) time: [n.a.]
Recalcification time: [n.a.]
Calcium corrects c.t.? [n.a.]

Inhib. normal plasma? [n.a.]
In vivo synthesis: [n.a.]
In vivo catabolism: [n.a.]

Evaluation of isolated patient fibrinogen
Thrombin time: [n.a.]
Reptilase time: [n.a.]
Ancrod (Arvin) time: [n.a.]

Abnormal subunit? [n.a.]
Abnormal FDPs? [n.a.]

Remarks
[1]Review article only; D. Heaton, personal communication.

References

1. Henschen, A., Kehl, M. and Southan, C. Genetically abnormal fibrinogens — strategies for structure elucidation, including fibrinopeptide analysis. In: *Variants of Human Fibrinogen*, E.A. Beck and M. Furlan (eds.), Hans Huber Publ., Berne, pp. 273-320, **1984**.

FIBRINOGEN CHRISTCHURCH II

Last update [1 December 1990]
Alphacode [CHRIST02]
Ref. type [Article]

Structural defect [Bβ(14) Arg → Cys]
Mutation [n.a.]

Family studies
Homozygote? [No]
Pedigree published? [No]

Functional defect(s)
FpA release: [Normal]
FpB release: [Abnormal]
Polymerization: [n.a.]
Stabilization: [n.a.]

Clinical manifestation(s) Bleeding? [Yes[1]] Thrombosis? [No]

Clinical laboratory results
Plasma fibrinogen concentration (mg/dL)
Chronometric: [n.a.]
Rate-indep'nt: [n.a.]
Immunologic: [n.a.]

*Hypo*dysfibrinogen? [n.a.]

Thrombin time:	[38s/(20s)]
Reptilase (batroxobin) time:	[26s/(18s)]
Prothrombin time:	[n.a.]
Partial thromboplastin time:	[n.a.]
Euglobulin lysis time:	[n.a.]
Bleeding time:	[n.a.]
Immunoelectrophoresis:	[n.a.]
Platelet aggregation:	[n.a.]

Other results with patient plasma
Ancrod (Arvin) time: [n.a.]
Recalcification time: [n.a.]
Calcium corrects c.t.? [n.a.]

Inhib. normal plasma? [n.a.]
In vivo synthesis: [n.a.]
In vivo catabolism: [n.a.]

Evaluation of isolated patient fibrinogen
Thrombin time: [n.a.]
Reptilase time: [n.a.]
Ancrod (Arvin) time: [n.a.]

Abnormal subunit? [No]
Abnormal FDPs? [n.a.]

Remarks
[1]Recurrent epistaxis in the proposita was reported.

References

1. Kaudewitz, H., Henschen, A., Soria, C., Soria, J., Bertrand, O. and Heaton, D. The molecular defect of the genetically abnormal fibrinogen Christchurch II. In: *Fibrinogen and Its Derivatives*, G. Muller-Berghaus, V. Scheefers-Borchel, E. Selmayr and A. Henschen (eds.), Elsevier, Amsterdam. pp. 31-36, **1986**.

FIBRINOGEN CLERMONT-FERRAND I

Last update	[1 December 1990]	**Structural defect**	[Aα(16) Arg → His]
Alphacode	[CLERMO01]	**Mutation**	[n.a.]
Ref. type	[Article]		

Family studies
Homozygote? [n.a.]
Pedigree published? [No]

Functional defect(s)
FpA release: [n.a.]
FpB release: [n.a.]
Polymerization: [Abnormal]
Stabilization: [Abnormal]

Clinical manifestation(s) Bleeding? [n.a.] Thrombosis? [n.a.]

Clinical laboratory results

Plasma fibrinogen concentration (mg/dL)
Chronometric: [n.a.]
Rate-indep'nt: [n.a.]
Immunologic: [n.a.]

*Hypo*dysfibrinogen? [n.a.]

Thrombin time:	[n.a.]
Reptilase (batroxobin) time:	[n.a.]
Prothrombin time:	[n.a.]
Partial thromboplastin time:	[n.a.]
Euglobulin lysis time:	[n.a.]
Bleeding time:	[n.a.]
Immunoelectrophoresis:	[n.a.]
Platelet aggregation:	[n.a.]

Other results with patient plasma

Ancrod (Arvin) time:	[n.a.]	Inhib. normal plasma?	[n.a.]
Recalcification time:	[n.a.]	In vivo synthesis:	[n.a.]
Calcium corrects c.t.?	[n.a.]	In vivo catabolism:	[n.a.]

Evaluation of isolated patient fibrinogen

Thrombin time:	[n.a.]	Abnormal subunit?	[n.a.]
Reptilase time:	[n.a.]	Abnormal FDPs?	[No]
Ancrod (Arvin) time:	[n.a.]		

Remarks

Results are from review articles; Soria et al. (1975) is not on file.

References

1. Soria, J., Soria, C., Samama, M. and Caen, J. Study of ten cases of congenital dysfibrinogenemia. Clinical and molecular biological aspects. In: *Fibrinogen — Structural Variants and Interactions*, A. Henschen, B. Hessel, J. McDonagh and T. Saldeen (eds.), Walter de Gruyter, Berlin. pp. 165-183, **1985**.

2. Haverkate, F., Timan, G., Soria, J., Soria, C. and Samama, M.M. Studies on the structure of the fragment D moiety of abnormal fibrinogens: Influence of calcium ions. *Thromb. Res.* **13**:689-692, **1978**.

3. Soria, J., Soria, C., Bezou, M.J., Picot, J., Bernard-Griffiths, I. and Coulet, M. [Dysfibrinogenemia with defective aggregation of fibrin monomers: fibrinogen Clermont-Ferrand]. *Proc. I Congr. Franc. Hematol.* p. 66, **1975**.

FIBRINOGEN CLEVELAND I

Last update [10 January 1994]
Alphacode [CLEVEL01]
Ref. type [Article]

Family studies
Homozygote? [n.a.]
Pedigree published? [Yes]

Structural defect [n.a.]
Mutation [n.a.]

Functional defect(s)
FpA release: [Normal]
FpB release: [Normal]
Polymerization: [Abnormal]
Stabilization: [Normal]

Clinical manifestation(s) Bleeding? [No[1]] Thrombosis? [No[1]]

Clinical laboratory results
Plasma fibrinogen concentration (mg/dL)
Chronometric: [n.a.]
Rate-indep'nt: [332/(177-415)]
Immunologic: [n.a.]

*Hypo*dysfibrinogen? [No]

Thrombin time:	[80s/(26-34s)]
Reptilase (batroxobin) time:	[165s/(70-80s)]
Prothrombin time:	[16.5s/(12-14s)]
Partial thromboplastin time:	[119s/(60-100s)]
Euglobulin lysis time:	[>180m/(>180m)]
Bleeding time:	[Normal]
Immunoelectrophoresis:	[Abnormal]
Platelet aggregation:	[Normal]

Other results with patient plasma
Ancrod (Arvin) time: [n.a.]
Recalcification time: [n.a.]
Calcium corrects c.t.? [No]

Inhib. normal plasma? [Yes]
In vivo synthesis: [n.a.]
In vivo catabolism: [n.a.]

Evaluation of isolated patient fibrinogen
Thrombin time: [n.a.]
Reptilase time: [n.a.]
Ancrod (Arvin) time: [n.a.]

Abnormal subunit? [Yes[2]]
Abnormal FDPs? [n.a.]

Remarks
[1]The patient exhibited surgical wound dehiscence that was treated successfully with ε-aminocaproic acid.
[2]The Aα-chain was about 3,000 Da smaller than normal.

References

1. Forman, W.B. and Kraus, J. Transurethral resection in a patient with a dysfibrinogen: fibrinogen Cleveland I. *J. Urol.* **118**:885-885, **1977**.

2. Forman, W.B. and Hadady, M. A simplified method for isolation of the S-carboxymethyl derivative chains of normal fibrinogen and fibrinogen Cleveland I. *Thromb. Res.* **8**:731-736, **1976**.

3. Forman, W.B., Ratnoff, O.D. and Boyer, M.H. An inherited qualitative abnormality in plasma fibrinogen: fibrinogen Cleveland. *J. Lab. Clin. Med.* **72**:455-472, **1968**.

4. Forman, W.B., Boyer, M.H. and Ratnoff, O.D. A hereditary defect in the coagulation of fibrinogen by thrombin: studies in a family with fibrinogen Cleveland. *Blood* **30**:863, **1967**. ABSTRACT

FIBRINOGEN CLEVELAND II

Last update [10 January 1994]
Alphacode [CLEVEL02]
Ref. type [Article]

Family studies
Homozygote? [n.a.]
Pedigree published? [Yes]

Structural defect [n.a.]
Mutation [n.a.]

Functional defect(s)
FpA release: [Abnormal]
FpB release: [Normal]
Polymerization: [Abnormal]
Stabilization: [Abnormal]

Clinical manifestation(s) Bleeding? [No] Thrombosis? [No]

Clinical laboratory results
Plasma fibrinogen concentration (mg/dL)
Chronometric: [n.a.]
Rate-indep'nt: [289/(177-415)]
Immunologic: [n.a.]

*Hypo*dysfibrinogen? [No]

Thrombin time:	[68s/(30s)]
Reptilase (batroxobin) time:	[50s/(21s)]
Prothrombin time:	[16.8s/(13.4s)]
Partial thromboplastin time:	[53.6s/(52.7s)]
Euglobulin lysis time:	[n.a.]
Bleeding time:	[Normal]
Immunoelectrophoresis:	[Normal]
Platelet aggregation:	[Normal]

Other results with patient plasma
Ancrod (Arvin) time: [n.a.]
Recalcification time: [n.a.]
Calcium corrects c.t.? [Yes]

Inhib. normal plasma? [Yes]
In vivo synthesis: [n.a.]
In vivo catabolism: [n.a.]

Evaluation of isolated patient fibrinogen
Thrombin time: [77s/(27.4s)]
Reptilase time: [196s/(84s)]
Ancrod (Arvin) time: [>1200s/(33.3s)]

Abnormal subunit? [No]
Abnormal FDPs? [n.a.]

Remarks

References

1. Crum, E.D., Shainoff, J.R., Graham, R.C. and Ratnoff, O.D. Fibrinogen Cleveland II. An abnormal fibrinogen with defective release of fibrinopeptide A. *J. Clin. Invest.* **53**:1308-1319, **1974**.

2. Crum, E.D., Shainoff, J.R. and Ratnoff, O.D. Fibrinogen Cleveland II. *Clin. Res.* **21**:550, **1973**. ABSTRACT

FIBRINOGEN COPENHAGEN I

Last update [1 December 1990]
Alphacode [COPENH01]
Ref. type [Article]

Family studies
Homozygote? [n.a.]
Pedigree published? [Yes]

Structural defect [n.a.]
Mutation [n.a.]

Functional defect(s)
FpA release: [Abnormal]
FpB release: [n.a.]
Polymerization: [Abnormal]
Stabilization: [n.a.]

Clinical manifestation(s) Bleeding? [No] Thrombosis? [Yes[1]]

Clinical laboratory results
Plasma fibrinogen concentration (mg/dL)
Chronometric: [n.a.]
Rate-indep'nt: [Normal[2]]
Immunologic: [Normal[2]]

*Hypo*dysfibrinogen? [No]

Thrombin time:	[30s/(13-17s)]
Reptilase (batroxobin) time:	[n.a.]
Prothrombin time:	[n.a.]
Partial thromboplastin time:	[n.a.]
Euglobulin lysis time:	[Normal]
Bleeding time:	[n.a.]
Immunoelectrophoresis:	[Normal]
Platelet aggregation:	[n.a.]

Other results with patient plasma
Ancrod (Arvin) time: [63s/(18-33s)]
Recalcification time: [n.a.]
Calcium corrects c.t.? [No]

Inhib. normal plasma? [No]
In vivo synthesis: [n.a.]
In vivo catabolism: [n.a.]

Evaluation of isolated patient fibrinogen
Thrombin time: [n.a.]
Reptilase time: [n.a.]
Ancrod (Arvin) time: [n.a.]

Abnormal subunit? [No]
Abnormal FDPs? [n.a.]

Remarks
[1]Three myocardial infarctions during a 2-year period were reported in the 53 year-old proposita.
[2]Data not reported.

References

1. Henschen, A., Kehl, M., Southan, C., Lottspeich, F. and Georgopoulos, D. Genetically abnormal fibrinogens — some current characterisation strategies. In: *Fibrinogen —Structure, Functional Aspects, Metabolism*, F. Haverkate, A. Henschen, W. Nieuwenhuizen and P.W. Straub (eds.), Walter de Gruyter, Berlin. pp. 125-144, **1983**.

2. Hansen, S.M., Clemmensen, I. and Wither, D. Fibrinogen Copenhagen; an abnormal fibrinogen with defective polymerization and release of fibrinopeptide A, but normal adsorption of plasminogen. *Scand. J. Clin. Lab. Invest.* **40**:221-226, **1980**.

FIBRINOGEN COPENHAGEN II

Last update [1 December 1990]
Alphacode [COPENH02]
Ref. type [Article]

Family studies
Homozygote? [n.a.]
Pedigree published? [No]

Structural defect [n.a.]
Mutation [n.a.]

Functional defect(s)
FpA release: [n.a.]
FpB release: [n.a.]
Polymerization: [Abnormal]
Stabilization: [n.a.]

Clinical manifestation(s) Bleeding? [No] Thrombosis? [Yes[1]]

Clinical laboratory results

Plasma fibrinogen concentration (mg/dL)
Chronometric: [n.a.]
Rate-indep'nt: [n.a.]
Immunologic: [1071/(204-442)]

*Hypo*dysfibrinogen? [No]

Thrombin time:	[22s/(13-17s)]
Reptilase (batroxobin) time:	[31s/(16s)]
Prothrombin time:	[n.a.]
Partial thromboplastin time:	[Normal[2]]
Euglobulin lysis time:	[5.3h/(2-4h)]
Bleeding time:	[n.a.]
Immunoelectrophoresis:	[Normal[3]]
Platelet aggregation:	[n.a.]

Other results with patient plasma
Ancrod (Arvin) time: [n.a.]
Recalcification time: [n.a.]
Calcium corrects c.t.? [n.a.]

Inhib. normal plasma? [n.a.]
In vivo synthesis: [n.a.]
In vivo catabolism: [n.a.]

Evaluation of isolated patient fibrinogen
Thrombin time: [33s/(18s)]
Reptilase time: [n.a.]
Ancrod (Arvin) time: [n.a.]

Abnormal subunit? [n.a.]
Abnormal FDPs? [n.a.]

Remarks
[1]Renal vein thrombosis in the 25 year-old propositus was reported.
[2]Data not reported.
[3]This result is inconsistent with the finding of increased sialic acid content.

References

1. Hansen, M.S. and Schousboe, I. An abnormal fibrinogen (Copenhagen II) with increased sialic acid content associated with thrombotic tendency and normal liver function. *Scand. J. Haematol.* **33**:9-14, **1984**.

FIBRINOGEN DATE I

Last update [10 January 1994]
Alphacode [DATE01]
Ref. type [Article]

Family studies
Homozygote? [n.a.]
Pedigree published? [Yes]

Structural defect [n.a.]
Mutation [n.a.]

Functional defect(s)
FpA release: [Normal]
FpB release: [Normal]
Polymerization: [Abnormal]
Stabilization: [n.a.]

Clinical manifestation(s) Bleeding? [No] Thrombosis? [Yes[1]]

Clinical laboratory results
Plasma fibrinogen concentration (mg/dL)
Chronometric: [45/(200-400)]
Rate-indep'nt: [n.a.]
Immunologic: [106/(180-460)]

*Hypo*dysfibrinogen? [Yes]

Thrombin time:	[48.5s/(13.5-20.4s)]
Reptilase (batroxobin) time:	[n.a.]
Prothrombin time:	[16.8/(10.3-11.5)]
Partial thromboplastin time:	[n.a.]
Euglobulin lysis time:	[n.a.]
Bleeding time:	[n.a.]
Immunoelectrophoresis:	[n.a.]
Platelet aggregation:	[n.a.]

Other results with patient plasma
Ancrod (Arvin) time: [n.a.]
Recalcification time: [n.a.]
Calcium corrects c.t.? [No]

Inhib. normal plasma? [n.a.]
In vivo synthesis: [n.a.]
In vivo catabolism: [n.a.]

Evaluation of isolated patient fibrinogen
Thrombin time: [32.3s/(<20.5s)]
Reptilase time: [n.a.]
Ancrod (Arvin) time: [n.a.]

Abnormal subunit? [No]
Abnormal FDPs? [No[2]]

Remarks
[1]Arterial and venous thrombosis were reported.
[2]Decreased t-PA binding to patient fibrin was reported; see also NIJMEGEN I.

References

1. Ieko, M., Sawada, K.-I., Sakurama, S., Yamagishi, I., Isogawa, S., Nakagawa, S., Satoh, M., Yasukouchi, T. and Matsuda, M. Fibrinogen Date: Congenital hypodysfibrinogenemia associated with decreased binding of tissue-plasminogen activator. *Am. J. Hematol.* **37**:228-233, **1991**.

FIBRINOGEN DETROIT I

Last update [1 December 1990]
Alphacode [DETROI01]
Ref. type [Article]

Family studies
Homozygote? [Yes]
Pedigree published? [Yes]

Structural defect [Aα(19) Arg → Ser]
Mutation [n.a.]

Functional defect(s)
FpA release: [Normal[1]]
FpB release: [Abnormal[1]]
Polymerization: [Abnormal]
Stabilization: [Normal]

Clinical manifestation(s) Bleeding? [Yes[2]] Thrombosis? [No]

Clinical laboratory results

Plasma fibrinogen concentration (mg/dL)
Chronometric: [0/(200-300)]
Rate-indep'nt: [300/(200-350)]
Immunologic: [960/(397-641)]

*Hypo*dysfibrinogen? [No]

Thrombin time:	[>60s/(14.5s)]
Reptilase (batroxobin) time:	[n.a.[3]]
Prothrombin time:	[>30s/(12.6s)]
Partial thromboplastin time:	[>600s/(50-70s)]
Euglobulin lysis time:	[>180m/(>180m)]
Bleeding time:	[Normal]
Immunoelectrophoresis:	[Anodal]
Platelet aggregation:	[n.a.]

Other results with patient plasma
Ancrod (Arvin) time: [n.a.]
Recalcification time: [>600s/(80-120s)]
Calcium corrects c.t.? [No]

Inhib. normal plasma? [Yes]
In vivo synthesis: [n.a.]
In vivo catabolism: [n.a.]

Evaluation of isolated patient fibrinogen
Thrombin time: [n.a.]
Reptilase time: [n.a.[3]]
Ancrod (Arvin) time: [n.a.]

Abnormal subunit? [No]
Abnormal FDPs? [n.a.]

Remarks

[1]The rate of *total* fibrinopeptide release was reduced, and indirect evidence indicated that no fibrinopeptide B was released. The authors concluded that fibrinopeptide A was released at the normal rate, but that fibrinopeptide B was not released.

[2]Menorrhagia in the 17 year-old proposita was reported.

[3]The *rate* of fibrinopeptide A release by Reptilase was normal.

FIBRINOGEN DETROIT I

References

1. Hawiger, J., Hammond, D.K., Timmons, S. and Budzynski, A.Z. Interaction of human fibrinogen with Staphylococci: Presence of a binding region on normal and abnormal fibrinogen variants and fibrinogen derivatives. *Blood* **51**:799-812, **1978**.

2. Kudryk, B., Blombäck, B. and Blombäck, M. Fibrinogen Detroit — an abnormal fibrinogen with non-functional NH2-terminal polymerization domain. *Thromb. Res.* **9**:25-36, **1976**.

3. Blombäck, B. and Blombäck, M. Molecular defects and variants of fibrinogen. *Nouv. Rev. Fr. Hematol.* **10**:671-678, **1970**.

4. Blombäck, M. and Blombäck, B. Fibrinogen Detroit — a molecular defect in the N-terminal disulphide knot. In: *Hemophilia and New Hemorrhagic States*, K.M. Brinkhous (ed.), Univ. of North Carolina Press, Chapel Hill. pp. 242-246, **1970**.

5. Mammen, E.F., Prasad, A.S., Barnhart, M.I. and Au, C.C. Fibrinogen Detroit. In: *Hemophilia and New Hemorrhagic States*, K.M. Brinkhous (ed.), Univ. of North Carolina Press, Chapel Hill. pp. 233-241, **1970**.

6. Mammen, E.F., Prasad, A.S., Barnhart, M.I. and Au, C.C. Congenital dysfibrinogenemia: fibrinogen Detroit. *J. Clin. Invest.* **48**:235-249, **1969**.

7. Blombäck, M., Blombäck, B., Mammen, E.F. and Prasad, A.S. Fibrinogen Detroit — a molecular defect in the N-terminal disulphide knot of human fibrinogen. *Nature* **218**:134-137, **1968**.

8. Mammen, E.F., Prasad, A.S. and Au, C.C. Studies on a family with dysfibrinogenemia. *Thromb. Diath. Haemorrh.* **19**:603-604, **1968**.

9. Mammen, E.F. and Prasad, A.S. [Familial dysfibrinogenemia—"Detroit fibrinogen"]. *Verh. Dtsch. Ges. Inn. Med.* **74**:140-144, **1968**.

FIBRINOGEN DUSART I[1]

Last update	[10 January 1994]	**Structural defect**	[Aα(554) Arg → Cys[2]]
Alphacode	[DUSART01]	**Mutation**	[CGT → TGT]
Ref. type	[Article]		

Family studies
Homozygote? [No]
Pedigree published? [Yes]

Functional defect(s)
FpA release: [Normal[3]]
FpB release: [Normal[3]]
Polymerization: [Abnormal]
Stabilization: [Normal]

Clinical manifestation(s) Bleeding? [No] Thrombosis? [Yes[4]]

Clinical laboratory results

Plasma fibrinogen concentration (mg/dL)
Chronometric: [165/(200-400)]
Rate-indep'nt: [n.a.]
Immunologic: [190/(200-400)]

*Hypo*dysfibrinogen? [No]

Thrombin time:	[35s/(20s)]
Reptilase (batroxobin) time:	[29.5s/(20s)]
Prothrombin time:	[17.5s/(12s)]
Partial thromboplastin time:	[n.a.]
Euglobulin lysis time:	[n.a.]
Bleeding time:	[n.a.]
Immunoelectrophoresis:	[n.a.]
Platelet aggregation:	[Normal]

Other results with patient plasma

Ancrod (Arvin) time:	[n.a.]	Inhib. normal plasma?	[n.a.]
Recalcification time:	[n.a.]	In vivo synthesis:	[n.a.]
Calcium corrects c.t.?	[n.a.]	In vivo catabolism:	[n.a.]

Evaluation of isolated patient fibrinogen

Thrombin time:	[22s/(12s)]	Abnormal subunit?	[No]
Reptilase time:	[27s/(18s)]	Abnormal FDPs?	[No[5]]
Ancrod (Arvin) time:	[n.a.]		

Remarks

Disulfide-linked fibrinogen-albumin complexes were reported.

[1]Also known as "DUSAR<u>D</u> I and "PARIS V." The preferred title is "DUSART I." In violation of the usual naming conventions, this variant was named after the family in whom it was discovered.

[2]The structural defect was determined with the PCR method.

[3]The rate of *total* fibrinopeptide release was normal.

[4]Recurrent venous thrombosis and fatal pulmonary embolism were reported. Caen (1990) reported recurrent pulmonary embolism despite anticoagulant therapy. Koopman et al. (1993) give a comprehensive family history.

[5]Defective lysis by plasmin, presumably due to a reduced rate of t-PA activation in the presence of the variant fibrin, was reported. Collet et al. (1993) describe "Dusart syndrome," a condition characterized by high incidence of thrombotic emboli due to the reduced fibrinolysis and increased clot "brittleness" associated with abnormal clot architecture.

FIBRINOGEN DUSART I

References

1. Collet, J.P., Soria, J., Mirshahi, M., Hirsch, M., Dagonnet, F.B., Caen, J. and Soria, C. Dusart syndrome: A new concept of the relationship between fibrin clot architecture and fibrin clot degradability: Hypofibrinolysis related to an abnormal clot structure. *Blood* **82**:2462-2469, **1993**.

2.. Koopman, J., Haverkate, F., Grimbergen, J., Lord, S.T., Mosesson, M.W., DiOrio, J.P., Siebenlist, K.S., Legrand, C., Soria, J., Soria, C. and Caen, J.P. Molecular basis for fibrinogen Dusart (Aα 554 Arg→Cys) and its association with abnormal fibrin polymerization and thrombophilia. *J. Clin. Invest.* **91**:1637-1643, **1993**.

3. Siebenlist, K.R., Mosesson, M.W., DiOrio, J.P., Soria, J., Soria, C. and Caen, J.P. The polymerization of fibrinogen Dusart (Aα 554 Arg → Cys) after removal of carboxy terminal regions of the Aα-chains. *Blood Coag. & Fibrinol.* **4**:61-65, **1993**.

4. Caen, J. Dusard syndrome in 1990. *Proc. X Intl. Fgen. Wkshp.*, **1990** ABSTRACT.

5. Soria, C., Soria, J., Mirshahi, M., Desvignes, P., Bonnet, P. and Caen, J.P. [Importance of the structure of the clot in thrombolysis]. *Ann. Biol. Clin. (Paris)* **45**:207-211, **1987**.

6. Lijnen, H.R., Soria, J., Soria, C., Collen, D. and Caen, J.P. Dysfibrinogenemia (fibrinogen Dusard) associated with impaired fibrin-enhanced plasminogen activation. *Thromb. Haemostas.* **51**:108-109, **1984**.

7. Soria, J., Soria, C. and Caen, P. A new type of congenital dysfibrinogenaemia with defective fibrin lysis—Dusard syndrome: possible relation to thrombosis. *Br. J. Haematol.* **53**:575-586, **1983**.

8. Caen, J.P., Soria, J. and Soria, C. [Structural anomaly of the fibrin clot with reduction of lys-plasminogen binding, as a cause of familial thrombosis]. *C. R. Seances. Acad. Sci. [III]* **294**:695-697, **1982**.

FIBRINOGEN ERFURT I

Last update [10 January 1994]
Alphacode [ERFURT01]
Ref. type [Article]

Family studies
Homozygote? [No]
Pedigree published? [Yes]

Structural defect [n.a.]
Mutation [n.a.]

Functional defect(s)
FpA release: [Normal]
FpB release: [Normal]
Polymerization: [n.a.]
Stabilization: [n.a.]

Clinical manifestation(s) Bleeding? [No] Thrombosis? [No]

Clinical laboratory results
Plasma fibrinogen concentration (mg/dL)
Chronometric: [193[1]]
Rate-indep'nt: [198[1]]
Immunologic: [n.a.]

*Hypo*dysfibrinogen? [No]

Thrombin time:	[Normal[2]]
Reptilase (batroxobin) time:	[Normal[2]]
Prothrombin time:	[Normal[2]]
Partial thromboplastin time:	[Normal[2]]
Euglobulin lysis time:	[n.a.]
Bleeding time:	[n.a.]
Immunoelectrophoresis:	[n.a.]
Platelet aggregation:	[n.a.]

Other results with patient plasma
Ancrod (Arvin) time: [n.a.]
Recalcification time: [n.a.]
Calcium corrects c.t.? [n.a.]

Inhib. normal plasma? [n.a.]
In vivo synthesis: [n.a.]
In vivo catabolism: [n.a.]

Evaluation of isolated patient fibrinogen
Thrombin time: [n.a.]
Reptilase time: [n.a.]
Ancrod (Arvin) time: [n.a.]

Abnormal subunit? [Yes[3]]
Abnormal FDPs? [n.a.]

Remarks
[1]Normal range not reported.
[2]Data not reported.
[3]High-resolution 2D electrophoresis was used to demonstrate the presence of a Bβ-chain with a slight decrease in m.w. (see also NEW YORK I). Detection of this undersized Bβ-chain in plasma and platelet fibrinogen was advanced as evidence for a common origin of these fibrinogen pools.

References

1. Meyer, M., Schellenberg, I., Vogel, G. and Bischoff, I. A new genetic fibrinogen variant (Fibrinogen Erfurt I) structurally characterized by an abnormal Bβ-chain and present both in plasma and platelets. *Thromb. Haemostas.* **59**:138-142, **1988**.

2. Meyer, M., Vogel, G., Gromnica-Ihle, E., Schellenberg, I. and Ostermann, G. Hereditary dysfibrinogenaemia: structural and functional studies on three fibrinogen variants. *Folia Haematol. (Leipz.)* **115**:499-502, **1988**.

FIBRINOGEN ERFURT II

Last update [1 December 1990]
Alphacode [ERFURT02]
Ref. type [Article]

Structural defect [n.a.]
Mutation [n.a.]

Family studies
Homozygote? [No]
Pedigree published? [No]

Functional defect(s)
FpA release: [Abnormal[1]]
FpB release: [Normal]
Polymerization: [n.a.]
Stabilization: [n.a.]

Clinical manifestation(s) Bleeding? [Yes[2]] Thrombosis? [No]

Clinical laboratory results
Plasma fibrinogen concentration (mg/dL)
Chronometric: [n.a.]
Rate-indep'nt: [n.a.]
Immunologic: [n.a.]

*Hypo*dysfibrinogen? [n.a.]

Thrombin time:	[Abnormal[3]]
Reptilase (batroxobin) time:	[n.a.]
Prothrombin time:	[n.a.]
Partial thromboplastin time:	[n.a.]
Euglobulin lysis time:	[n.a.]
Bleeding time:	[n.a.]
Immunoelectrophoresis:	[n.a.]
Platelet aggregation:	[n.a.]

Other results with patient plasma
Ancrod (Arvin) time: [n.a.]
Recalcification time: [n.a.]
Calcium corrects c.t.? [n.a.]

Inhib. normal plasma? [n.a.]
In vivo synthesis: [n.a.]
In vivo catabolism: [n.a.]

Evaluation of isolated patient fibrinogen
Thrombin time: [n.a.]
Reptilase time: [n.a.]
Ancrod (Arvin) time: [n.a.]

Abnormal subunit? [No]
Abnormal FDPs? [n.a.]

Remarks
[1]High-resolution two-dimensional electrophoresis indicated that fibrinopeptide A was not released.
[2]"Occasional bleeding" was reported.
[3]Data not reported.

References

1. Meyer, M., Vogel, G., Gromnica-Ihle, E., Schellenberg, I. and Ostermann, G. Hereditary dysfibrinogenaemia: structural and functional studies on three fibrinogen variants. *Folia Haematol. (Leipz.)* **115**:499-502, **1988**.

FIBRINOGEN ESSEN I

Last update [1 December 1990]
Alphacode [ESSEN01]
Ref. type [Article]

Family studies
Homozygote? [No]
Pedigree published? [No]

Structural defect [γ(275) Arg → His]
Mutation [n.a.]

Functional defect(s)
FpA release: [Normal]
FpB release: [Normal]
Polymerization: [Abnormal]
Stabilization: [n.a.]

Clinical manifestation(s) Bleeding? [No[1]] Thrombosis? [No[1]]

Clinical laboratory results
Plasma fibrinogen concentration (mg/dL)
Chronometric: [10/(200)]
Rate-indep'nt: [240/(200)]
Immunologic: [200/(200)]

*Hypo*dysfibrinogen? [No]

Thrombin time:	[46.4s/(12.5s)]
Reptilase (batroxobin) time:	[53.8s/(17.6s)]
Prothrombin time:	[n.a.]
Partial thromboplastin time:	[n.a.]
Euglobulin lysis time:	[n.a.]
Bleeding time:	[n.a.]
Immunoelectrophoresis:	[n.a.]
Platelet aggregation:	[n.a.]

Other results with patient plasma
Ancrod (Arvin) time: [n.a.]
Recalcification time: [n.a.]
Calcium corrects c.t.? [n.a.]

Inhib. normal plasma? [n.a.]
In vivo synthesis: [n.a.]
In vivo catabolism: [n.a.]

Evaluation of isolated patient fibrinogen
Thrombin time: [n.a.]
Reptilase time: [n.a.]
Ancrod (Arvin) time: [n.a.]

Abnormal subunit? [n.a.]
Abnormal FDPs? [n.a.]

Remarks
[1]Case reports for fibrinogens Essen and Perugia (same molecular defect) are negative for thrombotic or bleeding tendency. However, a thrombotic tendency has been described for fibrinogen Bergamo II, which also contains the γ(275) Arg → His substitution.

References

1. Reber, P., Furlan, M., Henschen, A. and Beck, E.A. Three new fibrinogen variants with defective polymerization sites in the γ-chain. In: *Fibrinogen and Its Derivatives. Biochemistry, Physiology and Pathophysiology*, G. Müller-Berghaus, U. Scheefers-Borchel, E. Selmayr and A. Henschen (eds.), Excerpta Medica, Amsterdam. pp. 41-42, **1986**.

2. Reber, P., Furlan, M., Henschen, A., Kaudewitz, H., Barbui, T., Hilgard, P., Nenci, G.G., Berrettini, M. and Beck, E.A. Three abnormal fibrinogen variants with the same amino acid substitution (γ-275 Arg → His): fibrinogens Bergamo II, Essen and Perugia. *Thromb. Haemostas.* **56**:401-406, **1986**.

FIBRINOGEN FRANKFURT I

Last update [1 December 1990]
Alphacode [FRANKF01]
Ref. type [Article]

Family studies
Homozygote? [n.a.]
Pedigree published? [No]

Structural defect [n.a.]
Mutation [n.a.]

Functional defect(s)
FpA release: [Normal]
FpB release: [Normal]
Polymerization: [Abnormal]
Stabilization: [n.a.]

Clinical manifestation(s) Bleeding? [No] Thrombosis? [Yes[1]]

Clinical laboratory results

Plasma fibrinogen concentration (mg/dL)
Chronometric: [27.5/(200-400)[2]]
Rate-indep'nt: [180/(160-320)[2]]
Immunologic: [162/(160-300)[2]]

*Hypo*dysfibrinogen? [No]

Thrombin time:	[60s/(<22s)]
Reptilase (batroxobin) time:	[>85s/(<20s)[2]]
Prothrombin time:	[22s/(16s)[2]]
Partial thromboplastin time:	[37.5s/(20-40s)[2]]
Euglobulin lysis time:	[n.a.]
Bleeding time:	[Normal]
Immunoelectrophoresis:	[n.a.[3]]
Platelet aggregation:	[Normal]

Other results with patient plasma
Ancrod (Arvin) time: [n.a.]
Recalcification time: [n.a.]
Calcium corrects c.t.? [n.a.]

Inhib. normal plasma? [No]
In vivo synthesis: [n.a.]
In vivo catabolism: [n.a.]

Evaluation of isolated patient fibrinogen
Thrombin time: [n.a.]
Reptilase time: [n.a.]
Ancrod (Arvin) time: [n.a.]

Abnormal subunit? [n.a.]
Abnormal FDPs? [n.a.]

Remarks
[1]Pulmonary embolism in the father of the proposita was reported.
[2]I. Scharrer, personal communication.
[3]An abnormal pattern was found on 2-dimensional immunoelectrophoresis.

References

1. Henschen, A., Kehl, M., Southan, C., Lottspeich, F. and Georgopoulos, D. Genetically abnormal fibrinogens — some current characterisation strategies. In: *Fibrinogen —Structure, Functional Aspects, Metabolism*, F. Haverkate, A. Henschen, W. Nieuwenhuizen and P.W. Straub (eds.), Walter de Gruyter, Berlin. pp. 125-144, **1983**.

2. Scharrer, I., Kirchmaier, C. and Maas, C. [Experimental study of congenital dysfibrinogenemia ("Fibrinogen Frankfurt")]. In: *Fibrinogen, Fibrin und Fibrinkleber*, K.I. Schimpf (ed.), F.K. Schattauer, Stuttgart, New York. pp. 165-173, **1980**.

3. Scharrer, I., Kirchmaier, C. and Maas, C. [Experimental study of congenital dysfibrinogenemia ("Fibrinogen Frankfurt")]. *Blut* **38**:62-62, **1979**. ABSTRACT

FIBRINOGEN FRANKFURT II

Last update [1 December 1990]
Alphacode [FRANKF02]
Ref. type [Article]

Family studies
Homozygote? [n.a.]
Pedigree published? [No]

Structural defect [n.a.]
Mutation [n.a.]

Functional defect(s)
FpA release: [Abnormal[1]]
FpB release: [n.a.]
Polymerization: [Abnormal[2]]
Stabilization: [n.a.]

Clinical manifestation(s) Bleeding? [Yes] Thrombosis? [No]

Clinical laboratory results
Plasma fibrinogen concentration (mg/dL)
Chronometric: [44/(200-400)]
Rate-indep'nt: [240/(160-320)]
Immunologic: [286/(160-300)]

*Hypo*dysfibrinogen? [No]

Thrombin time:	[52s/(<22s)[2]]
Reptilase (batroxobin) time:	[>55s/(<20s)[2]]
Prothrombin time:	[19s/(16s)[2]]
Partial thromboplastin time:	[38s/(20-40s)]
Euglobulin lysis time:	[n.a.]
Bleeding time:	[Normal]
Immunoelectrophoresis:	[n.a.[3]]
Platelet aggregation:	[Normal]

Other results with patient plasma
Ancrod (Arvin) time: [n.a.]
Recalcification time: [n.a.]
Calcium corrects c.t.? [n.a.]

Inhib. normal plasma? [No]
In vivo synthesis: [n.a.]
In vivo catabolism: [n.a.]

Evaluation of isolated patient fibrinogen
Thrombin time: [n.a.]
Reptilase time: [n.a.]
Ancrod (Arvin) time: [n.a.]

Abnormal subunit? [n.a.]
Abnormal FDPs? [n.a.]

Remarks
[1]Only half the normal amount of fibrinopeptide A was released.
[2]I. Scharrer, personal communication.
[3]An abnormal pattern was found on 2-dimensional immunoelectrophoresis.

References

1. Henschen, A., Kehl, M., Southan, C., Lottspeich, F. and Georgopoulos, D. Genetically abnormal fibrinogens — some current characterisation strategies. In: *Fibrinogen —Structure, Functional Aspects, Metabolism*, F. Haverkate, A. Henschen, W. Nieuwenhuizen and P.W. Straub (eds.), Walter de Gruyter, Berlin. pp. 125-144, **1983.**

2. Scharrer, I., Kirchmaier, C. and Maas, C. [Experimental study of congenital dysfibrinogenemia ("Fibrinogen Frankfurt")]. In: *Fibrinogen, Fibrin und Fibrinkleber*, K.I. Schimpf (ed.), F.K. Schattauer, Stuttgart, New York. pp. 165-173, **1980.**

3. Scharrer, I., Kirchmaier, C. and Maas, C. [Experimental study of congenital dysfibrinogenemia ("Fibrinogen Frankfurt")]. *Blut* **38**:62-62, **1979.** ABSTRACT

FIBRINOGEN FRANKFURT III

Last update	[1 December 1990]	**Structural defect**	[n.a.]
Alphacode	[FRANKF03]	**Mutation**	[n.a.]
Ref. type	[Article[1]]		

Family studies
Homozygote? [n.a.]
Pedigree published? [No]

Functional defect(s)
FpA release: [Abnormal[2]]
FpB release: [n.a.]
Polymerization: [Abnormal[3]]
Stabilization: [n.a.]

Clinical manifestation(s) Bleeding? [Yes[3]] Thrombosis? [No[3]]

Clinical laboratory results

Plasma fibrinogen concentration (mg/dL)
Chronometric: [36/(200-400)[3]]
Rate-indep'nt: [180/(160-320)[3]]
Immunologic: [308/(160-300)[3]]

*Hypo*dysfibrinogen? [No[3]]

Thrombin time:	[48s/(<22s)[3]]
Reptilase (batroxobin) time:	[71s/(<20s)[3]]
Prothrombin time:	[21s/(16s)[3]]
Partial thromboplastin time:	[39s/(20-40s)[3]]
Euglobulin lysis time:	[n.a.]
Bleeding time:	[Normal[3]]
Immunoelectrophoresis:	[n.a.]
Platelet aggregation:	[Normal[3]]

Other results with patient plasma

Ancrod (Arvin) time:	[n.a.]	Inhib. normal plasma?	[No[3]]
Recalcification time:	[n.a.]	In vivo synthesis:	[n.a.]
Calcium corrects c.t.?	[n.a.]	In vivo catabolism:	[n.a.]

Evaluation of isolated patient fibrinogen

Thrombin time:	[n.a.]	Abnormal subunit?	[n.a.]
Reptilase time:	[n.a.]	Abnormal FDPs?	[n.a.]
Ancrod (Arvin) time:	[n.a.]		

Remarks
[1]Review article only.
[2]Only half the normal amount of fibrinopeptide A was released.
[3]I. Scharrer, personal communication.

References

1. Henschen, A., Kehl, M., Southan, C., Lottspeich, F. and Georgopoulos, D. Genetically abnormal fibrinogens — some current characterisation strategies. In: *Fibrinogen —Structure, Functional Aspects, Metabolism*, F. Haverkate, A. Henschen, W. Nieuwenhuizen and P.W. Straub (eds.), Walter de Gruyter, Berlin. pp. 125-144, **1983**.

FIBRINOGEN FRANKFURT IV^Unp

Last update [1 December 1990]
Alphacode [FRANKF04]
Ref. type [Unpublished[1]]

Family studies
Homozygote? [n.a.]
Pedigree published? [No]

Structural defect [n.a.]
Mutation [n.a.]

Functional defect(s)
FpA release: [n.a.]
FpB release: [n.a.]
Polymerization: [Abnormal]
Stabilization: [n.a.]

Clinical manifestation(s) Bleeding? [No] Thrombosis? [Yes]

Clinical laboratory results
Plasma fibrinogen concentration (mg/dL)
Chronometric: [n.a.]
Rate-indep'nt: [n.a.]
Immunologic: [n.a.]

*Hypo*dysfibrinogen? [n.a.]

Thrombin time:	[40s/<22s)]
Reptilase (batroxobin) time:	[n.a.]
Prothrombin time:	[n.a.]
Partial thromboplastin time:	[n.a.]
Euglobulin lysis time:	[n.a.]
Bleeding time:	[n.a.]
Immunoelectrophoresis:	[n.a.]
Platelet aggregation:	[n.a.]

Other results with patient plasma
Ancrod (Arvin) time: [n.a.]
Recalcification time: [n.a.]
Calcium corrects c.t.? [n.a.]

Inhib. normal plasma? [n.a.]
In vivo synthesis: [n.a.]
In vivo catabolism: [n.a.]

Evaluation of isolated patient fibrinogen
Thrombin time: [n.a.]
Reptilase time: [n.a.]
Ancrod (Arvin) time: [n.a.]

Abnormal subunit? [n.a.]
Abnormal FDPs? [n.a.]

Remarks
[1]I. Scharrer, personal communication.

References

FIBRINOGEN FRANKFURT V^{Unp}

Last update [1 December 1990]
Alphacode [FRANKF05]
Ref. type [Unpublished[1]]

Family studies
Homozygote? [n.a.]
Pedigree published? [No]

Structural defect [n.a.]
Mutation [n.a.]

Functional defect(s)
FpA release: [n.a.]
FpB release: [n.a.]
Polymerization: [Abnormal]
Stabilization: [n.a.]

Clinical manifestation(s) Bleeding? [No] Thrombosis? [Yes]

Clinical laboratory results
Plasma fibrinogen concentration (mg/dL)
Chronometric: [n.a.]
Rate-indep'nt: [n.a.]
Immunologic: [n.a.]

*Hypo*dysfibrinogen? [n.a.]

Thrombin time: [>120s/(22s)]
Reptilase (batroxobin) time: [n.a.]
Prothrombin time: [n.a.]
Partial thromboplastin time: [n.a.]
Euglobulin lysis time: [n.a.]
Bleeding time: [n.a.]
Immunoelectrophoresis: [n.a.]
Platelet aggregation: [n.a.]

Other results with patient plasma
Ancrod (Arvin) time: [n.a.]
Recalcification time: [n.a.]
Calcium corrects c.t.? [n.a.]

Inhib. normal plasma? [n.a.]
In vivo synthesis: [n.a.]
In vivo catabolism: [n.a.]

Evaluation of isolated patient fibrinogen
Thrombin time: [n.a.]
Reptilase time: [n.a.]
Ancrod (Arvin) time: [n.a.]

Abnormal subunit? [n.a.]
Abnormal FDPs? [n.a.]

Remarks
[1]I. Scharrer, personal communication.

References

FIBRINOGEN FRANKFURT XIII[1]

Last update	[10 January 1994]	**Structural defect**	[Aα(16) Arg → Cys[2]]
Alphacode	[FRANKF13]	**Mutation**	[n.a.[3]]
Ref. type	[Article]		

Family studies

Homozygote?	[No]
Pedigree published?	[Yes]

Functional defect(s)

FpA release:	[Abnormal]
FpB release:	[Normal]
Polymerization:	[Abnormal]
Stabilization:	[n.a.]

Clinical manifestation(s) Bleeding? [No] Thrombosis? [No]

Clinical laboratory results

Plasma fibrinogen concentration (mg/dL)

Chronometric: [35[4]]
Rate-indep'nt: [n.a.]
Immunologic: [n.a.]

*Hypo*dysfibrinogen? [No]

Thrombin time:	[n.a.]
Reptilase (batroxobin) time:	[n.a.]
Prothrombin time:	[Abnormal]
Partial thromboplastin time:	[Abnormal]
Euglobulin lysis time:	[n.a.]
Bleeding time:	[n.a.]
Immunoelectrophoresis:	[n.a.]
Platelet aggregation:	[n.a.]

Other results with patient plasma

Ancrod (Arvin) time:	[n.a.]	Inhib. normal plasma?	[n.a.]
Recalcification time:	[n.a.]	In vivo synthesis:	[n.a.]
Calcium corrects c.t.?	[n.a.]	In vivo catabolism:	[n.a.]

Evaluation of isolated patient fibrinogen

Thrombin time:	[n.a.]	Abnormal subunit?	[No]
Reptilase time:	[n.a.]	Abnormal FDPs?	[n.a.]
Ancrod (Arvin) time:	[n.a.]		

Remarks

The father and mother exhibited different clinical laboratory results and clinical manifestations. The authors conclude that a second mutation may explain the disparate results observed among their four children. Results summarized here reflect data from the father and one daughter whose presentations appear not to have been influenced by the putative second mutation.

[1]This variant is out of sequence. Fibrinogens Frankfurt VI—XII have not been reported.
[2]The structural defect was determined with the PCR method.
[3]Results confirming the codon sequence change were not reported.
[4]Normal range not reported.

References

1. Galanakis, D., Spitzer, S. and Scharrer, I. Unusual Aα16Arg→Cys dysfibrinogenaemic family: absence of normal Aα-chains in fibrinogen from two of four heterozygous siblings. *Blood Coag. & Fibrinol.* 4:67-71, **1993**.

FIBRINOGEN FREIBURG I

Last update [1 December 1990]
Alphacode [FREIBU01]
Ref. type [Article]

Structural defect [n.a.]
Mutation [n.a.]

Family studies
Homozygote? [n.a.]
Pedigree published? [No]

Functional defect(s)
FpA release: [Abnormal]
FpB release: [n.a.]
Polymerization: [Abnormal]
Stabilization: [n.a.]

Clinical manifestation(s) Bleeding? [Yes[1]] Thrombosis? [No]

Clinical laboratory results
Plasma fibrinogen concentration (mg/dL)
Chronometric: [10-20[2]]
Rate-indep'nt: [n.a.]
Immunologic: [Subnormal[3]]

*Hypo*dysfibrinogen? [Yes]

Thrombin time:	[Abnormal[3]]
Reptilase (batroxobin) time:	[Abnormal[3]]
Prothrombin time:	[n.a.]
Partial thromboplastin time:	[n.a.]
Euglobulin lysis time:	[n.a.]
Bleeding time:	[n.a.]
Immunoelectrophoresis:	[n.a.]
Platelet aggregation:	[n.a.]

Other results with patient plasma
Ancrod (Arvin) time: [n.a.]
Recalcification time: [n.a.]
Calcium corrects c.t.? [Yes]

Inhib. normal plasma? [Yes]
In vivo synthesis: [n.a.]
In vivo catabolism: [n.a.]

Evaluation of isolated patient fibrinogen
Thrombin time: [n.a.]
Reptilase time: [n.a.]
Ancrod (Arvin) time: [n.a.]

Abnormal subunit? [No]
Abnormal FDPs? [n.a.]

Remarks
[1]One of four affected individuals had a "...major bleeding episode after trauma." Otherwise, no major bleeding problems were reported.
[2]Normal range not reported.
[3]Data not reported.

References

1. Hasler, K., Böttcher, D., Köttgen, E. and Neumann, H. [Defective stabilization of fibrin in a family with hypodysfibrinogenemia]. In: *Fibrinolyse, Thrombose, Hamostase*, E. Deutsch and K. Lechner (eds.), F.K. Schattauer, Stuttgart, New York. pp. 538-541, **1980**.

2. Böttcher, D., Hasler, K., Köttgen, E. and Maurath, J. Hereditary hypodysfibrinogenemia with defective release of fibrinogenopeptide A (Fibrinogen Freiburg). *Thromb. Haemostas.* **42**:78, **1979**. ABSTRACT

FIBRINOGEN GENEVA I

Last update [1 December 1990]
Alphaсode [GENEVA01]
Ref. type [Article]

Structural defect [Aα(16) Arg → Cys]
Mutation [n.a.]

Family studies
Homozygote? [No]
Pedigree published? [Yes]

Functional defect(s)
FpA release: [Abnormal[1]]
FpB release: [Normal]
Polymerization: [Abnormal]
Stabilization: [n.a.]

Clinical manifestation(s) Bleeding? [No[2]] Thrombosis? [No[2]]

Clinical laboratory results

Plasma fibrinogen concentration (mg/dL)
Chronometric: [14/(150-400)]
Rate-indep'nt: [180/(150-400)]
Immunologic: [180/(150-400)]

*Hypo*dysfibrinogen? [No]

Thrombin time:	[38.9s/(12-15s)]
Reptilase (batroxobin) time:	[60s/(16-18s)]
Prothrombin time:	[66%/(100%)]
Partial thromboplastin time:	[27.6s/(25-30s)]
Euglobulin lysis time:	[n.a.]
Bleeding time:	[n.a.]
Immunoelectrophoresis:	[n.a.]
Platelet aggregation:	[n.a.]

Other results with patient plasma
Ancrod (Arvin) time: [n.a.]
Recalcification time: [n.a.]
Calcium corrects c.t.? [n.a.]

Inhib. normal plasma? [n.a.]
In vivo synthesis: [n.a.]
In vivo catabolism: [n.a.]

Evaluation of isolated patient fibrinogen
Thrombin time: [n.a.]
Reptilase time: [n.a.]
Ancrod (Arvin) time: [n.a.]

Abnormal subunit? [No]
Abnormal FDPs? [n.a.]

Remarks
[1]Only half the normal amount of fibrinopeptide A was released.
[2]Recurrent spontaneous abortions were reported.

References

1. Furlan, M., Bögli, C., Hofer, A., Bouvier, C.A., and de Moerloose, P. Fibrinogen Geneva, a new case of Aα 16 Arg → Cys dysfibrinogenaemia. *Blood Coag. & Fibrinol.* **1**:139-144, **1990**.

FIBRINOGEN GENOVA I

Last update	[1 December 1990]	**Structural defect**	[n.a.]
Alphacode	[GENOVA01]	**Mutation**	[n.a.]
Ref. type	[Article]		

Functional defect(s)

FpA release:	[Normal[1]]
FpB release:	[Normal[1]]
Polymerization:	[Abnormal]
Stabilization:	[n.a.]

Family studies

Homozygote?	[n.a.]
Pedigree published?	[Yes]

Clinical manifestation(s) Bleeding? [No] Thrombosis? [No]

Clinical laboratory results

Plasma fibrinogen concentration (mg/dL)

Chronometric:	[140/(200-400)]
Rate-indep'nt:	[n.a.]
Immunologic:	[350/(200-450)]

*Hypo*dysfibrinogen? [No]

Thrombin time:	[58s/(18s)]
Reptilase (batroxobin) time:	[61.5s/(17s)]
Prothrombin time:	[18.5s/(14s)]
Partial thromboplastin time:	[Normal[2]]
Euglobulin lysis time:	[n.a.]
Bleeding time:	[n.a.]
Immunoelectrophoresis:	[n.a.]
Platelet aggregation:	[n.a.]

Other results with patient plasma

Ancrod (Arvin) time:	[n.a.]	Inhib. normal plasma?	[n.a.]
Recalcification time:	[n.a.]	In vivo synthesis:	[n.a.]
Calcium corrects c.t.?	[Yes]	In vivo catabolism:	[n.a.]

Evaluation of isolated patient fibrinogen

Thrombin time:	[116s/(17s)]	Abnormal subunit?	[No]
Reptilase time:	[90s/(20s)]	Abnormal FDPs?	[No]
Ancrod (Arvin) time:	[n.a.]		

Remarks

[1]The rate of *total* fibrinopeptide release was normal.
[2]Data not reported.

References

1. Hassan, H.J., Orlando, M., Tonini, G.P., Casalbore, P., Sarti, A., Boeri, E., Giacchino, R., Tentori, L. and Mori, P.G. An abnormal inherited fibrinogen (fibrinogen Genova) with delayed fibrin aggregation. *Scand. J. Haematol.* **29**:287-294, **1982**.

FIBRINOGEN GENOVA II

Last update [1 December 1990]
Alphacode [GENOVA02]
Ref. type [Article]

Family studies
Homozygote? [n.a.]
Pedigree published? [No]

Structural defect [n.a.]
Mutation [n.a.]

Functional defect(s)
FpA release: [Normal]
FpB release: [Normal]
Polymerization: [Abnormal]
Stabilization: [Abnormal[1]]

Clinical manifestation(s) Bleeding? [No] Thrombosis? [No]

Clinical laboratory results
Plasma fibrinogen concentration (mg/dL)
Chronometric: [59/(200-400)]
Rate-indep'nt: [370/(180-400)]
Immunologic: [350/(200-450)]

*Hypo*dysfibrinogen? [No]

Thrombin time: [43s/(13-17s)]
Reptilase (batroxobin) time: [61s/(15-20s)]
Prothrombin time: [16.8s/(12-14s)]
Partial thromboplastin time: [35s/(27-33s)]
Euglobulin lysis time: [n.a.]
Bleeding time: [Normal]
Immunoelectrophoresis: [Normal]
Platelet aggregation: [n.a.]

Other results with patient plasma
Ancrod (Arvin) time: [87s/(12-18s)]
Recalcification time: [n.a.]
Calcium corrects c.t.? [No]

Inhib. normal plasma? [Yes]
In vivo synthesis: [n.a.]
In vivo catabolism: [n.a.]

Evaluation of isolated patient fibrinogen
Thrombin time: [36s/(15-20s)]
Reptilase time: [n.a.]
Ancrod (Arvin) time: [n.a.]

Abnormal subunit? [No]
Abnormal FDPs? [No]

Remarks
[1]A reduced rate of factor XIII-catalyzed crosslinking was reported.

References

1. Rodeghiero, F., Castaman, G.C., Dal Belin Peruffo, A., Dini, E., Galletti, A., Barone, E. and Gastaldi, G. Fibrinogen Vicenza and Genova II: two new cases of congenital dysfibrinogenemia with isolated defect of fibrin monomer polymerization and inhibitory activity on normal coagulation. *Thromb. Haemostas.* **57**:252-258, **1987**.

FIBRINOGEN GENOVA III^{Abs}

Last update [1 December 1990]
Alphacode [GENOVA03]
Ref. type [Abstract]

Structural defect [n.a.]
Mutation [n.a.]

Family studies
Homozygote? [n.a.]
Pedigree published? [No]

Functional defect(s)
FpA release: [Normal]
FpB release: [Normal]
Polymerization: [Abnormal]
Stabilization: [Normal]

Clinical manifestation(s) Bleeding? [Yes] Thrombosis? [No]

Clinical laboratory results
Plasma fibrinogen concentration (mg/dL)
Chronometric: [Subnormal[1]]
Rate-indep'nt: [Normal[1]]
Immunologic: [Normal[1]]

*Hypo*dysfibrinogen? [No]

Thrombin time:	[Abnormal[1]]
Reptilase (batroxobin) time:	[Abnormal[1]]
Prothrombin time:	[n.a.]
Partial thromboplastin time:	[n.a.]
Euglobulin lysis time:	[n.a.]
Bleeding time:	[n.a.]
Immunoelectrophoresis:	[n.a.]
Platelet aggregation:	[n.a.]

Other results with patient plasma
Ancrod (Arvin) time: [n.a.]
Recalcification time: [n.a.]
Calcium corrects c.t.? [n.a.]

Inhib. normal plasma? [Yes]
In vivo synthesis: [n.a.]
In vivo catabolism: [n.a.]

Evaluation of isolated patient fibrinogen
Thrombin time: [n.a.]
Reptilase time: [n.a.]
Ancrod (Arvin) time: [n.a.]

Abnormal subunit? [No]
Abnormal FDPs? [Yes]

Remarks
[1]Data not reported.

References

1. Castaman, G., Rodeghiero, F., Galletti, A., Barone, E. and Gastaldi, G. Fibrinogen Genova III: A new congenital dysfibrinogenemia with bleeding diathesis and defective lysis by plasmin. *Thromb. Haemostas.* **58**:149, **1987**. ABSTRACT

FIBRINOGEN GIESSEN I

Last update [1 December 1990]
Alphacode [GIESSE01]
Ref. type [Article]

Family studies
Homozygote? [Yes]
Pedigree published? [No[2]]

Structural defect [Aα(16) Arg → His]
Mutation [n.a.]

Functional defect(s)
FpA release: [Abnormal]
FpB release: [Normal[1]]
Polymerization: [Abnormal]
Stabilization: [n.a.]

Clinical manifestation(s) Bleeding? [Yes[3]] Thrombosis? [No]

Clinical laboratory results
Plasma fibrinogen concentration (mg/dL)
Chronometric: [45/(200)]
Rate-indep'nt: [160/(200)]
Immunologic: [215/(240)]

*Hypo*dysfibrinogen? [No]

Thrombin time:	[>120s/(11-14s)]
Reptilase (batroxobin) time:	[>120s/(11-14s)]
Prothrombin time:	[28.4s/(11-14s)]
Partial thromboplastin time:	[37.7s/(22-34s)]
Euglobulin lysis time:	[Normal]
Bleeding time:	[Normal]
Immunoelectrophoresis:	[Normal]
Platelet aggregation:	[Normal]

Other results with patient plasma
Ancrod (Arvin) time: [n.a.]
Recalcification time: [n.a.]
Calcium corrects c.t.? [No]

Inhib. normal plasma? [n.a.]
In vivo synthesis: [n.a.]
In vivo catabolism: [n.a.]

Evaluation of isolated patient fibrinogen
Thrombin time: [n.a.]
Reptilase time: [n.a.]
Ancrod (Arvin) time: [n.a.]

Abnormal subunit? [No]
Abnormal FDPs? [No]

Remarks
[1]Other dysfibrinogens with this molecular defect exhibit delayed fibrinopeptide A and B release plus delayed polymerization of fibrin monomers.
[2]The index patient was adopted. Her only daughter was heterozygous for the trait.
[3]Excessive postpartum bleeding was reported; otherwise the proposita has normal hemostasis.

FIBRINOGEN GIESSEN I

References

1. Alving, B.M. and Henschen, A.H. Fibrinogen Giessen I: a congenital homozygously expressed dysfibrinogenemia with Aα-16 Arg — His substitution. *Am. J. Hematol.* **25**:479-482, **1987**.

2. Henschen, A. and Alving, B. Fibrinogen Giessen I, a classical dysfibrinogen: The molecular defect. In: *Fibrinogen and Its Derivatives. Biochemistry, Physiology, and Pathophysiology*, G. Muller-Berghaus, U. Scheefers-Borchel, E. Selmayr and A. Henschen (eds.), Excerpta Medica, Amsterdam. pp. 23-24, **1986**.

3. Mosesson, M.W., Natale, P.D., Amrani, D.L., Sherman, L.A., Joist, J.H. and Krause, W.H. Comparison of plasmic hydrolysis of normal fibrinogen and fibrinogen Giessen I. *Thromb. Res.* **12**:693-696, **1978**.

4. Bleyl, H. and Krause, W.H. Studies on the degradation of fibrinogen Giessen I. *Thromb. Res.* **9**:329-334, **1976**.

5. Krause, W.H. and Bleyl, H. Investigation on plasmin-proteolysis of abnormal fibrinogen (fibrinogen Giessen). *Thromb. Res.* **2**:361-364, **1973**.

6. Krause, W.H., Heene, D.L. and Lasch, H.G. Congenital dysfibrinogenemia (fibrinogen Giessen). *Thromb. Diath. Haemorrh.* **29**:547-561, **1973**.

7. Krause, W.H., Heene, D., Heinrich, D., Roka, L. and Lasch, H.G. [A new case of dysfibrinogenemia]. *Verh. Dtsch. Ges. Inn. Med.* **78**:1651-1653, **1972**.

8. Krause, W.H. and Zimmermann, P. [Quantitative electron microscopic studies on fibrin structure in dysfibrinogenemia]. *Klin. Wochenschr.* **50**:557-561, **1972**.

9. Krause, W.H., Heene, D. and Lasch, H.G. [A new case of dysfibrinogenemia]. *Klin. Wochenschr.* **49**:806-808, **1971**.

FIBRINOGEN GIESSEN II

Last update [1 December 1990]
Alphacode [GIESSE02]
Ref. type [Article]

Family studies
Homozygote? [n.a.]
Pedigree published? [No]

Structural defect [n.a.]
Mutation [n.a.]

Functional defect(s)
FpA release: [Abnormal]
FpB release: [n.a.]
Polymerization: [Abnormal]
Stabilization: [n.a.]

Clinical manifestation(s) Bleeding? [Yes[1]] Thrombosis? [No]

Clinical laboratory results

Plasma fibrinogen concentration (mg/dL)
Chronometric: [0/(250)]
Rate-indep'nt: [33/(260)]
Immunologic: [50/(300)]

*Hypo*dysfibrinogen? [Yes]

Thrombin time:	[222s/(18s)]
Reptilase (batroxobin) time:	[277s/(20s)]
Prothrombin time:	[15%/(80%)]
Partial thromboplastin time:	[67s/(45s)]
Euglobulin lysis time:	[n.a.]
Bleeding time:	[Normal]
Immunoelectrophoresis:	[Normal]
Platelet aggregation:	[n.a.]

Other results with patient plasma
Ancrod (Arvin) time: [298s/(20s)]
Recalcification time: [n.a.]
Calcium corrects c.t.? [n.a.]

Inhib. normal plasma? [Yes]
In vivo synthesis: [n.a.]
In vivo catabolism: [Increased]

Evaluation of isolated patient fibrinogen
Thrombin time: [n.a.]
Reptilase time: [n.a.]
Ancrod (Arvin) time: [n.a.]

Abnormal subunit? [n.a.]
Abnormal FDPs? [No[2]]

Remarks
[1]Menorrhagia in the 19 year-old proposita was reported.
[2]A reduced *rate* of FDP formation was reported.

References

1. Krause, W.H., Heene, D.L., Lasch, H.G. and Huth, K. [Congenital dysfibrinogenemia: fibrinogen Giessen II]. *Verh. Dtsch. Ges. Inn. Med.* **82**:1646-1649, **1976**.

2. Krause, W.H., Huth, K., Heene, D.L. and Lasch, H.G. [Hypodysfibrinogenemia: Fibrinogen Giessen II]. *Klin. Wochenschr.* **53**:781-782, **1975**.

FIBRINOGEN GIESSEN III

Last update [1 December 1990]
Alphacode [GIESSE03]
Ref. type [Article]

Structural defect [n.a.]
Mutation [n.a.]

Family studies
Homozygote? [n.a.]
Pedigree published? [No]

Functional defect(s)
FpA release: [n.a.]
FpB release: [n.a.]
Polymerization: [Abnormal]
Stabilization: [n.a.]

Clinical manifestation(s) Bleeding? [No] Thrombosis? [No]

Clinical laboratory results

Plasma fibrinogen concentration (mg/dL)
Chronometric: [180/(345)]
Rate-indep'nt: [160/(262)]
Immunologic: [304/(345)]

*Hypo*dysfibrinogen? [No]

Thrombin time:	[40.4s/(19-24s)]
Reptilase (batroxobin) time:	[54.2s/(20-25s)]
Prothrombin time:	[100%/(70-120%)]
Partial thromboplastin time:	[48s/(37-50s)]
Euglobulin lysis time:	[n.a.]
Bleeding time:	[Normal]
Immunoelectrophoresis:	[Normal]
Platelet aggregation:	[Abnormal]

Other results with patient plasma
Ancrod (Arvin) time: [n.a.]
Recalcification time: [n.a.]
Calcium corrects c.t.? [Yes]

Inhib. normal plasma? [n.a.]
In vivo synthesis: [n.a.]
In vivo catabolism: [n.a.]

Evaluation of isolated patient fibrinogen
Thrombin time: [n.a.]
Reptilase time: [n.a.]
Ancrod (Arvin) time: [n.a.]

Abnormal subunit? [n.a.]
Abnormal FDPs? [n.a.]

Remarks

References

1. Matthias, F.R., Krause, W.H., Ganssert, S., Mueller, K. and Lasch, H.G. [Dysfibrinogenemia. A new case: dysfibrinogenemia Giessen III]. *Klin. Wochenschr.* **55**:539-543, **1977**.

FIBRINOGEN GRAND RAPIDS I

Last update [1 December 1990]
Alphacode [GRANDR01]
Ref. type [Article]

Family studies
Homozygote? [No]
Pedigree published? [No]

Structural defect [n.a.]
Mutation [n.a.]

Functional defect(s)
FpA release: [Abnormal]
FpB release: [Abnormal]
Polymerization: [Abnormal]
Stabilization: [Abnormal[1]]

Clinical manifestation(s) Bleeding? [No] Thrombosis? [No]

Clinical laboratory results
Plasma fibrinogen concentration (mg/dL)
Chronometric: [48/(280)]
Rate-indep'nt: [93/(280)]
Immunologic: [120/(280)]

*Hypo*dysfibrinogen? [Yes]

Thrombin time:	[16.8s/(7.6s)]
Reptilase (batroxobin) time:	[n.a.]
Prothrombin time:	[14.5s/(10.5s)]
Partial thromboplastin time:	[32.2s/(27.5s)]
Euglobulin lysis time:	[n.a.]
Bleeding time:	[n.a.]
Immunoelectrophoresis:	[n.a.]
Platelet aggregation:	[n.a.]

Other results with patient plasma
Ancrod (Arvin) time: [n.a.]
Recalcification time: [n.a.]
Calcium corrects c.t.? [n.a.]

Inhib. normal plasma? [n.a.]
In vivo synthesis: [n.a.]
In vivo catabolism: [n.a.]

Evaluation of isolated patient fibrinogen
Thrombin time: [n.a.]
Reptilase time: [n.a.]
Ancrod (Arvin) time: [n.a.]

Abnormal subunit? [No]
Abnormal FDPs? [No]

Remarks
[1]A reduced *rate* of γ-γ crosslinking by factor XIII was reported.

References

1. Higgins, D.L., Lewis, S.D., Penner, J.A. and Shafer, J.A. A kinetic method for characterization of heterogenous fibrinogen and its application to fibrinogen Grand Rapids, a congenital dysfibrinogenemia. *Thromb. Haemostas.* **48**:182-186, **1982**.

FIBRINOGEN GRENOBLE I

Last update [1 December 1990]
Alphacode [GRENOB01]
Ref. type [Article]

Structural defect [n.a.]
Mutation [n.a.]

Family studies
Homozygote? [No]
Pedigree published? [No]

Functional defect(s)
FpA release: [n.a.]
FpB release: [n.a.]
Polymerization: [Abnormal]
Stabilization: [n.a.]

Clinical manifestation(s) Bleeding? [No[1]] Thrombosis? [No[1]]

Clinical laboratory results
Plasma fibrinogen concentration (mg/dL)
Chronometric: [50/(200-400)]
Rate-indep'nt: [120/(200-400)]
Immunologic: [210/(200-400)]

*Hypo*dysfibrinogen? [No]

Thrombin time:	[n.a.]
Reptilase (batroxobin) time:	[n.a.]
Prothrombin time:	[n.a.]
Partial thromboplastin time:	[n.a.]
Euglobulin lysis time:	[n.a.]
Bleeding time:	[n.a.]
Immunoelectrophoresis:	[n.a.]
Platelet aggregation:	[n.a.]

Other results with patient plasma
Ancrod (Arvin) time: [n.a.]
Recalcification time: [n.a.]
Calcium corrects c.t.? [n.a.]

Inhib. normal plasma? [n.a.]
In vivo synthesis: [n.a.]
In vivo catabolism: [n.a.]

Evaluation of isolated patient fibrinogen
Thrombin time: [n.a.]
Reptilase time: [n.a.]
Ancrod (Arvin) time: [n.a.]

Abnormal subunit? [Yes[2]]
Abnormal FDPs? [n.a.]

Remarks
[1]The index patient underwent pelvic surgery for prolapse with urinary incontinence; authors reported no complications and normal wound healing.
[2]Two-dimensional electrophoresis disclosed a γ-chain with an apparent M_R 1200-1300 higher than normal.

References

1. Polack, B., Valiron, O., Concord, E., Freyssinet, J.M. and Hudry-Clergeon, G. Molecular characterization of an abnormal fibrinogen by two-dimensional electrophoresis. *Clin. Chem.* **30**:2093-2097, **1984**.

FIBRINOGEN GUADELOUPE I

Last update [1 December 1990]
Alphacode [GUADEL01]
Ref. type [Article]

Family studies
Homozygote? [n.a.]
Pedigree published? [No]

Structural defect [n.a.]
Mutation [n.a.]

Functional defect(s)
FpA release: [n.a.]
FpB release: [n.a.]
Polymerization: [n.a.]
Stabilization: [n.a.]

Clinical manifestation(s) Bleeding? [n.a.] Thrombosis? [n.a.]

Clinical laboratory results

Plasma fibrinogen concentration (mg/dL)
Chronometric: [80[1]]
Rate-indep'nt: [265[1]]
Immunologic: [220[1]]

*Hypo*dysfibrinogen? [No]

Thrombin time:	[40s/(20s)]
Reptilase (batroxobin) time:	[36s/(23s)]
Prothrombin time:	[64%/(>70%)]
Partial thromboplastin time:	[40s/(38s)]
Euglobulin lysis time:	[n.a.]
Bleeding time:	[n.a.]
Immunoelectrophoresis:	[n.a.]
Platelet aggregation:	[Normal]

Other results with patient plasma
Ancrod (Arvin) time: [n.a.]
Recalcification time: [n.a.]
Calcium corrects c.t.? [n.a.]
Inhib. normal plasma? [n.a.]
In vivo synthesis: [n.a.]
In vivo catabolism: [n.a.]

Evaluation of isolated patient fibrinogen
Thrombin time: [n.a.]
Reptilase time: [n.a.]
Ancrod (Arvin) time: [n.a.]
Abnormal subunit? [n.a.]
Abnormal FDPs? [n.a.]

Remarks
[1]Normal range not reported.

References

1. Corrihons, G., Soria, J., Soria, C., Conard, J., Horellou, M.H. and Samama, M. [Congenital dysfibrinogenemia. Apropos of 13 cases]. *Sem. Hop. Paris* **59**:2517-2523, **1983**.

FIBRINOGEN HAARLEM I

Last update [1 December 1990]
Alphacode [HAARLE01]
Ref. type [Article]

Family studies
Homozygote? [No]
Pedigree published? [Yes]

Structural defect [n.a.]
Mutation [n.a.]

Functional defect(s)
FpA release: [Normal]
FpB release: [n.a.]
Polymerization: [Abnormal]
Stabilization: [n.a.]

Clinical manifestation(s) Bleeding? [No] Thrombosis? [No]

Clinical laboratory results

Plasma fibrinogen concentration (mg/dL)
Chronometric: [50/(200-400)]
Rate-indep'nt: [n.a.]
Immunologic: [240/(200-400)]

*Hypo*dysfibrinogen? [No]

Thrombin time:	[11s/(<8s)]
Reptilase (batroxobin) time:	[24s/(<20s)]
Prothrombin time:	[14s/(<13s)]
Partial thromboplastin time:	[45s/(<40s)]
Euglobulin lysis time:	[n.a.]
Bleeding time:	[Normal]
Immunoelectrophoresis:	[n.a.]
Platelet aggregation:	[n.a.]

Other results with patient plasma
Ancrod (Arvin) time: [n.a.]
Recalcification time: [n.a.]
Calcium corrects c.t.? [Yes]

Inhib. normal plasma? [n.a.]
In vivo synthesis: [n.a.]
In vivo catabolism: [n.a.]

Evaluation of isolated patient fibrinogen
Thrombin time: [21s/(18s)]
Reptilase time: [>180s/(30s)]
Ancrod (Arvin) time: [n.a.]

Abnormal subunit? [No]
Abnormal FDPs? [No]

Remarks

References

1. Hensen, A., Brommer, E.J., Gravesen, M. and Haverkate, F. [Familial dysfibrinogenemia; fibrinogen Haarlem I and II]. *Ned. Tijdschr. Geneeskd.* **125**:734-737, **1981**.

FIBRINOGEN HAARLEM II

Last update [1 December 1990]
Alphacode [HAARLE02]
Ref. type [Article]

Family studies
Homozygote? [No]
Pedigree published? [No]

Structural defect [n.a.]
Mutation [n.a.]

Functional defect(s)
FpA release: [Abnormal]
FpB release: [n.a.]
Polymerization: [Normal]
Stabilization: [n.a.]

Clinical manifestation(s) Bleeding? [No] Thrombosis? [No]

Clinical laboratory results
Plasma fibrinogen concentration (mg/dL)
Chronometric: [85/(200-400)]
Rate-indep'nt: [n.a.]
Immunologic: [260/(200-400)]

*Hypo*dysfibrinogen? [No]

Thrombin time:	[12s/(12s)]
Reptilase (batroxobin) time:	[n.a.]
Prothrombin time:	[13s/(13s)]
Partial thromboplastin time:	[43s/(43s)]
Euglobulin lysis time:	[n.a.]
Bleeding time:	[Normal]
Immunoelectrophoresis:	[n.a.]
Platelet aggregation:	[n.a.]

Other results with patient plasma
Ancrod (Arvin) time: [n.a.]
Recalcification time: [n.a.]
Calcium corrects c.t.? [Yes]

Inhib. normal plasma? [n.a.]
In vivo synthesis: [n.a.]
In vivo catabolism: [n.a.]

Evaluation of isolated patient fibrinogen
Thrombin time: [29s/(18s)]
Reptilase time: [43s/(30s)]
Ancrod (Arvin) time: [n.a.]

Abnormal subunit? [No]
Abnormal FDPs? [No]

Remarks

References

1. Hensen, A., Brommer, E.J., Gravesen, M. and Haverkate, F. [Familial dysfibrinogenemia; fibrinogen Haarlem I and II]. *Ned. Tijdschr. Geneeskd.* **125**:734-737, **1981**.

FIBRINOGEN HAIFA I

Last update	[1 December 1990]	**Structural defect**	[γ(275) Arg → His]
Alphacode	[HAIFA01]	**Mutation**	[n.a.]
Ref. type	[Article]		

Functional defect(s)

FpA release:	[Normal[1]]
FpB release:	[Normal[1]]
Polymerization:	[Abnormal]
Stabilization:	[Normal]

Family studies

Homozygote?	[n.a.]
Pedigree published?	[No]

Clinical manifestation(s) Bleeding? [No] Thrombosis? [Yes[2]]

Clinical laboratory results

Plasma fibrinogen concentration (mg/dL)

Chronometric:	[n.a.]
Rate-indep'nt:	[260/(150-500)]
Immunologic:	[n.a.]

*Hypo*dysfibrinogen? [No]

Thrombin time:	[33s/(11s)]
Reptilase (batroxobin) time:	[28s/(14s)]
Prothrombin time:	[15.5s/(14s)]
Partial thromboplastin time:	[28.5s/(26s)]
Euglobulin lysis time:	[Normal]
Bleeding time:	[Normal]
Immunoelectrophoresis:	[n.a.]
Platelet aggregation:	[Normal]

Other results with patient plasma

Ancrod (Arvin) time:	[n.a.]	Inhib. normal plasma?	[n.a.]
Recalcification time:	[n.a.]	In vivo synthesis:	[n.a.]
Calcium corrects c.t.?	[Yes]	In vivo catabolism:	[n.a.]

Evaluation of isolated patient fibrinogen

Thrombin time:	[36s/(16s)]	Abnormal subunit?	[No]
Reptilase time:	[30s/(16s)]	Abnormal FDPs?	[Yes[3]]
Ancrod (Arvin) time:	[n.a.]		

Remarks

[1]The rate of *total* fibrinopeptide release was normal.
[2]The proposita presented with peripheral arterial thrombosis.
[3]Calcium failed to protect fragment D from further proteolysis by plasmin.

FIBRINOGEN HAIFA I

References

1. Siebenlist, K.R., Mosesson, M.W., Di Orio, J.P., Tavori, S., Tatarsky, I. and Rimon, A. The polymerization of fibrin prepared from fibrinogen Haifa (γ_{275}Arg → His). *Thromb. Haemostas.* **62**:875-879, **1989**.

2. Siebenlist, K.R., Mosesson, M.W., DiOrio, J.P., Tavori, S., Tatarsky, I. and Rimon, A. Studies on the polymerization of fibrin Haifa (γ275 Arg → His). In: *Fibrinogen 3. Biochemistry, Biological Functions, Gene Regulation and Expression*, M.W. Mosesson, D.L. Amrani, K.R. Siebenlist and J.P. DiOrio (eds.), Elsevier Science Publ., B.V., Amsterdam. pp. 271-274, **1988**.

3. Soria, J., Soria, C., Samama, M., Tabori, S., Kehl, M., Henschen, A., Nieuwenhuizen, W., Rimon, A. and Tatarski, I. Fibrinogen Haifa: fibrinogen variant with absence of protective effect of calcium on plasmin degradation of γ chains. *Thromb. Haemostas.* **57**:310-313, **1987**.

4. Soria, J., Soria, C., Samama, M. and Caen, J. Study of ten cases of congenital dysfibrinogenemia. Clinical and molecular biological aspects. In: *Fibrinogen — Structural Variants and Interactions*, A. Henschen, B. Hessel, J. McDonagh and T. Saldeen (eds.), Walter de Gruyter, Berlin. pp. 165-183, **1985**.

5. Brook, J.G., Tabori, S., Tatarsky, I., Hashmonai, M. and Schramek, A. Fibrinogen "Haifa:" a new fibrinogen variant. A case report. *Haemostas.* **13**:277-281, **1983**.

6. Tavori, S., Brook, J.G., Hashmonai, M. and Tatarsky, I. A new variant of hereditary dysfibrinogenemia: a possible causal relationship to arterial thrombosis. *Adv. Pathol.* **1**:407-411, **1982**.

FIBRINOGEN HANNOVER I

Last update [1 December 1990]
Alphacode [HANNOV01]
Ref. type [Article]

Family studies
Homozygote? [n.a.]
Pedigree published? [No]

Structural defect [n.a.]
Mutation [n.a.]

Functional defect(s)
FpA release: [n.a.]
FpB release: [n.a.]
Polymerization: [n.a.]
Stabilization: [n.a.]

Clinical manifestation(s) Bleeding? [Yes[1]] Thrombosis? [No]

Clinical laboratory results
Plasma fibrinogen concentration (mg/dL)
Chronometric: [57/(200-280)]
Rate-indep'nt: [124/(180-280)]
Immunologic: [240/(210-320)]

*Hypo*dysfibrinogen? [No]

Thrombin time:	[34s/(17-23s)]
Reptilase (batroxobin) time:	[87s/(13-20s)]
Prothrombin time:	[76%/(90-112%)]
Partial thromboplastin time:	[44s/(35-45s)]
Euglobulin lysis time:	[n.a.]
Bleeding time:	[Normal]
Immunoelectrophoresis:	[n.a.]
Platelet aggregation:	[n.a.]

Other results with patient plasma
Ancrod (Arvin) time: [n.a.]
Recalcification time: [n.a.]
Calcium corrects c.t.? [Yes]

Inhib. normal plasma? [Yes]
In vivo synthesis: [n.a.]
In vivo catabolism: [n.a.]

Evaluation of isolated patient fibrinogen
Thrombin time: [n.a.]
Reptilase time: [n.a.]
Ancrod (Arvin) time: [n.a.]

Abnormal subunit? [n.a.]
Abnormal FDPs? [n.a.]

Remarks
[1]Excessive post-surgical bleeding was reported.

References

1. Barthels, M. and Sandvoss, G. [Fibrinogen "Hannover:" a further abnormal fibrinogen]. *Blut* **34**:99-106, **1977**.

FIBRINOGEN HERSHEY I

Last update [1 December 1990]
Alphacode [HERSHE01]
Ref. type [Article]

Family studies
Homozygote? [n.a.]
Pedigree published? [Yes]

Structural defect [n.a.]
Mutation [n.a.]

Functional defect(s)
FpA release: [Normal]
FpB release: [Normal]
Polymerization: [Abnormal]
Stabilization: [Normal]

Clinical manifestation(s) Bleeding? [No[1]] Thrombosis? [Yes[1]]

Clinical laboratory results
Plasma fibrinogen concentration (mg/dL)
Chronometric: [275/(176-377)]
Rate-indep'nt: [480/(200-450)[2]]
Immunologic: [630/(215-400)[2]]

*Hypo*dysfibrinogen? [No]

Thrombin time:	[26s/(20s)]
Reptilase (batroxobin) time:	[60s/(49s)]
Prothrombin time:	[16s/(12s)]
Partial thromboplastin time:	[66s/(42s)]
Euglobulin lysis time:	[Normal]
Bleeding time:	[n.a.]
Immunoelectrophoresis:	[Normal]
Platelet aggregation:	[Normal]

Other results with patient plasma
Ancrod (Arvin) time: [n.a.]
Recalcification time: [n.a.]
Calcium corrects c.t.? [Yes]

Inhib. normal plasma? [Yes]
In vivo synthesis: [n.a.]
In vivo catabolism: [n.a.]

Evaluation of isolated patient fibrinogen
Thrombin time: [n.a.]
Reptilase time: [60s/(49s)]
Ancrod (Arvin) time: [n.a.]

Abnormal subunit? [No]
Abnormal FDPs? [n.a.]

Remarks
[1]Proposita had lupus anticoagulant.
[2]Evidence is consistent with hyperfibrinogenemia in this patient.

References

1. Al-Mondhiry, H. and Galanakis, D. Dysfibrinogenemia and lupus anticoagulant in a patient with recurrent thrombosis. *J. Lab. Clin. Med.* **110**:726-733, **1987**.

FIBRINOGEN HERSHEY II

Last update [1 December 1990]
Alphacode [HERSHE02]
Ref. type [Article]

Structural defect [Aα(16) Arg → Cys[1]]
Mutation [CGT → TGT]

Family studies
Homozygote? [No]
Pedigree published? [No]

Functional defect(s)
FpA release: [Abnormal[2]]
FpB release: [n.a.]
Polymerization: [Abnormal]
Stabilization: [Normal]

Clinical manifestation(s) Bleeding? [No] Thrombosis? [Yes[3]]

Clinical laboratory results
Plasma fibrinogen concentration (mg/dL)
Chronometric: [38-112/(200-399)[4]]
Rate-indep'nt: [n.a.]
Immunologic: [664/(200-399)[4]]

*Hypo*dysfibrinogen? [No]

Thrombin time:	[70s/(20s)[4]]
Reptilase (batroxobin) time:	[n.a.]
Prothrombin time:	[12.8s/(12s)[4]]
Partial thromboplastin time:	[31s/(42s)[4]]
Euglobulin lysis time:	[Normal]
Bleeding time:	[n.a.]
Immunoelectrophoresis:	[Normal[4]]
Platelet aggregation:	[Normal[4]]

Other results with patient plasma
Ancrod (Arvin) time: [n.a.]
Recalcification time: [n.a.]
Calcium corrects c.t.? [n.a.]

Inhib. normal plasma? [Yes[4]]
In vivo synthesis: [n.a.]
In vivo catabolism: [n.a.]

Evaluation of isolated patient fibrinogen
Thrombin time: [n.a.]
Reptilase time: [62s/(25s)[4]]
Ancrod (Arvin) time: [n.a.]

Abnormal subunit? [No]
Abnormal FDPs? [n.a.]

Remarks
[1]The structural defect was determined with the PCR method.
[2]Only half the normal amount of fibrinopeptide A was released.
[3]Proposita was a diabetic with a history of CNS ischaemic attacks, left brachial artery occlusion, and myocardial infarction. Arterial thrombosis at age 68 was reported.
[4]H. Al-Mondhiry, personal communication.

References

1. Galanakis, D.K., Henschen, A., Schubach, W., Lord, S. and Al-Mondhiry, H. Determination of abnormal structure and heterozygosity by amplification of genomic DNA using the polymerase chain reaction and by amino acid sequence analyses. In: *Fibrinogen 4. Current Basic and Clinical Aspects*, M. Matsuda, S. Iwanaga, A. Takada and A. Henschen (eds.), Elsevier Science Publ., B.V., Amsterdam. pp. 173-178, **1990**.

FIBRINOGEN HOMBURG I

Last update	[1 December 1990]	**Structural defect**	[n.a.]
Alphacode	[HOMBUR01]	**Mutation**	[n.a.]
Ref. type	[Article]		

Family studies
Homozygote? [No]
Pedigree published? [Yes]

Functional defect(s)
FpA release: [Abnormal]
FpB release: [n.a.]
Polymerization: [Abnormal]
Stabilization: [Normal]

Clinical manifestation(s) Bleeding? [No] Thrombosis? [No]

Clinical laboratory results

Plasma fibrinogen concentration (mg/dL)
Chronometric: [58/(150-430)]
Rate-indep'nt: [250/(180-360)]
Immunologic: [270/(190-450)]

*Hypo*dysfibrinogen? [No]

Thrombin time:	[44s/(<23s)]
Reptilase (batroxobin) time:	[58s/(<18s)]
Prothrombin time:	[47%/(>75%)]
Partial thromboplastin time:	[43s/(<39s)]
Euglobulin lysis time:	[n.a.]
Bleeding time:	[Normal]
Immunoelectrophoresis:	[Normal[2]]
Platelet aggregation:	[Abnormal[2]]

Other results with patient plasma

Ancrod (Arvin) time:	[n.a.]	Inhib. normal plasma?	[No]
Recalcification time:	[n.a.]	In vivo synthesis:	[n.a.]
Calcium corrects c.t.?	[No[2]]	In vivo catabolism:	[n.a.]

Evaluation of isolated patient fibrinogen

Thrombin time:	[n.a.]	Abnormal subunit?	[n.a.]
Reptilase time:	[n.a.]	Abnormal FDPs?	[n.a.]
Ancrod (Arvin) time:	[n.a.]		

Remarks
[1]Three unexamined siblings of index patient are alleged to have had bleeding diathesis.
[2]U.T. Seyfert & E. Wenzel, personal communication.

References

1. Miyashita, C., Nienhaus, K.-H., Wenzel, E., Kohler, M. and Hellstern, P. Observation on a new variant of hereditary dysfibrinogenemia (Homburg I) with delayed fibrin polymerisation and without clinical abnormality. In: *Fibrinogen — Recent Biochemical and Medical Aspects*, A. Henschen, H. Graeff and F. Lottspeich (eds.), W. de Gruyter, Berlin. pp. 193-200, **1982**.

2. Nienhaus, K.H., Wenzel, E., Taubert, W., Vief, B., Podolsak, B., Dreher, B., Giannitsis, D., Hoffsymmer, B. and Hess, H. [A clinically asymptomatic, new form of dysfibrinogenemia, fibrinogen 'Homburg']. In: *Fibrinogen, Fibrin, und Fibrinkleber*, K.I. Schimpf (ed.), F.K. Schattauer, Stuttgart, New York. pp. 185-190, **1980**.

3. Wenzel, E., Seyfert, U.T., Weier, B., Bohnerth, St., Pindur, G., Gu, L., Jung, F., Mrowietz, Ch., Harbauer, G. and Kotitschke, R. Clinical, rheological and haemostaseological aspects of dysfibrinogenemia. In: *Fibrinogen 4. Current Basic and Clinical Aspects*, M. Matsuda, S. Iwanaga, A. Takada and A. Henschen (eds.), Elsevier Science Publ., B.V., Amsterdam. pp. 153-158, **1990**.

FIBRINOGEN HOMBURG II

Last update [1 December 1990]
Alphacode [HOMBUR02]
Ref. type [Article]

Structural defect [Aα(16) Arg → Cys]
Mutation [n.a.]

Family studies
Homozygote? [No]
Pedigree published? [Yes]

Functional defect(s)
FpA release: [Abnormal[1]]
FpB release: [n.a.]
Polymerization: [Abnormal[1]]
Stabilization: [Normal]

Clinical manifestation(s) Bleeding? [No] Thrombosis? [No]

Clinical laboratory results
Plasma fibrinogen concentration (mg/dL)
Chronometric: [88/(150-430)[1]]
Rate-indep'nt: [282/(180-360)[1]]
Immunologic: [210/(190-450)[1]]

*Hypo*dysfibrinogen? [No]

Thrombin time:	[42s/(<23s)[1]]
Reptilase (batroxobin) time:	[54s/(<18s)[1]]
Prothrombin time:	[48%/(>75%)[1]]
Partial thromboplastin time:	[44s/(<39s)[1]]
Euglobulin lysis time:	[n.a.]
Bleeding time:	[Normal]
Immunoelectrophoresis:	[Normal]
Platelet aggregation:	[Normal]

Other results with patient plasma
Ancrod (Arvin) time: [n.a.]
Recalcification time: [n.a.]
Calcium corrects c.t.? [No[1]]

Inhib. normal plasma? [No[1]]
In vivo synthesis: [n.a.]
In vivo catabolism: [n.a.]

Evaluation of isolated patient fibrinogen
Thrombin time: [n.a.]
Reptilase time: [n.a.]
Ancrod (Arvin) time: [n.a.]

Abnormal subunit? [n.a.]
Abnormal FDPs? [n.a.]

Remarks
[1]U.T. Seyfert & E. Wenzel, personal communication.

References

1. Miyashita, C., Schwamborn, J., von Blohn, G., Wenzel, E. and Hellstern, P. Preliminary report concerning two new cases of congenital dysfibrinogenemia (Homburg II and Homburg III). In: *Fibrinogen — Structural Variants and Interactions*, A. Henschen, B. Hessel, J. McDonagh and T. Saldeen (eds.), Walter de Gruyter, Berlin. pp. 237-246, **1985**.

2. Wenzel, E., Seyfert, U.T., Weier, B., Bohnerth, St., Pindur, G., Gu, L., Jung, F., Mrowietz, Ch., Harbauer, G. and Kotitschke, R. Clinical, rheological and haemostaseological aspects of dysfibrinogenemia. In: *Fibrinogen 4. Current Basic and Clinical Aspects*, M. Matsuda, S. Iwanaga, A. Takada and A. Henschen (eds.), Elsevier Science Publ., B.V., Amsterdam. pp. 153-158, **1990**.

FIBRINOGEN HOMBURG III

Last update [1 December 1990]
Alphacode [HOMBUR03]
Ref. type [Article]

Structural defect [Aα(16) Arg → Cys]
Mutation [n.a.]

Family studies
Homozygote? [No]
Pedigree published? [Yes]

Functional defect(s)
FpA release: [Abnormal[1]]
FpB release: [Abnormal[1]]
Polymerization: [Abnormal[1]]
Stabilization: [Normal]

Clinical manifestation(s) Bleeding? [Yes[2]] Thrombosis? [No]

Clinical laboratory results
Plasma fibrinogen concentration (mg/dL)
Chronometric: [55/(150-430)[1]]
Rate-indep'nt: [275/(180-360)[1]]
Immunologic: [240/(190-450)[1]]

*Hypo*dysfibrinogen? [No]

Thrombin time:	[42s/(<23s)[1]]
Reptilase (batroxobin) time:	[80s/(<18s)[1]]
Prothrombin time:	[50%/(>75%)[1]]
Partial thromboplastin time:	[35s/(<39s)]
Euglobulin lysis time:	[n.a.]
Bleeding time:	[Normal]
Immunoelectrophoresis:	[Normal]
Platelet aggregation:	[Abnormal]

Other results with patient plasma
Ancrod (Arvin) time: [n.a.]
Recalcification time: [n.a.]
Calcium corrects c.t.? [No[1]]

Inhib. normal plasma? [No]
In vivo synthesis: [n.a.]
In vivo catabolism: [n.a.]

Evaluation of isolated patient fibrinogen
Thrombin time: [n.a.]
Reptilase time: [n.a.]
Ancrod (Arvin) time: [n.a.]

Abnormal subunit? [n.a.]
Abnormal FDPs? [n.a.]

Remarks
[1]U.T. Seyfert & E. Wenzel, personal communication.
[2]Two spontaneous abortions, excessive postpartum bleeding, and abnormal bleeding following dental extraction in the 22 year-old proposita were reported.

References

1. Miyashita, C., Schwamborn, J., von Blohn, G., Wenzel, E. and Hellstern, P. Preliminary report concerning two new cases of congenital dysfibrinogenemia (Homburg II and Homburg III). In: *Fibrinogen —Structural Variants and Interactions*, A. Henschen, B. Hessel, J. McDonagh and T. Saldeen (eds.), Walter de Gruyter, Berlin. pp. 237-246, **1985**.

2. Wenzel, E., Seyfert, U.T., Weier, B., Bohnerth, St., Pindur, G., Gu, L., Jung, F., Mrowietz, Ch., Harbauer, G. and Kotitschke, R. Clinical, rheological and haemostaseological aspects of dysfibrinogenemia. In: *Fibrinogen 4. Current Basic and Clinical Aspects*, M. Matsuda, S. Iwanaga, A. Takada and A. Henschen (eds.), Elsevier Science Publ., B.V., Amsterdam. pp. 153-158, **1990**.

FIBRINOGEN HOMBURG IV

Last update [10 January 1994]
Alphacode [HOMBUR04]
Ref. type [Article]

Family studies
Homozygote? [No[1]]
Pedigree published? [No]

Structural defect [n.a.]
Mutation [n.a.]

Functional defect(s)
FpA release: [Normal]
FpB release: [Normal[1]]
Polymerization: [Abnormal]
Stabilization: [Normal[1]]

Clinical manifestation(s) Bleeding? [No] Thrombosis? [No]

Clinical laboratory results

Plasma fibrinogen concentration (mg/dL)
Chronometric: [64/(150-430)[1]]
Rate-indep'nt: [230/(180-360)[1]]
Immunologic: [180/(190-450)[1]]

*Hypo*dysfibrinogen? [No]

Thrombin time:	[29s/(<23s)[1]]
Reptilase (batroxobin) time:	[40.5s/(<18s)[1]]
Prothrombin time:	[46%/(>75%)[1]]
Partial thromboplastin time:	[42s/(<39s)[1]]
Euglobulin lysis time:	[n.a.]
Bleeding time:	[Normal[1]]
Immunoelectrophoresis:	[n.a.]
Platelet aggregation:	[n.a.]

Other results with patient plasma
Ancrod (Arvin) time: [n.a.]
Recalcification time: [n.a.]
Calcium corrects c.t.? [No[1]]

Inhib. normal plasma? [No[1]]
In vivo synthesis: [n.a.]
In vivo catabolism: [n.a.]

Evaluation of isolated patient fibrinogen
Thrombin time: [n.a.]
Reptilase time: [n.a.]
Ancrod (Arvin) time: [n.a.]

Abnormal subunit? [n.a.]
Abnormal FDPs? [n.a.]

Remarks
[1]U.T. Seyfert & E. Wenzel, personal communication.

References

1. Wenzel, E., Seyfert, U.T., Weier, B., Bohnerth, St., Pindur, G., Gu, L., Jung, F., Mrowietz, Ch., Harbauer, G. and Kotitschke, R. Clinical, rheological and haemostaseological aspects of dysfibrinogenemia. In: *Fibrinogen 4. Current Basic and Clinical Aspects*, M. Matsuda, S. Iwanaga, A. Takada and A. Henschen (eds.), Elsevier Science Publ., B.V., Amsterdam. pp. 153-158, **1990**.

FIBRINOGEN HOMBURG V

Last update [10 January 1994]
Alphacode [HOMBUR05]
Ref. type [Article]

Family studies
Homozygote? [No[1]]
Pedigree published? [No]

Structural defect [n.a.]
Mutation [n.a.]

Functional defect(s)
FpA release: [Abnormal]
FpB release: [Abnormal[1]]
Polymerization: [Abnormal]
Stabilization: [Normal[1]]

Clinical manifestation(s) Bleeding? [No] Thrombosis? [No]

Clinical laboratory results
Plasma fibrinogen concentration (mg/dL)
Chronometric: [29/(150-430)[1]]
Rate-indep'nt: [180/(180-360)[1]]
Immunologic: [388/(190-450)[1]]

*Hypo*dysfibrinogen? [No]

Thrombin time:	[40s/(<23s)[1]]
Reptilase (batroxobin) time:	[49s/(<18s)[1]]
Prothrombin time:	[54%/(>75%)[1]]
Partial thromboplastin time:	[41s/(<39s)[1]]
Euglobulin lysis time:	[n.a.]
Bleeding time:	[Normal[1]]
Immunoelectrophoresis:	[n.a.]
Platelet aggregation:	[n.a.]

Other results with patient plasma
Ancrod (Arvin) time: [n.a.]
Recalcification time: [n.a.]
Calcium corrects c.t.? [n.a.]

Inhib. normal plasma? [n.a.]
In vivo synthesis: [n.a.]
In vivo catabolism: [n.a.]

Evaluation of isolated patient fibrinogen
Thrombin time: [n.a.]
Reptilase time: [n.a.]
Ancrod (Arvin) time: [n.a.]

Abnormal subunit? [n.a.]
Abnormal FDPs? [n.a.]

Remarks
[1]U.T. Seyfert & E. Wenzel, personal communication.

References

1. Wenzel, E., Seyfert, U.T., Weier, B., Bohnerth, St., Pindur, G., Gu, L., Jung, F., Mrowietz, Ch., Harbauer, G. and Kotitschke, R. Clinical, rheological and haemostaseological aspects of dysfibrinogenemia. In: *Fibrinogen 4. Current Basic and Clinical Aspects*, M. Matsuda, S. Iwanaga, A. Takada and A. Henschen (eds.), Elsevier Science Publ., B.V., Amsterdam. pp. 153-158, **1990**.

FIBRINOGEN HOMBURG VI

Last update [1 December 1990]
Alphacode [HOMBUR06]
Ref. type [Article]

Structural defect [n.a.]
Mutation [n.a.]

Family studies
Homozygote? [n.a.]
Pedigree published? [No]

Functional defect(s)
FpA release: [n.a.]
FpB release: [n.a.]
Polymerization: [n.a.]
Stabilization: [n.a.]

Clinical manifestation(s) Bleeding? [No] Thrombosis? [No]

Clinical laboratory results

Plasma fibrinogen concentration (mg/dL)
Chronometric: [48/(150-430)[1]]
Rate-indep'nt: [120/(180-360)[1]]
Immunologic: [543/(190-450)[1]]

*Hypo*dysfibrinogen? [n.a.]

Thrombin time:	[38s/(<23s)[1]]
Reptilase (batroxobin) time:	[42s/(<18s)[1]]
Prothrombin time:	[59%/(>75%)[1]]
Partial thromboplastin time:	[39s/(<39s)[1]]
Euglobulin lysis time:	[n.a.]
Bleeding time:	[Normal[1]]
Immunoelectrophoresis:	[n.a.]
Platelet aggregation:	[Abnormal[1]]

Other results with patient plasma
Ancrod (Arvin) time: [n.a.]
Recalcification time: [n.a.]
Calcium corrects c.t.? [No[1]]

Inhib. normal plasma? [No[1]]
In vivo synthesis: [n.a.]
In vivo catabolism: [n.a.]

Evaluation of isolated patient fibrinogen
Thrombin time: [n.a.]
Reptilase time: [n.a.]
Ancrod (Arvin) time: [n.a.]

Abnormal subunit? [n.a.]
Abnormal FDPs? [n.a.]

Remarks
[1]U.T. Seyfert & E. Wenzel, personal communication.

References

1. Wenzel, E., Seyfert, U.T., Weier, B., Bohnerth, St., Pindur, G., Gu, L., Jung, F., Mrowietz, Ch., Harbauer, G. and Kotitschke, R. Clinical, rheological and haemostaseological aspects of dysfibrinogenemia. In: *Fibrinogen 4. Current Basic and Clinical Aspects*, M. Matsuda, S. Iwanaga, A. Takada and A. Henschen (eds.), Elsevier Science Publ., B.V., Amsterdam. pp. 153-158, **1990**.

FIBRINOGEN HOUSTON I

Last update [1 December 1990]
Alphacode [HOUSTO01]
Ref. type [Article]

Structural defect [n.a.]
Mutation [n.a.]

Family studies
Homozygote? [n.a.]
Pedigree published? [No]

Functional defect(s)
FpA release: [Normal[1]]
FpB release: [Normal[1]]
Polymerization: [Abnormal[2]]
Stabilization: [Normal]

Clinical manifestation(s) Bleeding? [Yes[3]] Thrombosis? [No]

Clinical laboratory results
Plasma fibrinogen concentration (mg/dL)
Chronometric: [n.a.]
Rate-indep'nt: [n.a.]
Immunologic: [640/(150-350)]

*Hypo*dysfibrinogen? [No]

Thrombin time:	[32s/(18-22s)]
Reptilase (batroxobin) time:	[21s/(21-22s)]
Prothrombin time:	[27s/(11-13s)]
Partial thromboplastin time:	[87s/(<35s)]
Euglobulin lysis time:	[n.a.]
Bleeding time:	[Normal]
Immunoelectrophoresis:	[Normal]
Platelet aggregation:	[Normal]

Other results with patient plasma
Ancrod (Arvin) time: [n.a.]
Recalcification time: [>1800s/(<135s)]
Calcium corrects c.t.? [No]

Inhib. normal plasma? [Yes[3]]
In vivo synthesis: [n.a.]
In vivo catabolism: [n.a.]

Evaluation of isolated patient fibrinogen
Thrombin time: [21s/(20-22s)]
Reptilase time: [n.a.]
Ancrod (Arvin) time: [n.a.]

Abnormal subunit? [No]
Abnormal FDPs? [Yes]

Remarks
[1]The rate of *total* fibrinopeptide release was normal.
[2]Fibrin monomers formed after Reptilase treatment polymerized normally; those formed after thrombin treatment polymerized abnormally. This suggests a defect in fibrinopeptide B release or in the B polymerization site.
[3]The index patient was positive for a circulating anticoagulant.

References

1. Weinger, R.S., Rudy, C., Moake, J.L., Conlon, C.L. and Cimo, P.L. Fibrinogen Houston: A dysfibrinogen exhibiting defective fibrin monomer aggregation and α-chain cross-linkages. *Am. J. Hematol.* **9**:237-248, **1980**.

FIBRINOGEN HOUSTON II

Last update	[1 December 1990]	**Structural defect**	[n.a.]
Alphacode	[HOUSTO02]	**Mutation**	[n.a.]
Ref. type	[Article]		

Family studies
Homozygote? [n.a.]
Pedigree published? [No]

Functional defect(s)
FpA release: [n.a.]
FpB release: [n.a.]
Polymerization: [n.a.]
Stabilization: [n.a.]

Clinical manifestation(s) Bleeding? [Yes[1]] Thrombosis? [No]

Clinical laboratory results
Plasma fibrinogen concentration (mg/dL)
Chronometric: [n.a.]
Rate-indep'nt: [n.a.]
Immunologic: [n.a.]

*Hypo*dysfibrinogen? [n.a.]

Thrombin time:	[27s/(<19s)]
Reptilase (batroxobin) time:	[n.a.]
Prothrombin time:	[13s/(11-12s)]
Partial thromboplastin time:	[42s/(24-36s)]
Euglobulin lysis time:	[n.a.]
Bleeding time:	[Normal]
Immunoelectrophoresis:	[n.a.]
Platelet aggregation:	[n.a.]

Other results with patient plasma

Ancrod (Arvin) time:	[n.a.]	Inhib. normal plasma?	[n.a.]
Recalcification time:	[n.a.]	In vivo synthesis:	[n.a.]
Calcium corrects c.t.?	[n.a.]	In vivo catabolism:	[n.a.]

Evaluation of isolated patient fibrinogen

Thrombin time:	[n.a.]	Abnormal subunit?	[n.a.]
Reptilase time:	[n.a.]	Abnormal FDPs?	[n.a.]
Ancrod (Arvin) time:	[n.a.]		

Remarks

[1]Severe post-surgical bleeding, corrected by administration of cryoprecipitate and fresh-frozen plasma, was reported (W.E. Walker, personal communication).

This variant was not named in the publication by Vander Woude et al. (1988). The name was assigned in consultation with J.C. Vander Woude, J.D. Milam, and W.E. Walker.

References

1. Vander Woude, J.C., Milam, J.D., Walker, W.E., Houchin, D.P., Weiland, A.P., and Cooley, D.A. Cardiovascular surgery in patients with congenital plasma coagulopathies. *Ann. Thorac. Surg.* **46**:283-288, **1988**.

FIBRINOGEN IJMUIDEN I

Last update [10 January 1994]
Alphacode [IJMUID01]
Ref. type [Article]

Family studies
Homozygote? [No]
Pedigree published? [No]

Structural defect [Bβ(14) Arg → Cys[1]]
Mutation [CGT → TGT]

Functional defect(s)
FpA release: [n.a.]
FpB release: [Abnormal[2]]
Polymerization: [Abnormal]
Stabilization: [n.a.]

Clinical manifestation(s) Bleeding? [No] Thrombosis? [Yes]

Clinical laboratory results
Plasma fibrinogen concentration (mg/dL)
Chronometric: [90/(180-490)]
Rate-indep'nt: [n.a.]
Immunologic: [270/(160-500)]

*Hypo*dysfibrinogen? [No]

Thrombin time:	[25.0s/(18.5s)]
Reptilase (batroxobin) time:	[26.0s/(20s)]
Prothrombin time:	[n.a.]
Partial thromboplastin time:	[n.a.]
Euglobulin lysis time:	[n.a.]
Bleeding time:	[n.a.]
Immunoelectrophoresis:	[n.a.]
Platelet aggregation:	[n.a.]

Other results with patient plasma
Ancrod (Arvin) time: [n.a.]
Recalcification time: [n.a.]
Calcium corrects c.t.? [n.a.]

Inhib. normal plasma? [n.a.]
In vivo synthesis: [n.a.]
In vivo catabolism: [n.a.]

Evaluation of isolated patient fibrinogen
Thrombin time: [n.a.]
Reptilase time: [n.a.]
Ancrod (Arvin) time: [n.a.]

Abnormal subunit? [n.a.]
Abnormal FDPs? [n.a.[3]]

Remarks
Abnormal high-molecular-weight fibrinogen complexes and disulfide-linked fibrinogen-albumin complexes were reported.
[1]The structural defect was determined with the PCR method.
[2]Only half the normal amount of FpB was released.
[3]A reduced rate of t-PA-induced plasminogen activation was reported.

References

1. Koopman, J., Haverkate, F., Grimbergen, J., Engesser, L., Nováková, I., Kerst, A.F.J.A. and Lord, S.T. Abnormal fibrinogens IJmuiden (BβArg_{14}→Cys) and Nijmegen (BβArg_{44}→Cys) form disulfide-linked fibrinogen-albumin complexes. *Proc. Natl. Acad. Sci. USA* **89**:3478-3482, **1992**.

2. Koopman, J. and Haverkate, F. Structure-function relationships in abnormal fibrinogens. Defects at the DNA level. In: *Fibrinogen 4. Current Basic and Clinical Aspects*, M. Matsuda, S. Iwanaga, A. Takada and A. Henschen (eds.), Elsevier Science Publ., B.V., Amsterdam. pp. 179-183, **1990**.

3. Koopman, J., Engesser, L., Nieveen, M., Haverkate, F. and Brommer, E.J.P. Fibrin polymerization associated with tissue-type plasminogen activator (t-PA) induced glu-plasminogen activation. In: *Fibrinogen and Its Derivatives*, G. Müller-Berghaus, U. Scheefers-Borchel, E. Selmayr and A. Henschen (eds.), Excerpta Medica, Amsterdam. pp. 315-318, **1986**.

FIBRINOGEN INDIANAPOLIS I

Last update [10 January 1994]
Alphacode [INDIAN01]
Ref. type [Article]

Structural defect [Aα(554) Arg → Leu[1]]
Mutation [CGT → CTT]

Family studies
Homozygote? [No]
Pedigree published? [Yes]

Functional defect(s)
FpA release: [n.a.]
FpB release: [n.a.]
Polymerization: [n.a.]
Stabilization: [n.a.]

Clinical manifestation(s) Bleeding? [No[2]] Thrombosis? [No[2]]

Clinical laboratory results

Plasma fibrinogen concentration (mg/dL)
Chronometric: [n.a.]
Rate-indep'nt: [n.a.]
Immunologic: [n.a.]

*Hypo*dysfibrinogen? [n.a.]

Thrombin time:	[n.a.]
Reptilase (batroxobin) time:	[n.a.]
Prothrombin time:	[n.a.]
Partial thromboplastin time:	[n.a.]
Euglobulin lysis time:	[n.a.]
Bleeding time:	[n.a.]
Immunoelectrophoresis:	[n.a.]
Platelet aggregation:	[n.a.]

Other results with patient plasma
Ancrod (Arvin) time: [n.a.]
Recalcification time: [n.a.]
Calcium corrects c.t.? [n.a.]

Inhib. normal plasma? [n.a.]
In vivo synthesis: [n.a.]
In vivo catabolism: [n.a.]

Evaluation of isolated patient fibrinogen
Thrombin time: [n.a.]
Reptilase time: [n.a.]
Ancrod (Arvin) time: [n.a.]

Abnormal subunit? [n.a.]
Abnormal FDPs? [n.a.]

Remarks

[1]The structural defect was determined with the PCR method.

[2]Fatal renal amyloidosis was reported for the propositus and some affected family members. The demise of the propositus (originally from Peru) precluded further functional analyses. See also fibrinogens Indianapolis II and III.

References

1. Benson, M.D., Liepnieks, J., Uemichi, T., Wheeler, G. and Correa, R. Hereditary renal amyloidosis associated with a mutant fibrinogen α-chain. *Nature Genet.* **3**:252-255, **1993**.

FIBRINOGEN INDIANAPOLIS II

Last update [10 January 1994]
Alphacode [INDIAN02]
Ref. type [Article]

Structural defect [Aα(526) Val → Glu]
Mutation [GAG → GTG]

Family studies
Homozygote? [No]
Pedigree published? [Yes]

Functional defect(s)
FpA release: [n.a.]
FpB release: [n.a.]
Polymerization: [n.a.]
Stabilization: [n.a.]

Clinical manifestation(s) Bleeding? [No[1]] Thrombosis? [No[1]]

Clinical laboratory results

Plasma fibrinogen concentration (mg/dL)
Chronometric: [Normal]
Rate-indep'nt: [n.a.]
Immunologic: [Normal]

*Hypo*dysfibrinogen? [No]

Thrombin time:	[Normal]
Reptilase (batroxobin) time:	[Normal]
Prothrombin time:	[n.a.]
Partial thromboplastin time:	[n.a.]
Euglobulin lysis time:	[n.a.]
Bleeding time:	[n.a.]
Immunoelectrophoresis:	[n.a.]
Platelet aggregation:	[n.a.]

Other results with patient plasma
Ancrod (Arvin) time: [n.a.]
Recalcification time: [n.a.]
Calcium corrects c.t.? [n.a.]

Inhib. normal plasma? [n.a.]
In vivo synthesis: [n.a.]
In vivo catabolism: [n.a.]

Evaluation of isolated patient fibrinogen
Thrombin time: [n.a.]
Reptilase time: [n.a.]
Ancrod (Arvin) time: [n.a.]

Abnormal subunit? [n.a.]
Abnormal FDPs? [n.a.]

Remarks

[1]Variants with this mutation have been associated with hereditary renal amyloidosis (see also fibrinogens Indianapolis I and III). Note that the thrombin time is not prolonged and the variant fibrinogen appears to be fully functional in terms of coagulability.

The assistance of J.J. Liepnieks and M.D. Benson in communicating unpublished results is acknowledged with appreciation.

References

1. Uemichi, T., Liepnieks, J.J. and Benson, M.D. Hereditary renal amyloidosis with a novel variant fibrinogen. *J. Clin. Invest.* **93**:731-736, **1994**.

FIBRINOGEN INDIANAPOLIS III

Last update [10 January 1994]
Alphacode [INDIAN03]
Ref. type [Article]

Structural defect [Aα(526) Val → Glu]
Mutation [GAG → GTG]

Family studies
Homozygote? [No]
Pedigree published? [Yes]

Functional defect(s)
FpA release: [n.a.]
FpB release: [n.a.]
Polymerization: [n.a.]
Stabilization: [n.a.]

Clinical manifestation(s) Bleeding? [No[1]] Thrombosis? [No[1]]

Clinical laboratory results
Plasma fibrinogen concentration (mg/dL)
Chronometric: [Normal]
Rate-indep'nt: [n.a.]
Immunologic: [Normal]

*Hypo*dysfibrinogen? [No]

Thrombin time:	[Normal]
Reptilase (batroxobin) time:	[Normal]
Prothrombin time:	[n.a.]
Partial thromboplastin time:	[n.a.]
Euglobulin lysis time:	[n.a.]
Bleeding time:	[n.a.]
Immunoelectrophoresis:	[n.a.]
Platelet aggregation:	[n.a.]

Other results with patient plasma
Ancrod (Arvin) time: [n.a.]
Recalcification time: [n.a.]
Calcium corrects c.t.? [n.a.]

Inhib. normal plasma? [n.a.]
In vivo synthesis: [n.a.]
In vivo catabolism: [n.a.]

Evaluation of isolated patient fibrinogen
Thrombin time: [n.a.]
Reptilase time: [n.a.]
Ancrod (Arvin) time: [n.a.]

Abnormal subunit? [n.a.]
Abnormal FDPs? [n.a.]

Remarks
[1]Variants with this mutation have been associated with hereditary renal amyloidosis (see also fibrinogens Indianapolis I and II). Note that the thrombin time is not prolonged and the variant fibrinogen appears to be fully functional in terms of coagulability.

The assistance of J.J. Liepnieks and M.D. Benson in communicating unpublished results is acknowledged with appreciation.

References

1. Uemichi, T., Liepnieks, J.J. and Benson, M.D. Hereditary renal amyloidosis with a novel variant fibrinogen. *J. Clin. Invest.* **93**:731-736, **1994**.

FIBRINOGEN IOWA CITY I

Last update [1 December 1990]
Alphacode [IOWACI01]
Ref. type [Article]

Family studies
Homozygote? [n.a.]
Pedigree published? [No]

Structural defect [n.a.]
Mutation [n.a.]

Functional defect(s)
FpA release: [n.a.]
FpB release: [n.a.]
Polymerization: [n.a.]
Stabilization: [Normal]

Clinical manifestation(s) Bleeding? [No[1]] Thrombosis? [No[1]]

Clinical laboratory results

Plasma fibrinogen concentration (mg/dL)
Chronometric: [71[2]]
Rate-indep'nt: [141[2]]
Immunologic: [238[2]]

*Hypo*dysfibrinogen? [No]

Thrombin time:	[278s/(34-38s)]
Reptilase (batroxobin) time:	[173s/(18s)]
Prothrombin time:	[n.a.]
Partial thromboplastin time:	[n.a.]
Euglobulin lysis time:	[n.a.]
Bleeding time:	[Normal]
Immunoelectrophoresis:	[Normal]
Platelet aggregation:	[Normal]

Other results with patient plasma
Ancrod (Arvin) time: [8-10h/(10s)]
Recalcification time: [n.a.]
Calcium corrects c.t.? [No]

Inhib. normal plasma? [n.a.]
In vivo synthesis: [n.a.]
In vivo catabolism: [n.a.]

Evaluation of isolated patient fibrinogen
Thrombin time: [n.a.]
Reptilase time: [n.a.]
Ancrod (Arvin) time: [n.a.]

Abnormal subunit? [n.a.]
Abnormal FDPs? [n.a.]

Remarks

[1]The index patient had a history of alcoholism, drug abuse, and pyromania.
[2]Normal range not reported.

References

1. Jacobsen, C.D. and Hoak, J.C. Fibrinogen Iowa City: An abnormal fibrinogen with no clinical symptoms. *Thromb. Res.* **2**:261-270, **1973**.

FIBRINOGEN IRVINE I

Last update [1 December 1990]
Alphacode [IRVINE01]
Ref. type [Article]

Structural defect [n.a.]
Mutation [n.a.]

Family studies
Homozygote? [n.a.]
Pedigree published? [Yes]

Functional defect(s)
FpA release: [Abnormal]
FpB release: [n.a.]
Polymerization: [n.a.]
Stabilization: [Normal]

Clinical manifestation(s) Bleeding? [No] Thrombosis? [Yes[1]]

Clinical laboratory results
Plasma fibrinogen concentration (mg/dL)
Chronometric: [170/(200-370)]
Rate-indep'nt: [290/(200-370)]
Immunologic: [300/(200-370)]

*Hypo*dysfibrinogen? [No]

Thrombin time:	[Abnormal[2]]
Reptilase (batroxobin) time:	[n.a.]
Prothrombin time:	[Normal[2]]
Partial thromboplastin time:	[Normal[2]]
Euglobulin lysis time:	[n.a.]
Bleeding time:	[n.a.]
Immunoelectrophoresis:	[Cathodal]
Platelet aggregation:	[n.a.]

Other results with patient plasma
Ancrod (Arvin) time: [n.a.]
Recalcification time: [n.a.]
Calcium corrects c.t.? [n.a.]

Inhib. normal plasma? [n.a.]
In vivo synthesis: [n.a.]
In vivo catabolism: [n.a.]

Evaluation of isolated patient fibrinogen
Thrombin time: [n.a.]
Reptilase time: [n.a.]
Ancrod (Arvin) time: [n.a.]

Abnormal subunit? [n.a.]
Abnormal FDPs? [n.a.]

Remarks
[1]Propositus exhibited predisposition to visceral vein thrombosis.
[2]Data not reported.

References

1. Lehmer, R.R., Elias, A.N., Capdeville, M.J., Brown, D.R. and Branson, H.E. Fibrinogen Irvine: a qualitatively abnormal fibrinogen associated with the predisposition to recurrent visceral and peripheral venous thrombosis. *J. Natl. Med. Assoc.* **78**:561-565, **1985**.

FIBRINOGEN ISE I

Last update	[10 January 1994]	**Structural defect**	[Bβ(15) Gly → Cys]
Alphacode	[ISE01]	**Mutation**	[n.a.]
Ref. type	[Article]		

Family studies
Homozygote? [No]
Pedigree published? [Yes]

Functional defect(s)
FpA release: [Normal]
FpB release: [Abnormal[1]]
Polymerization: [Abnormal[2]]
Stabilization: [n.a.]

Clinical manifestation(s) Bleeding? [No] Thrombosis? [No]

Clinical laboratory results

Plasma fibrinogen concentration (mg/dL)
Chronometric: [129/(150-350)]
Rate-indep'nt: [277/(150-350)]
Immunologic: [256/(150-350)]

*Hypo*dysfibrinogen? [No]

Thrombin time:	[22.4s/(12-13.8s)]
Reptilase (batroxobin) time:	[n.a.]
Prothrombin time:	[Normal[3]]
Partial thromboplastin time:	[Normal[3]]
Euglobulin lysis time:	[n.a.]
Bleeding time:	[Normal]
Immunoelectrophoresis:	[n.a.]
Platelet aggregation:	[Normal]

Other results with patient plasma

Ancrod (Arvin) time:	[n.a.]	Inhib. normal plasma?	[n.a.]
Recalcification time:	[n.a.]	In vivo synthesis:	[n.a.]
Calcium corrects c.t.?	[n.a.]	In vivo catabolism:	[n.a.]

Evaluation of isolated patient fibrinogen

Thrombin time:	[12.5s/(5.2-7.2s)]	Abnormal subunit?	[No]
Reptilase time:	[16.3s/(14.8-19.9s)]	Abnormal FDPs?	[No]
Ancrod (Arvin) time:	[n.a.]		

Remarks

[1]Only half the normal amount of fibrinopeptide B was released.

[2]Fibrin polymerization was abnormal when initiated by thrombin, but the polymerization curve was the same as normal when initiated by Reptilase.

[3]Data not reported.

References

1. Yoshida, N., Hirata, H., Asakura, S., Yamazumi, K., Matsuda, M., Wada, H., Shirakawa, S. and Okuma, M. Calcium binding to abnormal fibrinogens with a single amino acid replacement in the NH2-terminal region of fibrin α- or β-chain. *Thromb. Res.* **67**:613-618, **1992**.

2. Yoshida, N., Wada, H., Morita, K., Hirata, H., Matsuda, M., Yamazumi, K., Asakura, S. and Shirakawa, S. A new congenital abnormal fibrinogen Ise characterized by the replacement of Bβ Glycine-15 by cysteine. *Blood* **77**:1958-1963, **1991**.

FIBRINOGEN ISTANBUL I

Last update	[1 December 1990]	**Structural defect**	[n.a.]
Alphacode	[ISTANB01]	**Mutation**	[n.a.]
Ref. type	[Article]		

Family studies
Homozygote? [n.a.]
Pedigree published? [No]

Functional defect(s)
FpA release: [n.a.]
FpB release: [n.a.]
Polymerization: [n.a.]
Stabilization: [n.a.]

Clinical manifestation(s) Bleeding? [No] Thrombosis? [Yes[1]]

Clinical laboratory results

Plasma fibrinogen concentration (mg/dL)
Chronometric: [0/(200-300)]
Rate-indep'nt: [260/(200-300)[1]]
Immunologic: [320/(240)]

*Hypo*dysfibrinogen? [No]

Thrombin time:	[120s/(10s)]
Reptilase (batroxobin) time:	[80s/(14s)]
Prothrombin time:	[>120s/(12s)]
Partial thromboplastin time:	[300s/(45s)]
Euglobulin lysis time:	[No clot]
Bleeding time:	[n.a.]
Immunoelectrophoresis:	[Normal]
Platelet aggregation:	[Abnormal]

Other results with patient plasma

Ancrod (Arvin) time:	[n.a.]	Inhib. normal plasma?	[No]
Recalcification time:	[360s/(90s)]	In vivo synthesis:	[n.a.]
Calcium corrects c.t.?	[No]	In vivo catabolism:	[n.a.]

Evaluation of isolated patient fibrinogen

Thrombin time:	[n.a.]	Abnormal subunit?	[Yes]
Reptilase time:	[n.a.]	Abnormal FDPs?	[n.a.]
Ancrod (Arvin) time:	[n.a.]		

Remarks
[1]O.N. Ulutin, personal communication.

References

1. Ulutin, O.N. *The Platelets. Fundamentals and Clinical Applications*, pp. 288-289, **1976**

2. Ulutin, O.N. and Ulutin, S.B. Fibrinogen Istanbul — a new case of dysfibrinogenemia. *Second Meeting of the European and African Division of the International Society of Haematology* p. 252, **1973**. ABSTRACT

3. Ulutin, O.N. and Ulutin, S.B. [Fibrinogen Istanbul]. *Hematoloji, Turkey* 1:153-167, **1970**.

FIBRINOGEN ISTANBUL II^{Unp}

Last update [1 December 1990]
Alphacode [ISTANB02]
Ref. type [Unpublished[1]]

Family studies
Homozygote? [n.a.]
Pedigree published? [No]

Structural defect [n.a.]
Mutation [n.a.]

Functional defect(s)
FpA release: [Abnormal]
FpB release: [Abnormal]
Polymerization: [Normal]
Stabilization: [n.a.]

Clinical manifestation(s) Bleeding? [Yes] Thrombosis? [No]

Clinical laboratory results

Plasma fibrinogen concentration (mg/dL)
Chronometric: [n.a.]
Rate-indep'nt: [n.a.]
Immunologic: [n.a.]

*Hypo*dysfibrinogen? [n.a.]

Thrombin time:	[35s/(11s)]
Reptilase (batroxobin) time:	[n.a.]
Prothrombin time:	[n.a.]
Partial thromboplastin time:	[n.a.]
Euglobulin lysis time:	[n.a.]
Bleeding time:	[n.a.]
Immunoelectrophoresis:	[n.a.]
Platelet aggregation:	[n.a.]

Other results with patient plasma
Ancrod (Arvin) time: [n.a.]
Recalcification time: [n.a.]
Calcium corrects c.t.? [n.a.]

Inhib. normal plasma? [n.a.]
In vivo synthesis: [n.a.]
In vivo catabolism: [n.a.]

Evaluation of isolated patient fibrinogen
Thrombin time: [n.a.]
Reptilase time: [n.a.]
Ancrod (Arvin) time: [n.a.]

Abnormal subunit? [n.a.]
Abnormal FDPs? [n.a.]

Remarks
[1]O.N. Ulutin, personal communication.

References

FIBRINOGEN JENA I

Last update	[1 December 1990]	**Structural defect**	[n.a.]
Alphacode	[JENA01]	**Mutation**	[n.a.]
Ref. type	[Article]		

Family studies
Homozygote? [No]
Pedigree published? [Yes]

Functional defect(s)
FpA release: [Abnormal[1]]
FpB release: [n.a.]
Polymerization: [n.a.]
Stabilization: [n.a.]

Clinical manifestation(s) Bleeding? [No] Thrombosis? [No]

Clinical laboratory results

Plasma fibrinogen concentration (mg/dL)
Chronometric: [n.a.]
Rate-indep'nt: [186[2]]
Immunologic: [436[2]]

*Hypo*dysfibrinogen? [No]

Thrombin time:	[26s[2]]
Reptilase (batroxobin) time:	[60s[3]]
Prothrombin time:	[34%[3]]
Partial thromboplastin time:	[40s[2]]
Euglobulin lysis time:	[n.a.]
Bleeding time:	[n.a.]
Immunoelectrophoresis:	[n.a.]
Platelet aggregation:	[n.a.]

Other results with patient plasma

Ancrod (Arvin) time:	[n.a.]	Inhib. normal plasma?	[n.a.]
Recalcification time:	[n.a.]	In vivo synthesis:	[n.a.]
Calcium corrects c.t.?	[n.a.]	In vivo catabolism:	[n.a.]

Evaluation of isolated patient fibrinogen

Thrombin time:	[n.a.]	Abnormal subunit?	[n.a.]
Reptilase time:	[n.a.]	Abnormal FDPs?	[n.a.]
Ancrod (Arvin) time:	[n.a.]		

Remarks
[1]Only half the normal amount of fibrinopeptide A was released.
[2]Normal range not reported; this value is normal.
[3]Normal range not reported; this value is abnormal.

References

1. Maak, B. Hereditary dysfibrinogenaemia (fibrinogen Jena)—report of a family study. *Folia Haematol. (Leipz.)* **115**:519-522, **1988**.

FIBRINOGEN KANAZAWA I

Last update [10 January 1994]
Alphacode [KANAZA01]
Ref. type [Article]

Family studies
Homozygote? [No]
Pedigree published? [Yes]

Structural defect [Aα(18) Pro → Leu]
Mutation [n.a.]

Functional defect(s)
FpA release: [n.a.[1]]
FpB release: [n.a.[1]]
Polymerization: [Abnormal]
Stabilization: [n.a.]

Clinical manifestation(s) Bleeding? [No] Thrombosis? [No]

Clinical laboratory results

Plasma fibrinogen concentration (mg/dL)
Chronometric: [65/(150-350)]
Rate-indep'nt: [337/(150-350)] *Hypo*dysfibrinogen? [No]
Immunologic: [371/(150-350)]

Thrombin time:	[18.4s/(10.5s)]
Reptilase (batroxobin) time:	[187s/(31.3s)]
Prothrombin time:	[Normal]
Partial thromboplastin time:	[Normal]
Euglobulin lysis time:	[Normal]
Bleeding time:	[Normal]
Immunoelectrophoresis:	[n.a.]
Platelet aggregation:	[Normal]

Other results with patient plasma
Ancrod (Arvin) time: [n.a.]
Recalcification time: [n.a.]
Calcium corrects c.t.? [No]
Inhib. normal plasma? [n.a.]
In vivo synthesis: [n.a.]
In vivo catabolism: [n.a.]

Evaluation of isolated patient fibrinogen
Thrombin time: [n.a.]
Reptilase time: [n.a.]
Ancrod (Arvin) time: [n.a.]
Abnormal subunit? [No]
Abnormal FDPs? [n.a.]

Remarks
[1]Normal *amounts* of fibrinopeptides were released, but the rate was not determined.

Plasma concentrations of antithrombin-III, proteins C and S, plasminogen, α_2-plasmin inhibitor, plasmin-α_2-plasmin inhibitor complexes, and t-PA were normal.

References

1. Uotani, C., Miyata, T., Kumabashiri, I., Asakura, H., Saito, M., Matsuda, T., Kajiyama, S. and Iwanaga, S. Fibrinogen Kanazawa: a congenital dysfibrinogenaemia with delayed polymerization having a replacement of proline-18 by leucine in the Aα-chain. *Blood Coag. & Fibrinol.* **2**:413-417, **1991**.

FIBRINOGEN KASSEL I

Last update	[1 December 1990]	**Structural defect**	[n.a.]
Alphacode	[KASSEL01]	**Mutation**	[n.a.]
Ref. type	[Article[1]]		

Functional defect(s)

FpA release:	[Normal]
FpB release:	[Normal]
Polymerization:	[n.a.]
Stabilization:	[n.a.]

Family studies

Homozygote?	[n.a.]
Pedigree published?	[No]

Clinical manifestation(s) Bleeding? [n.a.] Thrombosis? [n.a.]

Clinical laboratory results

Plasma fibrinogen concentration (mg/dL)

Chronometric: [n.a.]
Rate-indep'nt: [n.a.]
Immunologic: [n.a.]

*Hypo*dysfibrinogen? [n.a.]

Thrombin time:	[n.a.]
Reptilase (batroxobin) time:	[n.a.]
Prothrombin time:	[n.a.]
Partial thromboplastin time:	[n.a.]
Euglobulin lysis time:	[n.a.]
Bleeding time:	[n.a.]
Immunoelectrophoresis:	[n.a.]
Platelet aggregation:	[n.a.]

Other results with patient plasma

Ancrod (Arvin) time:	[n.a.]	Inhib. normal plasma?	[n.a.]
Recalcification time:	[n.a.]	In vivo synthesis:	[n.a.]
Calcium corrects c.t.?	[n.a.]	In vivo catabolism:	[n.a.]

Evaluation of isolated patient fibrinogen

Thrombin time:	[n.a.]	Abnormal subunit?	[n.a.]
Reptilase time:	[n.a.]	Abnormal FDPs?	[n.a.]
Ancrod (Arvin) time:	[n.a.]		

Remarks

[1]Review article only; Janzarik et al., personal communication.

References

1. Henschen, A., Kehl, M. and Southan, C. Genetically abnormal fibrinogens — strategies for structure elucidation, including fibrinopeptide analysis. In: *Variants of Human Fibrinogen*, E.A. Beck and M. Furlan (eds.), Hans Huber Publ., Berne, pp. 273-320, **1984**.

FIBRINOGEN KAWAGUCHI I

Last update [1 December 1990]
Alphacode [KAWAGU01]
Ref. type [Article]

Family studies
Homozygote? [No]
Pedigree published? [Yes]

Structural defect [Aα(16) Arg → Cys]
Mutation [n.a.]

Functional defect(s)
FpA release: [Abnormal[1]]
FpB release: [n.a.]
Polymerization: [Abnormal]
Stabilization: [n.a.]

Clinical manifestation(s) Bleeding? [No] Thrombosis? [No]

Clinical laboratory results
Plasma fibrinogen concentration (mg/dL)
Chronometric: [<40/(200-400)]
Rate-indep'nt: [230/(200-400)]
Immunologic: [262/(200-400)]

*Hypo*dysfibrinogen? [No]

Thrombin time:	[55.1s/(13s)]
Reptilase (batroxobin) time:	[114s/(23.6s)]
Prothrombin time:	[19.1s/(11.4s)]
Partial thromboplastin time:	[29.9s/(24.8s)]
Euglobulin lysis time:	[n.a.]
Bleeding time:	[Normal]
Immunoelectrophoresis:	[n.a.]
Platelet aggregation:	[Normal]

Other results with patient plasma
Ancrod (Arvin) time: [n.a.]
Recalcification time: [n.a.]
Calcium corrects c.t.? [n.a.]

Inhib. normal plasma? [Yes]
In vivo synthesis: [n.a.]
In vivo catabolism: [n.a.]

Evaluation of isolated patient fibrinogen
Thrombin time: [n.a.]
Reptilase time: [n.a.]
Ancrod (Arvin) time: [n.a.]

Abnormal subunit? [No]
Abnormal FDPs? [n.a.]

Remarks
[1]Approximately 50% of fibrinopeptide A was not released.

The presence of an inter-chain disulfide bond at the site of the mutation was demonstrated; from this the authors concluded that Aα-chains assume a parallel configuration. This observation also provided direct demonstration that the variant fibrinogen was synthesized as a homodimer (i.e., both variant Aα-chains are present in the same molecule). See also Osaka I.

FIBRINOGEN KAWAGUCHI I

References

1. Miyata, T., Terukina, S., Matsuda, M., Kasamatsu, A., Takeda, Y., Murakami, T. and Iwanaga, S. Fibrinogens Kawaguchi and Osaka: an amino acid substitution of Aα arginine-16 to cysteine which forms an extra interchain disulfide bridge between the two Aα-chains. *J. Biochem. (Tokyo)* **102**:93-101, **1987**.

2. Matsuda, M., Terukina, S., Miyata, T. and Iwanaga, S. Defective release of fibrinopeptide A due to substitution of Aα-arginine-16 by cysteine in two abnormal fibrinogens Kawaguchi and Osaka. In: *Fibrinogen and Its Derivatives; Biochemistry, Physiology, and Pathophysiology*, Excerpta Medica, Amsterdam, New York, Oxford. pp. 37-40, **1986**.

3. Matsuda, M., Saeki, E., Kasamatsu, A., Nakamikawa, C., Manabe, S. and Samejima, Y. Fibrinogen Kawaguchi: An abnormal fibrinogen characterized by defective release of fibrinopeptide A. *Thromb. Res.* **37**:379-390, **1985**.

4. Saeki, E., Matsuda, M., Ichinose, A., Samejima, Y., Kasamatsu, A., Ara, R., Mitsuno, K., Kihara, T. and Hara, Y. ["Fibrinogen Kawaguchi": a hereditary dysfibrinogenemia characterized by defective release of fibrinopeptide A associated with altered polymerization of fibrin monomers]. *Nippon Ketsueki Gakkai Zasshi* **48**:1229-1235, **1985**.

FIBRINOGEN KENDAL I

Last update [1 December 1990]
Alphacode [KENDAL01]
Ref. type [Article[1]]

Family studies
Homozygote? [n.a.]
Pedigree published? [No]

Structural defect [Aα(16) Arg → His]
Mutation [n.a.]

Functional defect(s)
FpA release: [n.a.]
FpB release: [n.a.]
Polymerization: [n.a.]
Stabilization: [n.a.]

Clinical manifestation(s) Bleeding? [n.a.] Thrombosis? [n.a.]

Clinical laboratory results
Plasma fibrinogen concentration (mg/dL)
Chronometric: [n.a.]
Rate-indep'nt: [n.a.]
Immunologic: [n.a.]

*Hypo*dysfibrinogen? [Yes]

Thrombin time:	[n.a.]
Reptilase (batroxobin) time:	[n.a.]
Prothrombin time:	[n.a.]
Partial thromboplastin time:	[n.a.]
Euglobulin lysis time:	[n.a.]
Bleeding time:	[n.a.]
Immunoelectrophoresis:	[n.a.]
Platelet aggregation:	[n.a.]

Other results with patient plasma
Ancrod (Arvin) time: [n.a.]
Recalcification time: [n.a.]
Calcium corrects c.t.? [n.a.]

Inhib. normal plasma? [n.a.]
In vivo synthesis: [n.a.]
In vivo catabolism: [n.a.]

Evaluation of isolated patient fibrinogen
Thrombin time: [n.a.]
Reptilase time: [n.a.]
Ancrod (Arvin) time: [n.a.]

Abnormal subunit? [n.a.]
Abnormal FDPs? [n.a.]

Remarks
[1]Review article only; D. Gorst and D. Tabener, personal communication.

References

1. Lane, D.A., Thompson, E. and Southan, C. Rapid screening method of fibrinopeptide analysis applied to congenital dysfibrinogenaemia: Summary of 23 cases. In: *Fibrinogen 2. Biochemistry, Physiology and Clinical Relevance*, G.D.O. Lowe, J.T. Douglas, C.D. Forbes and A. Henschen (eds.), Elsevier, Amsterdam. pp. 71-74, **1987**.

FIBRINOGEN KIEL I

Last update [10 January 1994]
Alphacode [KIEL01]
Ref. type [Article]

Structural defect [Aα(16) Arg → His]
Mutation [n.a.]

Family studies
Homozygote? [No]
Pedigree published? [Yes]

Functional defect(s)
FpA release: [Abnormal[1]]
FpB release: [n.a.]
Polymerization: [n.a.]
Stabilization: [n.a.]

Clinical manifestation(s) Bleeding? [No] Thrombosis? [No]

Clinical laboratory results
Plasma fibrinogen concentration (mg/dL)
Chronometric: [87/(200-450)]
Rate-indep'nt: [177/(200-450)]
Immunologic: [258/(200-450)]

*Hypo*dysfibrinogen? [No]

Thrombin time:	[18s/(9-10.5s)]
Reptilase (batroxobin) time:	[n.a.]
Prothrombin time:	[89%/(70-100%)]
Partial thromboplastin time:	[31.7s/(<42s)]
Euglobulin lysis time:	[n.a.]
Bleeding time:	[n.a.]
Immunoelectrophoresis:	[n.a.]
Platelet aggregation:	[n.a.]

Other results with patient plasma
Ancrod (Arvin) time: [n.a.]
Recalcification time: [n.a.]
Calcium corrects c.t.? [n.a.]

Inhib. normal plasma? [n.a.]
In vivo synthesis: [n.a.]
In vivo catabolism: [n.a.]

Evaluation of isolated patient fibrinogen
Thrombin time: [n.a.]
Reptilase time: [n.a.]
Ancrod (Arvin) time: [n.a.]

Abnormal subunit? [n.a.]
Abnormal FDPs? [n.a.]

Remarks
[1]Only half the normal amount of fibrinopeptide A was released; the rate was not determined.

References

1. Seydewitz, H.H, Gram, J., Bruhn, H.D. and Witt, I. Fibrinogen Kiel: a congenital dysfibrinogenaemia with (Aα-16 Arg → His) substitution characterized by HPLC without prior isolation of fibrinogen. *Blood Coag. & Fibrinol.* **2**:501-506, **1991**.

FIBRINOGEN KYOTO I

Last update [10 January 1994]
Alphacode [KYOTO01]
Ref. type [Article]

Family studies
Homozygote? [No]
Pedigree published? [Yes]

Structural defect [γ(308) Asn → Lys[1]]
Mutation [AAT → AAG]

Functional defect(s)
FpA release: [Normal]
FpB release: [Normal]
Polymerization: [Abnormal]
Stabilization: [Normal]

Clinical manifestation(s) Bleeding? [No[2]] Thrombosis? [No[2]]

Clinical laboratory results
Plasma fibrinogen concentration (mg/dL)
Chronometric: [77/(150-350)]
Rate-indep'nt: [150/(150-350)]
Immunologic: [210/(150-350)]

*Hypo*dysfibrinogen? [No]

Thrombin time:	[47.6s/(16-18s)]
Reptilase (batroxobin) time:	[>200/(13-18s)]
Prothrombin time:	[Normal[3]]
Partial thromboplastin time:	[Normal[3]]
Euglobulin lysis time:	[n.a.]
Bleeding time:	[n.a.]
Immunoelectrophoresis:	[n.a.]
Platelet aggregation:	[n.a.]

Other results with patient plasma
Ancrod (Arvin) time: [n.a.]
Recalcification time: [n.a.]
Calcium corrects c.t.? [Yes]

Inhib. normal plasma? [n.a.]
In vivo synthesis: [n.a.]
In vivo catabolism: [n.a.]

Evaluation of isolated patient fibrinogen
Thrombin time: [179s/(17-18s)]
Reptilase time: [n.a.]
Ancrod (Arvin) time: [n.a.]

Abnormal subunit? [Yes[4]]
Abnormal FDPs? [Yes[5]]

Remarks
[1]The molecular defect was confirmed by the PCR method. See also fibrinogen Bicêtre II.
[2]Family history is positive for thrombosis and abnormal bleeding, but these symptoms were not evident in the propositus.
[3]Data not reported.
[4]SDS-PAGE disclosed a variant γ-chain with a subnormal molecular weight.
[5]This amino acid replacement results in *accelerated* cleavage of fragment D_1 by plasmin and the generation of a new plasmin cleavage site.

FIBRINOGEN KYOTO I

References

1. Mimuro, J., Muramatsu, S., Maekawa, H., Sakata, Y., Kaneko, M., Yoshitake, S., Okuma, M., Ito, Y., Takeda, Y. and Matsuda, M. Gene analyses of abnormal fibrinogens with a mutation in the γ chain. *Intl. J. Hematol.* **56**:129-134, **1992**.

2. Muramatsu, S., Mimuro, J., Maekawa, H., Sakata, Y., Matsuda, M., Yoshitake, S. and Okuma, M. Gene analysis of abnormal fibrinogens characterized by a mutation in the γ chain. *Thromb. Haemostas.* **65**:821, **1991**. ABSTRACT

3. Yoshida, N., Terukina, S., Okuma, M., Moroi, M., Aoki, N. and Matsuda, M. Characterization of an apparently lower molecular weight γ-chain variant in fibrinogen Kyoto I. The replacement of γ-asparagine 308 by lysine which causes accelerated cleavage of fragment D1 by plasmin and the generation of a new plasmin cleavage site. *J. Biol. Chem.* **263**:13848-13856, **1988**.

4. Yoshida, N., Okuma, M., Moroi, M. and Matsuda, M. A lower molecular weight γ-chain variant in a congenital abnormal fibrinogen (Kyoto). *Blood* **68**:703-707, **1986**.

FIBRINOGEN KYOTO II

Last update [10 January 1994]
Alphacode [KYOTO02]
Ref. type [Article]

Family studies
Homozygote? [n.a.]
Pedigree published? [No]

Structural defect [Aα(18) Pro → Leu]
Mutation [n.a.]

Functional defect(s)
FpA release: [Normal]
FpB release: [Normal]
Polymerization: [Abnormal]
Stabilization: [n.a.]

Clinical manifestation(s) Bleeding? [Yes[1]] Thrombosis? [No]

Clinical laboratory results

Plasma fibrinogen concentration (mg/dL)
Chronometric: [64/(150-350)]
Rate-indep'nt: [201/(150-350)]
Immunologic: [216/(150-350)]

*Hypo*dysfibrinogen? [No]

Thrombin time:	[22.3s/(11.7-12.7)]
Reptilase (batroxobin) time:	[>100s/(11.2-14.3s)]
Prothrombin time:	[Abnormal[2]]
Partial thromboplastin time:	[Abnormal[2]]
Euglobulin lysis time:	[n.a.]
Bleeding time:	[n.a.]
Immunoelectrophoresis:	[n.a.]
Platelet aggregation:	[n.a.]

Other results with patient plasma
Ancrod (Arvin) time: [n.a.]
Recalcification time: [n.a.]
Calcium corrects c.t.? [n.a.]

Inhib. normal plasma? [n.a.]
In vivo synthesis: [n.a.]
In vivo catabolism: [n.a.]

Evaluation of isolated patient fibrinogen
Thrombin time: [>100s/(10.2s)]
Reptilase time: [>100s/(11.7s)]
Ancrod (Arvin) time: [n.a.]

Abnormal subunit? [No]
Abnormal FDPs? [No]

Remarks
[1]Excessive postpartum bleeding was reported. Endometrial curettage was performed without complications.
[2]Data not reported.

References

1. Yoshida, N., Hirata, H., Asakura, S., Yamazumi, K., Matsuda, M., Wada, H., Shirakawa, S. and Okuma, M. Calcium binding to abnormal fibrinogens with a single amino acid replacement in the NH2-terminal region of fibrin α- or β-chain. *Thromb. Res.* **67**:613-618, **1992**.

2. Yoshida, N., Okuma, M., Hirata, H., Matsuda, M., Yamazumi, K. and Asakura, S. Fibrinogen Kyoto II, a new congenitally abnormal molecule, characterized by the replacement of Aα proline-18 by leucine. *Blood* **78**:149-153, **1991**.

3. Matsuda, M., Yoshida, N., Terukina, S., Yamazumi, K. and Maekawa, H. Molecular abnormalities of fibrinogen — The present status of structure elucidation. In: *Fibrinogen 4. Current Basic and Clinical Aspects*, M. Matsuda, S. Iwanaga, A. Takada and A. Henschen (eds.), Elsevier Science Publ. B.V., Amsterdam. pp. 139-152, **1990**.

FIBRINOGEN KYOTO III

Last update [10 January 1994]
Alphacode [KYOTO03]
Ref. type [Article]

Family studies
Homozygote? [No]
Pedigree published? [No]

Structural defect [γ(330) Asp → Tyr[1]]
Mutation [GAT → TAT]

Functional defect(s)
FpA release: [Normal]
FpB release: [Normal]
Polymerization: [Abnormal]
Stabilization: [Normal]

Clinical manifestation(s) Bleeding? [No] Thrombosis? [No]

Clinical laboratory results

Plasma fibrinogen concentration (mg/dL)
Chronometric: [68/(200-400)]
Rate-indep'nt: [n.a.]
Immunologic: [290/(200-400)]

*Hypo*dysfibrinogen? [No]

Thrombin time:	[20.4s(10.1s)]
Reptilase (batroxobin) time:	[n.a.]
Prothrombin time:	[13.9s/(10.9s)]
Partial thromboplastin time:	[Normal[2]]
Euglobulin lysis time:	[n.a.]
Bleeding time:	[n.a.]
Immunoelectrophoresis:	[n.a.]
Platelet aggregation:	[n.a.]

Other results with patient plasma
Ancrod (Arvin) time: [34.1s/(17s)]
Recalcification time: [n.a.]
Calcium corrects c.t.? [Yes]

Inhib. normal plasma? [n.a.]
In vivo synthesis: [n.a.]
In vivo catabolism: [n.a.]

Evaluation of isolated patient fibrinogen
Thrombin time: [135s/(11.1s)]
Reptilase time: [n.a.]
Ancrod (Arvin) time: [>300s/(15.3s)]

Abnormal subunit? [Yes[3]]
Abnormal FDPs? [Yes]

Remarks
[1]The molecular defect was confirmed with the PCR method.
[2]Data not reported.
[3]SDS-PAGE disclosed a γ-chain about 1500 Da smaller than normal.

FIBRINOGEN KYOTO III

References

1. Mimuro, J., Muramatsu, S., Maekawa, H., Sakata, Y., Kaneko, M., Yoshitake, S., Okuma, M., Ito, Y., Takeda, Y. and Matsuda, M. Gene analyses of abnormal fibrinogens with a mutation in the γ chain. *Intl. J. Hematol.* **56**:129-134, **1992**.

2. Muramatsu, S., Mimuro, J., Maekawa, H., Sakata, Y., Matsuda, M., Yoshitake, S. and Okuma, M. Gene analysis of abnormal fibrinogens characterized by a mutation in the γ chain. *Thromb. Haemostas.* **65**:821, **1991**. ABSTRACT

3. Terukina, S., Yamazumi, K., Okamoto, K., Yamashita, H., Ito, Y. and Matsuda, M. Fibrinogen Kyoto III: a congenital dysfibrinogen with a γ aspartic acid-330 to tyrosine substitution. *Blood* **74**:2681-2687, **1989**.

4. Terukina, S., Yamazumi, K., Maekawa, H., Okamoto, K., Akasaka, K., Yamashita, H., Ito, Y. and Matsuda, M. Fibrinogen Kyoto III: a replacement of γ Asp-330 by Tyr. In: *Fibrinogen 4. Current Basic and Clinical Aspects*, M. Matsuda, S. Iwanaga, A. Takada and A. Henschen (eds.), Elsevier Science Publ., B.V., Amsterdam. pp. 171-171, **1990**.

FIBRINOGEN LA CEVAINA I^{Unp}

Last update [10 January 1994]
Alphacode [LACEVA01]
Ref. type [Unpublished[1]]

Structural defect [n.a.]
Mutation [n.a.]

Family studies
Homozygote? [n.a.]
Pedigree published? [No]

Functional defect(s)
FpA release: [Normal]
FpB release: [Normal]
Polymerization: [Abnormal]
Stabilization: [Normal]

Clinical manifestation(s) Bleeding? [No] Thrombosis? [No]

Clinical laboratory results

Plasma fibrinogen concentration (mg/dL)
Chronometric: [n.a.]
Rate-indep'nt: [n.a.]
Immunologic: [n.a.]

*Hypo*dysfibrinogen? [No]

Thrombin time:	[60s/(15-18s)]
Reptilase (batroxobin) time:	[n.a.]
Prothrombin time:	[n.a.]
Partial thromboplastin time:	[n.a.]
Euglobulin lysis time:	[n.a.]
Bleeding time:	[n.a.]
Immunoelectrophoresis:	[n.a.]
Platelet aggregation:	[n.a.]

Other results with patient plasma
Ancrod (Arvin) time: [n.a.]
Recalcification time: [n.a.]
Calcium corrects c.t.? [n.a.]

Inhib. normal plasma? [n.a.]
In vivo synthesis: [n.a.]
In vivo catabolism: [n.a.]

Evaluation of isolated patient fibrinogen
Thrombin time: [n.a.]
Reptilase time: [n.a.]
Ancrod (Arvin) time: [n.a.]

Abnormal subunit? [n.a.]
Abnormal FDPs? [n.a.]

Remarks
[1]C.L. Arocha-Pinango & A. Torres, personal communication.

References

FIBRINOGEN LA GUAIRA I

Last update	[10 January 1994]	**Structural defect**	[n.a.]
Alphacode	[LAGUAI01]	**Mutation**	[n.a.]
Ref. type	[Article]		

Family studies
Homozygote? [n.a.]
Pedigree published? [No]

Functional defect(s)
FpA release: [Normal]
FpB release: [Normal]
Polymerization: [Abnormal]
Stabilization: [Normal]

Clinical manifestation(s) Bleeding? [No] Thrombosis? [No]

Clinical laboratory results

Plasma fibrinogen concentration (mg/dL)
Chronometric: [85[1]]
Rate-indep'nt: [340[1]]
Immunologic: [350[1]]

*Hypo*dysfibrinogen? [No]

Thrombin time:	[Abnormal[2]]
Reptilase (batroxobin) time:	[Abnormal[2]]
Prothrombin time:	[n.a.]
Partial thromboplastin time:	[n.a.]
Euglobulin lysis time:	[n.a.]
Bleeding time:	[n.a.]
Immunoelectrophoresis:	[Normal]
Platelet aggregation:	[n.a.]

Other results with patient plasma

Ancrod (Arvin) time:	[n.a.]	Inhib. normal plasma?	[No]
Recalcification time:	[n.a.]	In vivo synthesis:	[n.a.]
Calcium corrects c.t.?	[Yes]	In vivo catabolism:	[n.a.]

Evaluation of isolated patient fibrinogen

Thrombin time:	[n.a.]	Abnormal subunit?	[n.a.]
Reptilase time:	[n.a.]	Abnormal FDPs?	[No[3]]
Ancrod (Arvin) time:	[n.a.]		

Remarks

[1]Normal range not reported.
[2]Data not reported; thrombin and Reptilase times were, respectively, 38s and 50s longer than normal.
[3]An *increased* rate of FDP formation was reported.

Electron microscopy of patient fibrinogen and fibrin (Marchi et al., 1990) disclosed no differences from normal.

References

1. Arocha-Piñango, C.L., Bosch, N., Torres, A., Caires-Tronchoni, D., Marchi, R., Vidal, H. and Rizzo, M.G. Dysfibrinogenemias in Latin America. A cooperative study group. *Rev. Iberoamer. Tromb. Hemostasia* **3**:110-122, **1990**.

2. Marchi, R., Arocha-Piñango, C.L. and Gil, F. Electron microscopy studies of 7 patients with dysfibrinogenemia and some of their relatives. *Rev. Iberoamer. Tromb. Hemostasia* **3**:185-190, **1990**.

FIBRINOGEN LA PLATA I

Last update [10 January 1994]
Alphacode [LAPLAT01]
Ref. type [Article]

Family studies
Homozygote? [n.a.]
Pedigree published? [No]

Structural defect [n.a.]
Mutation [n.a.]

Functional defect(s)
FpA release: [Normal]
FpB release: [Normal]
Polymerization: [Abnormal]
Stabilization: [Normal[1]]

Clinical manifestation(s) Bleeding? [No] Thrombosis? [No]

Clinical laboratory results

Plasma fibrinogen concentration (mg/dL)
Chronometric: [n.a.]
Rate-indep'nt: [230[2]]
Immunologic: [230[2]]

*Hypo*dysfibrinogen? [No]

Thrombin time:	[28s/(15-18s)[1]]
Reptilase (batroxobin) time:	[Abnormal[3]]
Prothrombin time:	[n.a.]
Partial thromboplastin time:	[n.a.]
Euglobulin lysis time:	[n.a.]
Bleeding time:	[n.a.]
Immunoelectrophoresis:	[Normal]
Platelet aggregation:	[n.a.]

Other results with patient plasma
Ancrod (Arvin) time: [n.a.]
Recalcification time: [n.a.]
Calcium corrects c.t.? [No]

Inhib. normal plasma? [No]
In vivo synthesis: [n.a.]
In vivo catabolism: [n.a.]

Evaluation of isolated patient fibrinogen
Thrombin time: [n.a.]
Reptilase time: [n.a.]
Ancrod (Arvin) time: [n.a.]

Abnormal subunit? [n.a.]
Abnormal FDPs? [No]

Remarks
[1]C.L. Arocha-Piñango & H. Vidal, personal communication.
[2]Normal range not reported.
[3]Data not reported; Reptilase time was 15s longer than normal.

References

1. Arocha-Piñango, C.L., Bosch, N., Torres, A., Caires-Tronchoni, D., Marchi, R., Vidal, H. and Rizzo, M.G. Dysfibrinogenemias in Latin America. A cooperative study group. *Rev. Iberoamer. Tromb. Hemostasia* **3**:110-122, **1990**.

FIBRINOGEN LEDYARD I

Last update [10 January 1994]
Alphacode [LEDYAR01]
Ref. type [Article]

Family studies
Homozygote? [No]
Pedigree published? [No]

Structural defect [Aα(16) Arg → Cys]
Mutation [n.a.]

Functional defect(s)
FpA release: [Abnormal[1]]
FpB release: [Abnormal]
Polymerization: [Abnormal]
Stabilization: [n.a.]

Clinical manifestation(s) Bleeding? [Yes[2]] Thrombosis? [No]

Clinical laboratory results
Plasma fibrinogen concentration (mg/dL)
Chronometric: [40/(150-350)]
Rate-indep'nt: [n.a.]
Immunologic: [315/(150-350)]

*Hypo*dysfibrinogen? [No]

Thrombin time:	[62.3s/(16-20s)]
Reptilase (batroxobin) time:	[30.2s/(13-16.9s)]
Prothrombin time:	[13.2s/(9.6-12s)]
Partial thromboplastin time:	[28.8s/(25.6-35.2s)]
Euglobulin lysis time:	[n.a.]
Bleeding time:	[n.a.]
Immunoelectrophoresis:	[n.a.]
Platelet aggregation:	[n.a.[3]]

Other results with patient plasma
Ancrod (Arvin) time: [n.a.]
Recalcification time: [n.a.]
Calcium corrects c.t.? [n.a.]

Inhib. normal plasma? [n.a.]
In vivo synthesis: [n.a.]
In vivo catabolism: [n.a.]

Evaluation of isolated patient fibrinogen
Thrombin time: [n.a.]
Reptilase time: [n.a.]
Ancrod (Arvin) time: [n.a.]

Abnormal subunit? [n.a.]
Abnormal FDPs? [n.a.]

Remarks
[1]Only half the normal amount of fibrinopeptide A was released.
[2]Spontaneous epistaxis and excessive post-traumatic bleeding in the 10 year-old propositus was reported.
[3]Normal *support* of platelet aggregation was reported. See also STONY BROOK I.

Biochemical studies were performed on the proband's father.

References

1. Lee, M.H., Kaczmarek, E., Chin, D.T., Oda, A., McIntosh, S., Bauer, K.A., Clyne, L.P. and McDonagh, J. Fibrinogen Ledyard (AαArg_{16} → Cys): Biochemical and physiologic characterization. *Blood* **78**:1744-1752, **1991**.

FIBRINOGEN LEITCHFIELD I

Last update [1 December 1990]
Alphacode [LEITCH01]
Ref. type [Article[1]]

Structural defect [Aα(16) Arg → His]
Mutation [n.a.]

Family studies
Homozygote? [No]
Pedigree published? [n.a.]

Functional defect(s)
FpA release: [n.a.]
FpB release: [n.a.]
Polymerization: [n.a.]
Stabilization: [n.a.]

Clinical manifestation(s) Bleeding? [n.a.] Thrombosis? [n.a.]

Clinical laboratory results
Plasma fibrinogen concentration (mg/dL)
Chronometric: [n.a.]
Rate-indep'nt: [n.a.]
Immunologic: [n.a.]

*Hypo*dysfibrinogen? [n.a.]

Thrombin time:	[n.a.]
Reptilase (batroxobin) time:	[n.a.]
Prothrombin time:	[n.a.]
Partial thromboplastin time:	[n.a.]
Euglobulin lysis time:	[n.a.]
Bleeding time:	[n.a.]
Immunoelectrophoresis:	[n.a.]
Platelet aggregation:	[n.a.]

Other results with patient plasma
Ancrod (Arvin) time: [n.a.]
Recalcification time: [n.a.]
Calcium corrects c.t.? [n.a.]

Inhib. normal plasma? [n.a.]
In vivo synthesis: [n.a.]
In vivo catabolism: [n.a.]

Evaluation of isolated patient fibrinogen
Thrombin time: [n.a.]
Reptilase time: [n.a.]
Ancrod (Arvin) time: [n.a.]

Abnormal subunit? [n.a.]
Abnormal FDPs? [n.a.]

Remarks
[1]Review article only; D.K. Galanakis, personal communication.

References

1. Henschen, A., Kehl, M. and Southan, C. Genetically abnormal fibrinogens — strategies for structure elucidation, including fibrinopeptide analysis. In: *Variants of Human Fibrinogen*, E.A. Beck and M. Furlan (eds.), Hans Huber Publ., Berne, pp. 273-320, **1984**.

FIBRINOGEN LEOGAN I

Last update [1 December 1990]
Alphacode [LEOGAN01]
Ref. type [Article]

Structural defect [Aα(16) Arg → Cys[1]]
Mutation [CGT → TGT]

Family studies
Homozygote? [No]
Pedigree published? [No]

Functional defect(s)
FpA release: [Abnormal[2]]
FpB release: [n.a.]
Polymerization: [Abnormal]
Stabilization: [Normal]

Clinical manifestation(s) Bleeding? [No[3]] Thrombosis? [No[3]]

Clinical laboratory results
Plasma fibrinogen concentration (mg/dL)
Chronometric: [55[4]]
Rate-indep'nt: [n.a.]
Immunologic: [525[4]]

*Hypo*dysfibrinogen? [No]

Thrombin time:	[48s/(20s)]
Reptilase (batroxobin) time:	[n.a.]
Prothrombin time:	[n.a.]
Partial thromboplastin time:	[n.a.]
Euglobulin lysis time:	[Normal]
Bleeding time:	[n.a.]
Immunoelectrophoresis:	[n.a.]
Platelet aggregation:	[n.a.]

Other results with patient plasma
Ancrod (Arvin) time: [n.a.]
Recalcification time: [n.a.]
Calcium corrects c.t.? [n.a.]

Inhib. normal plasma? [n.a.]
In vivo synthesis: [n.a.]
In vivo catabolism: [n.a.]

Evaluation of isolated patient fibrinogen
Thrombin time: [n.a.]
Reptilase time: [n.a.]
Ancrod (Arvin) time: [n.a.]

Abnormal subunit? [No]
Abnormal FDPs? [n.a.]

Remarks
[1]The structural defect was determined with the PCR method.
[2]Only half the normal amount of fibrinopeptide A was released.
[3]The proposita is a 24 year-old black woman from Leogan, Haiti. Two spontaneous abortions and one full-term normal delivery were reported.
[4]Normal range not reported; the chronometric value is low and the immunologic value is normal.

References

1. Galanakis, D.K., Henschen, A., Schubach, W., Lord, S. and Al-Mondhiry, H. Determination of abnormal structure and heterozygosity by amplification of genomic DNA using the polymerase chain reaction and by amino acid sequence analyses. In: *Fibrinogen 4. Current Basic and Clinical Aspects*, M. Matsuda, S. Iwanaga, A. Takada and A. Henschen (eds.), Elsevier Science Publ., B.V., Amsterdam. pp. 173-178, **1990**.

FIBRINOGEN LEUVEN I

Last update [1 December 1990]
Alphacode [LEUVEN01]
Ref. type [Article]

Family studies
Homozygote? [n.a.]
Pedigree published? [Yes[1]]

Structural defect [n.a.]
Mutation [n.a.]

Functional defect(s)
FpA release: [n.a.]
FpB release: [n.a.]
Polymerization: [Abnormal]
Stabilization: [Normal]

Clinical manifestation(s) Bleeding? [No] Thrombosis? [No]

Clinical laboratory results
Plasma fibrinogen concentration (mg/dL)
Chronometric: [78/(200-400)]
Rate-indep'nt: [159/(200-400)]
Immunologic: [128/(200-400)]

*Hypo*dysfibrinogen? [Yes]

Thrombin time:	[29.2s/(19s)[2]]
Reptilase (batroxobin) time:	[47.2s/(20s)]
Prothrombin time:	[n.a.]
Partial thromboplastin time:	[Normal[3]]
Euglobulin lysis time:	[Normal[3]]
Bleeding time:	[Normal]
Immunoelectrophoresis:	[n.a.]
Platelet aggregation:	[n.a.]

Other results with patient plasma
Ancrod (Arvin) time: [110s/(27s)]
Recalcification time: [Normal[3]]
Calcium corrects c.t.? [No]

Inhib. normal plasma? [Yes]
In vivo synthesis: [n.a.]
In vivo catabolism: [n.a.]

Evaluation of isolated patient fibrinogen
Thrombin time: [n.a.]
Reptilase time: [n.a.]
Ancrod (Arvin) time: [n.a.]

Abnormal subunit? [No]
Abnormal FDPs? [n.a.]

Remarks
[1]Pedigree is incomplete.
[2]Thrombin time was unusually dependent on pH.
[3]Data not reported.

A brief discussion of fibrinogen Leuven I is published in *Thromb. Diath. Haemorrh.* **39**:331-338 (1970).

References

1. Verhaeghe, R., Verstraete, M., Vermylen, J. and Vermylen, C. Fibrinogen 'Leuven', another genetic variant. *Br. J. Haematol.* **26**:421-433, **1974**.

FIBRINOGEN LILLE I

Last update [10 January 1994]
Alphacode [LILLE01]
Ref. type [Article]

Structural defect [Aα(7) Asp → Asn]
Mutation [n.a.]

Family studies
Homozygote? [No]
Pedigree published? [No[2]]

Functional defect(s)
FpA release: [n.a.[1]]
FpB release: [n.a.[1]]
Polymerization: [Abnormal]
Stabilization: [Normal]

Clinical manifestation(s) Bleeding? [No] Thrombosis? [No]

Clinical laboratory results

Plasma fibrinogen concentration (mg/dL)
Chronometric: [<20/(410)]
Rate-indep'nt: [340/(375)]
Immunologic: [505/(420)]

*Hypo*dysfibrinogen? [No]

Thrombin time:	[No clot]
Reptilase (batroxobin) time:	[No clot]
Prothrombin time:	[55s/(15s)]
Partial thromboplastin time:	[88s/(50s)]
Euglobulin lysis time:	[n.a.]
Bleeding time:	[Normal]
Immunoelectrophoresis:	[Normal]
Platelet aggregation:	[n.a.]

Other results with patient plasma
Ancrod (Arvin) time: [n.a.]
Recalcification time: [190s/(130s)]
Calcium corrects c.t.? [n.a.]

Inhib. normal plasma? [No]
In vivo synthesis: [n.a.]
In vivo catabolism: [n.a.]

Evaluation of isolated patient fibrinogen
Thrombin time: [19m/(24s)]
Reptilase time: [No clot]
Ancrod (Arvin) time: [n.a.]

Abnormal subunit? [No]
Abnormal FDPs? [Yes[3]]

Remarks
[1]The rate of *total* fibrinopeptide release was reduced; individual fibrinopeptide release was not reported.
[2]The proposita was adopted; family studies were not possible.
[3]Abnormal fragment E presumably was due to the presence of unreleased fibrinopeptide A.

FIBRINOGEN LILLE I

References

1. Zheng, Z., Ashton, R.W., Ni, F. and Scheraga, H.A. Thrombin hydrolysis of an N-terminal peptide from fibrinogen Lille: Kinetic and NMR studies. *Biochemistry* **31**:4426-4431, **1992**.

2. Morris, S., Denninger, M.H., Finlayson, J.S. and Ménaché, D. Fibrinogen Lille: A (alpha) 7 ASP → ASN. *Thromb. Haemostas.* **46**:104, **1981**. ABSTRACT

3. Denninger, M.H., Finlayson, J.S., Reamer, L.A., Parquet-Gernez, A., Goudemand, M. and Ménaché, D. Congenital dysfibrinogenemia: Fibrinogen Lille (Errata). *Thromb. Res.* **15**:291-293, **1979**.

4. Denninger, M.H., Finlayson, J.S., Reamer, L.A., Parquet-Gernez, A., Goudemand, M. and Ménaché, D. Congenital dysfibrinogenemia: fibrinogen Lille. *Thromb. Res.* **13**:453-466, **1978**.

5. Denninger, M.H., Parquet-Gernez, A., Goudemand, M. and Ménaché, D. [A new case of dysfibrinogenemia: Fibrinogen Lille]. *Nouv. Rev. Fr. Hematol.* **18**:519, **1977**. ABSTRACT

FIBRINOGEN LIMA I

Last update [10 January 1994]
Alphacode [LIMA01]
Ref. type [Article]

Structural defect [Aα(141) Arg → Ser[1]]
Mutation [n.a.]

Family studies
Homozygote? [Yes]
Pedigree published? [No[2]]

Functional defect(s)
FpA release: [n.a.]
FpB release: [n.a.]
Polymerization: [Abnormal[3]]
Stabilization: [n.a.]

Clinical manifestation(s) Bleeding? [Yes[4]] Thrombosis? [No]

Clinical laboratory results
Plasma fibrinogen concentration (mg/dL)
Chronometric: [50[5]]
Rate-indep'nt: [240[5]]
Immunologic: [n.a.]

*Hypo*dysfibrinogen? [No]

Thrombin time:	[38.4s/(12.2)]
Reptilase (batroxobin) time:	[Abnormal[6]]
Prothrombin time:	[n.a.]
Partial thromboplastin time:	[n.a.]
Euglobulin lysis time:	[n.a.]
Bleeding time:	[n.a.]
Immunoelectrophoresis:	[Anodal]
Platelet aggregation:	[n.a.]

Other results with patient plasma
Ancrod (Arvin) time: [28.4s/(11.5)]
Recalcification time: [n.a.]
Calcium corrects c.t.? [Yes]

Inhib. normal plasma? [n.a.]
In vivo synthesis: [n.a.]
In vivo catabolism: [n.a.]

Evaluation of isolated patient fibrinogen
Thrombin time: [n.a.]
Reptilase time: [n.a.]
Ancrod (Arvin) time: [n.a.]

Abnormal subunit? [Yes[7]]
Abnormal FDPs? [No[8]]

Remarks
[1]This mutation yields a new glycosylation site. See also ASAHI I, CARACAS II, and PONTOISE I.
[2]There is evidence of consanguinity.
[3]The polymerization delay was corrected by desialylation.
[4]Transient microhematuria was reported in the 10-year-old proposita.
[5]Normal range not reported.
[6]Data not reported.
[7]Aα chains *larger* than normal (due to glycosylation at Aα Asn^{139}) were reported.
[8]"Slow plasmin degradation" was reported. This variant exhibits normal t-PA binding and plasminogen activation, a finding that is not consistent with the putative location of a plasminogen binding site at Aα (148-160).

FIBRINOGEN LIMA I

References

1. Maekawa, H., Yamazumi, K., Muramatsu, S., Kaneko, M., Hirata, H., Takahashi, N., Arocha-Piñango, C.L., Rodriguez, S., Nagy, H., Perez-Requejo, J.L. and Matsuda, M. Fibrinogen Lima: A homozygous dysfibrinogen with an Aα-arginine-141 to serine substitution associated with extra N-glycosylation at Aα-asparagine-139. Impaired fibrin gel formation but normal fibrin-facilitated plasminogen activation catalyzed by tissue-type plasminogen activator. *J. Clin. Invest.* **90**:67-76, **1992**.

2. Arocha-Piñango, C.L., Rodríguez, S., Naggy, H., and Perez-Requejo, J.L. Fibrinogen Lima. A new dysfibrinogenaemia with a high-molecular-weight α-chain and effective polymerization. *Blood Coag. & Fibrinol.* 1:561-565, **1990**.

3. Maekawa, H., Yamazumi, K., Muramatsu, S., Matsuda, C.L., Arocha-Piñango, C.L., Rodríguez, S., Naggy, H., and Perez-Requejo, J.L. Fibrinogen Lima with a replacement of Aα Arg-141 by Ser identified in the Aα chain part of the D domain. *Proc. X Intl. Fgen. Wkshp.*, **1990** ABSTRACT.

4. Arocha-Piñango, C.L., Rodríguez, S., Naggy, H., and Perez-Requejo, J.L. Fibrinogen Lima. A new dysfibrinogenemia with abnormal polymerization and slow plasmin degradation. *Proc. X Intl. Fgen. Wkshp.*, **1990** ABSTRACT.

FIBRINOGEN LOGROÑO I

Last update [1 December 1990]
Alphacode [LOGRON01]
Ref. type [Article]

Family studies
Homozygote? [No]
Pedigree published? [Yes]

Structural defect [n.a.]
Mutation [n.a.]

Functional defect(s)
FpA release: [n.a.]
FpB release: [n.a.]
Polymerization: [Abnormal]
Stabilization: [n.a.]

Clinical manifestation(s) Bleeding? [No] Thrombosis? [No]

Clinical laboratory results
Plasma fibrinogen concentration (mg/dL)
Chronometric: [n.a.]
Rate-indep'nt: [40/(200-400)]
Immunologic: [170/(150-350)]

*Hypo*dysfibrinogen? [No]

Thrombin time:	[54s/(18-20s)]
Reptilase (batroxobin) time:	[127s/(15-18s)]
Prothrombin time:	[18s/(11-13s)]
Partial thromboplastin time:	[43s/(35-40s)]
Euglobulin lysis time:	[210m/(>180m)]
Bleeding time:	[Normal]
Immunoelectrophoresis:	[Normal]
Platelet aggregation:	[Normal]

Other results with patient plasma
Ancrod (Arvin) time: [n.a.]
Recalcification time: [n.a.]
Calcium corrects c.t.? [n.a.]

Inhib. normal plasma? [Yes]
In vivo synthesis: [n.a.]
In vivo catabolism: [n.a.]

Evaluation of isolated patient fibrinogen
Thrombin time: [n.a.]
Reptilase time: [n.a.]
Ancrod (Arvin) time: [n.a.]

Abnormal subunit? [No]
Abnormal FDPs? [No]

Remarks

References

1. Rocha, E., Lasierra, J., Narvaiza, M.J., Vilades, E., Palacios, E. and Fernández, J. Fibrinogen Logroño. A new case of congenital dysfibrinogenemia. *Ric. Clin. Lab.* **14**:663-672, **1984**.

FIBRINOGEN LONDON I

Last update	[1 December 1990]	**Structeral defect**	[n.a.]
Alphacode	[LONDON01]	**Mutation**	[n.a.]
Ref. type	[Article]		

Functional defect(s)

FpA release:	[Normal]
FpB release:	[Normal]
Polymerization:	[Abnormal]
Stabilization:	[n.a.]

Family studies

Homozygote?	[n.a.]
Pedigree published?	[Yes]

Clinical manifestation(s) Bleeding? [No] Thrombosis? [Yes[1]]

Clinical laboratory results

Plasma fibrinogen concentration (mg/dL)

Chronometric:	[n.a.]
Rate-indep'nt:	[239/(230)]
Immunologic:	[400/(400)]

*Hypo*dysfibrinogen? [No]

Thrombin time:	[91s/(10.6s)[2]]
Reptilase (batroxobin) time:	[45s/(15.6s)]
Prothrombin time:	[n.a.]
Partial thromboplastin time:	[80.8s/(50.6s)]
Euglobulin lysis time:	[n.a.]
Bleeding time:	[n.a.]
Immunoelectrophoresis:	[Normal]
Platelet aggregation:	[n.a.]

Other results with patient plasma

Ancrod (Arvin) time:	[n.a.]	Inhib. normal plasma?	[Yes]
Recalcification time:	[n.a.]	In vivo synthesis:	[n.a.]
Calcium corrects c.t.?	[No]	In vivo catabolism:	[n.a.]

Evaluation of isolated patient fibrinogen

Thrombin time:	[65s/(5.2s)[2]]	Abnormal subunit?	[No]
Reptilase time:	[n.a.]	Abnormal FDPs?	[n.a.]
Ancrod (Arvin) time:	[n.a.]		

Remarks

[1]Angina and myocardial infarction in the 44 year-old propositus were reported.

[2]Thrombin time was unusually dependent on pH.

FIBRINOGEN LONDON I

References

1. Ruf, W., Bender, A., Lane, D.A., Preissner, K.T., Selmayr, E. and Muller-Berghaus, G. Thrombin-induced fibrinopeptide B release from normal and variant fibrinogens: influence of inhibitors of fibrin polymerization. *Biochim. Biophys. Acta* **965**:169-175, **1988**.

2. Ruf, W., Preissner, K.T., Lane, D.A. and Muller-Berghaus, G. Decreased rate of fibrinopeptide B release from fibrinogen London I. In: *Fibrinogen 2. Biochemistry, Physiology and Clinical Relevance*, G.D.O. Lowe, J.T. Douglas, C.D. Forbes and A. Henschen (eds.), Elsevier, Amsterdam. pp. 67-70, **1987**.

3. Lane, D.A., Ireland, H., Thompson, E., Southan, C. and Henschen, A. Fibrinogens London I - IV, Manchester, Sydney I and II. Cleavage of fibrinopeptides by thrombin and expression of their polymerisation abnormalities. In: *Fibrinogen — Structural Variants and Interactions*, A. Henschen, B. Hessel, J. McDonagh and T. Saldeen (eds.), W. de Gruyter, Berlin. pp. 197-206, **1985**.

4. Henschen, A., Kehl, M., Southan, C., Lottspeich, F. and Georgopoulos, D. Genetically abnormal fibrinogens — some current characterisation strategies. In: *Fibrinogen —Structure, Functional Aspects, Metabolism*, F. Haverkate, A. Henschen, W. Nieuwenhuizen and P.W. Straub (eds.), Walter de Gruyter, Berlin. pp. 125-144, **1983**.

5. Lane, D.A., Allen, A.K., Markwick, J., Thompson, E. and Mackie, I. Carbohydrate in abnormal fibrinogens. In: *Fibrinogen — Recent Biochemical and Medical Aspects*, A. Henschen, H. Graeff and F. Lottspeich (eds.), W. deGruyter, Berlin. pp. 183-192, **1982**.

6. Lane, D.A., Cuddigan, B., VanRoss, M. and Kakkar, V.V. Dysfibrinogenaemia characterized by abnormal fibrin monomer polymerization and normal fibrinopeptide A release. *Br. J. Haematol.* **44**:483-494, **1980**.

FIBRINOGEN LONDON II

Last update [1 December 1990]
Alphacode [LONDON02]
Ref. type [Article]

Structural defect [n.a.]
Mutation [n.a.]

Family studies
Homozygote? [n.a.]
Pedigree published? [No]

Functional defect(s)
FpA release: [Normal]
FpB release: [n.a.]
Polymerization: [Abnormal]
Stabilization: [n.a.]

Clinical manifestation(s) Bleeding? [No] Thrombosis? [Yes]

Clinical laboratory results
Plasma fibrinogen concentration (mg/dL)
Chronometric: [100/(220)]
Rate-indep'nt: [n.a.]
Immunologic: [130/(220-550)]

*Hypo*dysfibrinogen? [Yes]

Thrombin time:	[30-180s/(15s)]
Reptilase (batroxobin) time:	[45s/(11s)]
Prothrombin time:	[14s/(12s)]
Partial thromboplastin time:	[44s/(33s)]
Euglobulin lysis time:	[n.a.]
Bleeding time:	[n.a.]
Immunoelectrophoresis:	[n.a.]
Platelet aggregation:	[n.a.]

Other results with patient plasma
Ancrod (Arvin) time: [n.a.]
Recalcification time: [n.a.]
Calcium corrects c.t.? [n.a.]

Inhib. normal plasma? [n.a.]
In vivo synthesis: [n.a.]
In vivo catabolism: [Normal]

Evaluation of isolated patient fibrinogen
Thrombin time: [30-180s/(12.6s)]
Reptilase time: [n.a.]
Ancrod (Arvin) time: [n.a.]

Abnormal subunit? [n.a.]
Abnormal FDPs? [n.a.]

Remarks

References

1. Lane, D.A., Ireland, H., Thompson, E., Southan, C. and Henschen, A. Fibrinogens London I - IV, Manchester, Sydney I and II. Cleavage of fibrinopeptides by thrombin and expression of their polymerisation abnormalities. In: *Fibrinogen —Structural Variants and Interactions*, A. Henschen, B. Hessel, J. McDonagh and T. Saldeen (eds.), W. de Gruyter, Berlin. pp. 197-206, **1985**.

FIBRINOGEN LONDON III

Last update [1 December 1990]
Alphacode [LONDON03]
Ref. type [Article]

Family studies
Homozygote? [Yes]
Pedigree published? [No]

Structural defect [n.a.]
Mutation [n.a.]

Functional defect(s)
FpA release: [Abnormal[1]]
FpB release: [Abnormal]
Polymerization: [Abnormal]
Stabilization: [n.a.]

Clinical manifestation(s) Bleeding? [No] Thrombosis? [No]

Clinical laboratory results
Plasma fibrinogen concentration (mg/dL)
Chronometric: [n.a.]
Rate-indep'nt: [110/(200-400)]
Immunologic: [420/(200-400)]

*Hypo*dysfibrinogen? [No]

Thrombin time:	[25s/(9-12s)]
Reptilase (batroxobin) time:	[n.a.]
Prothrombin time:	[Normal[2]]
Partial thromboplastin time:	[43s/(38-41s)]
Euglobulin lysis time:	[n.a.]
Bleeding time:	[n.a.]
Immunoelectrophoresis:	[n.a.]
Platelet aggregation:	[n.a.]

Other results with patient plasma
Ancrod (Arvin) time: [n.a.]
Recalcification time: [n.a.]
Calcium corrects c.t.? [n.a.]

Inhib. normal plasma? [No]
In vivo synthesis: [n.a.]
In vivo catabolism: [n.a.]

Evaluation of isolated patient fibrinogen
Thrombin time: [95s/(20s)]
Reptilase time: [n.a.]
Ancrod (Arvin) time: [n.a.]

Abnormal subunit? [No]
Abnormal FDPs? [n.a.]

Remarks
[1]Only half the normal amount of fibrinopeptide A was released.
[2]Data not reported; prothrombin time ratio was 1.1.

FIBRINOGEN LONDON III

References

1. Lane, D.A., Ireland, H., Thompson, E., Southan, C. and Henschen, A. Fibrinogens London I - IV, Manchester, Sydney I and II. Cleavage of fibrinopeptides by thrombin and expression of their polymerisation abnormalities. In: *Fibrinogen — Structural Variants and Interactions*, A. Henschen, B. Hessel, J. McDonagh and T. Saldeen (eds.), W. de Gruyter, Berlin. pp. 197-206, **1985**.

2. Henschen, A., Kehl, M., Southan, C., Lottspeich, F. and Georgopoulos, D. Genetically abnormal fibrinogens — some current characterisation strategies. In: *Fibrinogen —Structure, Functional Aspects, Metabolism*, F. Haverkate, A. Henschen, W. Nieuwenhuizen and P.W. Straub (eds.), Walter de Gruyter, Berlin. pp. 125-144, **1983**.

3. Southan, C., Lane, D.A. and Henschen, A. Functional characterisation and protein chemical analysis of two new cases of dysfibrinogenemia, London III and IV. In: *Fibrinogen —Structure, Functional Aspects, Metabolism*, F. Haverkate, A. Henschen, W. Nieuwenhuizen and P.W. Straub (eds.), Walter de Gruyter, Berlin. pp. 167-182, **1983**.

4. Lane, D.A., Ireland, H., Thompson, E., Frost, T.J. and Cuddigan, B. Two more abnormal fibrinogens (London III and Sydney) with impaired fibrinopeptide release. *Thromb. Res.* **28**:821-824, **1982**.

FIBRINOGEN LONDON IV

Last update [1 December 1990]
Alphacode [LONDON04]
Ref. type [Article]

Family studies
Homozygote? [n.a.]
Pedigree published? [No]

Structural defect [n.a.]
Mutation [n.a.]

Functional defect(s)
FpA release: [Abnormal]
FpB release: [Abnormal]
Polymerization: [Abnormal]
Stabilization: [n.a.]

Clinical manifestation(s) Bleeding? [No] Thrombosis? [No]

Clinical laboratory results
Plasma fibrinogen concentration (mg/dL)
Chronometric: [n.a.]
Rate-indep'nt: [260/(200-400)]
Immunologic: [n.a.]

*Hypo*dysfibrinogen? [No]

Thrombin time:	[19s/(9-12s)]
Reptilase (batroxobin) time:	[38s/(18s)]
Prothrombin time:	[Normal[1]]
Partial thromboplastin time:	[57s/(38-41s)]
Euglobulin lysis time:	[n.a.]
Bleeding time:	[Normal]
Immunoelectrophoresis:	[n.a.]
Platelet aggregation:	[n.a.]

Other results with patient plasma
Ancrod (Arvin) time: [n.a.]
Recalcification time: [n.a.]
Calcium corrects c.t.? [n.a.]

Inhib. normal plasma? [No]
In vivo synthesis: [n.a.]
In vivo catabolism: [n.a.]

Evaluation of isolated patient fibrinogen
Thrombin time: [30s/(20s)]
Reptilase time: [n.a.]
Ancrod (Arvin) time: [n.a.]

Abnormal subunit? [No]
Abnormal FDPs? [No]

Remarks
[1]Data not reported; prothrombin time ratio was 1.1.

References

1. Lane, D.A., Ireland, H., Thompson, E., Southan, C. and Henschen, A. Fibrinogens London I - IV, Manchester, Sydney I and II. Cleavage of fibrinopeptides by thrombin and expression of their polymerisation abnormalities. In: *Fibrinogen — Structural Variants and Interactions*, A. Henschen, B. Hessel, J. McDonagh and T. Saldeen (eds.), W. de Gruyter, Berlin. pp. 197-206, **1985**.

2. Southan, C., Lane, D.A. and Henschen, A. Functional characterisation and protein chemical analysis of two new cases of dysfibrinogenemia, London III and IV. In: *Fibrinogen — Structure, Functional Aspects, Metabolism*, F. Haverkate, A. Henschen, W. Nieuwenhuizen and P.W. Straub (eds.), Walter de Gruyter, Berlin. pp. 167-182, **1983**.

FIBRINOGEN LONDON V

Last update [1 December 1990]
Alphaconde [LONDON05]
Ref. type [Article]

Family studies
Homozygote? [n.a.]
Pedigree published? [No]

Structural defect [n.a.]
Mutation [n.a.]

Functional defect(s)
FpA release: [Normal]
FpB release: [Normal]
Polymerization: [Abnormal]
Stabilization: [n.a.]

Clinical manifestation(s) Bleeding? [No] Thrombosis? [Yes[1]]

Clinical laboratory results
Plasma fibrinogen concentration (mg/dL)
Chronometric: [n.a.]
Rate-indep'nt: [n.a.]
Immunologic: [n.a.[2]]

*Hypo*dysfibrinogen? [Yes]

Thrombin time:	[n.a.]
Reptilase (batroxobin) time:	[n.a.]
Prothrombin time:	[44s/(14s)]
Partial thromboplastin time:	[n.a.]
Euglobulin lysis time:	[n.a.]
Bleeding time:	[n.a.]
Immunoelectrophoresis:	[n.a.]
Platelet aggregation:	[n.a.]

Other results with patient plasma
Ancrod (Arvin) time: [n.a.]
Recalcification time: [n.a.]
Calcium corrects c.t.? [n.a.]

Inhib. normal plasma? [n.a.]
In vivo synthesis: [n.a.]
In vivo catabolism: [n.a.]

Evaluation of isolated patient fibrinogen
Thrombin time: [n.a.]
Reptilase time: [n.a.]
Ancrod (Arvin) time: [n.a.]

Abnormal subunit? [n.a.]
Abnormal FDPs? [n.a.]

Remarks
[1]Venous thrombosis was reported.
[2]Immunologically low plasma fibrinogen was noted; actual result was not reported.

References

1. Southan, C., Thompson, E. and Lane, D.A. Direct analysis of plasma fibrinogen-derived fibrinopeptides by high-performance liquid chromatography: investigation of nine congenital fibrinogen abnormalities. *Br. J. Haematol.* **65**:469-473, **1987**.

FIBRINOGEN LONDON VI

Last update [1 December 1990]
Alphacode [LONDON06]
Ref. type [Article]

Family studies
Homozygote? [No]
Pedigree published? [No]

Structural defect [n.a.]
Mutation [n.a.]

Functional defect(s)
FpA release: [Abnormal[1]]
FpB release: [n.a.]
Polymerization: [n.a.]
Stabilization: [n.a.]

Clinical manifestation(s) Bleeding? [n.a.] Thrombosis? [n.a.]

Clinical laboratory results
Plasma fibrinogen concentration (mg/dL)
Chronometric: [n.a.]
Rate-indep'nt: [90[2]]
Immunologic: [n.a.]

*Hypo*dysfibrinogen? [Yes]

Thrombin time:	[25s/(11s)]
Reptilase (batroxobin) time:	[n.a.]
Prothrombin time:	[n.a.]
Partial thromboplastin time:	[n.a.]
Euglobulin lysis time:	[n.a.]
Bleeding time:	[n.a.]
Immunoelectrophoresis:	[n.a.]
Platelet aggregation:	[n.a.]

Other results with patient plasma
Ancrod (Arvin) time: [n.a.]
Recalcification time: [n.a.]
Calcium corrects c.t.? [n.a.]

Inhib. normal plasma? [n.a.]
In vivo synthesis: [n.a.]
In vivo catabolism: [n.a.]

Evaluation of isolated patient fibrinogen
Thrombin time: [n.a.]
Reptilase time: [n.a.]
Ancrod (Arvin) time: [n.a.]

Abnormal subunit? [n.a.]
Abnormal FDPs? [n.a.]

Remarks
[1]Only half the normal amount of fibrinopeptide A was released.
[2]Normal range not reported.

References

1. Southan, C., Thompson, E. and Lane, D.A. Direct analysis of plasma fibrinogen-derived fibrinopeptides by high-performance liquid chromatography: investigation of nine congenital fibrinogen abnormalities. *Br. J. Haematol.* **65**:469-473, **1987**.

FIBRINOGEN LONG BEACH I[Abs]

Last update [1 December 1990]
Alphacode [LONGBE01]
Ref. type [Abstract]

Structural defect [Aα(16) Arg → His]
Mutation [n.a.]

Family studies
Homozygote? [n.a.]
Pedigree published? [No]

Functional defect(s)
FpA release: [n.a.]
FpB release: [n.a.]
Polymerization: [n.a.]
Stabilization: [n.a.]

Clinical manifestation(s) Bleeding? [n.a.] Thrombosis? [n.a.]

Clinical laboratory results
Plasma fibrinogen concentration (mg/dL)
Chronometric: [n.a.]
Rate-indep'nt: [n.a.]
Immunologic: [n.a.]

*Hypo*dysfibrinogen? [No]

Thrombin time: [n.a.]
Reptilase (batroxobin) time: [n.a.]
Prothrombin time: [n.a.]
Partial thromboplastin time: [n.a.]
Euglobulin lysis time: [n.a.]
Bleeding time: [n.a.]
Immunoelectrophoresis: [n.a.]
Platelet aggregation: [n.a.]

Other results with patient plasma
Ancrod (Arvin) time: [n.a.]
Recalcification time: [n.a.]
Calcium corrects c.t.? [n.a.]

Inhib. normal plasma? [n.a.]
In vivo synthesis: [n.a.]
In vivo catabolism: [n.a.]

Evaluation of isolated patient fibrinogen
Thrombin time: [n.a.]
Reptilase time: [n.a.]
Ancrod (Arvin) time: [n.a.]

Abnormal subunit? [n.a.]
Abnormal FDPs? [n.a.]

Remarks

References

1. Pirkle, H., Theodor, I., Vukasin, P., Nandi, B., Miyada, D., Baker, J. and Dukes, M. Fibrinogen Long Beach. *Thromb. Haemostas.* **58**:148, **1987**. ABSTRACT

FIBRINOGEN LOS ANGELES I[Abs]

Last update [1 December 1990]
Alphacode [LOSANG01]
Ref. type [Abstract]

Family studies
Homozygote? [n.a.]
Pedigree published? [No]

Structural defect [n.a.]
Mutation [n.a.]

Functional defect(s)
FpA release: [n.a.]
FpB release: [n.a.]
Polymerization: [Abnormal]
Stabilization: [Normal]

Clinical manifestation(s) Bleeding? [No] Thrombosis? [No]

Clinical laboratory results
Plasma fibrinogen concentration (mg/dL)
Chronometric: [Subnormal[1]]
Rate-indep'nt: [Normal[1]]
Immunologic: [Normal[1]]

*Hypo*dysfibrinogen? [No]

Thrombin time:	[Abnormal[1]]
Reptilase (batroxobin) time:	[n.a.]
Prothrombin time:	[Abnormal[1]]
Partial thromboplastin time:	[Normal[1]]
Euglobulin lysis time:	[n.a.]
Bleeding time:	[n.a.]
Immunoelectrophoresis:	[Abnormal]
Platelet aggregation:	[n.a.]

Other results with patient plasma
Ancrod (Arvin) time: [n.a.]
Recalcification time: [n.a.]
Calcium corrects c.t.? [Yes]

Inhib. normal plasma? [Yes]
In vivo synthesis: [n.a.]
In vivo catabolism: [n.a.]

Evaluation of isolated patient fibrinogen
Thrombin time: [n.a.]
Reptilase time: [n.a.]
Ancrod (Arvin) time: [n.a.]

Abnormal subunit? [n.a.]
Abnormal FDPs? [n.a.]

Remarks
[1]Data not reported

References

1. Zietz, B.H. and Scott, J.L. An inherited defect in fibrinogen polymerization: fibrinogen Los Angeles. *Clin. Res.* **18**:179, **1970**. ABSTRACT

FIBRINOGEN LOUISVILLE I

Last update [1 December 1990]
Alphacode [LOUISV01]
Ref. type [Article]

Family studies
Homozygote? [No]
Pedigree published? [Yes]

Structural defect [Aα(16) Arg → His]
Mutation [n.a.]

Functional defect(s)
FpA release: [Abnormal[1]]
FpB release: [n.a.]
Polymerization: [Normal]
Stabilization: [n.a.]

Clinical manifestation(s) Bleeding? [Yes[2]] Thrombosis? [No]

Clinical laboratory results
Plasma fibrinogen concentration (mg/dL)
Chronometric: [60-80[3]]
Rate-indep'nt: [n.a.]
Immunologic: [Normal[4]]

*Hypo*dysfibrinogen? [No]

Thrombin time:	[Abnormal[4]]
Reptilase (batroxobin) time:	[n.a.]
Prothrombin time:	[n.a.]
Partial thromboplastin time:	[n.a.]
Euglobulin lysis time:	[n.a.]
Bleeding time:	[n.a.]
Immunoelectrophoresis:	[n.a.]
Platelet aggregation:	[n.a.[5]]

Other results with patient plasma
Ancrod (Arvin) time: [n.a.]
Recalcification time: [n.a.]
Calcium corrects c.t.? [n.a.]

Inhib. normal plasma? [Yes]
In vivo synthesis: [n.a.]
In vivo catabolism: [n.a.]

Evaluation of isolated patient fibrinogen
Thrombin time: [Abnormal[4]]
Reptilase time: [n.a.]
Ancrod (Arvin) time: [n.a.]

Abnormal subunit? [No]
Abnormal FDPs? [n.a.]

Remarks
[1]Only half the normal amount of fibrinopeptide A was released.
[2]Easy bruising and excessive post-surgical bleeding in the 54 year-old propositus were reported.
[3]Normal range not reported.
[4]Data not reported.
[5]The variant fibrinogen exhibited normal *support* of platelet aggregation.

References

1. Galanakis, D.K., Henschen, A., Keeling, M., Kehl, M., Dismore, R. and Peerschke, E.I. Fibrinogen Louisville: an Aα-16 Arg → His defect that forms no hybrid molecules in heterozygous individuals and inhibits aggregation of normal fibrin monomers. *Ann. N. Y. Acad. Sci.* **408**:644-648, **1983.**

2. Henschen, A., Kehl, M., Southan, C., Lottspeich, F. and Georgopoulos, D. Genetically abnormal fibrinogens — some current characterisation strategies. In: *Fibrinogen —Structure, Functional Aspects, Metabolism*, F. Haverkate, A. Henschen, W. Nieuwenhuizen and P.W. Straub (eds.), Walter de Gruyter, Berlin. pp. 125-144, **1983.**

3. Kehl, M., Lottspeich, F. and Henschen, A. Genetically abnormal fibrinogens releasing abnormal fibrinopeptides as characterised by high-performance liquid chromatography. In: *Fibrinogen — Structure, Functional Aspects, Metabolism*, F. Haverkate, A. Henschen, W. Nieuwenhuizen and P.W. Straub (eds.), Walter de Gruyter, Berlin. pp. 183-193, **1983.**

FIBRINOGEN MAASTRICHT I[Abs]

Last update [10 January 1994]
Alphacode [MAASTR01]
Ref. type [Abstract]

Family studies
Homozygote? [n.a.]
Pedigree published? [No]

Structural defect [n.a.]
Mutation [n.a.]

Functional defect(s)
FpA release: [n.a.]
FpB release: [n.a.]
Polymerization: [n.a.]
Stabilization: [n.a.]

Clinical manifestation(s) Bleeding? [Yes[1]] Thrombosis? [No]

Clinical laboratory results
Plasma fibrinogen concentration (mg/dL)
Chronometric: [20[2]]
Rate-indep'nt: [n.a.]
Immunologic: [n.a.]

*Hypo*dysfibrinogen? [n.a.[2]]

Thrombin time:	[n.a.]
Reptilase (batroxobin) time:	[n.a.]
Prothrombin time:	[n.a.]
Partial thromboplastin time:	[n.a.]
Euglobulin lysis time:	[n.a.]
Bleeding time:	[n.a.]
Immunoelectrophoresis:	[n.a.]
Platelet aggregation:	[n.a.]

Other results with patient plasma
Ancrod (Arvin) time: [n.a.]
Recalcification time: [n.a.]
Calcium corrects c.t.? [n.a.]

Inhib. normal plasma? [n.a.]
In vivo synthesis: [n.a.]
In vivo catabolism: [n.a.]

Evaluation of isolated patient fibrinogen
Thrombin time: [n.a.]
Reptilase time: [n.a.]
Ancrod (Arvin) time: [n.a.]

Abnormal subunit? [n.a.]
Abnormal FDPs? [n.a.]

Remarks
[1]Umbilical bleeding in the 1 month-old proposita was reported.
[2]Authors suggest *hypo*dysfibrinogenemia; however, this is not substantiated by plasma fibrinogen determinations using methods that do not rely on the rate of coagulation. Until such data become available, this variant will not be classified as a hypodysfibrinogen.

References

1. Hamulyak, K., Muller, A.D. and Hemker, H.C. A new case of congenital combined hypo-dysfibrinogenemia? *Thromb. Haemostas.* **58**:148-148, **1987**. ABSTRACT

FIBRINOGEN MADRID I

Last update [1 December 1990]
Alphacode [MADRID01]
Ref. type [Article]

Family studies
Homozygote? [n.a.]
Pedigree published? [No]

Structural defect [n.a.]
Mutation [n.a.]

Functional defect(s)
FpA release: [Normal]
FpB release: [Abnormal]
Polymerization: [Normal]
Stabilization: [n.a.]

Clinical manifestation(s) Bleeding? [No] Thrombosis? [No]

Clinical laboratory results

Plasma fibrinogen concentration (mg/dL)
Chronometric: [59[1]]
Rate-indep'nt: [248[1]]
Immunologic: [300[1]]

*Hypo*dysfibrinogen? [No]

Thrombin time:	[60s/(17s)]
Reptilase (batroxobin) time:	[42s/(16s)]
Prothrombin time:	[85%[2]]
Partial thromboplastin time:	[39s/(45s)]
Euglobulin lysis time:	[n.a.]
Bleeding time:	[n.a.]
Immunoelectrophoresis:	[Normal]
Platelet aggregation:	[n.a.]

Other results with patient plasma
Ancrod (Arvin) time: [n.a.]
Recalcification time: [n.a.]
Calcium corrects c.t.? [n.a.]

Inhib. normal plasma? [n.a.]
In vivo synthesis: [n.a.]
In vivo catabolism: [n.a.]

Evaluation of isolated patient fibrinogen
Thrombin time: [n.a.]
Reptilase time: [n.a.]
Ancrod (Arvin) time: [n.a.]

Abnormal subunit? [n.a.]
Abnormal FDPs? [n.a.]

Remarks
[1]Normal range not reported.
[2]Within normal limits.

References

1. Borrell, M., Vila, L., Sola, J., Coll, I., Gómez, N., González, N. and Rutllant, M.L. Two cases of dysfibrinogenemia characterized by abnormal FPB release: Fibrinogen Madrid I & II. *Thromb. Res.* **45**:591-599, **1987**.

FIBRINOGEN MADRID II

Last update [1 December 1990]
Alphacode [MADRID02]
Ref. type [Article]

Family studies
Homozygote? [No]
Pedigree published? [No]

Structural defect [n.a.]
Mutation [n.a.]

Functional defect(s)
FpA release: [Abnormal[1]]
FpB release: [Abnormal]
Polymerization: [Normal]
Stabilization: [n.a.]

Clinical manifestation(s) Bleeding? [No] Thrombosis? [No]

Clinical laboratory results
Plasma fibrinogen concentration (mg/dL)
Chronometric: [45[2]]
Rate-indep'nt: [266[2]]
Immunologic: [260[2]]

*Hypo*dysfibrinogen? [No]

Thrombin time:	[Abnormal[3]]
Reptilase (batroxobin) time:	[58s/(16s)]
Prothrombin time:	[43%[2]]
Partial thromboplastin time:	[n.a.]
Euglobulin lysis time:	[n.a.]
Bleeding time:	[n.a.]
Immunoelectrophoresis:	[Normal]
Platelet aggregation:	[n.a.]

Other results with patient plasma
Ancrod (Arvin) time: [n.a.]
Recalcification time: [n.a.]
Calcium corrects c.t.? [n.a.]

Inhib. normal plasma? [n.a.]
In vivo synthesis: [n.a.]
In vivo catabolism: [n.a.]

Evaluation of isolated patient fibrinogen
Thrombin time: [65s/(18s)]
Reptilase time: [n.a.]
Ancrod (Arvin) time: [n.a.]

Abnormal subunit? [n.a.]
Abnormal FDPs? [n.a.]

Remarks
[1]Only half the normal amount of fibrinopeptide A was released.
[2]Normal range not reported.
[3]Data not reported.

References

1. Borrell, M., Vila, L., Sola, J., Coll, I., Gómez, N., González, N. and Rutllant, M.L. Two cases of dysfibrinogenemia characterized by abnormal FPB release: Fibrinogen Madrid I & II. *Thromb. Res.* **45**:591-599, **1987**.

2. Southan, C., Thompson, E. and Lane, D.A. Direct analysis of plasma fibrinogen-derived fibrinopeptides by high-performance liquid chromatography: investigation of nine congenital fibrinogen abnormalities. *Br. J. Haematol.* **65**:469-473, **1987**.

FIBRINOGEN MADRID III

Last update [1 December 1990]
Alphacode [MADRID03]
Ref. type [Article]

Family studies
Homozygote? [No]
Pedigree published? [No]

Structural defect [n.a.]
Mutation [n.a.]

Functional defect(s)
FpA release: [Abnormal[1]]
FpB release: [n.a.]
Polymerization: [Normal]
Stabilization: [Normal]

Clinical manifestation(s) Bleeding? [No] Thrombosis? [No]

Clinical laboratory results
Plasma fibrinogen concentration (mg/dL)
Chronometric: [70/(200-400)]
Rate-indep'nt: [n.a.]
Immunologic: [248/(200-400)]

*Hypo*dysfibrinogen? [No]

Thrombin time:	[32s/(18-20s)]
Reptilase (batroxobin) time:	[35s/(15-18s)]
Prothrombin time:	[16s/(12-14s)]
Partial thromboplastin time:	[40s/(35-45s)]
Euglobulin lysis time:	[>180m/(>180m)[2]]
Bleeding time:	[Normal[2]]
Immunoelectrophoresis:	[n.a.]
Platelet aggregation:	[Normal[2]]

Other results with patient plasma
Ancrod (Arvin) time: [n.a.]
Recalcification time: [n.a.]
Calcium corrects c.t.? [No]

Inhib. normal plasma? [Yes]
In vivo synthesis: [n.a.]
In vivo catabolism: [n.a.]

Evaluation of isolated patient fibrinogen
Thrombin time: [n.a.]
Reptilase time: [n.a.]
Ancrod (Arvin) time: [n.a.]

Abnormal subunit? [No[2]]
Abnormal FDPs? [No[2]]

Remarks
[1]Only half the normal amount of fibrinopeptide A was released.
[2]F.J. Fernández, personal communication.

References

1. Fernández, J., de la Torre, S., Losada, G., Villar, J.M., Paramo, J.A., Cuesta, B. and Rocha, E. Two cases of congenital dysfibrinogenemia. Fibrinogens Madrid III and Malaga. In: *Fibrinogen 3. Biochemistry, Biological Functions, Gene Regulation and Expression*, M.W. Mosesson, D.L. Amrani, K.R. Siebenlist and J.P. DiOrio (eds.), Elsevier Science Publ., B.V., Amsterdam. pp. 255-258, **1988**.

FIBRINOGEN MAGDEBURG II[Abs]

Last update [10 January 1994]
Alphacode [MAGDEB02]
Ref. type [Abstract]

Family studies
Homozygote? [n.a.]
Pedigree published? [No]

Structural defect [n.a.]
Mutation [n.a.]

Functional defect(s)
FpA release: [n.a.]
FpB release: [n.a.]
Polymerization: [n.a.]
Stabilization: [n.a.]

Clinical manifestation(s) Bleeding? [Yes[1]] Thrombosis? [No]

Clinical laboratory results

Plasma fibrinogen concentration (mg/dL)
Chronometric: [Subnormal[2]]
Rate-indep'nt: [Normal[2]]
Immunologic: [n.a.]

*Hypo*dysfibrinogen? [No]

Thrombin time:	[n.a.]
Reptilase (batroxobin) time:	[n.a.]
Prothrombin time:	[Abnormal[2]]
Partial thromboplastin time:	[n.a.]
Euglobulin lysis time:	[n.a.]
Bleeding time:	[n.a.]
Immunoelectrophoresis:	[n.a.]
Platelet aggregation:	[n.a.]

Other results with patient plasma
Ancrod (Arvin) time: [n.a.]
Recalcification time: [n.a.]
Calcium corrects c.t.? [n.a.]

Inhib. normal plasma? [n.a.]
In vivo synthesis: [n.a.]
In vivo catabolism: [n.a.]

Evaluation of isolated patient fibrinogen
Thrombin time: [n.a.]
Reptilase time: [n.a.]
Ancrod (Arvin) time: [n.a.]

Abnormal subunit? [n.a.]
Abnormal FDPs? [n.a.]

Remarks
[1]A mild bleeding tendency was reported.
[2]Data not reported.

This is the first report of a variant fibrinogen from Magdeburg; it is not clear why it was designated Magdeburg "II."

References

1. Meyer, M., Lutze, G. and Gromnica-Ilhe, E. Dysfibrinogenemia: abnormalities in the Bβ chains of fibrinogens Berlin II and Magdeburg II. *Thromb. Haemostas.* **65**:903, **1991**. ABSTRACT

FIBRINOGEN MALAGA I

Last update [1 December 1990]
Alphacode [MALAGA01]
Ref. type [Article]

Structural defect [n.a.]
Mutation [n.a.]

Family studies
Homozygote? [No]
Pedigree published? [No]

Functional defect(s)

FpA release:	[Abnormal[1]]
FpB release:	[n.a.]
Polymerization:	[Abnormal]
Stabilization:	[Normal]

Clinical manifestation(s) Bleeding? [No] Thrombosis? [No]

Clinical laboratory results

Plasma fibrinogen concentration (mg/dL)
Chronometric: [55/(200-400)]
Rate-indep'nt: [n.a.]
Immunologic: [164/(200-400)]

*Hypo*dysfibrinogen? [No]

Thrombin time:	[31s/(18-20s)]
Reptilase (batroxobin) time:	[23s/(15-18s)]
Prothrombin time:	[16s/(12-14s)]
Partial thromboplastin time:	[46s/(35-45s)]
Euglobulin lysis time:	[>180/(>180)[2]]
Bleeding time:	[Normal[2]]
Immunoelectrophoresis:	[n.a.]
Platelet aggregation:	[Normal[2]]

Other results with patient plasma

Ancrod (Arvin) time:	[n.a.]	Inhib. normal plasma?	[Yes]
Recalcification time:	[n.a.]	In vivo synthesis:	[n.a.]
Calcium corrects c.t.?	[No]	In vivo catabolism:	[n.a.]

Evaluation of isolated patient fibrinogen

Thrombin time:	[n.a.]	Abnormal subunit?	[No[2]]
Reptilase time:	[n.a.]	Abnormal FDPs?	[No[2]]
Ancrod (Arvin) time:	[n.a.]		

Remarks
[1]Only half the normal amount of fibrinopeptide A was released.
[2]F.J. Fernández, personal communication.

References

1. Fernández, J., de la Torre, S., Losada, G., Villar, J.M., Paramo, J.A., Cuesta, B. and Rocha, E. Two cases of congenital dysfibrinogenemia. Fibrinogens Madrid III and Malaga. In: *Fibrinogen 3. Biochemistry, Biological Functions, Gene Regulation and Expression*, M.W. Mosesson, D.L. Amrani, K.R. Siebenlist and J.P. DiOrio (eds.), Elsevier Science Publ., B.V., Amsterdam. pp. 255-258, **1988**.

FIBRINOGEN MALMÖE I

Last update [10 January 1994]
Alphacode [MALMOE01]
Ref. type [Article]

Family studies
Homozygote? [n.a.]
Pedigree published? [No]

Structural defect [n.a.]
Mutation [n.a.]

Functional defect(s)
FpA release: [Normal]
FpB release: [Normal]
Polymerization: [Abnormal]
Stabilization: [Normal]

Clinical manifestation(s) Bleeding? [No] Thrombosis? [Yes[1]]

Clinical laboratory results

Plasma fibrinogen concentration (mg/dL)
Chronometric: [n.a.]
Rate-indep'nt: [70[2]]
Immunologic: [n.a.]

*Hypo*dysfibrinogen? [Yes]

Thrombin time:	[25-30s/(<20s)]
Reptilase (batroxobin) time:	[22-24s/(19s)]
Prothrombin time:	[n.a.]
Partial thromboplastin time:	[n.a.]
Euglobulin lysis time:	[n.a.]
Bleeding time:	[n.a.]
Immunoelectrophoresis:	[n.a.]
Platelet aggregation:	[Normal]

Other results with patient plasma
Ancrod (Arvin) time: [n.a.]
Recalcification time: [n.a.]
Calcium corrects c.t.? [n.a.]

Inhib. normal plasma? [n.a.]
In vivo synthesis: [n.a.]
In vivo catabolism: [Normal]

Evaluation of isolated patient fibrinogen
Thrombin time: [20.5s/(15s)]
Reptilase time: [30s/(21s)]
Ancrod (Arvin) time: [n.a.]

Abnormal subunit? [No]
Abnormal FDPs? [No]

Remarks

[1]The proposita presented with deep vein thrombosis and pulmonary embolism while taking oral contraceptives. She also has experienced 3 first-trimester miscarriages. Transient episodes of increased plasma fibronectin were reported.

[2]Normal range not reported.

References

1. Soria, J., Soria, C., Hedner, U., Nilsson, I.M., Bergqvist, D. and Samama, M. Episodes of increased fibronectin level observed in a patient suffering from recurrent thrombosis related to congenital hypodysfibrinogenaemia (fibrinogen Malmöe). *Br. J. Haematol.* **61**:727-738, **1985**.

FIBRINOGEN MANCHESTER I

Last update [1 December 1990]
Alphacode [MANCHE01]
Ref. type [Article]

Family studies
Homozygote? [No]
Pedigree published? [Yes]

Structural defect [Aα(16) Arg → His[1]]
Mutation [CGT → CAT]

Functional defect(s)
FpA release: [Abnormal]
FpB release: [Abnormal]
Polymerization: [Abnormal]
Stabilization: [Normal]

Clinical manifestation(s) Bleeding? [No] Thrombosis? [No]

Clinical laboratory results

Plasma fibrinogen concentration (mg/dL)
Chronometric: [n.a.]
Rate-indep'nt: [562[2]]
Immunologic: [n.a.]

*Hypo*dysfibrinogen? [No]

Thrombin time:	[110s/(24s)]
Reptilase (batroxobin) time:	[n.a.]
Prothrombin time:	[21s/(14s)]
Partial thromboplastin time:	[36.5s/(34.5s)]
Euglobulin lysis time:	[n.a.]
Bleeding time:	[n.a.]
Immunoelectrophoresis:	[Normal]
Platelet aggregation:	[n.a.]

Other results with patient plasma
Ancrod (Arvin) time: [Abnormal[3]]
Recalcification time: [30s/(15s)]
Calcium corrects c.t.? [No]

Inhib. normal plasma? [No]
In vivo synthesis: [n.a.]
In vivo catabolism: [n.a.]

Evaluation of isolated patient fibrinogen
Thrombin time: [147s/(12.4s)]
Reptilase time: [n.a.]
Ancrod (Arvin) time: [n.a.]

Abnormal subunit? [No]
Abnormal FDPs? [No]

Remarks

[1]The structural defect was confirmed with the PCR method (Koopman et al., 1988).
[2]Normal range not reported.
[3]Data not reported.

The variant fibrinogen also was detected in platelet fibrinogen.

FIBRINOGEN MANCHESTER I

References

1. Koopman, J., Haverkate, F., Lane, D.A. and Lord, S.T. Sequence analysis of the fibrinogen Manchester Aα-chain gene after amplification of genomic DNA using the polymerase chain reaction (PCR). In: *Fibrinogen 3. Biochemistry, Biological Functions, Gene Regulation and Expression*, M.W. Mosesson, D.L. Amrani, K.R. Siebenlist and J.P. DiOrio (eds.), Elsevier Science Publ., B.V., Amsterdam. pp. 275-278, **1988**.

2. Lane, D.A., Ireland, H., Thompson, E., Southan, C. and Henschen, A. Fibrinogens London I - IV, Manchester, Sydney I and II. Cleavage of fibrinopeptides by thrombin and expression of their polymerisation abnormalities. In: *Fibrinogen —Structural Variants and Interactions*, A. Henschen, B. Hessel, J. McDonagh and T. Saldeen (eds.), W. de Gruyter, Berlin. pp. 197-206, **1985**.

3. Southan, C., Lane, D.A., Knight, I., Ireland, H. and Bottomley, J. Fibrinogen Manchester. Detection of a heterozygous phenotype in the intraplatelet pool. *Biochem. J.* **229**:723-730, **1985**.

4. Henschen, A., Kehl, M., Southan, C., Lottspeich, F. and Georgopoulos, D. Genetically abnormal fibrinogens — some current characterisation strategies. In: *Fibrinogen —Structure, Functional Aspects, Metabolism*, F. Haverkate, A. Henschen, W. Nieuwenhuizen and P.W. Straub (eds.), Walter de Gruyter, Berlin. pp. 125-144, **1983**.

5. Lane, D.A., Ireland, H., Southan, C., Kehl, M. and Henschen, A. The molecular abnormality of fibrinogen Manchester. In: *Fibrinogen — Structure, Functional Aspects, Metabolism*, F. Haverkate, A. Henschen, W. Nieuwenhuizen and P.W. Straub (eds.), Walter de Gruyter, Berlin. pp. 155-166, **1983**.

6. Lane, D.A., Southan, C., Ireland, H., Thompson, E., Kehl, M. and Henschen, A. Delayed release of an abnormal fibrinopeptide A from fibrinogen Manchester: effect of the Aα-16 Arg leads to His substitution upon fibrin monomer polymerization and the immunological crossreactivity of the peptide. *Br. J. Haematol.* **53**:587-597, **1983**.

7. Southan, C., Kehl, M., Henschen, A. and Lane, D.A. Fibrinogen Manchester: identification of an abnormal fibrinopeptide A with a C-terminal arginine leads to histidine substitution. *Br. J. Haematol.* **54**:143-151, **1983**.

8. Lane, D.A., Allen, A.K., Markwick, J., Thompson, E. and Mackie, I. Carbohydrate in abnormal fibrinogens. In: *Fibrinogen — Recent Biochemical and Medical Aspects*, A. Henschen, H. Graeff and F. Lottspeich (eds.), W. deGruyter, Berlin. pp. 183-192, **1982**.

9. Lane, D.A., VanRoss, M., Kakkar, V.V., Bottomley, K.J., Dhir, K., Holt, L.P. and MacIver, J.E. An abnormal fibrinogen with delayed fibrinopeptide A release. *Br. J. Haematol.* **46**:89-98, **1980**.

FIBRINOGEN MANNHEIM I

Last update [1 December 1990]
Alphacode [MANNHE01]
Ref. type [Article]

Structural defect [Aα(19) Arg → Gly]
Mutation [n.a.]

Family studies
Homozygote? [No]
Pedigree published? [Yes]

Functional defect(s)
FpA release: [Abnormal]
FpB release: [n.a.]
Polymerization: [Abnormal]
Stabilization: [Normal]

Clinical manifestation(s) Bleeding? [Yes[1]] Thrombosis? [No]

Clinical laboratory results

Plasma fibrinogen concentration (mg/dL)
Chronometric: [55-80[2]]
Rate-indep'nt: [n.a.]
Immunologic: [370-380[2]]

*Hypo*dysfibrinogen? [No]

Thrombin time:	[34.5s[3]]
Reptilase (batroxobin) time:	[57.5s[3]]
Prothrombin time:	[n.a.]
Partial thromboplastin time:	[n.a.]
Euglobulin lysis time:	[n.a.]
Bleeding time:	[Normal]
Immunoelectrophoresis:	[n.a.]
Platelet aggregation:	[Normal]

Other results with patient plasma
Ancrod (Arvin) time: [n.a.]
Recalcification time: [n.a.]
Calcium corrects c.t.? [n.a.]
Inhib. normal plasma? [n.a.]
In vivo synthesis: [n.a.]
In vivo catabolism: [n.a.]

Evaluation of isolated patient fibrinogen
Thrombin time: [n.a.]
Reptilase time: [n.a.]
Ancrod (Arvin) time: [n.a.]
Abnormal subunit? [No]
Abnormal FDPs? [n.a.[4]]

Remarks

[1]Excessive menstrual and postpartum bleeding, and easy bruising were reported. These symptoms were *not* observed in Aarhus I.

[2]Normal range not reported.

[3]This result is "prolonged;" normal range not reported.

[4]A reduced rate of tPA-induced plasminogen activation was reported.

Reptilase failed to clot the variant fibrinogen. This provided a convenient means of removing normal fibrinogen prior to structural analysis.

References

1. Dempfle, C.E.H. and Henschen, A. Fibrinogen Mannheim I — identification of an Aα19 Arg → Gly substitution in dysfibrinogenaemia associated with bleeding tendency. In: *Fibrinogen 4. Current Basic and Clinical Aspects*, M. Matsuda, S. Iwanaga, A. Takada and A. Henschen (eds.), Elsevier Science Publ. B.V., Amsterdam. pp. 159-166, **1990.**

2. Heene, D.L., Dempfle, C.E., Borck, P., Kirschstein, W., Harenberg, J. and Brossmer, R. Dysfibrinogenaemia with impaired release of fibrinopeptide A and t-PA-induced plasminogen activation: Fibrinogen Mannheim I. *Thromb. Haemostas.* **62**:75, **1989**. ABSTRACT

FIBRINOGEN MANNHEIM II[Abs]

Last update [1 December 1990]
Alphacode [MANNHE02]
Ref. type [Abstract]

Family studies
Homozygote? [n.a.]
Pedigree published? [No]

Structural defect [n.a.]
Mutation [n.a.]

Functional defect(s)
FpA release: [Normal]
FpB release: [n.a.]
Polymerization: [Abnormal]
Stabilization: [Normal]

Clinical manifestation(s) Bleeding? [Yes[1]] Thrombosis? [Yes[2]]

Clinical laboratory results
Plasma fibrinogen concentration (mg/dL)
Chronometric: [50-80[3]]
Rate-indep'nt: [n.a.]
Immunologic: [150-180[3]]

*Hypo*dysfibrinogen? [Yes]

Thrombin time: [27.5s[4]]
Reptilase (batroxobin) time: [22s[4]]
Prothrombin time: [n.a.]
Partial thromboplastin time: [n.a.]
Euglobulin lysis time: [85-110m[5]]
Bleeding time: [Normal]
Immunoelectrophoresis: [n.a.]
Platelet aggregation: [n.a.]

Other results with patient plasma
Ancrod (Arvin) time: [n.a.]
Recalcification time: [n.a.]
Calcium corrects c.t.? [n.a.]
Inhib. normal plasma? [n.a.]
In vivo synthesis: [n.a.]
In vivo catabolism: [n.a.]

Evaluation of isolated patient fibrinogen
Thrombin time: [n.a.]
Reptilase time: [n.a.]
Ancrod (Arvin) time: [n.a.]
Abnormal subunit? [No]
Abnormal FDPs? [n.a.[6]]

Remarks
[1]Excessive postpartum and post-traumatic bleeding was reported.
[2]Arterial thrombosis was reported.
[3]Normal range not reported.
[4]This result is "prolonged;" normal range not reported.
[5]This result is "reduced;" normal range not reported.
[6]A reduced rate of tPA-induced plasminogen activation was reported.

References

1. Dempfle, C.E., Kirschstein, W., Watzlawick, H., Brossmer, R., Simianer, S., Harenberg, J. and Heene, D.L. Hypodysfibrinogenaemia with impaired fibrin polymerization associated with excessive postpartum bleeding: fibrinogen Mannheim II. *Thromb. Haemostas.* **62**:159, **1989**. ABSTRACT

FIBRINOGEN MARBURG I

Last update [10 January 1994]
Alphacode [MARBUR01]
Ref. type [Article]

Family studies
Homozygote? [Yes]
Pedigree published? [Yes]

Structural defect [Aα(461) Lys → stop[1]]
Mutation [AAA → TAA]

Functional defect(s)
FpA release: [Normal]
FpB release: [Normal]
Polymerization: [Abnormal]
Stabilization: [Normal]

Clinical manifestation(s) Bleeding? [Yes[2]] Thrombosis? [Yes[3]]

Clinical laboratory results
Plasma fibrinogen concentration (mg/dL)
Chronometric: [<25/(250)]
Rate-indep'nt: [190/(280)]
Immunologic: [60/(250)[4]]

*Hypo*dysfibrinogen? [Yes[4]]

Thrombin time:	[240s/(20s)[5]]
Reptilase (batroxobin) time:	[>1 hr/(20s)]
Prothrombin time:	[31s/(15s)]
Partial thromboplastin time:	[78s/(40s)]
Euglobulin lysis time:	[>120m/(>120m)]
Bleeding time:	[Normal]
Immunoelectrophoresis:	[Normal]
Platelet aggregation:	[n.a.]

Other results with patient plasma
Ancrod (Arvin) time: [n.a.]
Recalcification time: [n.a.]
Calcium corrects c.t.? [No]

Inhib. normal plasma? [Yes]
In vivo synthesis: [n.a.]
In vivo catabolism: [n.a.]

Evaluation of isolated patient fibrinogen
Thrombin time: [640s/(20s)[5]]
Reptilase time: [n.a.]
Ancrod (Arvin) time: [n.a.]

Abnormal subunit? [Yes[6]]
Abnormal FDPs? [n.a.]

Remarks

[1]This mutation produces a deletion of Aα (461—610); nevertheless, α-chain crosslinking appears to be normal. Disulfide-linked fibrinogen-albumin complexes were detected. The structural defect was determined by PCR.

[2]Severe postpartum bleeding was reported for the proposita and her heterozygous sister.

[3]Recurrent pulmonary emboli and pelvic thromboses were reported.

[4]The proposita exhibited hypodysfibrinogenemia; heterozygotic family members exhibited low-normal plasma fibrinogen concentrations.

[5]The thrombin time was unusually dependent on pH.

[6]SDS-PAGE disclosed a Mr 47,000 Aα-chain.

FIBRINOGEN MARBURG I

References

1. Egbring, R., Seitz, R., Koopman, J., Haverkate, F., Fuchs, G., Appel, D. and Lerch, L. Bleeding complications in homozygous and heterozygous patients with hypodysfibrinogenemia (H-DF) Marburg (M). *Blood Coag. & Fibrinol.* **4**:821, **1993**. ABSTRACT

2. Sobel, J., Wu, H.Q., Trakht, I., Haverkate, F. and Egbring, R. Alpha chain crosslinking in fibrinogen Marburg (Aα #1-461). *Blood Coag. & Fibrinol.* **4**:812-813, **1993**. ABSTRACT

3. Koopman, J., Haverkate, F., Grimbergen, J., Egbring, R. and Lord, S.T. Fibrinogen Marburg: a homozygous case of dysfibrinogenemia, lacking amino acids Aα 461—610 (Lys 461 AAA → Stop TAA). *Blood* **80**:1972-1979, **1992**.

4. Koopman, J., Haverkate, F., Lord, S.T., and Grimbergen, J. Identification of structural defects in abnormal fibrinogens using the polymerase chain reaction. *Proc. X Intl. Fgen. Wkshp.* **1990** ABSTRACT.

5. Fuchs, G., Egbring, R. and Havemann, K. Fibrinogen Marburg. A new genetic variant of fibrinogen. *Blut* **34**:107-118, **1977**.

FIBRINOGEN MARSEILLE I

Last update	[1 December 1990]	**Structural defect**	[n.a.]
Alphacode	[MARSEI01]	**Mutation**	[n.a.]
Ref. type	[Article]		

Family studies
Homozygote? [n.a.]
Pedigree published? [No]

Functional defect(s)
FpA release: [Abnormal[1]]
FpB release: [Normal]
Polymerization: [Abnormal]
Stabilization: [Normal]

Clinical manifestation(s) Bleeding? [No] Thrombosis? [No]

Clinical laboratory results
Plasma fibrinogen concentration (mg/dL)
Chronometric: [25/(240)]
Rate-indep'nt: [n.a.]
Immunologic: [220/(240)]

*Hypo*dysfibrinogen? [No]

Thrombin time:	[73s/(25s)]
Reptilase (batroxobin) time:	[>60s/(19s)]
Prothrombin time:	[16.5s/(12s)]
Partial thromboplastin time:	[Normal[2]]
Euglobulin lysis time:	[Normal]
Bleeding time:	[Normal]
Immunoelectrophoresis:	[Normal]
Platelet aggregation:	[Abnormal[3]]

Other results with patient plasma

Ancrod (Arvin) time:	[n.a.]	Inhib. normal plasma?	[n.a.]
Recalcification time:	[n.a.]	In vivo synthesis:	[n.a.]
Calcium corrects c.t.?	[No]	In vivo catabolism:	[n.a.]

Evaluation of isolated patient fibrinogen

Thrombin time:	[46s/(20s)]	Abnormal subunit?	[No]
Reptilase time:	[46s/(15s)]	Abnormal FDPs?	[No]
Ancrod (Arvin) time:	[n.a.]		

Remarks
[1]Only half the normal amount of fibrinopeptide A was released.
[2]Data not reported.
[3]Authors concluded that hyperaggregation was not due to the variant fibrinogen.

References

1. Henschen, A., Kehl, M., Southan, C., Lottspeich, F. and Georgopoulos, D. Genetically abnormal fibrinogens — some current characterisation strategies. In: *Fibrinogen —Structure, Functional Aspects, Metabolism*, F. Haverkate, A. Henschen, W. Nieuwenhuizen and P.W. Straub (eds.), Walter de Gruyter, Berlin. pp. 125-144, **1983**.

2. Soria, J., Soria, C., Juhan, I., Perrimond, H., Haverkate, F. and Orsini, A. Fibrinogen Marseille. A new case of congenital dysfibrinogenaemia. *Haemostas.* **9**:214-225, **1980**.

3. Haverkate, F., Timan, G., Soria, J., Soria, C. and Samama, M.M. Studies on the structure of the fragment D moiety of abnormal fibrinogens: Influence of calcium ions. *Thromb. Res.* **13**:689-692, **1978**.

FIBRINOGEN METZ I

Last update	[1 December 1990]	**Structural defect**	[Aα(16) Arg → Cys]
Alphacode	[METZ01]	**Mutation**	[n.a.]
Ref. type	[Article]		

Functional defect(s)

FpA release:	[Abnormal[1]]
FpB release:	[Normal]
Polymerization:	[Abnormal]
Stabilization:	[Normal]

Family studies

Homozygote?	[Yes]
Pedigree published?	[Yes[2]]

Clinical manifestation(s) Bleeding? [Yes[3]] Thrombosis? [No]

Clinical laboratory results

Plasma fibrinogen concentration (mg/dL)

Chronometric:	[0/(300-450)]
Rate-indep'nt:	[250/(300-450)]
Immunologic:	[300/(200-400)]

*Hypo*dysfibrinogen? [No]

Thrombin time:	[No clot]
Reptilase (batroxobin) time:	[No clot]
Prothrombin time:	[No clot]
Partial thromboplastin time:	[No clot]
Euglobulin lysis time:	[120m/(240m)[4]]
Bleeding time:	[Normal]
Immunoelectrophoresis:	[Cathodal[5]]
Platelet aggregation:	[Abnormal[6]]

Other results with patient plasma

Ancrod (Arvin) time:	[No clot]	Inhib. normal plasma?	[n.a.]
Recalcification time:	[n.a.]	In vivo synthesis:	[n.a.]
Calcium corrects c.t.?	[No]	In vivo catabolism:	[n.a.]

Evaluation of isolated patient fibrinogen

Thrombin time:	[n.a.]	Abnormal subunit?	[Yes[5]]
Reptilase time:	[n.a.]	Abnormal FDPs?	[No]
Ancrod (Arvin) time:	[n.a.]		

Remarks

[1]Fibrinopeptide A is not released.
[2]There is evidence of consanguinity.
[3]A mild bleeding tendency and recurrent spontaneous abortions were reported.
[4]Bovine thrombin was used to clot the fibrinogen.
[5]The isolated α-chain exhibited increased anodal mobility on isoelectric focusing.
[6]The variant fibrinogen was not detected in platelet fibrinogen.

Fibrinogen Metz binds about four times more citrate than normal, and is clotted by human thrombin only in whole blood. Bovine thrombin will clot the purified fibrinogen.

FIBRINOGEN METZ I

References

1. Mosesson, M.W., DiOrio, J.P., Muller, M.F., Shainoff, J.R., Siebenlist, K.R., Amrani, D.L., Homandberg, G.A., Soria, J., Soria, C. and Samama, M. Studies on the ultrastructure of fibrin lacking fibrinopeptide B (β-fibrin). *Blood* **69**:1073-1081, **1987**.

2. Mosesson, M.W., Siebenlist, K.R., DiOrio, J.P., Hainfeld, J.F, Wall, J.S., Soria, J., Soria, C. and Samama, M. Evidence that proximal NH2-terminal portions of fibrinogen Metz (Aα 16 Arg → Cys) Aα chains are oriented in the same direction. In: *Fibrinogen and Its Derivatives. Biochemistry, Physiology, and Pathophysiology*, G. Muller-Berghaus, U. Scheefers-Borchel, E. Selmayr and A. Henschen (eds.). Excerpta Medica, Amsterdam; pp. 3-15, **1986**.

3. Soria, J., Soria, C., Samama, M. and Caen, J. Study of ten cases of congenital dysfibrinogenemia. Clinical and molecular biological aspects. In: *Fibrinogen – Structural Variants and Interactions*, A. Henschen, B. Hessel, J. McDonagh and T. Saldeen (eds.). Walter de Gruyter, Berlin; pp. 165-183, **1985**.

4. Corrihons, G., Soria, J., Soria, C., Conard, J., Horellou, M.H. and Samama, M. [Congenital dysfibrinogenemia. Apropos of 13 cases]. *Sem. Hop. Paris* **59**:2517-2523, **1983**.

5. Henschen, A., Kehl, M., Southan, C., Lottspeich, F. and Georgopoulos, D. Genetically abnormal fibrinogens – some current characterisation strategies. In: *Fibrinogen – Structure, Functional Aspects, Metabolism*, F. Haverkate, A. Henschen, W. Nieuwenhuizen and P.W. Straub (eds.). Walter de Gruyter, Berlin; pp. 125-144, **1983**.

6. Ladure, P., Ricordel, Y., Soria, J., Soria, C. and Samama, M. Binding of citrate to normal fibrinogen and to Metz fibrinogen. In: *Fibrinogen – Recent Biochemical and Medical Aspects*, A. Henschen, H. Graeff and F. Lottspeich (eds.). W. de Gruyter, Berlin; pp. 145-152, **1982**.

7. Soria, J., Soria, C., Samama, M., Henschen, A. and Southan, C. Detection of fibrinogen abnormality in dysfibrinogenemia: Special report on fibrinogen Metz characterized by an amino acid substitution located at the peptide bond cleaved by thrombin. In: *Fibrinogen – Recent Biochemical and Medical Aspects*, A. Henschen, H. Graeff and F. Lottspeich (eds.). W. de Gruyter, Berlin; pp. 129-144, **1982**.

8. Southan, C., Henschen, A. and Lottspeich, F. The search for molecular defects in abnormal fibrinogens. In: *Fibrinogen – Recent Biochemical and Medical Aspects*, A. Henschen, H. Graeff and F. Lottspeich (eds.). W. de Gruyter, Berlin; pp. 153-166, **1982**.

9. Henschen, A., Southan, C., Soria, J., Soria, C. and Samama, M. Structure abnormality of fibrinogen Metz and its relationship to the clotting defect. *Thromb. Haemostas.* **46**:103, **1981**. ABSTRACT

10. Haverkate, F., Timan, G., Soria, J., Soria, C. and Samama, M.M. Studies on the structure of the fragment D moiety of abnormal fibrinogens: Influence of calcium ions. *Thromb. Res.* **13**:689-692, **1978**.

11. Soria, J., Soria, C., Samama, M., Poirot, E. and Kling, C. Human platelet fibrinogen: a protein different from plasma fibrinogen. *Pathol. Biol. (Paris.)* **24**:15-17, **1976**.

12. Soria, C., Soria, J., Samama, M., Poirot, E. and Kling, C. Proceedings: Role of trisodium citrate in the unclottability by thrombin of fibrinogen Metz. *Thromb. Diath. Haemorrh.* **34**:571, **1975**. ABSTRACT

13. Soria, J., Soria, C., Samama, M., Poirot, E. and Kling, C. Fibrinogen Troyes – fibrinogen Metz. Two new cases of congenital dysfibrinogenemia. *Thromb. Diath. Haemorrh.* **27**:619-633, **1972**.

14. Soria, J., Soria, C. and Boulard, C. [Structural anomaly of Metz fibrinogen, localized on the (A) chain of the molecule]. *Biochimie* **54**:415-417, **1972**.

FIBRINOGEN MÉXICO DF I^{Abs}

Last update [10 January 1994]
Alphacode [MEXICO01]
Ref. type [Abstract]

Family studies
Homozygote? [n.a.]
Pedigree published? [No]

Structural defect [n.a.]
Mutation [n.a.]

Functional defect(s)
FpA release: [Abnormal]
FpB release: [Abnormal]
Polymerization: [Abnormal]
Stabilization: [n.a.]

Clinical manifestation(s) Bleeding? [No] Thrombosis? [No]

Clinical laboratory results
Plasma fibrinogen concentration (mg/dL)
Chronometric: [n.a.]
Rate-indep'nt: [n.a.]
Immunologic: [n.a.]

*Hypo*dysfibrinogen? [n.a.]

Thrombin time:	[n.a.]
Reptilase (batroxobin) time:	[n.a.]
Prothrombin time:	[n.a.]
Partial thromboplastin time:	[n.a.]
Euglobulin lysis time:	[n.a.]
Bleeding time:	[n.a.]
Immunoelectrophoresis:	[Normal]
Platelet aggregation:	[n.a.]

Other results with patient plasma
Ancrod (Arvin) time: [n.a.]
Recalcification time: [n.a.]
Calcium corrects c.t.? [n.a.]

Inhib. normal plasma? [n.a.]
In vivo synthesis: [n.a.]
In vivo catabolism: [n.a.]

Evaluation of isolated patient fibrinogen
Thrombin time: [n.a.]
Reptilase time: [n.a.]
Ancrod (Arvin) time: [n.a.]

Abnormal subunit? [n.a.]
Abnormal FDPs? [No]

Remarks

References

1. Gonzáles-Llaven, J., Vargas-Linares, M.E., Azaola-Espinoza, P., Gonzáles-Angulo, A. and Watanabe, C. An abnormal fibrinogen identified in a Mexican Family. *Proc. XVII Congr. Int. Soc. Hematol.* p. 938, **1978**. ABSTRACT

FIBRINOGEN MILAN I[1]

Last update	[1 December 1990]	**Structural defect**	[γ(330) Asp → Val]
Alphacode	[MILAN01]	**Mutation**	[n.a.]
Ref. type	[Article]		

Family studies
Homozygote? [No]
Pedigree published? [No]

Functional defect(s)
FpA release: [Normal]
FpB release: [Normal]
Polymerization: [Abnormal]
Stabilization: [n.a.]

Clinical manifestation(s) Bleeding? [No] Thrombosis? [No]

Clinical laboratory results

Plasma fibrinogen concentration (mg/dL)
Chronometric: [40/(150-300)]
Rate-indep'nt: [300/(150-300)]
Immunologic: [240/(150-300)]

*Hypo*dysfibrinogen? [No]

Thrombin time:	[21s/(11-14s)]
Reptilase (batroxobin) time:	[24.7s/(14-15s)]
Prothrombin time:	[n.a.]
Partial thromboplastin time:	[n.a.]
Euglobulin lysis time:	[n.a.]
Bleeding time:	[Normal]
Immunoelectrophoresis:	[n.a.]
Platelet aggregation:	[n.a.]

Other results with patient plasma

Ancrod (Arvin) time:	[n.a.]	Inhib. normal plasma?	[n.a.]
Recalcification time:	[n.a.]	In vivo synthesis:	[n.a.]
Calcium corrects c.t.?	[n.a.]	In vivo catabolism:	[n.a.]

Evaluation of isolated patient fibrinogen

Thrombin time:	[n.a.]	Abnormal subunit?	[Yes[2]]
Reptilase time:	[n.a.]	Abnormal FDPs?	[Yes]
Ancrod (Arvin) time:	[n.a.]		

Remarks

[1]Also known as "MILANO I."
[2]Increased cathodal mobility of the isolated γ-chain was reported.

The index patient was a female child from northern Italy. Laboratory results are those of her father, who was similarly afflicted.

References

1. Reber, P., Furlan, M., Rupp, C., Kehl, M., Henschen, A., Manucci, P.M. and Beck, E.A. Fibrinogen Milano I: abnormal fibrin polymerization related to a carboxy-terminal defect of the γ-chain (γ-330 Asp → Val). In: *Fibrinogen, Fibrin Formation and Fibrinolysis*, D.A. Lane, A. Henschen and M.K. Jasani (eds.), W. de Gruyter, Berlin. pp. 97-102, **1986**.

2. Reber, P., Furlan, M., Rupp, C., Kehl, M., Henschen, A., Mannucci, P.M. and Beck, E.A. Characterization of fibrinogen Milano I: amino acid exchange γ-330 Asp → Val impairs fibrin polymerization. *Blood* **67**:1751-1756, **1986**.

FIBRINOGEN MILAN II[1]

Last update	[10 January 1994]	**Structural defect**	[Bβ(68) Ala → Thr[2]]
Alphacode	[MILAN02]	**Mutation**	[GCT → ACT]
Ref. type	[Article]		

Family studies
Homozygote? [Yes[3]]
Pedigree published? [Yes[3]]

Functional defect(s)
FpA release: [Abnormal]
FpB release: [Abnormal]
Polymerization: [Normal]
Stabilization: [Normal]

Clinical manifestation(s) Bleeding? [No] Thrombosis? [Yes[4]]

Clinical laboratory results

Plasma fibrinogen concentration (mg/dL)
Chronometric: [170/(200-400)]
Rate-indep'nt: [320[5]]
Immunologic: [300/(200-400)]

*Hypo*dysfibrinogen? [No]

Thrombin time:	[>180s/(19.8s)]
Reptilase (batroxobin) time:	[21.8s/(22.1s)]
Prothrombin time:	[21s/(13s)]
Partial thromboplastin time:	[28s/(28-43s)[6]]
Euglobulin lysis time:	[167m/(281m)]
Bleeding time:	[Normal[6]]
Immunoelectrophoresis:	[n.a.]
Platelet aggregation:	[Normal]

Other results with patient plasma

Ancrod (Arvin) time:	[23s/(23s)]	Inhib. normal plasma?	[Yes[6]]
Recalcification time:	[n.a.]	In vivo synthesis:	[n.a.]
Calcium corrects c.t.?	[No]	In vivo catabolism:	[n.a.]

Evaluation of isolated patient fibrinogen

Thrombin time:	[90s/(23s)[7]]	Abnormal subunit?	[n.a.]
Reptilase time:	[38s/(65s)[8]]	Abnormal FDPs?	[n.a.]
Ancrod (Arvin) time:	[16s/(23s)[8]]		

Remarks

[1]Also known as "MILANO II" (home to one of the three patients) and "NAPLES I" (city where first studied). ▪[2]The structural defect was determined with the PCR method. ▪[3]There is evidence of consanguinity. ▪[4]The 21 year-old propositus exhibited thrombosis in the abdominal aorta; his 26 year-old sister exhibited occlusion of the right internal carotid artery; his brother experienced venous thrombosis after abdominal surgery. ▪[5]Normal range not reported. ▪[6]G. DiMinno and M. Colucci, personal communication. ▪[7]This result was obtained with bovine thrombin; the corresponding results with human thrombin were [190s/(18s)]. Defective binding of thrombin to patient fibrinogen was reported. ▪[8]This is the only variant with *shortened* Reptilase and ancrod times.

FIBRINOGEN MILAN II

References

1. Koopman, J., Haverkate, F., Lord, S.T., Grimbergen, J. and Mannucci, P.M. Molecular basis of fibrinogen Naples associated with defective thrombin binding and thrombophilia. Homozygous substitution of Bβ 68 Ala→Thr. *J. Clin. Invest.* **90**:238-244, **1992**.

2. Koopman, J., Grimbergen, J., Lord, S.T., Haverkate, F., and Mannucci, P.M. The functional and structural defect of fibrinogen Naples and its relation with thrombosis. *Proc. X Intl. Fgen. Wkshp.*, **1990** ABSTRACT.

3. Koopman, J., Haverkate, F., Lord, S.T., and Grimbergen, J. Identification of structural defects in abnormal fibrinogens using the polymerase chain reaction. *Proc. X Intl. Fgen. Wkshp.*, **1990** ABSTRACT.

4. Di Minno, G., Cerbone, A.M., Cirillo, F., Colucci, M., Semeraro, N., Di Santo, G., Mattioli, P.L., Mancini, M. and Quattrone, A. Abnormal fibrinogen (fibrinogen Naples) characterized by defective interaction with thrombin and plasmin in two young siblings with arterial thrombosis. *Thromb. Haemostas.* **58**:514-514, **1987**. ABSTRACT

5. Haverkate, F., Koopman, J., Kluft, C., D'Angelo, A., Cattaneo, M. and Mannucci, P.M. Fibrinogens "Milano II" and "Naples." *Thromb. Haemostas.* **57**:375, **1987**.

6. Haverkate, F., Koopman, J., Kluft, C., D'Angelo, A., Cattaneo, M. and Mannucci, P.M. Fibrinogen Milano II: a congenital dysfibrinogenaemia associated with juvenile arterial and venous thrombosis. *Thromb. Haemostas.* **55**:131-135, **1986**.

7. Haverkate, F., Koopman, J. and Kluft, C. Fibrinogen Milan II: a congenital dysfibrinogenaemia with a defective clotting by thrombin, normal clotting by arvin, Reptilase and prothrombin-staphylocoagulase complex, associated with thrombotic episodes. In: *Fibrinogen —Structural Variants and Interactions*, A. Henschen, B. Hessel, J. McDonagh and T. Saldeen (eds.), Walter de Gruyter, Berlin. pp. 223-236, **1985**.

8. Quattrone, A., Colucci, M., Donati, M.B., Meduri, M., Mussoni, L., Roncaglioni, M.C., Semeraro, N., Carlomagno, S. and Bonavita, V. Stroke in two young siblings with congenital dysfibrinogenemia. *Ital. J. Neurol. Sci.* **4**:229-232, **1983**.

9. Quattrone, A., Colucci, M., Donati, M.B., Roncaglioni, M.C., Semeraro, N., Carlomagno, S., and Bonavita, V. Cerebral thrombosis in two siblings with dysfibrinogenemia. *Neurosci. Lett.* **Suppl. 3**:S54, **1979**. ABSTRACT

FIBRINOGEN MILAN III[Abs1]

Last update [10 January 1994]
Alphacode [MILAN03]
Ref. type [Abstract]

Family studies
Homozygote? [Yes]
Pedigree published? [No]

Structural defect [n.a.]
Mutation [n.a.]

Functional defect(s)
FpA release: [n.a.]
FpB release: [n.a.]
Polymerization: [Abnormal]
Stabilization: [n.a.]

Clinical manifestation(s) Bleeding? [No] Thrombosis? [Yes[2]]

Clinical laboratory results
Plasma fibrinogen concentration (mg/dL)
Chronometric: [<20[3]]
Rate-indep'nt: [Normal[4]]
Immunologic: [Normal[4]]
*Hypo*dysfibrinogen? [No]

Thrombin time:	[Abnormal[4]]
Reptilase (batroxobin) time:	[Abnormal[4]]
Prothrombin time:	[n.a.]
Partial thromboplastin time:	[n.a.]
Euglobulin lysis time:	[n.a.]
Bleeding time:	[n.a.]
Immunoelectrophoresis:	[n.a.]
Platelet aggregation:	[n.a.]

Other results with patient plasma
Ancrod (Arvin) time: [n.a.]
Recalcification time: [n.a.]
Calcium corrects c.t.? [n.a.]
Inhib. normal plasma? [Yes]
In vivo synthesis: [n.a.]
In vivo catabolism: [n.a.]

Evaluation of isolated patient fibrinogen
Thrombin time: [n.a.]
Reptilase time: [n.a.]
Ancrod (Arvin) time: [n.a.]
Abnormal subunit? [Yes[5]]
Abnormal FDPs? [n.a.]

Remarks
[1]Also known as "MILANO III."
[2]Recurrent thrombophlebitis in the 13 year-old proposita was reported.
[3]Normal range not reported.
[4]Data not reported.
[5]An abnormal Aα-chain was detected by isoelectric focusing.

References

1. Bögli, C., Hofer, A., Furlan, M., Beck, E.A., Baudo, F. and Redaelli, R. Fibrinogen Milano III, a new abnormal hereditary fibrinogen variant with a defect in the Aα-chain. *Thromb. Haemostas.* **58**:515, **1987**. ABSTRACT

FIBRINOGEN MILAN IV[1]

Last update	[10 January 1994]	**Structural defect**	[Aα(16) Arg → His]
Alphacode	[MILAN04]	**Mutation**	[n.a.]
Ref. type	[Article]		

Family studies
Homozygote? [No]
Pedigree published? [No]

Functional defect(s)
FpA release: [Abnormal[2]]
FpB release: [n.a.]
Polymerization: [Abnormal]
Stabilization: [n.a.]

Clinical manifestation(s) Bleeding? [No[3]] Thrombosis? [No[3]]

Clinical laboratory results

Plasma fibrinogen concentration (mg/dL)
Chronometric: [35/(150-400)]
Rate-indep'nt: [180/(150-400)]
Immunologic: [187/(150-400)]

*Hypo*dysfibrinogen? [No]

Thrombin time:	[25s/(12-15s)]
Reptilase (batroxobin) time:	[>180s/(16-18s)]
Prothrombin time:	[n.a.]
Partial thromboplastin time:	[n.a.]
Euglobulin lysis time:	[n.a.]
Bleeding time:	[n.a.]
Immunoelectrophoresis:	[n.a.]
Platelet aggregation:	[n.a.]

Other results with patient plasma

Ancrod (Arvin) time:	[n.a.]	Inhib. normal plasma?	[n.a.]
Recalcification time:	[n.a.]	In vivo synthesis:	[n.a.]
Calcium corrects c.t.?	[n.a.]	In vivo catabolism:	[n.a.]

Evaluation of isolated patient fibrinogen

Thrombin time:	[n.a.]	Abnormal subunit?	[n.a.]
Reptilase time:	[n.a.]	Abnormal FDPs?	[n.a.]
Ancrod (Arvin) time:	[n.a.]		

Remarks

[1]Also known as "MILANO IV."
[2]Only half the normal amount of FpA was released.
[3]A single spontaneous abortion was reported for both the proposita and her mother.

References

1. Bögli, C., Hofer, A., Baudo, F., Redaelli, R. and Furlan, M. Fibrinogen Milano IV, another case of congenital dysfibrinogenemia with an abnormal fibrinopeptide A release (Aα 16 Arg → His). *Haemostas.* **22**:7-11, **1992**.

FIBRINOGEN MILAN VI[1]

Last update [1 December 1990]
Alphacode [MILAN06]
Ref. type [Article]

Structural defect [Aα(16) Arg → His]
Mutation [n.a.]

Family studies
Homozygote? [No]
Pedigree published? [Yes]

Functional defect(s)
FpA release: [n.a.]
FpB release: [n.a.]
Polymerization: [Abnormal]
Stabilization: [n.a.]

Clinical manifestation(s) Bleeding? [Yes[2]] Thrombosis? [No]

Clinical laboratory results

Plasma fibrinogen concentration (mg/dL)
Chronometric: [30/(230)]
Rate-indep'nt: [n.a.]
Immunologic: [190/(230)]

*Hypo*dysfibrinogen? [No]

Thrombin time:	[51s/(17s)]
Reptilase (batroxobin) time:	[51s/(20s)]
Prothrombin time:	[n.a.]
Partial thromboplastin time:	[n.a.]
Euglobulin lysis time:	[n.a.]
Bleeding time:	[Normal]
Immunoelectrophoresis:	[n.a.]
Platelet aggregation:	[Abnormal]

Other results with patient plasma
Ancrod (Arvin) time: [n.a.]
Recalcification time: [n.a.]
Calcium corrects c.t.? [n.a.]

Inhib. normal plasma? [n.a.]
In vivo synthesis: [n.a.]
In vivo catabolism: [n.a.]

Evaluation of isolated patient fibrinogen
Thrombin time: [n.a.]
Reptilase time: [n.a.]
Ancrod (Arvin) time: [n.a.]

Abnormal subunit? [No]
Abnormal FDPs? [n.a.]

Remarks

[1]Also known as MILANO VI. This variant is out of sequence; fibrinogen Milan V has not been reported.

[2]One episode of gastrointestinal bleeding was reported. No other abnormal bleeding (including post-tonsillectomy) was reported. A platelet aggregation abnormality may account for the observed G.I. bleeding.

References

1. Bögli, C., Cofrancesco, E., Cortellaro, M., Della Volpe, A., Hofer, A., Furlan, M. and Zanussi, C. Fibrinogen Milano. VI: A heterozygous dysfibrinogenemia (Aα 16 Arg → His) with bleeding tendency. *Eur. J. Haematol.* **45**:26-30, **1990**.

FIBRINOGEN MILAN VII[Abs1]

Last update [10 January 1994]
Alphacode [MILAN07]
Ref. type [Abstract]

Structural defect [γ(358) Ser → Cys[2]]
Mutation [TCT → TGT]

Family studies
Homozygote? [No]
Pedigree published? [No]

Functional defect(s)
FpA release: [Normal]
FpB release: [Normal]
Polymerization: [Abnormal[3]]
Stabilization: [n.a.]

Clinical manifestation(s) Bleeding? [No] Thrombosis? [No]

Clinical laboratory results
Plasma fibrinogen concentration (mg/dL)
Chronometric: [n.a.]
Rate-indep'nt: [n.a.]
Immunologic: [n.a.]

*Hypo*dysfibrinogen? [n.a.]

Thrombin time:	[Abnormal]
Reptilase (batroxobin) time:	[n.a.]
Prothrombin time:	[n.a.]
Partial thromboplastin time:	[n.a.]
Euglobulin lysis time:	[n.a.]
Bleeding time:	[n.a.]
Immunoelectrophoresis:	[n.a.]
Platelet aggregation:	[n.a.]

Other results with patient plasma
Ancrod (Arvin) time: [n.a.]
Recalcification time: [n.a.]
Calcium corrects c.t.? [n.a.]

Inhib. normal plasma? [n.a.]
In vivo synthesis: [n.a.]
In vivo catabolism: [n.a.]

Evaluation of isolated patient fibrinogen
Thrombin time: [n.a.]
Reptilase time: [n.a.]
Ancrod (Arvin) time: [n.a.]

Abnormal subunit? [n.a.]
Abnormal FDPs? [n.a.]

Remarks
[1]Also known as MILANO VII. This variant is out of sequence; fibrinogen Milan V has not been reported.
[2]The structural defect was determined with the PCR method.
[3]The authors concluded that disulfide-linked albumin did not interfere with fibrin monomer polymerization.

References

1. Steinmann, C., Bögli, C., Iungo, M., Lämmle, B., Heinemann, G., Wermuth, B., Redaelli, R., Baudo, F. and Furlan, M. A new substitution, γ-358 Ser → Cys, in fibrinogen Milano VII causes defective fibrin polymerization. *Thromb. Haemostas.* **69**:962, **1993**. ABSTRACT

2. Steinmann, C., Bögli, C., Lämmle, B., Heinemann, G., Wermuth, B., Baudo, F., Redaelli, R. and Furlan, M. A new substitution γ 358 Ser → Cys in fibrinogen Milano VII causes defective fibrin monomer polymerization. *Proc. XI Int'l. F'gen. Wkshop.* 7, **1992**. ABSTRACT

FIBRINOGEN MITAKA I[Abs]

Last update	[10 January 1994]	**Structural defect**	[n.a.]
Alphacode	[MITAKA01]	**Mutation**	[n.a.]
Ref. type	[Abstract]		

Family studies
Homozygote? [n.a.]
Pedigree published? [No]

Functional defect(s)
FpA release: [Normal]
FpB release: [Normal]
Polymerization: [Abnormal]
Stabilization: [Normal]

Clinical manifestation(s) Bleeding? [No] Thrombosis? [No]

Clinical laboratory results

Plasma fibrinogen concentration (mg/dL)
Chronometric: [67-156[1]]
Rate-indep'nt: [n.a.]
Immunologic: [125-174[1]]

*Hypo*dysfibrinogen? [Yes]

Thrombin time:	[Abnormal]
Reptilase (batroxobin) time:	[Abnormal]
Prothrombin time:	[Abnormal]
Partial thromboplastin time:	[Normal]
Euglobulin lysis time:	[n.a.]
Bleeding time:	[n.a.]
Immunoelectrophoresis:	[Anodal]
Platelet aggregation:	[n.a.]

Other results with patient plasma

Ancrod (Arvin) time:	[Abnormal]	Inhib. normal plasma?	[n.a.]
Recalcification time:	[n.a.]	In vivo synthesis:	[n.a.]
Calcium corrects c.t.?	[n.a.]	In vivo catabolism:	[n.a.]

Evaluation of isolated patient fibrinogen

Thrombin time:	[n.a.]	Abnormal subunit?	[No]
Reptilase time:	[n.a.]	Abnormal FDPs?	[n.a.]
Ancrod (Arvin) time:	[n.a.]		

Remarks

[1]Normal range not reported; authors considered these values to be subnormal.

References

1. Muraki, H., Ando, Y., Matsuda, S., Kikuchi, M., Hasegawa, M., Ono, F., Yamamoto, M., Suzuki, M., Nakamura, S. and Iwanaga, S. Fibrinogen 'Mitaka': a hereditary hypodysfibrinogenemia. *Proc. XVI Congr. Int. Soc. Hematol.* p. 310, **1976**. ABSTRACT

FIBRINOGEN MITAKA II

Last update [10 January 1994]
Alphacode [MITAKA02]
Ref. type [Article]

Structural defect [Aα(11) Glu → Gly]
Mutation [n.a.]

Family studies
Homozygote? [No]
Pedigree published? [No]

Functional defect(s)
FpA release: [Abnormal]
FpB release: [Abnormal]
Polymerization: [Normal]
Stabilization: [n.a.]

Clinical manifestation(s) Bleeding? [Yes[1]] Thrombosis? [No]

Clinical laboratory results
Plasma fibrinogen concentration (mg/dL)
Chronometric: [91/(350)]
Rate-indep'nt: [308/(350)]
Immunologic: [n.a.]

*Hypo*dysfibrinogen? [No]

Thrombin time:	[28.3s/(13.2s)]
Reptilase (batroxobin) time:	[n.a.]
Prothrombin time:	[77%[2]]
Partial thromboplastin time:	[42.6s/(27-40s)]
Euglobulin lysis time:	[n.a.]
Bleeding time:	[n.a.]
Immunoelectrophoresis:	[n.a.]
Platelet aggregation:	[n.a.]

Other results with patient plasma
Ancrod (Arvin) time: [18.7s/(20.1s)]
Recalcification time: [n.a.]
Calcium corrects c.t.? [No]

Inhib. normal plasma? [n.a.]
In vivo synthesis: [n.a.]
In vivo catabolism: [n.a.]

Evaluation of isolated patient fibrinogen
Thrombin time: [41.2s/(16.7s)[3]]
Reptilase time: [n.a.]
Ancrod (Arvin) time: [21.2s/(19.7s)]

Abnormal subunit? [No]
Abnormal FDPs? [n.a.]

Remarks
[1]The index patient was a 14 year old female with easy bruising and recurrent purpura.
[2]Within normal limits.
[3]Observation of reduced thrombin binding to fibrinogen Mitaka II supports conclusions from crystallographic analyses indicating that AαGlu^{11} forms a salt bridge with Arg^{173} of bovine and human α-thrombin.

References

1. Niwa, K., Yaginuma, A., Nakanishi, M., Wada, Y., Sugo, T., Asakura, S., Watanabe, N. and Matsuda, M. Fibrinogen Mitaka II: a hereditary dysfibrinogen with defective thrombin binding caused by an Aα Glu-11 to Gly substitution. *Blood* **82**:3658-3663, **1993**.

2. Niwa, K., Wada, Y., Asakura, S., Yaginuma, A., Watanabe, N. and Matsuda, M. Fibrinogen Mitaka II: a new type of hereditary abnormal fibrinogen with an Aα Glu-11 to Gly substitution characterized by impaired binding with thrombin. *Blood Coag. & Fibrinol.* **4**:819-820, **1993**. ABSTRACT

FIBRINOGEN MONTEVIDEO I

Last update	[10 January 1994]	**Structural defect**	[n.a.]
Alphacode	[MONTEV01]	**Mutation**	[n.a.]
Ref. type	[Article]		

Family studies

Homozygote?	[n.a.]
Pedigree published?	[No]

Functional defect(s)

FpA release:	[Normal]
FpB release:	[Normal]
Polymerization:	[Abnormal]
Stabilization:	[Normal]

Clinical manifestation(s) Bleeding? [Yes[1]] Thrombosis? [No]

Clinical laboratory results

Plasma fibrinogen concentration (mg/dL)

Chronometric: [60[2]]
Rate-indep'nt: [144[2]] *Hypo*dysfibrinogen? [Yes]
Immunologic: [109[2].]

Thrombin time:	[Abnormal[3]]
Reptilase (batroxobin) time:	[n.a.]
Prothrombin time:	[n.a.]
Partial thromboplastin time:	[n.a.]
Euglobulin lysis time:	[n.a.]
Bleeding time:	[n.a.]
Immunoelectrophoresis:	[Normal]
Platelet aggregation:	[n.a.]

Other results with patient plasma

Ancrod (Arvin) time:	[n.a.]	Inhib. normal plasma?	[No]
Recalcification time:	[n.a.]	In vivo synthesis:	[n.a.]
Calcium corrects c.t.?	[No]	In vivo catabolism:	[n.a.]

Evaluation of isolated patient fibrinogen

Thrombin time:	[n.a.]	Abnormal subunit?	[No]
Reptilase time:	[n.a.]	Abnormal FDPs?	[n.a.]
Ancrod (Arvin) time:	[n.a.]		

Remarks

[1]"Moderate" bleeding and a concomitant factor X deficiency were reported; details were not provided.
[2]Normal range not reported.
[3]Data not reported.

Electron microscopy of patient fibrinogen and fibrin (Marchi et al., 1990) disclosed no differences from normal.

References

1. Arocha-Piñango, C.L., Bosch, N., Torres, A., Caires-Tronchoni, D., Marchi, R., Vidal, H. and Rizzo, M.G. Dysfibrinogenemias in Latin America. A cooperative study group. *Rev. Iberoamer. Tromb. Hemostasia* **3**:110-122, **1990**.

2. Marchi, R., Arocha-Piñango, C.L. and Gil, F. Electron microscopy studies of 7 patients with dysfibrinogenemia and some of their relatives. *Rev. Iberoamer. Tromb. Hemostasia* **3**:185-190, **1990**.

FIBRINOGEN MONTREAL I

Last update [1 December 1990]
Alphacode [MONTRE01]
Ref. type [Article]

Family studies
Homozygote? [n.a.]
Pedigree published? [No]

Structural defect [n.a.]
Mutation [n.a.]

Functional defect(s)
FpA release: [Normal[1]]
FpB release: [Normal[1]]
Polymerization: [Abnormal]
Stabilization: [n.a.]

Clinical manifestation(s) Bleeding? [No] Thrombosis? [No]

Clinical laboratory results
Plasma fibrinogen concentration (mg/dL)
Chronometric: [170/(250-450)]
Rate-indep'nt: [110/(200-400)]
Immunologic: [360/(350-700)]

*Hypo*dysfibrinogen? [No]

Thrombin time:	[46s/(10s)[2]]
Reptilase (batroxobin) time:	[80s/(18s)]
Prothrombin time:	[18s/(12s)]
Partial thromboplastin time:	[n.a.]
Euglobulin lysis time:	[240m/(240m)]
Bleeding time:	[Abnormal]
Immunoelectrophoresis:	[Normal]
Platelet aggregation:	[n.a.]

Other results with patient plasma
Ancrod (Arvin) time: [n.a.]
Recalcification time: [n.a.]
Calcium corrects c.t.? [No]

Inhib. normal plasma? [n.a.]
In vivo synthesis: [n.a.]
In vivo catabolism: [n.a.]

Evaluation of isolated patient fibrinogen
Thrombin time: [n.a.]
Reptilase time: [n.a.]
Ancrod (Arvin) time: [n.a.]

Abnormal subunit? [Yes]
Abnormal FDPs? [n.a.]

Remarks
[1]The rate of *total* fibrinopeptide release was normal.
[2]Thrombin time was unusually dependent on pH.

References

1. Lacombe, M., Soria, J., Soria, C., D'Angelo, G., Lavallee, R. and Bonny, Y. Fibrinogen Montreal. A new case of congenital dysfibrinogenemia with defective aggregation of monomers. *Thromb. Diath. Haemorrh.* **29**:536-546, 1973.

FIBRINOGEN MONTREAL II[Abs]

Last update	[1 December 1990]	**Structural defect**	[n.a.]
Alphacode	[MONTRE02]	**Mutation**	[n.a.]
Ref. type	[Abstract]		

Family studies
Homozygote? [n.a.]
Pedigree published? [No]

Functional defect(s)
FpA release: [n.a.]
FpB release: [n.a.]
Polymerization: [Abnormal]
Stabilization: [n.a.]

Clinical manifestation(s) Bleeding? [Yes[1]] Thrombosis? [No]

Clinical laboratory results

Plasma fibrinogen concentration (mg/dL)
Chronometric: [n.a.]
Rate-indep'nt: [Normal[2]]
Immunologic: [Normal[2]]

*Hypo*dysfibrinogen? [No]

Thrombin time:	[Abnormal[2]]
Reptilase (batroxobin) time:	[Abnormal[2]]
Prothrombin time:	[Abnormal[2]]
Partial thromboplastin time:	[Abnormal[2]]
Euglobulin lysis time:	[n.a.]
Bleeding time:	[n.a.]
Immunoelectrophoresis:	[n.a.]
Platelet aggregation:	[n.a.]

Other results with patient plasma

Ancrod (Arvin) time:	[n.a.]	Inhib. normal plasma?	[No]
Recalcification time:	[n.a.]	In vivo synthesis:	[n.a.]
Calcium corrects c.t.?	[n.a.]	In vivo catabolism:	[n.a.]

Evaluation of isolated patient fibrinogen

Thrombin time:	[n.a.]	Abnormal subunit?	[n.a.]
Reptilase time:	[n.a.]	Abnormal FDPs?	[n.a.]
Ancrod (Arvin) time:	[n.a.]		

Remarks
[1]Excessive bleeding after dental extraction was reported.
[2]Data not reported.

References

1. D'Angelo, G., Lacombe, M., Lemay, J., Lavallee, R., Bonny, Y. and Boileau, J. A new congenital dysfibrinogenemia with hemorrhagic diathesis (Fibrinogen Montreal II). *Thromb. Diath. Haemorrh.* **39**:570, **1975**. ABSTRACT

FIBRINOGEN MONTREAL III^{Abs}

Last update [10 January 1994]
Alphacode [MONTRE03]
Ref. type [Abstract]

Structural defect [n.a.]
Mutation [n.a.]

Family studies
Homozygote? [n.a.]
Pedigree published? [No]

Functional defect(s)
FpA release: [n.a.]
FpB release: [n.a.]
Polymerization: [n.a.]
Stabilization: [n.a.]

Clinical manifestation(s) Bleeding? [No] Thrombosis? [No]

Clinical laboratory results
Plasma fibrinogen concentration (mg/dL)
Chronometric: [40-80[1]]
Rate-indep'nt: [n.a.]
Immunologic: [360[1]]

*Hypo*dysfibrinogen? [No]

Thrombin time:	[>3m/(15s)]
Reptilase (batroxobin) time:	[Abnormal]
Prothrombin time:	[Abnormal]
Partial thromboplastin time:	[n.a.]
Euglobulin lysis time:	[n.a.]
Bleeding time:	[n.a.]
Immunoelectrophoresis:	[n.a.]
Platelet aggregation:	[n.a.]

Other results with patient plasma
Ancrod (Arvin) time: [n.a.]
Recalcification time: [n.a.]
Calcium corrects c.t.? [n.a.]

Inhib. normal plasma? [n.a.]
In vivo synthesis: [n.a.]
In vivo catabolism: [n.a.]

Evaluation of isolated patient fibrinogen
Thrombin time: [n.a.]
Reptilase time: [n.a.]
Ancrod (Arvin) time: [n.a.]

Abnormal subunit? [n.a.]
Abnormal FDPs? [n.a.]

Remarks
[1]Normal range not reported.

The index patient had a history of heavy drinking, and no coagulation abnormalities were detected in one brother and two sisters. Thus, the authors were unable to determine if this dysfibrinogenemia was congenital or acquired.

References

1. Laurin, S. and Capet-Antonini, F.C. Evaluation of a non-hemorrhagic dysfibrinogenemia: fibrinogen 'Montreal III'. *Proc. XVI Congr. Int. Soc. Hematol.* p. 310, **1976** ABSTRACT

FIBRINOGEN MORIOKA I[Abs]

Last update [1 December 1990]
Alphacode [MORIOK01]
Ref. type [Abstract]

Structural defect [γ(275) Arg → Cys]
Mutation [n.a.]

Family studies
Homozygote? [No]
Pedigree published? [No]

Functional defect(s)
FpA release: [n.a.]
FpB release: [n.a.]
Polymerization: [Abnormal]
Stabilization: [Normal]

Clinical manifestation(s) Bleeding? [No] Thrombosis? [No]

Clinical laboratory results

Plasma fibrinogen concentration (mg/dL)
Chronometric: [n.a.]
Rate-indep'nt: [n.a.]
Immunologic: [n.a.]

*Hypo*dysfibrinogen? [n.a.]

Thrombin time:	[n.a.]
Reptilase (batroxobin) time:	[n.a.]
Prothrombin time:	[n.a.]
Partial thromboplastin time:	[n.a.]
Euglobulin lysis time:	[n.a.]
Bleeding time:	[n.a.]
Immunoelectrophoresis:	[n.a.]
Platelet aggregation:	[n.a.]

Other results with patient plasma
Ancrod (Arvin) time: [n.a.]
Recalcification time: [n.a.]
Calcium corrects c.t.? [n.a.]

Inhib. normal plasma? [n.a.]
In vivo synthesis: [n.a.]
In vivo catabolism: [n.a.]

Evaluation of isolated patient fibrinogen
Thrombin time: [n.a.]
Reptilase time: [n.a.]
Ancrod (Arvin) time: [n.a.]

Abnormal subunit? [Yes[1]]
Abnormal FDPs? [Yes]

Remarks

[1]SDS-PAGE disclosed a γ-chain approx. 500 Da larger than normal.

References

1. Terukina, S., Matsuda, M., Yoshida, N., Yamazumi, K., Takeda, Y. and Takano, T. Two abnormal fibrinogens designated as Osaka II and Morioka with a hitherto unidentified amino acid substitution; γ-Arg-275 by Cys. *Thromb. Haemostas.* **58**:515, **1987**. ABSTRACT

FIBRINOGEN MUNICH I[1]

Last update [1 December 1990]
Alphacode [MUNICH01]
Ref. type [Article]

Family studies
Homozygote? [n.a.]
Pedigree published? [No]

Structural defect [Aα(19) Arg → Asn]
Mutation [n.a.]

Functional defect(s)
FpA release: [Abnormal]
FpB release: [n.a.]
Polymerization: [Abnormal]
Stabilization: [n.a.]

Clinical manifestation(s) Bleeding? [Yes[2]] Thrombosis? [No]

Clinical laboratory results

Plasma fibrinogen concentration (mg/dL)
Chronometric: [n.a.]
Rate-indep'nt: [210/(150-400)]
Immunologic: [n.a.]

*Hypo*dysfibrinogen? [No]

Thrombin time:	[29s/(12-14s)]
Reptilase (batroxobin) time:	[>300s/(18-20s)]
Prothrombin time:	[51%/(>70%)]
Partial thromboplastin time:	[n.a.]
Euglobulin lysis time:	[n.a.]
Bleeding time:	[Normal]
Immunoelectrophoresis:	[n.a.]
Platelet aggregation:	[Normal]

Other results with patient plasma

Ancrod (Arvin) time:	[>300s/(11-12s)]	Inhib. normal plasma?	[n.a.]
Recalcification time:	[n.a.]	In vivo synthesis:	[n.a.]
Calcium corrects c.t.?	[n.a.]	In vivo catabolism:	[n.a.]

Evaluation of isolated patient fibrinogen

Thrombin time:	[n.a.]	Abnormal subunit?	[n.a.]
Reptilase time:	[n.a.]	Abnormal FDPs?	[n.a.]
Ancrod (Arvin) time:	[n.a.]		

Remarks
[1] Also known as MÜNCHEN I.
[2] A mild bleeding tendency (hematuria, hematoma, epistaxis) and abnormal bleeding during pregnancy in two sisters was reported.

References

1. Henschen, A., Kehl, M., Southan, C., Lottspeich, F. and Georgopoulos, D. Genetically abnormal fibrinogens - some current characterisation strategies. In: *Fibrinogen —Structure, Functional Aspects, Metabolism*, F. Haverkate, A. Henschen, W. Nieuwenhuizen and P.W. Straub (eds.), Walter de Gruyter, Berlin. pp. 125-144, **1983**.

2. Marx, R. and Schramm, W. On dysfibrinogenemia. In: *Fibrinogen —Recent Biochemical and Medical Aspects*, A. Henschen, H. Graeff and F. Lottspeich (eds.), W. de Gruyter, Berlin. pp. 123-128, **1982**.

3. Southan, C., Henschen, A. and Lottspeich, F. The search for molecular defects in abnormal fibrinogens. In: *Fibrinogen —Recent Biochemical and Medical Aspects*, A. Henschen, H. Graeff and F. Lottspeich (eds.), W. de Gruyter, Berlin. pp. 153-166, **1982**.

4. Marx, R. and Schramm, W. Diskussionsbeitrag zum Thema 'Fibrinogenopathien'. In: *Fibrinogen, Fibrin und Fibrinkleber*, K.I. Schimpf (ed.), F.K. Schattauer, Stuttgart. pp. 195-197, **1980**.

FIBRINOGEN MUNICH II[1]

Last update	[10 January 1994]	**Structural defect**	[n.a.]
Alphacode	[MUNICH02]	**Mutation**	[n.a.]
Ref. type	[Article]		

Family studies
Homozygote? [n.a.]
Pedigree published? [No]

Functional defect(s)
FpA release: [Abnormal]
FpB release: [n.a.]
Polymerization: [Abnormal]
Stabilization: [n.a.]

Clinical manifestation(s) Bleeding? [Yes] Thrombosis? [No]

Clinical laboratory results
Plasma fibrinogen concentration (mg/dL)
Chronometric: [37[2]]
Rate-indep'nt: [180[2]]
Immunologic: [n.a.]

*Hypo*dysfibrinogen? [No]

Thrombin time:	[31s[3]]
Reptilase (batroxobin) time:	[104s[3]]
Prothrombin time:	[45s[3]]
Partial thromboplastin time:	[47.5s[3]]
Euglobulin lysis time:	[Normal]
Bleeding time:	[Abnormal]
Immunoelectrophoresis:	[n.a.]
Platelet aggregation:	[n.a.]

Other results with patient plasma

Ancrod (Arvin) time:	[n.a.]	Inhib. normal plasma?	[n.a.]
Recalcification time:	[n.a.]	In vivo synthesis:	[n.a.]
Calcium corrects c.t.?	[n.a.]	In vivo catabolism:	[n.a.]

Evaluation of isolated patient fibrinogen

Thrombin time:	[n.a.]	Abnormal subunit?	[n.a.]
Reptilase time:	[n.a.]	Abnormal FDPs?	[n.a.]
Ancrod (Arvin) time:	[n.a.]		

Remarks
[1]Also known as MÜNCHEN II.
[2]Authors classified this result as normal; normal range not reported.
[3]Authors classified this result as abnormal; normal range not reported.

References

1. Marx, R. and Schramm, W. On dysfibrinogenemia. In: *Fibrinogen —Recent Biochemical and Medical Aspects*, A. Henschen, H. Graeff and F. Lottspeich (eds.), W. de Gruyter, Berlin. pp. 123-128, **1982**.

FIBRINOGEN MÜNSTER I^{Abs}

Last update [1 December 1990]
Alphacode [MUNSTE01]
Ref. type [Abstract]

Structural defect [n.a.]
Mutation [n.a.]

Family studies
Homozygote? [n.a.]
Pedigree published? [No]

Functional defect(s)
FpA release: [n.a.]
FpB release: [n.a.]
Polymerization: [n.a.]
Stabilization: [n.a.]

Clinical manifestation(s) Bleeding? [n.a.] Thrombosis? [n.a.]

Clinical laboratory results

Plasma fibrinogen concentration (mg/dL)
Chronometric: [n.a.]
Rate-indep'nt: [n.a.]
Immunologic: [n.a.]

*Hypo*dysfibrinogen? [n.a.]

Thrombin time:	[n.a.]
Reptilase (batroxobin) time:	[n.a.]
Prothrombin time:	[n.a.]
Partial thromboplastin time:	[n.a.]
Euglobulin lysis time:	[n.a.]
Bleeding time:	[n.a.]
Immunoelectrophoresis:	[n.a.]
Platelet aggregation:	[n.a.]

Other results with patient plasma
Ancrod (Arvin) time: [n.a.]
Recalcification time: [n.a.]
Calcium corrects c.t.? [n.a.]

Inhib. normal plasma? [n.a.]
In vivo synthesis: [n.a.]
In vivo catabolism: [n.a.]

Evaluation of isolated patient fibrinogen
Thrombin time: [n.a.]
Reptilase time: [n.a.]
Ancrod (Arvin) time: [n.a.]

Abnormal subunit? [n.a.]
Abnormal FDPs? [n.a.]

Remarks

References

1. Henschen, A., Kehl, M., Southan, C., Lottspeich, F. and Georgopoulos, D. Genetically abnormal fibrinogens — some current characterisation strategies. In: *Fibrinogen —Structure, Functional Aspects, Metabolism*, F. Haverkate, A. Henschen, W. Nieuwenhuizen and P.W. Straub (eds.), Walter de Gruyter, Berlin. pp. 125-144, **1983**.

FIBRINOGEN NAGOYA I

Last update [1 December 1990]
Alphacode [NAGOYA01]
Ref. type [Article]

Structural defect [γ(329) Gln → Arg]
Mutation [n.a.]

Family studies
Homozygote? [No]
Pedigree published? [No]

Functional defect(s)
FpA release: [Normal]
FpB release: [Normal]
Polymerization: [Abnormal]
Stabilization: [Normal]

Clinical manifestation(s) Bleeding? [No] Thrombosis? [No]

Clinical laboratory results
Plasma fibrinogen concentration (mg/dL)
Chronometric: [80/(180-360)]
Rate-indep'nt: [228/(200-400)]
Immunologic: [220/(200-400)]

*Hypo*dysfibrinogen? [No]

Thrombin time:	[20.8s/(10.2s)]
Reptilase (batroxobin) time:	[n.a.]
Prothrombin time:	[16.8s/(12.3s)]
Partial thromboplastin time:	[58s/(47-57s)]
Euglobulin lysis time:	[n.a.]
Bleeding time:	[Normal]
Immunoelectrophoresis:	[n.a.]
Platelet aggregation:	[Normal]

Other results with patient plasma
Ancrod (Arvin) time: [n.a.]
Recalcification time: [n.a.]
Calcium corrects c.t.? [No]

Inhib. normal plasma? [Yes]
In vivo synthesis: [n.a.]
In vivo catabolism: [n.a.]

Evaluation of isolated patient fibrinogen
Thrombin time: [n.a.]
Reptilase time: [n.a.]
Ancrod (Arvin) time: [n.a.]

Abnormal subunit? [Yes[1]]
Abnormal FDPs? [No]

Remarks
[1]SDS-PAGE disclosed a γ-chain with a m.w. about 1500 larger than normal. A charge abnormality in the γ-chain was detected by cation exchange chromatography.

References

1. Miyata, T., Furukawa, K., Iwanaga, S., Takamatsu, J. and Saito, H. Fibrinogen Nagoya, a replacement of glutamine-329 by arginine in the γ-chain that impairs the polymerization of fibrin monomer. *J. Biochem. (Tokyo)* **105**:10-14, **1989**.

2. Mizuochi, T., Taniguchi, T., Asami, Y., Takamatsu, J., Okude, M., Iwanaga, S. and Kobata, A. Comparative studies on the structures of the carbohydrate moieties of human fibrinogen and abnormal fibrinogen Nagoya. *J. Biochem. (Tokyo)* **92**:283-293, **1982**.

3. Takamatsu, J. and Iwanaga, S. [Studies on abnormal fibrinogen]. *Nippon Ketsueki Gakkai Zasshi* **43**:1203-1211, **1980**.

4. Takamatsu, J., Ogata, K., Kamiya, T. and Koie, K. A novel dysfibrinogenemia with abnormal γ-chain (Fibrinogen Nagoya). *Thromb. Haemostas.* **42**:78, **1979**. ABSTRACT

FIBRINOGEN NANCY I

Last update [10 January 1994]
Alphacode [NANCY01]
Ref. type [Article]

Structural defect [n.a.]
Mutation [n.a.]

Family studies
Homozygote? [n.a.]
Pedigree published? [No]

Functional defect(s)
FpA release: [n.a.[1]]
FpB release: [n.a.[1]]
Polymerization: [Abnormal]
Stabilization: [n.a.]

Clinical manifestation(s) Bleeding? [No] Thrombosis? [Yes[2]]

Clinical laboratory results

Plasma fibrinogen concentration (mg/dL)
Chronometric: [270[3]]
Rate-indep'nt: [380/(300-450)]
Immunologic: [290[3]]

*Hypo*dysfibrinogen? [No]

Thrombin time:	[75s/(23s)]
Reptilase (batroxobin) time:	[67s/(32s)]
Prothrombin time:	[77%[3]]
Partial thromboplastin time:	[n.a.]
Euglobulin lysis time:	[n.a.]
Bleeding time:	[Normal]
Immunoelectrophoresis:	[Anodal]
Platelet aggregation:	[n.a.]

Other results with patient plasma
Ancrod (Arvin) time: [n.a.]
Recalcification time: [n.a.]
Calcium corrects c.t.? [Yes]

Inhib. normal plasma? [No]
In vivo synthesis: [n.a.]
In vivo catabolism: [n.a.]

Evaluation of isolated patient fibrinogen
Thrombin time: [n.a.]
Reptilase time: [n.a.]
Ancrod (Arvin) time: [n.a.]

Abnormal subunit? [No[4]]
Abnormal FDPs? [n.a.]

Remarks
[1]The rate of *total* fibrinopeptide release was reduced; individual fibrinopeptide release was not reported.
[2]Patient died from pulmonary embolism at age 20 yrs.
[3]Normal range not reported.
[4]No abnormal subunits were detected by isoelectric focusing (only). The results of SDS-PAGE were not reported.

References

1. Soria, J., Soria, C., Durand, G. and Feger, J. [Electrofocusing of abnormal fibrinogens in polyacrylamide gel]. *Ann. Biol. Clin. (Paris)* **30**:161-165, **1972**.

2. Streiff, F., Alexandre, P., Vigneron, C., Soria, J., Soria, C. and Mester, L. [A new case of Congenital and familial dysfibrinogenemia without Hemorrhagic Diathesis]. *Thromb. Diath. Haemorrh.* **26**:565-576, **1971**.

FIBRINOGEN *NAPLES I*[1]

Last update [*10 January 1994*]
Alphacode [*NAPLES01*]
Ref. type [*Article*]

Structural defect [*Bβ(68) Ala → Thr*[2]]
Mutation [*GCT → ACT*]

Family studies
Homozygote? [*Yes*[3]]
Pedigree published? [*Yes*[3]]

Functional defect(s)
FpA release: [*Abnormal*]
FpB release: [*Abnormal*]
Polymerization: [*Normal*]
Stabilization: [*Normal*]

Clinical manifestation(s) Bleeding? [*No*] Thrombosis? [*Yes*[4]]

Clinical laboratory results
Plasma fibrinogen concentration (mg/dL)
Chronometric: [*170/(200-400)*]
Rate-indep'nt: [*320*[5]]
Immunologic: [*300/(200-400)*]
*Hypo*dysfibrinogen? [*No*]

Thrombin time:	[*>180s/(19.8s)*]
Reptilase (batroxobin) time:	[*21.8s/(22.1s)*]
Prothrombin time:	[*21s/(13s)*]
Partial thromboplastin time:	[*28s/(28-43s)*[6]]
Euglobulin lysis time:	[*167m/(281m)*]
Bleeding time:	[*Normal*[6]]
Immunoelectrophoresis:	[*n.a.*]
Platelet aggregation:	[*Normal*]

Other results with patient plasma
Ancrod (Arvin) time: [*23s/(23s)*]
Recalcification time: [*n.a.*]
Calcium corrects c.t.? [*No*]
Inhib. normal plasma? [*Yes*[6]]
In vivo synthesis: [*n.a.*]
In vivo catabolism: [*n.a.*]

Evaluation of isolated patient fibrinogen
Thrombin time: [*90s/(23s)*[7]]
Reptilase time: [*38s/(65s)*[8]]
Ancrod (Arvin) time: [*16s/(23s)*[8]]
Abnormal subunit? [*n.a.*]
Abnormal FDPs? [*n.a.*]

Remarks
[1]Also known as "MILAN II" or "MILANO II" (home to one of the three patients). "NAPLES" refers to the city in which this variant was first studied. Results are italicized to avoid duplication with MILAN II in summary tables. ▪[2]The structural defect was determined with the PCR method. ▪[3]There is evidence of consanguinity. ▪[4]The 21 year-old propositus exhibited thrombosis in the abdominal aorta; his 26 year-old sister exhibited occlusion of the right internal carotid artery; his brother experienced venous thrombosis after abdominal surgery. ▪[5]Normal range not reported. ▪[6]G. DiMinno and M. Colucci, personal communication. ▪[7]This result was obtained with bovine thrombin; the corresponding results with human thrombin were [190s/(18s)]. Defective binding of thrombin to patient fibrinogen was reported. ▪[8]This is the only variant with *shortened* Reptilase and ancrod times.

FIBRINOGEN *NAPLES I*

References

1. Koopman, J., Haverkate, F., Lord, S.T., Grimbergen, J. and Mannucci, P.M. Molecular basis of fibrinogen Naples associated with defective thrombin binding and thrombophilia. Homozygous substitution of Bβ 68 Ala→Thr. *J. Clin. Invest.* **90**:238-244, **1992**.

2. Koopman, J., Grimbergen, J., Lord, S.T., Haverkate, F., and Mannucci, P.M. The functional and structural defect of fibrinogen Naples and its relation with thrombosis. *Proc. X Intl. Fgen. Wkshp.*, **1990** ABSTRACT.

3. Koopman, J., Haverkate, F., Lord, S.T., and Grimbergen, J. Identification of structural defects in abnormal fibrinogens using the polymerase chain reaction. *Proc. X Intl. Fgen. Wkshp.*, **1990** ABSTRACT.

4. Di Minno, G., Cerbone, A.M., Cirillo, F., Colucci, M., Semeraro, N., Di Santo, G., Mattioli, P.L., Mancini, M. and Quattrone, A. Abnormal fibrinogen (Fibrinogen Naples) characterized by defective interaction with thrombin and plasmin in two young siblings with arterial thrombosis. *Thromb. Haemostas.* **58**:514-514, **1987**. ABSTRACT

5. Haverkate, F., Koopman, J., Kluft, C., D'Angelo, A., Cattaneo, M. and Mannucci, P.M. Fibrinogens "Milano II" and "Naples." *Thromb. Haemostas.* **57**:375, **1987**.

6. Haverkate, F., Koopman, J., Kluft, C., D'Angelo, A., Cattaneo, M. and Mannucci, P.M. Fibrinogen Milano II: a congenital dysfibrinogenaemia associated with juvenile arterial and venous thrombosis. *Thromb. Haemostas.* **55**:131-135, **1986**.

7. Haverkate, F., Koopman, J. and Kluft, C. Fibrinogen Milan II: A congenital dysfibrinogenaemia with a defective clotting by thrombin, normal clotting by arvin, Reptilase and prothrombin-staphylocoagulase complex, associated with thrombotic episodes. In: *Fibrinogen —Structural Variants and Interactions*, A. Henschen, B. Hessel, J. McDonagh and T. Saldeen (eds.), Walter de Gruyter, Berlin. pp. 223-236, **1985**.

8. Quattrone, A., Colucci, M., Donati, M.B., Meduri, M., Mussoni, L., Roncaglioni, M.C., Semeraro, N., Carlomagno, S. and Bonavita, V. Stroke in two young siblings with congenital dysfibrinogenemia. *Ital. J. Neurol. Sci.* **4**:229-232, **1983**.

9. Quattrone, A., Colucci, M., Donati, M.B., Roncaglioni, M.C., Semeraro, N., Carlomagno, S., and Bonavita, V. Cerebral thrombosis in two siblings with dysfibrinogenemia. *Neurosci. Lett.* **Suppl. 3**:S54, **1979**. ABSTRACT

FIBRINOGEN NEW ALBANY I

Last update [1 December 1990]
Alphacode [NEWALB01]
Ref. type [Article[1]]

Family studies
Homozygote? [No]
Pedigree published? [No]

Structural defect [Aα(16) Arg → His]
Mutation [n.a.]

Functional defect(s)
FpA release: [n.a.]
FpB release: [n.a.]
Polymerization: [n.a.]
Stabilization: [n.a.]

Clinical manifestation(s) Bleeding? [No] Thrombosis? [No]

Clinical laboratory results
Plasma fibrinogen concentration (mg/dL)
Chronometric: [n.a.]
Rate-indep'nt: [n.a.]
Immunologic: [n.a.]

*Hypo*dysfibrinogen? [n.a.]

Thrombin time:	[n.a.]
Reptilase (batroxobin) time:	[n.a.]
Prothrombin time:	[n.a.]
Partial thromboplastin time:	[n.a.]
Euglobulin lysis time:	[n.a.]
Bleeding time:	[n.a.]
Immunoelectrophoresis:	[n.a.]
Platelet aggregation:	[n.a.]

Other results with patient plasma
Ancrod (Arvin) time: [n.a.]
Recalcification time: [n.a.]
Calcium corrects c.t.? [n.a.]

Inhib. normal plasma? [n.a.]
In vivo synthesis: [n.a.]
In vivo catabolism: [n.a.]

Evaluation of isolated patient fibrinogen
Thrombin time: [n.a.]
Reptilase time: [n.a.]
Ancrod (Arvin) time: [n.a.]

Abnormal subunit? [n.a.]
Abnormal FDPs? [n.a.]

Remarks
[1]Review articles only; D.K. Galanakis, personal communication.

References

1. Henschen, A., Kehl, M. and Southan, C. Genetically abnormal fibrinogens — strategies for structure elucidation, including fibrinopeptide analysis. In: *Variants of Human Fibrinogen*, E.A. Beck and M. Furlan (eds.), Hans Huber Publ., Berne, pp. 273-320, **1984**.

2. Henschen, A., Kehl, M., Southan, C., Lottspeich, F. and Georgopoulos, D. Genetically abnormal fibrinogens — some current characterisation strategies. In: *Fibrinogen —Structure, Functional Aspects, Metabolism*, F. Haverkate, A. Henschen, W. Nieuwenhuizen and P.W. Straub (eds.), Walter de Gruyter, Berlin. pp. 125-144, **1983**.

FIBRINOGEN NEWARK I[Abs]

Last update	[1 December 1990]	**Structural defect**	[n.a.]
Alphacode	[NEWARK01]	**Mutation**	[n.a.]
Ref. type	[Abstract]		

Family studies
Homozygote? [n.a.]
Pedigree published? [No]

Functional defect(s)
FpA release: [n.a.]
FpB release: [n.a.]
Polymerization: [n.a.]
Stabilization: [n.a.]

Clinical manifestation(s) Bleeding? [Yes[1]] Thrombosis? [No]

Clinical laboratory results
Plasma fibrinogen concentration (mg/dL)
Chronometric: [230[2]]
Rate-indep'nt: [n.a.]
Immunologic: [140[2]]

*Hypo*dysfibrinogen? [No]

Thrombin time:	[n.a.]
Reptilase (batroxobin) time:	[n.a.]
Prothrombin time:	[n.a.]
Partial thromboplastin time:	[n.a.]
Euglobulin lysis time:	[Normal[3]]
Bleeding time:	[Normal]
Immunoelectrophoresis:	[Normal]
Platelet aggregation:	[Normal]

Other results with patient plasma

Ancrod (Arvin) time:	[n.a.]	Inhib. normal plasma?	[No]
Recalcification time:	[n.a.]	In vivo synthesis:	[n.a.]
Calcium corrects c.t.?	[n.a.]	In vivo catabolism:	[n.a.]

Evaluation of isolated patient fibrinogen

Thrombin time:	[n.a.]	Abnormal subunit?	[n.a.]
Reptilase time:	[n.a.]	Abnormal FDPs?	[Yes[4]]
Ancrod (Arvin) time:	[n.a.]		

Remarks
[1]Menorrhagia, hematomas, and excessive bleeding after dental extraction were reported.
[2]Normal range not reported.
[3]Data not reported.
[4]Immunoelectrophoresis disclosed an abnormal fragment D.

References

1. Stein, I.D., Poskitt, T.R., Arkel, Y. and Wu, H.V. Minimal dysfibrinogenemia. *Blood* **54 (Suppl. 1)**:196, **1979**. ABSTRACT

FIBRINOGEN NEW BRITAIN I[Abs]

Last update [10 January 1994]
Alphacode [NEWBRI01]
Ref. type [Abstract]

Family studies
Homozygote? [n.a.]
Pedigree published? [No]

Structural defect [Aα(16) Arg → His]
Mutation [n.a.]

Functional defect(s)
FpA release: [Abnormal]
FpB release: [n.a.]
Polymerization: [Abnormal]
Stabilization: [n.a.]

Clinical manifestation(s) Bleeding? [No] Thrombosis? [No]

Clinical laboratory results
Plasma fibrinogen concentration (mg/dL)
Chronometric: [120[1]]
Rate-indep'nt: [225[1]]
Immunologic: [n.a.]

*Hypo*dysfibrinogen? [No]

Thrombin time:	[Abnormal]
Reptilase (batroxobin) time:	[Abnormal]
Prothrombin time:	[n.a.]
Partial thromboplastin time:	[n.a.]
Euglobulin lysis time:	[n.a.]
Bleeding time:	[n.a.]
Immunoelectrophoresis:	[n.a.]
Platelet aggregation:	[n.a.]

Other results with patient plasma
Ancrod (Arvin) time: [n.a.]
Recalcification time: [n.a.]
Calcium corrects c.t.? [n.a.]

Inhib. normal plasma? [n.a.]
In vivo synthesis: [n.a.]
In vivo catabolism: [n.a.]

Evaluation of isolated patient fibrinogen
Thrombin time: [n.a.]
Reptilase time: [n.a.]
Ancrod (Arvin) time: [n.a.]

Abnormal subunit? [n.a.]
Abnormal FDPs? [n.a.]

Remarks
[1]Normal range not reported.

References

1. Webb, C.D., Hantgan, R.R., Byeff, P.D. and Owen, J. Fibrinogen New Britain: an Aα16 Arg → His substitution also showing abnormal polymerization. *Proc. XI Int'l. F'gen. Wkshop.* p. 11, **1992**. ABSTRACT

FIBRINOGEN NEW ORLEANS I

Last update [1 December 1990]
Alphacode [NEWORL01]
Ref. type [Article]

Family studies
Homozygote? [No]
Pedigree published? [Yes]

Structural defect [n.a.]
Mutation [n.a.]

Functional defect(s)
FpA release: [Abnormal[1]]
FpB release: [Abnormal[1]]
Polymerization: [Normal]
Stabilization: [Normal]

Clinical manifestation(s) Bleeding? [Yes[2]] Thrombosis? [No]

Clinical laboratory results
Plasma fibrinogen concentration (mg/dL)
Chronometric: [50-73/(200-400)]
Rate-indep'nt: [445/(180-290)]
Immunologic: [640/(200-450)]

*Hypo*dysfibrinogen? [No[3]]

Thrombin time:	[43.5s/(15s)]
Reptilase (batroxobin) time:	[1320s/(55s)]
Prothrombin time:	[15s/(11.5s)]
Partial thromboplastin time:	[58.5s/(30-39s)]
Euglobulin lysis time:	[n.a.]
Bleeding time:	[n.a.]
Immunoelectrophoresis:	[Anodal]
Platelet aggregation:	[n.a.]

Other results with patient plasma
Ancrod (Arvin) time: [50s/(31.5s)]
Recalcification time: [n.a.]
Calcium corrects c.t.? [n.a.]

Inhib. normal plasma? [Yes[4]]
In vivo synthesis: [n.a.]
In vivo catabolism: [n.a.]

Evaluation of isolated patient fibrinogen
Thrombin time: [125s/(26s)]
Reptilase time: [n.a.]
Ancrod (Arvin) time: [n.a.]

Abnormal subunit? [No]
Abnormal FDPs? [n.a.]

Remarks
[1]Determined by comparative SDS-PAGE of Aα and Bβ chains.
[2]Hematuria and excessive postpartum bleeding in the 30 year-old proposita were reported.
[3]The evidence is consistent with *hyper*fibrinogenemia.
[4]W.A. Andes, personal communication.

References

1. Andes, W.A., Chavin, S.I., Beltran, G. and Stuckey, W.J. Fibrinogen New Orleans: hereditary dysfibrinogenemia with an Aα-chain abnormality. *Thromb. Res.* **25**:41-50, **1982**.

FIBRINOGEN NEW ORLEANS II[Abs]

Last update [1 December 1990]
Alphacode [NEWORL02]
Ref. type [Abstract]

Structural defect [n.a.]
Mutation [n.a.]

Family studies
Homozygote? [n.a.]
Pedigree published? [No]

Functional defect(s)
FpA release: [n.a.]
FpB release: [n.a.]
Polymerization: [Normal]
Stabilization: [n.a.]

Clinical manifestation(s) Bleeding? [No] Thrombosis? [Yes]

Clinical laboratory results

Plasma fibrinogen concentration (mg/dL)
Chronometric: [95[1]]
Rate-indep'nt: [n.a.]
Immunologic: [262[1]]

*Hypo*dysfibrinogen? [No]

Thrombin time:	[34s/(19s)]
Reptilase (batroxobin) time:	[Normal[2]]
Prothrombin time:	[15.4s/(12s)]
Partial thromboplastin time:	[Normal[2]]
Euglobulin lysis time:	[n.a.]
Bleeding time:	[n.a.]
Immunoelectrophoresis:	[Normal]
Platelet aggregation:	[n.a.]

Other results with patient plasma
Ancrod (Arvin) time: [Normal[2]]
Recalcification time: [n.a.]
Calcium corrects c.t.? [n.a.]

Inhib. normal plasma? [No[3]]
In vivo synthesis: [n.a.]
In vivo catabolism: [n.a.]

Evaluation of isolated patient fibrinogen
Thrombin time: [Abnormal[3]]
Reptilase time: [n.a.]
Ancrod (Arvin) time: [n.a.]

Abnormal subunit? [n.a.]
Abnormal FDPs? [n.a.]

Remarks
[1]Normal range not reported.
[2]Data not reported.
[3]W.A. Andes, personal communication.

References

1. Andes, W.A. Fibrinogen New Orleans II: a new dysfibrinogenemia with venous thrombosis. *Thromb. Haemostas.* **50**:337, **1983**. ABSTRACT

2. Andes, W.A. Fibrinogen New Orleans II: a new dysfibrinogenemia with venous thrombosis. *Blood* **60 (Suppl. 1)**:206a, **1982**. ABSTRACT

FIBRINOGEN NEW YORK I

Last update [1 December 1990]
Alphacode [NEWYOR01]
Ref. type [Article]

Structural defect [Bβ(9-72) deletion[1]]
Mutation [Exon 2 deletion]

Family studies
Homozygote? [No]
Pedigree published? [Yes]

Functional defect(s)
FpA release: [Abnormal]
FpB release: [Abnormal]
Polymerization: [Abnormal]
Stabilization: [Normal]

Clinical manifestation(s) Bleeding? [No] Thrombosis? [Yes[2]]

Clinical laboratory results
Plasma fibrinogen concentration (mg/dL)
Chronometric: [n.a.]
Rate-indep'nt: [64/(200-450)]
Immunologic: [156/(200-450)]

*Hypo*dysfibrinogen? [No]

Thrombin time:	[72s/(7.5s)[3]]
Reptilase (batroxobin) time:	[73.5s/(33s)]
Prothrombin time:	[Abnormal[4]]
Partial thromboplastin time:	[n.a.[5]]
Euglobulin lysis time:	[>120m/(>120m)]
Bleeding time:	[n.a.]
Immunoelectrophoresis:	[Anodal]
Platelet aggregation:	[Normal]

Other results with patient plasma
Ancrod (Arvin) time: [n.a.]
Recalcification time: [n.a.]
Calcium corrects c.t.? [No]

Inhib. normal plasma? [No]
In vivo synthesis: [n.a.]
In vivo catabolism: [n.a.]

Evaluation of isolated patient fibrinogen
Thrombin time: [Abnormal]
Reptilase time: [n.a.]
Ancrod (Arvin) time: [n.a.]

Abnormal subunit? [Yes]
Abnormal FDPs? [n.a.]

Remarks
[1]This deletion corresponds exactly to exon 2 of the Bβ-chain gene.
[2]Recurrent venous thrombosis and fatal pulmonary embolism in the proposita were reported.
[3]The thrombin clotting time was unusually dependent on pH.
[4]PT was "3-4s" longer than normal; data not reported.
[5]Affected relatives of index patient had markedly prolonged PTT's. The PTT of the index patient was not reported.

References

1. Liu, C.Y., Wallen, P. and Handley, D.A. Fibrinogen New York I: The structural, functional, and genetic defects and an hypothesis of the role of fibrin in the regulation of coagulation and fibrinolysis. In: *Fibrinogen, Fibrin Formation and Fibrinolysis*, D.A. Lane, A. Henschen and M.K. Jasani (eds.), W. de Gruyter, Berlin. pp. 79-90, **1986**.

2. Liu, C.Y., Koehn, J.A. and Morgan, F.J. Characterization of fibrinogen New York 1. A dysfunctional fibrinogen with a deletion of Bβ (9-72) corresponding exactly to exon 2 of the gene. *J. Biol. Chem.* **260**:4390-4396, **1985**.

3. Al-Mondhiry, H., Bilezikian, S.B. and Nossel, H.L. Fibrinogen "New York" — an abnormal fibrinogen associated with thromboembolism: Functional evaluation. *Blood* **45**:607-619, **1975**.

FIBRINOGEN NEW YORK II

Last update [10 January 1994]
Alphacode [NEWYOR02]
Ref. type [Article]

Family studies
Homozygote? [n.a.]
Pedigree published? [No]

Structural defect [n.a.]
Mutation [n.a.]

Functional defect(s)
FpA release: [Abnormal]
FpB release: [Abnormal]
Polymerization: [Abnormal]
Stabilization: [n.a.]

Clinical manifestation(s) Bleeding? [Yes[1]] Thrombosis? [No]

Clinical laboratory results
Plasma fibrinogen concentration (mg/dL)
Chronometric: [n.a.]
Rate-indep'nt: [200/(200-400)]
Immunologic: [n.a.]

*Hypo*dysfibrinogen? [No]

Thrombin time:	[45.2s/(12-15s)]
Reptilase (batroxobin) time:	[80s/(17-23s)]
Prothrombin time:	[13s/(11-12.5s)]
Partial thromboplastin time:	[40.9s/(31-36s)]
Euglobulin lysis time:	[n.a.]
Bleeding time:	[n.a.]
Immunoelectrophoresis:	[n.a.]
Platelet aggregation:	[n.a.]

Other results with patient plasma
Ancrod (Arvin) time: [n.a.]
Recalcification time: [n.a.]
Calcium corrects c.t.? [No]

Inhib. normal plasma? [n.a.]
In vivo synthesis: [n.a.]
In vivo catabolism: [n.a.]

Evaluation of isolated patient fibrinogen
Thrombin time: [48.4s/(16s)]
Reptilase time: [n.a.]
Ancrod (Arvin) time: [n.a.]

Abnormal subunit? [No]
Abnormal FDPs? [n.a.]

Remarks
[1]Easy bruising in the 45 year-old propositus was reported.

References

1. Liu, C.Y. and Karp, G. Fibrinogen New York II, III, and IV: relationship between abnormal fibrin monomer polymerization, bleeding tendency, and thrombotic tendency. In: *Fibrinogen 2. Biochemistry, Physiology and Clinical Relevance*, G.D.O. Lowe, J.T. Douglas, C.D. Forbes and A. Henschen (eds.), Elsevier, Amsterdam. pp. 53-56, **1987**.

FIBRINOGEN NEW YORK III

Last update [10 January 1994]
Alphacode [NEWYOR03]
Ref. type [Article]

Family studies
Homozygote? [n.a.]
Pedigree published? [No]

Structural defect [n.a.]
Mutation [n.a.]

Functional defect(s)
FpA release: [Normal]
FpB release: [Normal]
Polymerization: [Abnormal]
Stabilization: [n.a.]

Clinical manifestation(s) Bleeding? [Yes[1]] Thrombosis? [No]

Clinical laboratory results

Plasma fibrinogen concentration (mg/dL)
Chronometric: [n.a.]
Rate-indep'nt: [195/(200-400)]
Immunologic: [n.a.]

*Hypo*dysfibrinogen? [No]

Thrombin time:	[32.9s/(12-15s)]
Reptilase (batroxobin) time:	[47.8s/(17-23s)]
Prothrombin time:	[13.1s/(11-12.5s)]
Partial thromboplastin time:	[56.3s/(31-36s)]
Euglobulin lysis time:	[n.a.]
Bleeding time:	[n.a.]
Immunoelectrophoresis:	[n.a.]
Platelet aggregation:	[n.a.]

Other results with patient plasma
Ancrod (Arvin) time: [n.a.]
Recalcification time: [n.a.]
Calcium corrects c.t.? [No]

Inhib. normal plasma? [n.a.]
In vivo synthesis: [n.a.]
In vivo catabolism: [n.a.]

Evaluation of isolated patient fibrinogen
Thrombin time: [n.a.]
Reptilase time: [n.a.]
Ancrod (Arvin) time: [n.a.]

Abnormal subunit? [No]
Abnormal FDPs? [n.a.]

Remarks

[1]Post traumatic hematuria in the 17 year-old propositus was reported.

References

1. Liu, C.Y. and Karp, G. Fibrinogen New York II, III, and IV: relationship between abnormal fibrin monomer polymerization, bleeding tendency, and thrombotic tendency. In: *Fibrinogen 2. Biochemistry, Physiology and Clinical Relevance*, G.D.O. Lowe, J.T. Douglas, C.D. Forbes and A. Henschen (eds.), Elsevier, Amsterdam. pp. 53-56, **1987**.

FIBRINOGEN NEW YORK IV

Last update [10 January 1994]
Alphacode [NEWYOR04]
Ref. type [Article]

Structural defect [n.a.]
Mutation [n.a.]

Family studies
Homozygote? [n.a.]
Pedigree published? [No]

Functional defect(s)
FpA release: [Normal]
FpB release: [Normal]
Polymerization: [Abnormal]
Stabilization: [n.a.]

Clinical manifestation(s) Bleeding? [Yes[1]] Thrombosis? [No]

Clinical laboratory results
Plasma fibrinogen concentration (mg/dL)
Chronometric: [n.a.]
Rate-indep'nt: [100/(200-400)]
Immunologic: [n.a.]

*Hypo*dysfibrinogen? [Yes]

Thrombin time:	[20.7s/(12-15s)]
Reptilase (batroxobin) time:	[180s/(17-23s)]
Prothrombin time:	[17.6s/(11-12.5s)]
Partial thromboplastin time:	[39.4s/(31-36s)]
Euglobulin lysis time:	[n.a.]
Bleeding time:	[n.a.]
Immunoelectrophoresis:	[n.a.]
Platelet aggregation:	[n.a.]

Other results with patient plasma
Ancrod (Arvin) time: [n.a.]
Recalcification time: [n.a.]
Calcium corrects c.t.? [Yes]

Inhib. normal plasma? [n.a.]
In vivo synthesis: [n.a.]
In vivo catabolism: [n.a.]

Evaluation of isolated patient fibrinogen
Thrombin time: [28.4s/(16s)]
Reptilase time: [n.a.]
Ancrod (Arvin) time: [n.a.]

Abnormal subunit? [No]
Abnormal FDPs? [n.a.]

Remarks
[1]Excessive bleeding after dental extraction in the 11 year-old proposita was reported.

References

1. Liu, C.Y. and Karp, G. Fibrinogen New York II, III, and IV: relationship between abnormal fibrin monomer polymerization, bleeding tendency, and thrombotic tendency. In: *Fibrinogen 2. Biochemistry, Physiology and Clinical Relevance*, G.D.O. Lowe, J.T. Douglas, C.D. Forbes and A. Henschen (eds.), Elsevier, Amsterdam. pp. 53-56, **1987**.

FIBRINOGEN NIJMEGEN I

Last update	[10 January 1994]	**Structural defect**	[Bβ(44) Arg → Cys[1]]
Alphacode	[NIJMEG01]	**Mutation**	[CGT → TGT]
Ref. type	[Article]		

Family studies
Homozygote? [No]
Pedigree published? [Yes]

Functional defect(s)
FpA release: [Normal]
FpB release: [Normal]
Polymerization: [Abnormal]
Stabilization: [n.a.]

Clinical manifestation(s) Bleeding? [No] Thrombosis? [Yes[2]]

Clinical laboratory results

Plasma fibrinogen concentration (mg/dL)
Chronometric: [120/(180-490)]
Rate-indep'nt: [n.a.]
Immunologic: [350/(160-500)]

*Hypo*dysfibrinogen? [No]

Thrombin time:	[20.2s/(18.5s)]
Reptilase (batroxobin) time:	[22.7s/(<20s)]
Prothrombin time:	[n.a.]
Partial thromboplastin time:	[n.a.]
Euglobulin lysis time:	[n.a.]
Bleeding time:	[n.a.]
Immunoelectrophoresis:	[n.a.]
Platelet aggregation:	[n.a.]

Other results with patient plasma

Ancrod (Arvin) time:	[n.a.]	Inhib. normal plasma?	[n.a.]
Recalcification time:	[n.a.]	In vivo synthesis:	[n.a.]
Calcium corrects c.t.?	[n.a.]	In vivo catabolism:	[n.a.]

Evaluation of isolated patient fibrinogen

Thrombin time:	[22.7s/(20s)]	Abnormal subunit?	[No]
Reptilase time:	[30s/(25s)]	Abnormal FDPs?	[n.a.[2]]
Ancrod (Arvin) time:	[n.a.]		

Remarks

[1]The structural defect was determined with the PCR method.

[2]Patient plasma exhibited abnormal *acceleration* of t-PA-catalyzed plasminogen activation.

Abnormal high-molecular-weight fibrinogen complexes and disulfide-linked fibrinogen-albumin complexes were reported.

FIBRINOGEN NIJMEGEN I

References

1. Koopman, J., Haverkate, F., Grimbergen, J., Engesser, L., Nováková, I., Kerst, A.F.J.A. and Lord, S.T. Abnormal fibrinogens IJmuiden (BβArg_{14}→Cys) and Nijmegen (BβArg_{44}→Cys) form disulfide-linked fibrinogen-albumin complexes. *Proc. Natl. Acad. Sci. USA* **89**:3478-3482, **1992**.

2. Koopman, J., Haverkate, F., Lord, S.T., and Grimbergen, J. Identification of structural defects in abnormal fibrinogens using the polymerase chain reaction. *Proc. X Intl. Fgen. Wkshp.*, **1990** ABSTRACT.

3. Engesser, L., Koopman, J., de Munk, G., Haverkate, F., Novakova, I., Verheijen, J.H., Briet, E. and Brommer, E.J.P. Fibrinogen Nijmegen: Congenital dysfibrinogenemia associated with impaired t-PA mediated plasminogen activation and decreased binding of t-PA. *Thromb. Haemostas.* **60**:113-120, **1988**.

4. Engesser, L., Koopman, J., DeMunk, G., Haverkate, F., Novakova, I., Verheijen, J.H., Briet, E. and Brommer, E.J.P. An abnormal fibrinogen (Fibrinogen Nijmegen) with a decreased binding of t-PA and a reduced acceleration of t-PA induced plasminogen activation. In: *Fibrinogen 3. Biochemistry, Biological Functions, Gene Regulation and Expression*, M.W. Mosesson, D.L. Amrani, K.R. Siebenlist and J.P. DiOrio (eds.), Elsevier Science Publ., B.V., Amsterdam. pp. 259-262, **1988**.

FIBRINOGEN NOTTINGHAM I

Last update [1 December 1990]
Alphacode [NOTTIN01]
Ref. type [Article[1]]

Structural defect [n.a.]
Mutation [n.a.]

Family studies
Homozygote? [n.a.]
Pedigree published? [No]

Functional defect(s)
FpA release: [n.a.]
FpB release: [n.a.]
Polymerization: [n.a.]
Stabilization: [n.a.]

Clinical manifestation(s) Bleeding? [n.a.] Thrombosis? [n.a.]

Clinical laboratory results

Plasma fibrinogen concentration (mg/dL)
Chronometric: [n.a.]
Rate-indep'nt: [n.a.]
Immunologic: [n.a.]

*Hypo*dysfibrinogen? [Yes]

Thrombin time:	[n.a.]
Reptilase (batroxobin) time:	[n.a.]
Prothrombin time:	[n.a.]
Partial thromboplastin time:	[n.a.]
Euglobulin lysis time:	[n.a.]
Bleeding time:	[n.a.]
Immunoelectrophoresis:	[n.a.]
Platelet aggregation:	[n.a.]

Other results with patient plasma
Ancrod (Arvin) time: [n.a.]
Recalcification time: [n.a.]
Calcium corrects c.t.? [n.a.]

Inhib. normal plasma? [n.a.]
In vivo synthesis: [n.a.]
In vivo catabolism: [n.a.]

Evaluation of isolated patient fibrinogen
Thrombin time: [n.a.]
Reptilase time: [n.a.]
Ancrod (Arvin) time: [n.a.]

Abnormal subunit? [n.a.]
Abnormal FDPs? [n.a.]

Remarks

[1]Review article only; P. Jones, personal communication.

References

1. Lane, D.A., Thompson, E. and Southan, C. Rapid screening method of fibrinopeptide analysis applied to congenital dysfibrinogenaemia: summary of 23 cases. In: *Fibrinogen 2. Biochemistry, Physiology and Clinical Relevance*, G.D.O. Lowe, J.T. Douglas, C.D. Forbes and A. Henschen (eds.), Elsevier, Amsterdam. pp. 71-74, **1987**.

FIBRINOGEN OKLAHOMA I

Last update [10 January 1994]
Alphacode [OKLAHO01]
Ref. type [Article]

Structural defect [n.a.]
Mutation [n.a.]

Family studies
Homozygote? [n.a.]
Pedigree published? [Yes]

Functional defect(s)
FpA release: [Normal[1]]
FpB release: [Normal[1]]
Polymerization: [Normal]
Stabilization: [Normal]

Clinical manifestation(s) Bleeding? [Yes[2]] Thrombosis? [No]

Clinical laboratory results
Plasma fibrinogen concentration (mg/dL)
Chronometric: [n.a.]
Rate-indep'nt: [237[3]]
Immunologic: [n.a.]

*Hypo*dysfibrinogen? [No]

Thrombin time:	[n.a.]
Reptilase (batroxobin) time:	[n.a.]
Prothrombin time:	[15s/(15-17s)]
Partial thromboplastin time:	[n.a.]
Euglobulin lysis time:	[2.5-7h/(21-30h)]
Bleeding time:	[Normal]
Immunoelectrophoresis:	[Normal]
Platelet aggregation:	[n.a.]

Other results with patient plasma
Ancrod (Arvin) time: [n.a.]
Recalcification time: [200s/(100-200s)]
Calcium corrects c.t.? [n.a.]

Inhib. normal plasma? [No]
In vivo synthesis: [n.a.]
In vivo catabolism: [Normal]

Evaluation of isolated patient fibrinogen
Thrombin time: [n.a.]
Reptilase time: [n.a.]
Ancrod (Arvin) time: [n.a.]

Abnormal subunit? [No]
Abnormal FDPs? [n.a.]

Remarks
[1]The rate of *total* fibrinopeptide release was normal.
[2]Excessive bleeding after dental extraction, easy bruising, poor wound healing, and menorrhagia were among the symptoms reported in 13 affected family members.
[3]Normal range not reported.

It has not been demonstrated conclusively that fibrinogen Oklahoma is functionally or structurally defective. This "dysfibrinogen" initially was described as a factor XIII variant (5,6), then as a fibrinogen variant (2-4). More recently (1), an evaluation of fibrinogen Oklahoma failed to disclose any functional, structural, or physicochemical abnormalities.

FIBRINOGEN OKLAHOMA I

References

1. Finlayson, J.S. "Fibrinogen Oklahoma: a study of interactions. *Ann. N. Y. Acad. Sci.* **408**:577-582, **1983**.

2. Hampton, J.W. Fibrinogen abnormality with defective cross-linkage. *Fed. Proc.* **29**:647, **1970**. ABSTRACT

3. Morton, R.O. and Hampton, J.W. Fibrinogen Oklahoma — Characterization of a familial bleeding diathesis. *Clin. Res.* **18**:533, **1970**. ABSTRACT

4. Hampton, J.W. and Bird, R.M. Qualitative fibrinogen defect associated with abnormal fibrin stabilization. *J. Lab. Clin. Med.* **72**:882, **1968**. ABSTRACT

5. Hampton, J.W., Cunningham, G.R. and Bird, R.M. The pattern of inheritance of defective fibrinase (Factor XIII). *J. Lab. Clin. Med.* **67**:914-921, **1966**

6. Hampton, J.W., Bird, R.M. and Hammarsten, D.M. Defective fibrinase activity in two brothers. *J. Lab. Clin. Med.* **65**:469-474, **1965**.

FIBRINOGEN ORLEANS I

Last update [1 December 1990]
Alphacode [ORLEAN01]
Ref. type [Article]

Family studies
Homozygote? [n.a.]
Pedigree published? [No]

Structural defect [n.a.]
Mutation [n.a.]

Functional defect(s)
FpA release: [n.a.[1]]
FpB release: [n.a.[1]]
Polymerization: [Abnormal]
Stabilization: [n.a.]

Clinical manifestation(s) Bleeding? [No] Thrombosis? [No]

Clinical laboratory results
Plasma fibrinogen concentration (mg/dL)
Chronometric: [50[2]]
Rate-indep'nt: [n.a.]
Immunologic: [370[2]]

*Hypo*dysfibrinogen? [No]

Thrombin time:	[58s/(20s)]
Reptilase (batroxobin) time:	[n.a.]
Prothrombin time:	[64%[3]]
Partial thromboplastin time:	[n.a.]
Euglobulin lysis time:	[n.a.]
Bleeding time:	[Normal]
Immunoelectrophoresis:	[Normal]
Platelet aggregation:	[n.a.]

Other results with patient plasma
Ancrod (Arvin) time: [n.a.]
Recalcification time: [n.a.]
Calcium corrects c.t.? [n.a.]

Inhib. normal plasma? [No]
In vivo synthesis: [n.a.]
In vivo catabolism: [n.a.]

Evaluation of isolated patient fibrinogen
Thrombin time: [n.a.]
Reptilase time: [n.a.]
Ancrod (Arvin) time: [n.a.]

Abnormal subunit? [n.a.]
Abnormal FDPs? [n.a.]

Remarks
[1]The rate of *total* fibrinopeptide release was reduced; individual fibrinopeptide release was not reported.
[2]Normal range not reported.
[3]Slightly prolonged.

References

1. Vaugier, G.L., Maze, A., Griffault, J., Vacher, J. and Plutino, C. [Fibrinogen Orleans. A new case of congenital dysfibrinogenemia (letter)]. *Presse. Med.* **12**:1079-1080, **1983**. ABSTRACT

FIBRINOGEN ORSAY I

Last update [1 December 1990]
Alphacode [ORSAY01]
Ref. type [Article]

Structural defect [n.a.]
Mutation [n.a.]

Family studies
Homozygote? [n.a.]
Pedigree published? [No]

Functional defect(s)
FpA release: [n.a.]
FpB release: [n.a.]
Polymerization: [n.a.]
Stabilization: [n.a.]

Clinical manifestation(s) Bleeding? [No] Thrombosis? [No]

Clinical laboratory results
Plasma fibrinogen concentration (mg/dL)
Chronometric: [275[1]]
Rate-indep'nt: [330[1]]
Immunologic: [350[1]]

*Hypo*dysfibrinogen? [No]

Thrombin time:	[50s/(19s)]
Reptilase (batroxobin) time:	[36s/(16s)]
Prothrombin time:	[48%/(>70%)]
Partial thromboplastin time:	[30s/(30s)]
Euglobulin lysis time:	[n.a.]
Bleeding time:	[n.a.]
Immunoelectrophoresis:	[n.a.]
Platelet aggregation:	[n.a.]

Other results with patient plasma
Ancrod (Arvin) time: [n.a.]
Recalcification time: [n.a.]
Calcium corrects c.t.? [n.a.]

Inhib. normal plasma? [n.a.]
In vivo synthesis: [n.a.]
In vivo catabolism: [n.a.]

Evaluation of isolated patient fibrinogen
Thrombin time: [n.a.]
Reptilase time: [n.a.]
Ancrod (Arvin) time: [n.a.]

Abnormal subunit? [n.a.]
Abnormal FDPs? [n.a.]

Remarks
[1]Normal range not reported.

References

1. Corrihons, G., Soria, J., Soria, C., Conard, J., Horellou, M.H. and Samama, M. [Congenital dysfibrinogenemia. Apropos of 13 cases]. *Sem. Hop. Paris* **59**:2517-2523, **1983**.

FIBRINOGEN OSAKA I

Last update [1 December 1990]
Alphacode [OSAKA01]
Ref. type [Article]

Family studies
Homozygote? [No]
Pedigree published? [No]

Structural defect [Aα(16) Arg → Cys]
Mutation [n.a.]

Functional defect(s)
FpA release: [Abnormal[1]]
FpB release: [n.a.]
Polymerization: [Abnormal[1]]
Stabilization: [n.a.]

Clinical manifestation(s) Bleeding? [No] Thrombosis? [No]

Clinical laboratory results
Plasma fibrinogen concentration (mg/dL)
Chronometric: [n.a.]
Rate-indep'nt: [n.a.]
Immunologic: [n.a.]

*Hypo*dysfibrinogen? [n.a.]

Thrombin time:	[n.a.]
Reptilase (batroxobin) time:	[n.a.]
Prothrombin time:	[n.a.]
Partial thromboplastin time:	[n.a.]
Euglobulin lysis time:	[n.a.]
Bleeding time:	[n.a.]
Immunoelectrophoresis:	[n.a.]
Platelet aggregation:	[n.a.]

Other results with patient plasma
Ancrod (Arvin) time: [n.a.]
Recalcification time: [n.a.]
Calcium corrects c.t.? [n.a.]

Inhib. normal plasma? [n.a.]
In vivo synthesis: [n.a.]
In vivo catabolism: [n.a.]

Evaluation of isolated patient fibrinogen
Thrombin time: [n.a.]
Reptilase time: [n.a.]
Ancrod (Arvin) time: [n.a.]

Abnormal subunit? [n.a.]
Abnormal FDPs? [n.a.]

Remarks
[1]Data not reported. Approximately 50% of fibrinopeptide A was not released.

The presence of an inter-chain disulfide bond at the site of the mutation was demonstrated; from this the authors concluded that Aα-chains assume a parallel configuration. This observation also provided direct demonstration that the variant fibrinogen was synthesized as a homodimer (i.e., both variant Aα-chains are present in the same molecule). See also Kawaguchi I.

References

1. Miyata, T., Terukina, S., Matsuda, M., Kasamatsu, A., Takeda, Y., Murakami, T. and Iwanaga, S. Fibrinogens Kawaguchi and Osaka: an amino acid substitution of Aα-arginine-16 to cysteine which forms an extra interchain disulfide bridge between the two Aα-chains. *J. Biochem. (Tokyo)* **102**:93-101, **1987**.

2. Matsuda, M., Terukina, S., Miyata, T. and Iwanaga, S. Defective release of fibrinopeptide A due to substitution of Aα arginine-16 by cysteine in two abnormal fibrinogens Kawaguchi and Osaka. In: *Fibrinogen and Its Derivatives; Biochemistry, Physiology, and Pathophysiology*, Excerpta Medica, Amsterdam, New York, Oxford. pp. 37-40, **1986**.

FIBRINOGEN OSAKA II

Last update	[10 January 1994]	**Structural defect**	[γ(275) Arg → Cys[1]]
Alphacode	[OSAKA02]	**Mutation**	[CGC → TGC]
Ref. type	[Article]		

Functional defect(s)

FpA release:	[Normal]
FpB release:	[Normal]
Polymerization:	[Abnormal]
Stabilization:	[Normal]

Family studies

Homozygote?	[No]
Pedigree published?	[No]

Clinical manifestation(s) Bleeding? [No] Thrombosis? [No]

Clinical laboratory results

Plasma fibrinogen concentration (mg/dL)

Chronometric:	[40/(200-400)]		
Rate-indep'nt:	[Normal[2]]	*Hypo*dysfibrinogen?	[No]
Immunologic:	[n.a.]		

Thrombin time:	[107.9s/(14.3s)]
Reptilase (batroxobin) time:	[n.a.]
Prothrombin time:	[n.a.]
Partial thromboplastin time:	[n.a.]
Euglobulin lysis time:	[n.a.]
Bleeding time:	[n.a.]
Immunoelectrophoresis:	[n.a.]
Platelet aggregation:	[n.a.]

Other results with patient plasma

Ancrod (Arvin) time:	[n.a.]	Inhib. normal plasma?	[n.a.]
Recalcification time:	[n.a.]	In vivo synthesis:	[n.a.]
Calcium corrects c.t.?	[n.a.]	In vivo catabolism:	[n.a.]

Evaluation of isolated patient fibrinogen

Thrombin time:	[>300s/(15.3s)]	Abnormal subunit?	[Yes[3]]
Reptilase time:	[n.a.]	Abnormal FDPs?	[Yes[4]]
Ancrod (Arvin) time:	[>300s/(17.6s)]		

Remarks

[1]The molecular defect was confirmed by the PCR method.

[2]Data not reported.

[3]SDS-PAGE disclosed an oversized γ-chain.

[4]An oversized γ-chain remnant from fragment D_1 was reported. The variant fragment D_1 failed to inhibit fibrin monomer polymerization, thus indicating that it contained an abnormal polymerization site.

The authors provide evidence that Cys_{275} forms a disulfide bond with cysteine.

FIBRINOGEN OSAKA II

References

1. Mimuro, J., Muramatsu, S., Maekawa, H., Sakata, Y., Kaneko, M., Yoshitake, S., Okuma, M., Ito, Y., Takeda, Y. and Matsuda, M. Gene analyses of abnormal fibrinogens with a mutation in the γ chain. *Intl. J. Hematol.* **56**:129-134, **1992**.

2. Muramatsu, S., Mimuro, J., Maekawa, H., Sakata, Y., Matsuda, M., Yoshitake, S. and Okuma, M. Gene analysis of abnormal fibrinogens characterized by a mutation in the γ chain. *Thromb. Haemostas.* **65**:821, **1991**. ABSTRACT

3. Matsuda, M., Terukina, S., Yoshida, N., Yamazumi, K. and Maekawa, H. Abnormal fibrinogens with two structural defects. *Adv. Exp. Med. Biol.* **281**:63-72, **1990**.

4. Terukina, S., Matsuda, M., Hirata, H., Takeda, Y., Miyata, T., Takao, T. and Shimonishi, Y. Substitution of γ Arg-275 by Cys in an abnormal fibrinogen, "fibrinogen Osaka II: evidence for a unique solitary cystine structure at the mutation site. *J. Biol. Chem.* **263**:13579-13587, **1988**.

5. Terukina, S., Matsuda, M., Yoshida, N., Yamazumi, K., Takeda, Y. and Takano, T. Two abnormal fibrinogens designated as Osaka II and Morioka with a hitherto unidentified amino acid substitution; γ Arg-275 by Cys. *Thromb. Haemostas.* **58**:515, **1987**. ABSTRACT

FIBRINOGEN OSAKA III

Last update [10 January 1994]
Alphacode [OSAKA03]
Ref. type [Article]

Structural defect [γ(275) Arg → His]
Mutation [n.a.]

Family studies
Homozygote? [No]
Pedigree published? [No]

Functional defect(s)
FpA release: [Normal]
FpB release: [Normal]
Polymerization: [Abnormal]
Stabilization: [Normal]

Clinical manifestation(s) Bleeding? [No] Thrombosis? [No]

Clinical laboratory results
Plasma fibrinogen concentration (mg/dL)
Chronometric: [93/(150-350)]
Rate-indep'nt: [181/(150-350)]
Immunologic: [270/(150-350)]

*Hypo*dysfibrinogen? [No]

Thrombin time:	[43.8s/(14.8-16.4s)]
Reptilase (batroxobin) time:	[>100s/(12.1-13.7s)]
Prothrombin time:	[15.2s/(11.3-12.1s)]
Partial thromboplastin time:	[n.a.]
Euglobulin lysis time:	[n.a.]
Bleeding time:	[Normal]
Immunoelectrophoresis:	[n.a.]
Platelet aggregation:	[n.a.]

Other results with patient plasma
Ancrod (Arvin) time: [n.a.]
Recalcification time: [n.a.]
Calcium corrects c.t.? [No]

Inhib. normal plasma? [n.a.]
In vivo synthesis: [n.a.]
In vivo catabolism: [n.a.]

Evaluation of isolated patient fibrinogen
Thrombin time: [>100s/(10.2-12s)]
Reptilase time: [n.a.]
Ancrod (Arvin) time: [n.a.]

Abnormal subunit? [Yes[1]]
Abnormal FDPs? [Yes[2]]

Remarks
[1]SDS-PAGE disclosed an apparently higher m.w. γ-chain.
[2]SDS-PAGE disclosed an apparently higher m.w. fragment D_1.

References

1. Yoshida, N., Imaoka, S., Hirata, H., Matsuda, M. and Asakura, S. Heterozygous abnormal fibrinogen Osaka III with the replacement of γ arginine-275 by histidine has an apparently higher molecular weight γ-chain variant. *Thromb. Haemost.* **68**:534-538, **1992**.

FIBRINOGEN OSAKA IV

Last update [10 January 1994]
Alphaco de [OSAKA04]
Ref. type [Article]

Family studies
Homozygote? [No]
Pedigree published? [Yes]

Structural defect [Aα(16) Arg → His]
Mutation [n.a.]

Functional defect(s)
FpA release: [Abnormal[1]]
FpB release: [Normal]
Polymerization: [Abnormal]
Stabilization: [n.a.]

Clinical manifestation(s) Bleeding? [No[2]] Thrombosis? [No[2]]

Clinical laboratory results
Plasma fibrinogen concentration (mg/dL)
Chronometric: [54/(150-350)]
Rate-indep'nt: [n.a.]
Immunologic: [335/(180-350)]
*Hypo*dysfibrinogen? [No]

Thrombin time:	[80.9s/(14.4s)]
Reptilase (batroxobin) time:	[106s/(20.9s)]
Prothrombin time:	[57%/(80-120%)]
Partial thromboplastin time:	[28s/(20-35s)]
Euglobulin lysis time:	[n.a.]
Bleeding time:	[n.a.]
Immunoelectrophoresis:	[n.a.]
Platelet aggregation:	[n.a.]

Other results with patient plasma
Ancrod (Arvin) time: [n.a.]
Recalcification time: [n.a.]
Calcium corrects c.t.? [No]
Inhib. normal plasma? [n.a.]
In vivo synthesis: [n.a.]
In vivo catabolism: [n.a.]

Evaluation of isolated patient fibrinogen
Thrombin time: [n.a.]
Reptilase time: [n.a.]
Ancrod (Arvin) time: [n.a.]
Abnormal subunit? [No]
Abnormal FDPs? [No[3]]

Remarks
[1]Only half the normal amount of FpA was released. Ancrod did not release the variant FpA.
[2]At age 42 the propositus underwent gastrectomy for adenocarcinoma of the stomach without complications. Intraoperative fibrinogen supplementation with cryoprecipitate was suboptimal due to apparently rapid clearance; whole blood transfusion was preferred (see Tsujinaka et al., 1988).
[3]Reduced binding of fragment D_1 to ancrod-treated fibrinogen Osaka IV, and elevated plasma FDPs were reported.

References

1. Yamazumi, K., Terukina, S., Matsuda, M., Kanbayashi, J., Sakon, M. and Tsujinaka, T. Fibrinogen Osaka IV: a congenital dysfibrinogenemia found in a patient originally reported in relation to surgery, now defined to have an Aα arginine-16 to histidine substitution. *Jpn. J. Surg.* **23**:45-50, **1993**.

2. Tsujinaka, T., Kambayashi, J., Kang, J., Sakon, M. and Mori, T. Intraoperative management of a dysfibrinogenemic patient with gastric cancer. *Jpn. J. Surg.* **18**:43-46, **1988**.

FIBRINOGEN OSAKA V

Last update	[10 January 1994]	**Structural defect**	[γ(375) Arg → Gly]
Alphacode	[OSAKA05]	**Mutation**	[n.a.]
Ref. type	[Article]		

Family studies
Homozygote? [No]
Pedigree published? [No]

Functional defect(s)
FpA release: [n.a.]
FpB release: [n.a.]
Polymerization: [Abnormal[1]]
Stabilization: [n.a.]

Clinical manifestation(s) Bleeding? [No] Thrombosis? [No]

Clinical laboratory results

Plasma fibrinogen concentration (mg/dL)
Chronometric: [90/(150-350)]
Rate-indep'nt: [218/(150-350)]
Immunologic: [250/(150-350)]

*Hypo*dysfibrinogen? [No]

Thrombin time:	[14.3s/(9.7s)]
Reptilase (batroxobin) time:	[n.a.]
Prothrombin time:	[n.a.]
Partial thromboplastin time:	[n.a.]
Euglobulin lysis time:	[n.a.]
Bleeding time:	[n.a.]
Immunoelectrophoresis:	[n.a.]
Platelet aggregation:	[n.a.]

Other results with patient plasma

Ancrod (Arvin) time:	[n.a.]	Inhib. normal plasma?	[n.a.]
Recalcification time:	[n.a.]	In vivo synthesis:	[n.a.]
Calcium corrects c.t.?	[Yes[2]]	In vivo catabolism:	[n.a.]

Evaluation of isolated patient fibrinogen

Thrombin time:	[23.7s/(8.7s)]	Abnormal subunit?	[Yes[3]]
Reptilase time:	[37.3s/(10s)]	Abnormal FDPs?	[Yes[4]]
Ancrod (Arvin) time:	[n.a.]		

Remarks

[1]Fibrin polymerization was abnormal at <0.1 mM Ca^{2+}, and normal at >5 mM Ca^{2+}.

[2]The authors concluded that the variant γ-chain lacks a high-affinity calcium binding site.

[3]Isoelectric focusing disclosed abnormal γ-chains; SDS-PAGE disclosed abnormal γ-chain mobility only in the presence of calcium (Yoshida et al., 1994).

[4]Calcium failed to protect fragment D_1 from further proteolysis by plasmin.

References

1. Yoshida, N., Hirata, H., Imaoka, S., Matsuda, M., Yamazumi, K. and Asakura, S. Effect of calcium on the mobility of γ-chain from fibrinogen Osaka V on sodium dodecyl sulfate-polyacrylamide gel electrophoresis. *Thromb. Res.* **73**:79-82, **1994**.

2. Yoshida, N., Hirata, H., Morigami, Y., Imaoka, S., Matsuda, M., Yamazumi, K. and Asakura, S. Characterization of an abnormal fibrinogen Osaka V with the replacement of γ-arginine 375 by glycine. The lack of high affinity calcium binding to D-domains and the lack of protective effect of calcium on fibrinolysis. *J. Biol. Chem.* **267**:2753-2759, **1992**.

3. Yoshida, N., and Matsuda, M. Fibrinogen Osaka V with a γ Arg-375 to Gly substitution is defective in the high-affinity but normal in the low-affinity calcium binding sites. *Proc. X Intl. Fgen. Wkshp.*, **1990** ABSTRACT.

FIBRINOGEN OSLO I

Last update [10 January 1994]
Alphacode [OSLO01]
Ref. type [Article]

Family studies
Homozygote? [No]
Pedigree published? [Yes]

Structural defect [n.a.]
Mutation [n.a.]

Functional defect(s)
FpA release: [n.a.[1]]
FpB release: [n.a.[1]]
Polymerization: [n.a.]
Stabilization: [n.a.]

Clinical manifestation(s) Bleeding? [No] Thrombosis? [Yes[2]]

Clinical laboratory results
Plasma fibrinogen concentration (mg/dL)
Chronometric: [n.a.]
Rate-indep'nt: [270/(195-330)] *Hypo*dysfibrinogen? [No]
Immunologic: [n.a.]

Thrombin time:	[24.5/(25-36)[3]]
Reptilase (batroxobin) time:	[n.a.]
Prothrombin time:	[15.3s/(12.6-17s)]
Partial thromboplastin time:	[56.9s/(54-60s)]
Euglobulin lysis time:	[n.a.]
Bleeding time:	[n.a.]
Immunoelectrophoresis:	[n.a.]
Platelet aggregation:	[n.a.[4]]

Other results with patient plasma
Ancrod (Arvin) time: [n.a.]
Recalcification time: [n.a.]
Calcium corrects c.t.? [n.a.]

Inhib. normal plasma? [n.a.]
In vivo synthesis: [n.a.]
In vivo catabolism: [n.a.]

Evaluation of isolated patient fibrinogen
Thrombin time: [n.a.]
Reptilase time: [n.a.]
Ancrod (Arvin) time: [n.a.]

Abnormal subunit? [Yes[5]]
Abnormal FDPs? [n.a.]

Remarks
[1]The rate of fibrinopeptide release was not reported; however, fibrinopeptides with normal mobility on RP-HPLC were detected.
[2]A high incidence of thromboembolic disorders including post-traumatic, post-surgical, and postpartum thrombophlebitis and pulmonary embolism in affected family members was reported.
[3]This is an *average* value for 5 affected family members. Note that the thrombin time was *shorter* than normal. Compare with fibrinogens Chapel Hill VI and Strasbourg I.
[4]Increased binding of the variant fibrinogen to platelets was reported.
[5]Bβ-chain variants (charge isomers) were detected by two-dimensional electrophoresis.

FIBRINOGEN OSLO I

References

1. Thorsen, L.I., Brosstad, F., Solum, N.O. and Stormorken, H. Increased binding to ADP-stimulated platelets and aggregation effect of the dysfibrinogen Oslo I as compared with normal fibrinogen. *Scand. J. Haematol.* **36**:203-210, **1986**.

2. Soria, J., Soria, C., Samama, M. and Caen, J. Study of ten cases of congenital dysfibrinogenemia. Clinical and molecular biological aspects. In: *Fibrinogen — Structural Variants and Interactions*, A. Henschen, B. Hessel, J. McDonagh and T. Saldeen (eds.), Walter de Gruyter, Berlin. pp. 165-183, **1985**.

3. Brosstad, F., Teige, B., Olaisen, B., Gravem, K., Godal, H.C. and Stormorken, H. Two-dimensional electrophoretic characterization (iso-dalt) of fibrinogen and fibrin subunit chains from four different genetic dysfibrinogen variants. In: *Fibrinogen — Structure, Functional Aspects, Metabolism*, F. Haverkate, A. Henschen, W. Nieuwenhuizen and P.W. Straub (eds.), Walter de Gruyter, Berlin. pp. 145-154, **1983**.

4. Henschen, A., Kehl, M., Southan, C., Lottspeich, F. and Georgopoulos, D. Genetically abnormal fibrinogens — some current characterisation strategies. In: *Fibrinogen — Structure, Functional Aspects, Metabolism*, F. Haverkate, A. Henschen, W. Nieuwenhuizen and P.W. Straub (eds.), Walter de Gruyter, Berlin. pp. 125-144, **1983**.

5. Egeberg, O. Inherited fibrinogen abnormality causing thrombophilia. *Thromb. Diath. Haemorrh.* **17**:176-187, **1967**.

FIBRINOGEN OSLO II

Last update [1 December 1990]
Alphacode [OSLO02]
Ref. type [Article]

Family studies
Homozygote? [n.a.]
Pedigree published? [Yes]

Structural defect [n.a.]
Mutation [n.a.]

Functional defect(s)
FpA release: [Normal]
FpB release: [Normal]
Polymerization: [Abnormal]
Stabilization: [n.a.]

Clinical manifestation(s) Bleeding? [No] Thrombosis? [No]

Clinical laboratory results
Plasma fibrinogen concentration (mg/dL)
Chronometric: [70/(200-400)]
Rate-indep'nt: [240/(200-400)]
Immunologic: [270/(200-400)]

*Hypo*dysfibrinogen? [No]

Thrombin time:	[41s/(18-23s)]
Reptilase (batroxobin) time:	[n.a.]
Prothrombin time:	[18s/(13-17s)]
Partial thromboplastin time:	[33s/(25-35s)]
Euglobulin lysis time:	[n.a.]
Bleeding time:	[n.a.]
Immunoelectrophoresis:	[n.a.]
Platelet aggregation:	[n.a.]

Other results with patient plasma
Ancrod (Arvin) time: [n.a.]
Recalcification time: [n.a.]
Calcium corrects c.t.? [No]

Inhib. normal plasma? [n.a.]
In vivo synthesis: [n.a.]
In vivo catabolism: [n.a.]

Evaluation of isolated patient fibrinogen
Thrombin time: [n.a.]
Reptilase time: [n.a.]
Ancrod (Arvin) time: [n.a.]

Abnormal subunit? [No]
Abnormal FDPs? [n.a.]

Remarks
The results are those from the affected mother of the index patient.

References

1. Brosstad, F., Teige, B., Olaisen, B., Gravem, K., Godal, H.C. and Stormorken, H. Two-dimensional electrophoretic characterization (iso-dalt) of fibrinogen and fibrin subunit chains from four different genetic dysfibrinogen variants. In: *Fibrinogen —Structure, Functional Aspects, Metabolism*, F. Haverkate, A. Henschen, W. Nieuwenhuizen and P.W. Straub (eds.), Walter de Gruyter, Berlin. pp. 145-154, **1983**.

2. Henschen, A., Kehl, M., Southan, C., Lottspeich, F. and Georgopoulos, D. Genetically abnormal fibrinogens — some current characterisation strategies. In: *Fibrinogen —Structure, Functional Aspects, Metabolism*, F. Haverkate, A. Henschen, W. Nieuwenhuizen and P.W. Straub (eds.), Walter de Gruyter, Berlin. pp. 125-144, **1983**.

3. Lane, D.A., Allen, A.K., Markwick, J., Thompson, E. and Mackie, I. Carbohydrate in abnormal fibrinogens. In: *Fibrinogen — Recent Biochemical and Medical Aspects*, A. Henschen, H. Graeff and F. Lottspeich (eds.), W. deGruyter, Berlin. pp. 183-192, **1982**.

4. Godal, H.C., Brosstad, F. and Kierulf, P. Three new cases of an inborn qualitative fibrinogen defect (fibrinogen Oslo II). *Scand. J. Haematol.* **20**:57-62, **1978**.

FIBRINOGEN OSLO III

Last update [1 December 1990]
Alphacode [OSLO03]
Ref. type [Article]

Structural defect [n.a.]
Mutation [n.a.]

Family studies
Homozygote? [No]
Pedigree published? [No]

Functional defect(s)
FpA release: [n.a.[1]]
FpB release: [n.a.[1]]
Polymerization: [n.a.]
Stabilization: [Normal]

Clinical manifestation(s) Bleeding? [No] Thrombosis? [No]

Clinical laboratory results
Plasma fibrinogen concentration (mg/dL)
Chronometric: [n.a.]
Rate-indep'nt: [n.a.]
Immunologic: [n.a.]

*Hypo*dysfibrinogen? [n.a.]

Thrombin time:	[n.a.]
Reptilase (batroxobin) time:	[n.a.]
Prothrombin time:	[n.a.]
Partial thromboplastin time:	[n.a.]
Euglobulin lysis time:	[n.a.]
Bleeding time:	[n.a.]
Immunoelectrophoresis:	[n.a.]
Platelet aggregation:	[n.a.]

Other results with patient plasma
Ancrod (Arvin) time: [n.a.]
Recalcification time: [n.a.]
Calcium corrects c.t.? [n.a.]

Inhib. normal plasma? [n.a.]
In vivo synthesis: [n.a.]
In vivo catabolism: [n.a.]

Evaluation of isolated patient fibrinogen
Thrombin time: [n.a.]
Reptilase time: [n.a.]
Ancrod (Arvin) time: [n.a.]

Abnormal subunit? [Yes[2]]
Abnormal FDPs? [n.a.]

Remarks
[1]Fibrinopeptides with normal mobility on RP-HPLC were detected; the *rate* of fibrinopeptide release was not determined.
[2]Larger-than-normal γ-chain variants were detected by two-dimensional electrophoresis.

References

1. Henschen, A., Kehl, M., Southan, C., Lottspeich, F. and Georgopoulos, D. Genetically abnormal fibrinogens — some current characterisation strategies. In: *Fibrinogen — Structure, Functional Aspects, Metabolism*, F. Haverkate, A. Henschen, W. Nieuwenhuizen and P.W. Straub (eds.), Walter de Gruyter, Berlin. pp. 125-144, **1983**.

2. Brosstad, F., Teige, B., Olaisen, B., Gravem, K., Godal, H.C. and Stormorken, H. Two-dimensional electrophoretic characterization (iso-dalt) of fibrinogen and fibrin subunit chains from four different genetic dysfibrinogen variants. In: *Fibrinogen — Structure, Functional Aspects, Metabolism*, F. Haverkate, A. Henschen, W. Nieuwenhuizen and P.W. Straub (eds.), Walter de Gruyter, Berlin. pp. 145-154, **1983**.

FIBRINOGEN OSLO IV

Last update [1 December 1990]
Alphacode [OSLO04]
Ref. type [Article]

Family studies
Homozygote? [n.a.]
Pedigree published? [Yes]

Structural defect [n.a.]
Mutation [n.a.]

Functional defect(s)
FpA release: [n.a.[1]]
FpB release: [n.a.[1]]
Polymerization: [Abnormal]
Stabilization: [n.a.]

Clinical manifestation(s) Bleeding? [No] Thrombosis? [No]

Clinical laboratory results
Plasma fibrinogen concentration (mg/dL)
Chronometric: [48/(170-374)]
Rate-indep'nt: [150/(170-374)]
Immunologic: [n.a.]

*Hypo*dysfibrinogen? [Yes]

Thrombin time:	[40.7s/(16-19s)]
Reptilase (batroxobin) time:	[38.5s/(15-18s)]
Prothrombin time:	[17.5s/(15-18s)]
Partial thromboplastin time:	[31s/(25-35s)]
Euglobulin lysis time:	[6h/(>2.5h)]
Bleeding time:	[Normal]
Immunoelectrophoresis:	[n.a.]
Platelet aggregation:	[Normal]

Other results with patient plasma
Ancrod (Arvin) time: [n.a.]
Recalcification time: [n.a.]
Calcium corrects c.t.? [n.a.]

Inhib. normal plasma? [n.a.]
In vivo synthesis: [n.a.]
In vivo catabolism: [n.a.]

Evaluation of isolated patient fibrinogen
Thrombin time: [n.a.]
Reptilase time: [n.a.]
Ancrod (Arvin) time: [n.a.]

Abnormal subunit? [n.a.]
Abnormal FDPs? [n.a.]

Remarks
[1]Fibrinopeptides with normal mobility on RP-HPLC were detected. The rate of fibrinopeptide release was not determined.

References

1. Brosstad, F., Teige, B., Olaisen, B., Gravem, K., Godal, H.C. and Stormorken, H. Two-dimensional electrophoretic characterization (iso-dalt) of fibrinogen and fibrin subunit chains from four different genetic dysfibrinogen variants. In: *Fibrinogen —Structure, Functional Aspects, Metabolism*, F. Haverkate, A. Henschen, W. Nieuwenhuizen and P.W. Straub (eds.), Walter de Gruyter, Berlin. pp. 145-154, **1983**.

2. Henschen, A., Kehl, M., Southan, C., Lottspeich, F. and Georgopoulos, D. Genetically abnormal fibrinogens — some current characterisation strategies. In: *Fibrinogen —Structure, Functional Aspects, Metabolism*, F. Haverkate, A. Henschen, W. Nieuwenhuizen and P.W. Straub (eds.), Walter de Gruyter, Berlin. pp. 125-144, **1983**.

3. Stormorken, H., Brosstad, F. and Seim, H. A new dysfibrinogenemia: fibrinogen Oslo IV. *Thromb. Haemostas.* **49**:120-122, **1983**.

FIBRINOGEN OVIEDO I

Last update [1 December 1990]
Alphacode [OVIEDO01]
Ref. type [Article]

Family studies
Homozygote? [n.a.]
Pedigree published? [No[1]]

Structural defect [n.a.]
Mutation [n.a.]

Functional defect(s)
FpA release: [Normal]
FpB release: [Normal]
Polymerization: [Abnormal]
Stabilization: [Normal]

Clinical manifestation(s) Bleeding? [No] Thrombosis? [No]

Clinical laboratory results

Plasma fibrinogen concentration (mg/dL)
Chronometric: [74/(200-400)]
Rate-indep'nt: [n.a.]
Immunologic: [370/(200-400)]

*Hypo*dysfibrinogen? [No]

Thrombin time:	[43s/(17-20s)]
Reptilase (batroxobin) time:	[50s/(15-18s)]
Prothrombin time:	[13s/(11-13s)]
Partial thromboplastin time:	[45s/(40-45s)]
Euglobulin lysis time:	[180m/(180m)]
Bleeding time:	[n.a.]
Immunoelectrophoresis:	[Normal]
Platelet aggregation:	[n.a.]

Other results with patient plasma
Ancrod (Arvin) time: [n.a.]
Recalcification time: [n.a.]
Calcium corrects c.t.? [Yes]

Inhib. normal plasma? [Yes]
In vivo synthesis: [n.a.]
In vivo catabolism: [n.a.]

Evaluation of isolated patient fibrinogen
Thrombin time: [Abnormal[2]]
Reptilase time: [n.a.]
Ancrod (Arvin) time: [n.a.]

Abnormal subunit? [No]
Abnormal FDPs? [No]

Remarks
[1]Five family members also were affected.
[2]Data not reported.

Plasma concentrations of antithrombin III and plasminogen were within normal limits.

References

1. Fernández, F.J., Rodríguez Pinto, C., Páramo, J., Cuesta, B., Collado, M., and Rocha, E. Fibrinogen Oviedo I. A new Spanish dysfibrinogenaemia. *Blood Coag. & Fibrinol.* **1**:571-575, **1990**.

2. Fernández, J., Rodriguez Pinto, C., Rocha, E., Fernández Urgelles, M., Páramo, J.A. and Romo, M. Fibrinogens Oviedo I, Oviedo II and Oviedo III: three new cases of dysfibrinogenemia with abnormal fibrin aggregation. *Thromb. Haemostas.* **54**:159, **1985**. ABSTRACT

FIBRINOGEN OVIEDO II[Abs]

Last update [1 December 1990]
Alphacode [OVIEDO02]
Ref. type [Abstract]

Structural defect [n.a.]
Mutation [n.a.]

Family studies
Homozygote? [n.a.]
Pedigree published? [No]

Functional defect(s)
FpA release: [Normal]
FpB release: [Normal]
Polymerization: [Abnormal]
Stabilization: [Normal]

Clinical manifestation(s) Bleeding? [No] Thrombosis? [No]

Clinical laboratory results
Plasma fibrinogen concentration (mg/dL)
Chronometric: [Subnormal[1]]
Rate-indep'nt: [n.a.]
Immunologic: [Normal[1]]

*Hypo*dysfibrinogen? [No]

Thrombin time:	[Abnormal[1]]
Reptilase (batroxobin) time:	[Abnormal[1]]
Prothrombin time:	[n.a.]
Partial thromboplastin time:	[n.a.]
Euglobulin lysis time:	[n.a.]
Bleeding time:	[n.a.]
Immunoelectrophoresis:	[Normal]
Platelet aggregation:	[n.a.]

Other results with patient plasma
Ancrod (Arvin) time: [n.a.]
Recalcification time: [n.a.]
Calcium corrects c.t.? [Yes]

Inhib. normal plasma? [Yes]
In vivo synthesis: [n.a.]
In vivo catabolism: [n.a.]

Evaluation of isolated patient fibrinogen
Thrombin time: [Abnormal[1]]
Reptilase time: [n.a.]
Ancrod (Arvin) time: [n.a.]

Abnormal subunit? [No]
Abnormal FDPs? [n.a.]

Remarks
[1]Data not reported.

References

1. Fernández, J., Rodriguez Pinto, C., Rocha, E., Fernández Urgelles, M., Páramo, J.A. and Romo, M. Fibrinogens Oviedo I, Oviedo II and Oviedo III: three new cases of dysfibrinogenemia with abnormal fibrin aggregation. *Thromb. Haemostas.* **54**:159, **1985**. ABSTRACT

FIBRINOGEN OVIEDO III[Abs]

Last update [1 December 1990]
Alphacode [OVIEDO03]
Ref. type [Abstract]

Structural defect [n.a.]
Mutation [n.a.]

Family studies
Homozygote? [n.a.]
Pedigree published? [No]

Functional defect(s)
FpA release: [Normal]
FpB release: [Normal]
Polymerization: [Abnormal]
Stabilization: [Normal]

Clinical manifestation(s) Bleeding? [No] Thrombosis? [No]

Clinical laboratory results

Plasma fibrinogen concentration (mg/dL)
Chronometric: [Subnormal[1]]
Rate-indep'nt: [n.a.]
Immunologic: [Normal[1]]

*Hypo*dysfibrinogen? [No]

Thrombin time:	[Abnormal[1]]
Reptilase (batroxobin) time:	[Abnormal[1]]
Prothrombin time:	[n.a.]
Partial thromboplastin time:	[n.a.]
Euglobulin lysis time:	[n.a.]
Bleeding time:	[n.a.]
Immunoelectrophoresis:	[Normal]
Platelet aggregation:	[n.a.]

Other results with patient plasma
Ancrod (Arvin) time: [n.a.]
Recalcification time: [n.a.]
Calcium corrects c.t.? [Yes]

Inhib. normal plasma? [Yes]
In vivo synthesis: [n.a.]
In vivo catabolism: [n.a.]

Evaluation of isolated patient fibrinogen
Thrombin time: [Abnormal[1]]
Reptilase time: [n.a.]
Ancrod (Arvin) time: [n.a.]

Abnormal subunit? [No]
Abnormal FDPs? [n.a.]

Remarks
[1]Data not reported.

References

1. Fernández, J., Rodriguez Pinto, C., Rocha, E., Fernández Urgelles, M., Páramo, J.A. and Romo, M. Fibrinogens Oviedo I, Oviedo II and Oviedo III: three new cases of dysfibrinogenemia with abnormal fibrin aggregation. *Thromb. Haemostas.* **54**:159, **1985**. ABSTRACT

FIBRINOGEN PAMPLONA I

Last update [1 December 1990]
Alphacode [PAMPLO01]
Ref. type [Article]

Family studies
Homozygote? [No]
Pedigree published? [Yes]

Structural defect [n.a.]
Mutation [n.a.]

Functional defect(s)
FpA release: [n.a.]
FpB release: [n.a.]
Polymerization: [Abnormal]
Stabilization: [Normal]

Clinical manifestation(s) Bleeding? [No] Thrombosis? [No]

Clinical laboratory results
Plasma fibrinogen concentration (mg/dL)
Chronometric: [n.a.]
Rate-indep'nt: [124/(200-400)]
Immunologic: [200/(200-400)]

*Hypo*dysfibrinogen? [No]

Thrombin time:	[75s/(18-20s)]
Reptilase (batroxobin) time:	[72s/(15-18s)]
Prothrombin time:	[17s/(11-13s)]
Partial thromboplastin time:	[58s/(35-45s)]
Euglobulin lysis time:	[>180m/(>180m)]
Bleeding time:	[Normal]
Immunoelectrophoresis:	[Cathodal]
Platelet aggregation:	[Normal]

Other results with patient plasma
Ancrod (Arvin) time: [n.a.]
Recalcification time: [n.a.]
Calcium corrects c.t.? [n.a.]

Inhib. normal plasma? [Yes]
In vivo synthesis: [n.a.]
In vivo catabolism: [n.a.]

Evaluation of isolated patient fibrinogen
Thrombin time: [180s/(15-20s)]
Reptilase time: [n.a.]
Ancrod (Arvin) time: [n.a.]

Abnormal subunit? [No]
Abnormal FDPs? [No[1]]

Remarks
[1]A reduced *rate* of FDP formation was reported.

References

1. Gastearena, J., Rocha, E., Orue, M.T., Narvaiza, M.J., Perez Equiza, E. and Fernández, J. [Fibrinogen Pamplona. A new molecular variant]. *Sangre (Barc.)* **26**:575-587, **1981**.

FIBRINOGEN PAMPLONA II

Last update	[1 December 1990]	**Structural defect**	[n.a.]
Alphacode	[PAMPLO02]	**Mutation**	[n.a.]
Ref. type	[Article]		

Family studies
Homozygote? [No[1]]
Pedigree published? [No]

Functional defect(s)
FpA release: [Normal]
FpB release: [Abnormal[1]]
Polymerization: [Abnormal]
Stabilization: [Normal]

Clinical manifestation(s) Bleeding? [No] Thrombosis? [Yes[2]]

Clinical laboratory results

Plasma fibrinogen concentration (mg/dL)
Chronometric: [145/(200-400)]
Rate-indep'nt: [340/(200-400)]
Immunologic: [310/(200-400)]

*Hypo*dysfibrinogen? [No]

Thrombin time:	[63s/(18-20s)]
Reptilase (batroxobin) time:	[13s/(15-18s)]
Prothrombin time:	[15s/(11-13s)]
Partial thromboplastin time:	[40s/(35-40s)]
Euglobulin lysis time:	[200m/(>180m)]
Bleeding time:	[Normal[1]]
Immunoelectrophoresis:	[Normal[1]]
Platelet aggregation:	[Normal[1]]

Other results with patient plasma

Ancrod (Arvin) time:	[n.a.]	Inhib. normal plasma?	[No[1]]
Recalcification time:	[n.a.]	In vivo synthesis:	[n.a.]
Calcium corrects c.t.?	[Yes[1]]	In vivo catabolism:	[n.a.]

Evaluation of isolated patient fibrinogen

Thrombin time:	[n.a.[3]]	Abnormal subunit?	[No]
Reptilase time:	[n.a.]	Abnormal FDPs?	[No]
Ancrod (Arvin) time:	[n.a.]		

Remarks
[1]F.J. Fernández, personal communication.
[2]Bilateral deep vein thrombosis in the proposita was reported.
[3]Reduced binding of thrombin to fibrin was reported.

References

1. Fernández, J., Páramo, J.A., Cuesta, B., Aranda, A. and Rocha, E. Fibrinogen Pamplona II. A new congenital dysfibrinogenemia with abnormal fibrin-enhanced plasminogen activation and defective binding of thrombin to fibrin. In: *Fibrinogen and Its Derivatives. Biochemistry, Physiology and Pathophysiology*, G. Müller-Berghaus, U. Scheefers-Borchel, E. Selmayr and A. Henschen (eds.), Excerpta Medica, Amsterdam. pp. 25-30, **1986**.

FIBRINOGEN PARIS I

Last update [10 January 1994]
Alphacode [PARIS01]
Ref. type [Article]

Family studies
Homozygote? [No]
Pedigree published? [No]

Structural defect [γ(351) Gly → Insertion[1]]
Mutation [GGT → GTT...[1]]

Functional defect(s)
FpA release: [Normal[2]]
FpB release: [Normal[2]]
Polymerization: [Abnormal]
Stabilization: [Abnormal]

Clinical manifestation(s) Bleeding? [No] Thrombosis? [No]

Clinical laboratory results
Plasma fibrinogen concentration (mg/dL)
Chronometric: [n.a.]
Rate-indep'nt: [n.a.]
Immunologic: [n.a.]

*Hypo*dysfibrinogen? [n.a.]

Thrombin time:	[No clot]
Reptilase (batroxobin) time:	[40s/(18s)]
Prothrombin time:	[No clot]
Partial thromboplastin time:	[n.a.]
Euglobulin lysis time:	[n.a.]
Bleeding time:	[Normal]
Immunoelectrophoresis:	[Normal]
Platelet aggregation:	[n.a.]

Other results with patient plasma
Ancrod (Arvin) time: [n.a.]
Recalcification time: [150s/(150s)]
Calcium corrects c.t.? [No[3]]

Inhib. normal plasma? [Yes]
In vivo synthesis: [n.a.]
In vivo catabolism: [n.a.]

Evaluation of isolated patient fibrinogen
Thrombin time: [150s/(15s)[3]]
Reptilase time: [n.a.]
Ancrod (Arvin) time: [n.a.]

Abnormal subunit? [Yes[4]]
Abnormal FDPs? [Yes[5]]

Remarks

[1]A 45 bp fragment inserted between exons 8 and 9 encodes a 15 amino acid insert between γ(350) Gln and γ(351) Gly — with the following sequence: Val-Met-Cys-Gly-Glu-Ala-Leu-Pro-Met-Leu-Lys-Asp-Pro-Cys-Tyr. Alternative mRNA splicing yields a γ(351) Gly → Ser substitution at $\gamma_{\text{Paris I}}$ (365), the point at which the original sequence resumes. The structural defect was determined with the PCR method.

[2]The rate of *total* fibrinopeptide release was normal.

[3]Calcium was required to obtain a clot in the presence of thrombin.

[4]The γ-chains were about 2,500 Da larger than normal.

[5]An abnormal fragment D was reported.

FIBRINOGEN PARIS I

References

1. Rosenberg, J.B., Newman, P.J., Mosesson, M.W., Guillin, M.-C. and Amrani, D.L. Paris I dysfibrinogenemia: a point mutation in intron 8 results in insertion of a 15 amino acid sequence in the fibrinogen γ-chain. *Thromb. Haemost.* **69**:217-220, **1993**.

2. Finlayson, J.S., Reamer, L.A., Mosesson, M.W. and Ménaché, D. Fibrinopeptide release from fibrinogen Paris I. *Thromb. Res.* **17**:577-579, **1980**.

3. Mosesson, M.W., Feldmann, G. and Ménaché, D. Electron microscopy of fibrin Paris I. *Blood* **56**:80-83, **1980**.

4. Jandrot-Perrus, M., Mosesson, M.W., Denninger, M.H. and Ménaché, D. Studies of platelet fibrinogen from a subject with a congenital plasma fibrinogen abnormality (fibrinogen Paris I). *Blood* **54**:1109-1116, **1979**.

5. Hawiger, J., Hammond, D.K., Timmons, S. and Budzynski, A.Z. Interaction of human fibrinogen with Staphylococci: presence of a binding region on normal and abnormal fibrinogen variants and fibrinogen derivatives. *Blood* **51**:799-812, **1978**.

6. Budzynski, A.Z. and Marder, V.J. Plasmic degradation of fibrinogen Paris I. *J. Lab. Clin. Med.* **88**:817-825, **1976**.

7. Mosesson, M.W., Denninger, M.H. and Ménaché, D. Hydrolysis of fibrinogen Paris I by plasmin. *Thromb. Res.* **9**:115-121, **1976**.

8. Mosesson, M.W., Amrani, D.L. and Ménaché, D. Studies on the structural abnormality of fibrinogen Paris I. *J. Clin. Invest.* **57**:782-790, **1976**.

9. Budzynski, A.Z., Marder, V.J., Ménaché, D. and Guillin, M.C. Proceedings: Structural abnormality in the γ polypeptide chain of Paris I fibrinogen. *Thromb. Diath. Haemorrh.* **34**:329, **1975**. ABSTRACT

10. Budzynski, A.Z., Marder, V.J., Ménaché, D. and Guillin, M.C. Defect in the γ polypeptide chain of a congenital abnormal fibrinogen (Paris I). *Nature* **252**:66-68, **1974**.

11. Guillin, M.-C. and Ménaché, D. Fetal fibrinogen and fibrinogen Paris I: comparative fibrin monomers aggregation studies. *Thromb. Res.* **3**:117-135, **1973**.

12. Mester, L. and Szabados, L. Differences constitutionneles et fonctionnelles entre les fragments glucidiques du fibrinogene humain normal et d'un fibrinogene humaine anormal. *Bull. Soc. Chim. Biol.* **50**:2561-2566, **1968**.

13. Ménaché, D. Constitutional and familial abnormal fibrinogen. *Thromb. Diath. Haemorrh.* **Suppl. 13**:173-185, **1964**.

14. Ménaché, D. Dysfibrinogenemie constitutionnelle at familiale. In: *Proc. 9th Congr. Europ. Soc. Haemat., Lisbon 1963*, R. Fauvert and J.P. Soulier (eds.). S. Karger, New York; pp. 1255-1259, **1963**.

FIBRINOGEN PARIS II

Last update [1 December 1990]
Alphacode [PARIS02]
Ref. type [Article]

Family studies
Homozygote? [n.a.]
Pedigree published? [Yes]

Structural defect [n.a.]
Mutation [n.a.]

Functional defect(s)
FpA release: [Normal[1]]
FpB release: [Normal[1]]
Polymerization: [Abnormal]
Stabilization: [n.a.]

Clinical manifestation(s) Bleeding? [No] Thrombosis? [Yes[2]]

Clinical laboratory results
Plasma fibrinogen concentration (mg/dL)
Chronometric: [90[3]]
Rate-indep'nt: [270[3]]
Immunologic: [300[3]]

*Hypo*dysfibrinogen? [No]

Thrombin time:	[85s/(20s)[4]]
Reptilase (batroxobin) time:	[60s/(18s)]
Prothrombin time:	[18s/(12s)]
Partial thromboplastin time:	[n.a.]
Euglobulin lysis time:	[n.a.]
Bleeding time:	[Normal]
Immunoelectrophoresis:	[Normal]
Platelet aggregation:	[n.a.]

Other results with patient plasma
Ancrod (Arvin) time: [180s/(4s)]
Recalcification time: [n.a.]
Calcium corrects c.t.? [No]

Inhib. normal plasma? [No]
In vivo synthesis: [n.a.]
In vivo catabolism: [n.a.]

Evaluation of isolated patient fibrinogen
Thrombin time: [n.a.[4]]
Reptilase time: [n.a.]
Ancrod (Arvin) time: [n.a.]

Abnormal subunit? [n.a.]
Abnormal FDPs? [n.a.]

Remarks
[1]The rate of *total* fibrinopeptide release was normal.
[2]F. Haverkate, personal communication.
[3]Normal range not reported.
[4]The thrombin time was unusually dependent on pH.

References

1. Corrihons, G., Soria, J., Soria, C., Conard, J., Horellou, M.H. and Samama, M. [Congenital dysfibrinogenemia. Apropos of 13 cases]. *Sem. Hop. Paris* **59**:2517-2523, **1983**.

2. Samama, M., Soria, J., Soria, C. and Bousser, J. [Congenital and familial dysfibrinogenemia without hemorrhagic tendency]. *Nouv. Rev. Fr. Hematol.* **9**:817-832, **1969**.

FIBRINOGEN PARIS III

Last update [1 December 1990]
Alphacode [PARIS03]
Ref. type [Article]

Family studies
Homozygote? [n.a.]
Pedigree published? [No]

Structural defect [n.a.]
Mutation [n.a.]

Functional defect(s)
FpA release: [Normal[1]]
FpB release: [Normal[1]]
Polymerization: [Abnormal]
Stabilization: [Normal]

Clinical manifestation(s) Bleeding? [No] Thrombosis? [No]

Clinical laboratory results
Plasma fibrinogen concentration (mg/dL)
Chronometric: [240/(250-400)]
Rate-indep'nt: [300/(250-400)]
Immunologic: [300/(250-400)]

*Hypo*dysfibrinogen? [No]

Thrombin time:	[50s/(20s)]
Reptilase (batroxobin) time:	[45s/(18s)]
Prothrombin time:	[15s/(12s)]
Partial thromboplastin time:	[n.a.]
Euglobulin lysis time:	[>3h/(>3h)]
Bleeding time:	[Normal]
Immunoelectrophoresis:	[Normal]
Platelet aggregation:	[Normal]

Other results with patient plasma
Ancrod (Arvin) time: [n.a.]
Recalcification time: [n.a.]
Calcium corrects c.t.? [n.a.]

Inhib. normal plasma? [n.a.]
In vivo synthesis: [n.a.]
In vivo catabolism: [n.a.]

Evaluation of isolated patient fibrinogen
Thrombin time: [n.a.]
Reptilase time: [n.a.]
Ancrod (Arvin) time: [n.a.]

Abnormal subunit? [No]
Abnormal FDPs? [No]

Remarks
[1]The rate of *total* fibrinopeptide release was normal.

References

1. Haverkate, F., Timan, G., Soria, J., Soria, C. and Samama, M.M. Studies on the structure of the fragment D moiety of abnormal fibrinogens: influence of calcium ions. *Thromb. Res.* **13**:689-692, **1978**.

2. Soria, J. and Soria, C. [Familial dysfibrinogenemia with abnormal monomer aggregation Paris III fibrinogen]. *Pathol. Biol. (Paris)* **22**:72-79, **1974**.

FIBRINOGEN PARIS IV

Last update [1 December 1990]
Alphacode [PARIS04]
Ref. type [Article]

Family studies
Homozygote? [n.a.]
Pedigree published? [No]

Structural defect [n.a.]
Mutation [n.a.]

Functional defect(s)
FpA release: [n.a.]
FpB release: [n.a.]
Polymerization: [Abnormal]
Stabilization: [n.a.]

Clinical manifestation(s) Bleeding? [No] Thrombosis? [No]

Clinical laboratory results
Plasma fibrinogen concentration (mg/dL)
Chronometric: [55/(200-450)]
Rate-indep'nt: [315/(200-450)]
Immunologic: [300/(200-450)]

*Hypo*dysfibrinogen? [No]

Thrombin time:	[72s/(18-29s)]
Reptilase (batroxobin) time:	[45s/(18-22s)]
Prothrombin time:	[50%]
Partial thromboplastin time:	[n.a.]
Euglobulin lysis time:	[n.a.]
Bleeding time:	[Normal]
Immunoelectrophoresis:	[n.a.]
Platelet aggregation:	[n.a.]

Other results with patient plasma
Ancrod (Arvin) time: [n.a.]
Recalcification time: [n.a.]
Calcium corrects c.t.? [n.a.]

Inhib. normal plasma? [No]
In vivo synthesis: [n.a.]
In vivo catabolism: [n.a.]

Evaluation of isolated patient fibrinogen
Thrombin time: [n.a.]
Reptilase time: [n.a.]
Ancrod (Arvin) time: [n.a.]

Abnormal subunit? [n.a.]
Abnormal FDPs? [No]

Remarks

References

1. Corrihons, G., Soria, J., Soria, C., Conard, J., Horellou, M.H. and Samama, M. [Congenital dysfibrinogenemia. Apropos of 13 cases]. *Sem. Hop. Paris* **59**:2517-2523, **1983**.

2. Amsellem, M., Samama, M., Conard, J., Levyne, S. and Ohlgiesser, C. [Congenital dysfibrinogenaemia. Two new cases]. *Nouv. Presse Med.* **7**:3745-3748, **1978**.

3. Haverkate, F., Timan, G., Soria, J., Soria, C. and Samama, M.M. Studies on the structure of the fragment D moiety of abnormal fibrinogens: influence of calcium ions. *Thromb. Res.* **13**:689-692, **1978**.

FIBRINOGEN *PARIS V*[1]

Last update [*10 January 1994*]
Alphacode [*PARIS05*]
Ref. type [*Article*]

Family studies
Homozygote? [*No*]
Pedigree published? [*Yes*]

Structural defect [*Aα(554) Arg → Cys*[2]]
Mutation [*CGT → TGT*]

Functional defect(s)
FpA release: [*Normal*[3]]
FpB release: [*Normal*[3]]
Polymerization: [*Abnormal*]
Stabilization: [*Normal*]

Clinical manifestation(s) Bleeding? [*No*] Thrombosis? [*Yes*[4]]

Clinical laboratory results
Plasma fibrinogen concentration (mg/dL)
Chronometric: [*165/(200-400)*]
Rate-indep'nt: [*n.a.*]
Immunologic: [*190/(200-400)*]

*Hypo*dysfibrinogen? [*No*]

Thrombin time:	[*35s/(20s)*]
Reptilase (batroxobin) time:	[*29.5s/(20s)*]
Prothrombin time:	[*17.5s/(12s)*]
Partial thromboplastin time:	[*n.a.*]
Euglobulin lysis time:	[*n.a.*]
Bleeding time:	[*n.a.*]
Immunoelectrophoresis:	[*n.a.*]
Platelet aggregation:	[*Normal*]

Other results with patient plasma
Ancrod (Arvin) time: [*n.a.*]
Recalcification time: [*n.a.*]
Calcium corrects c.t.? [*n.a.*]

Inhib. normal plasma? [*n.a.*]
In vivo synthesis: [*n.a.*]
In vivo catabolism: [*n.a.*]

Evaluation of isolated patient fibrinogen
Thrombin time: [*22s/(12s)*]
Reptilase time: [*27s/(18s)*]
Ancrod (Arvin) time: [*n.a.*]

Abnormal subunit? [*No*]
Abnormal FDPs? [*No*[5]]

Remarks

Disulfide-linked fibrinogen-albumin complexes were reported.

[1]Also known as "DUSARD I," and "DUSART I." The preferred title is "DUSART I." Results are italicized to avoid duplication with DUSART I in summary tables. In violation of the usual naming conventions, this variant was named after the family in whom it was discovered.

[2]The structural defect was determined with the PCR method.

[3]The rate of *total* fibrinopeptide release was normal.

[4]Recurrent thrombophlebitis and fatal pulmonary embolism were reported. Caen (1990) reported recurrent pulmonary embolism despite anticoagulant therapy. Koopman et al. (1993) give a comprehensive family history.

[5]Defective lysis by plasmin, presumably due to a reduced rate of t-PA activation in the presence of the variant fibrin, was reported.

FIBRINOGEN *PARIS V*

References

1. Koopman, J., Haverkate, F., Grimbergen, J., Lord, S.T., Mosesson, M.W., DiOrio, J.P., Siebenlist, K.S., Legrand, C., Soria, J., Soria, C. and Caen, J.P. Molecular basis for fibrinogen Dusart (Aα 554 Arg→Cys) and its association with abnormal fibrin polymerization and thrombophilia. *J. Clin. Invest.* **91**:1637-1643, **1993**.

2. Siebenlist, K.R., Mosesson, M.W., DiOrio, J.P., Soria, J., Soria, C. and Caen, J.P. The polymerization of fibrinogen Dusart (Aα 554 Arg → Cys) after removal of carboxy terminal regions of the Aα-chains. *Blood Coag. & Fibrinol.* **4**:61-65, **1993**.

3. Caen, J. Dusard syndrome in 1990. *Proc. X Intl. Fgen. Wkshp.*, **1990** ABSTRACT.

4. Soria, C., Soria, J., Mirshahi, M., Desvignes, P., Bonnet, P. and Caen, J.P. [Importance of the structure of the clot in thrombolysis]. *Ann. Biol. Clin. (Paris)* **45**:207-211, **1987**.

5. Lijnen, H.R., Soria, J., Soria, C., Collen, D. and Caen, J.P. Dysfibrinogenemia (fibrinogen Dusard) associated with impaired fibrin-enhanced plasminogen activation. *Thromb. Haemostas.* **51**:108-109, **1984**.

6. Soria, J., Soria, C. and Caen, P. A new type of congenital dysfibrinogenaemia with defective fibrin lysis — Dusard syndrome: possible relation to thrombosis. *Br. J. Haematol.* **53**:575-586, **1983**.

7. Caen, J.P., Soria, J. and Soria, C. [Structural anomaly of the fibrin clot with reduction of lys-plasminogen binding, as a cause of familial thrombosis]. *C. R. Seances. Acad. Sci. [III]* **294**:695-697, **1982**.

FIBRINOGEN PARIS VI

Last update	[1 December 1990]	**Structural defect**	[Aα(16) Arg → His[1]]
Alphacode	[PARIS06]	**Mutation**	[n.a.]
Ref. type	[Article]		

Functional defect(s)

FpA release:	[n.a.[2]]
FpB release:	[n.a.[2]]
Polymerization:	[n.a.[2]]
Stabilization:	[n.a.]

Family studies

Homozygote?	[No]
Pedigree published?	[No]

Clinical manifestation(s) Bleeding? [n.a.] Thrombosis? [n.a.]

Clinical laboratory results

Plasma fibrinogen concentration (mg/dL)

Chronometric:	[n.a.]
Rate-indep'nt:	[250[3]]
Immunologic:	[n.a.]

*Hypo*dysfibrinogen? [No]

Thrombin time:	[54s/(20s)]
Reptilase (batroxobin) time:	[60s/(22s)]
Prothrombin time:	[n.a.]
Partial thromboplastin time:	[n.a.]
Euglobulin lysis time:	[n.a.]
Bleeding time:	[n.a.]
Immunoelectrophoresis:	[n.a.]
Platelet aggregation:	[n.a.]

Other results with patient plasma

Ancrod (Arvin) time:	[n.a.]	Inhib. normal plasma?	[n.a.]
Recalcification time:	[n.a.]	In vivo synthesis:	[n.a.]
Calcium corrects c.t.?	[n.a.]	In vivo catabolism:	[n.a.]

Evaluation of isolated patient fibrinogen

Thrombin time:	[n.a.]	Abnormal subunit?	[n.a.]
Reptilase time:	[n.a.]	Abnormal FDPs?	[n.a.]
Ancrod (Arvin) time:	[n.a.]		

Remarks

[1]This substitution was inferred from the fibrinopeptide A elution position on RP-HPLC.

[2]Rates of fibrinopeptide release and fibrin monomer polymerization were not reported. Other dysfibrinogens with this molecular defect exhibit delayed fibrinopeptide A and B release plus delayed polymerization of fibrin monomers.

[3]Normal range not reported.

References

1. Southan, C., Thompson, E. and Lane, D.A. Direct analysis of plasma fibrinogen-derived fibrinopeptides by high-performance liquid chromatography: investigation of nine congenital fibrinogen abnormalities. *Br. J. Haematol.* **65**:469-473, **1987**.

2. Corrihons, G., Soria, J., Soria, C., Conard, J., Horellou, M.H. and Samama, M. [Congenital dysfibrinogenemia. Apropos of 13 cases]. *Sem. Hop. Paris* **59**:2517-2523, **1983**.

FIBRINOGEN PARMA I

Last update [10 January 1994]
Alphacode [PARMA01]
Ref. type [Article]

Family studies
Homozygote? [n.a.]
Pedigree published? [Yes]

Structural defect [n.a.]
Mutation [n.a.]

Functional defect(s)
FpA release: [n.a.]
FpB release: [n.a.]
Polymerization: [n.a.]
Stabilization: [n.a.]

Clinical manifestation(s) Bleeding? [Yes] Thrombosis? [No]

Clinical laboratory results
Plasma fibrinogen concentration (mg/dL)
Chronometric: [n.a.]
Rate-indep'nt: [60[1]]
Immunologic: [n.a.]

*Hypo*dysfibrinogen? [Yes]

Thrombin time:	[n.a.]
Reptilase (batroxobin) time:	[n.a.]
Prothrombin time:	[28s/(16s)]
Partial thromboplastin time:	[n.a.]
Euglobulin lysis time:	[n.a.]
Bleeding time:	[Normal]
Immunoelectrophoresis:	[n.a.]
Platelet aggregation:	[Normal]

Other results with patient plasma
Ancrod (Arvin) time: [n.a.]
Recalcification time: [180s/(100-120s)]
Calcium corrects c.t.? [n.a.]

Inhib. normal plasma? [n.a.]
In vivo synthesis: [Decreased]
In vivo catabolism: [Normal]

Evaluation of isolated patient fibrinogen
Thrombin time: [n.a.]
Reptilase time: [n.a.]
Ancrod (Arvin) time: [n.a.]

Abnormal subunit? [n.a.]
Abnormal FDPs? [n.a.]

Remarks
[1]Normal range not reported.

This is the first reported case of dysfibrinogenemia. Initially, it was thought to be a case of hypofibrinogenemia; it now appears to represent an example of hypodysfibrinogenemia.

References

1. Imperato, C. and Dettori, A.G. Ipofibrinogenemia congenita con fibroastenia. *Helvet. Paediat. Acta* **13**:380-399, **1958**.

FIBRINOGEN PERUGIA I

Last update [1 December 1990]
Alphacode [PERUGI01]
Ref. type [Article]

Structural defect [γ(275) Arg → His]
Mutation [n.a.]

Family studies
Homozygote? [No]
Pedigree published? [No]

Functional defect(s)
FpA release: [Normal]
FpB release: [Normal]
Polymerization: [Abnormal]
Stabilization: [n.a.]

Clinical manifestation(s) Bleeding? [No] Thrombosis? [No]

Clinical laboratory results
Plasma fibrinogen concentration (mg/dL)
Chronometric: [28/(200)]
Rate-indep'nt: [150/(200)]
Immunologic: [150/(200)]

*Hypo*dysfibrinogen? [No]

Thrombin time:	[26.1s/(12.5s)]
Reptilase (batroxobin) time:	[31.6s/(17.6s)]
Prothrombin time:	[n.a.]
Partial thromboplastin time:	[n.a.]
Euglobulin lysis time:	[n.a.]
Bleeding time:	[n.a.]
Immunoelectrophoresis:	[n.a.]
Platelet aggregation:	[n.a.]

Other results with patient plasma
Ancrod (Arvin) time: [n.a.]
Recalcification time: [n.a.]
Calcium corrects c.t.? [n.a.]

Inhib. normal plasma? [n.a.]
In vivo synthesis: [n.a.]
In vivo catabolism: [n.a.]

Evaluation of isolated patient fibrinogen
Thrombin time: [n.a.]
Reptilase time: [n.a.]
Ancrod (Arvin) time: [n.a.]

Abnormal subunit? [n.a.]
Abnormal FDPs? [n.a.]

Remarks

References

1. Reber, P., Furlan, M., Henschen, A. and Beck, E.A. Three new fibrinogen variants with defective polymerization site in the γ-chain. In: *Fibrinogen and Its Derivatives. Biochemistry, Physiology and Pathophysiology*, G. Muller-Berghaus, U. Scheefers-Borchel, E. Selmayr and A. Henschen (eds.), Excerpta Medica, Amsterdam. pp. 41-42, **1986**.

2. Reber, P., Furlan, M., Henschen, A., Kaudewitz, H., Barbui, T., Hilgard, P., Nenci, G.G., Berrettini, M. and Beck, E.A. Three abnormal fibrinogen variants with the same amino acid substitution (γ-275 Arg → His): fibrinogens Bergamo II, Essen and Perugia. *Thromb. Haemostas.* **56**:401-406, **1986**.

FIBRINOGEN PETOSKEY I

Last update [1 December 1990]
Alphacode [PETOSK01]
Ref. type [Article]

Structural defect [Aα(16) Arg → His[1]]
Mutation [n.a.]

Family studies
Homozygote? [No]
Pedigree published? [Yes]

Functional defect(s)
FpA release: [Abnormal]
FpB release: [Abnormal]
Polymerization: [Abnormal]
Stabilization: [Normal]

Clinical manifestation(s) Bleeding? [No] Thrombosis? [No]

Clinical laboratory results
Plasma fibrinogen concentration (mg/dL)
Chronometric: [96/(>200)]
Rate-indep'nt: [298/(>200)]
Immunologic: [n.a.]

*Hypo*dysfibrinogen? [No]

Thrombin time:	[13.6s/(8-9s)]
Reptilase (batroxobin) time:	[n.a.]
Prothrombin time:	[11s/(13s)]
Partial thromboplastin time:	[30.1s/(35s)]
Euglobulin lysis time:	[n.a.]
Bleeding time:	[n.a.]
Immunoelectrophoresis:	[n.a.]
Platelet aggregation:	[n.a.]

Other results with patient plasma
Ancrod (Arvin) time: [n.a.]
Recalcification time: [n.a.]
Calcium corrects c.t.? [n.a.]

Inhib. normal plasma? [No]
In vivo synthesis: [n.a.]
In vivo catabolism: [n.a.]

Evaluation of isolated patient fibrinogen
Thrombin time: [n.a.]
Reptilase time: [Abnormal[2]]
Ancrod (Arvin) time: [n.a.]

Abnormal subunit? [No]
Abnormal FDPs? [No]

Remarks
[1]Fibrinogen Petoskey I was the first in which an Arg → His substitution was identified at Aα(16).
[2]Data not reported.

References

1. Higgins, D.L. and Shafer, J.A. Fibrinogen Petoskey, a dysfibrinogenemia characterized by replacement of Arg-Aα 16 by a histidyl residue. *J. Biol. Chem.* **256**:12013-12017, **1981**.

2. Higgins, D.L., Penner, J.A. and Shafer, J.A. Fibrinogen Petoskey: identification of a new dysfibrinogenemia characterized by altered release of fibrinopeptide A. *Thromb. Res.* **23**:491-504, **1981**.

FIBRINOGEN PHILADELPHIA I

Last update [1 December 1990]
Alphacode [PHILAD01]
Ref. type [Article]

Structural defect [n.a.]
Mutation [n.a.]

Family studies
Homozygote? [n.a.]
Pedigree published? [Yes]

Functional defect(s)
FpA release: [Normal[1]]
FpB release: [Normal[1]]
Polymerization: [Abnormal]
Stabilization: [n.a.]

Clinical manifestation(s) Bleeding? [Yes[2]] Thrombosis? [No]

Clinical laboratory results
Plasma fibrinogen concentration (mg/dL)
Chronometric: [73/(232-444)]
Rate-indep'nt: [78/(160-380)]
Immunologic: [78[3]]

*Hypo*dysfibrinogen? [Yes]

Thrombin time:	[83.6s/(18-22s)]
Reptilase (batroxobin) time:	[300s/(38.5s)]
Prothrombin time:	[16s/(11.5-13.5s)]
Partial thromboplastin time:	[76s/(45-90s)]
Euglobulin lysis time:	[120m/(>120m)]
Bleeding time:	[Normal]
Immunoelectrophoresis:	[Normal]
Platelet aggregation:	[n.a.]

Other results with patient plasma
Ancrod (Arvin) time: [n.a.]
Recalcification time: [n.a.]
Calcium corrects c.t.? [No]

Inhib. normal plasma? [Yes]
In vivo synthesis: [Normal[4]]
In vivo catabolism: [Increased]

Evaluation of isolated patient fibrinogen
Thrombin time: [n.a.]
Reptilase time: [n.a.]
Ancrod (Arvin) time: [n.a.]

Abnormal subunit? [No]
Abnormal FDPs? [n.a.]

Remarks
[1]The rate of *total* fibrinopeptide release was normal.
[2]Excessive bleeding after surgery, trauma, or dental extraction in the 46 year-old proposita was reported.
[3]Normal range not reported.
[4]Two affected patients were studied; one had a normal synthetic rate, the other's was slightly below normal.

References

1. Gralnick, H.R., Coller, B.S., Fratantoni, J.C. and Martinez, J. Fibrinogen Bethesda III: a hypodysfibrinogenemia. *Blood* **53**:28-46, **1979**.

2. Martinez, J., Holburn, R.R., Shapiro, S.S. and Erslev, A.J. Fibrinogen Philadelphia. A hereditary hypodysfibrinogenemia characterized by fibrinogen hypercatabolism. *J. Clin. Invest.* **53**:600-611, **1974**.

FIBRINOGEN PHILADELPHIA II

Last update [1 December 1990]
Alphacode [PHILAD02]
Ref. type [Article]

Family studies
Homozygote? [n.a.]
Pedigree published? [No]

Structural defect [n.a.]
Mutation [n.a.]

Functional defect(s)
FpA release: [n.a.[1]]
FpB release: [n.a.[1]]
Polymerization: [n.a.]
Stabilization: [n.a.]

Clinical manifestation(s) Bleeding? [n.a.] Thrombosis? [n.a.]

Clinical laboratory results
Plasma fibrinogen concentration (mg/dL)
Chronometric: [n.a.]
Rate-indep'nt: [n.a.]
Immunologic: [n.a.]

*Hypo*dysfibrinogen? [n.a.]

Thrombin time:	[n.a.]
Reptilase (batroxobin) time:	[n.a.]
Prothrombin time:	[n.a.]
Partial thromboplastin time:	[n.a.]
Euglobulin lysis time:	[n.a.]
Bleeding time:	[n.a.]
Immunoelectrophoresis:	[n.a.]
Platelet aggregation:	[n.a.]

Other results with patient plasma
Ancrod (Arvin) time: [n.a.]
Recalcification time: [n.a.]
Calcium corrects c.t.? [n.a.]

Inhib. normal plasma? [n.a.]
In vivo synthesis: [n.a.]
In vivo catabolism: [n.a.]

Evaluation of isolated patient fibrinogen
Thrombin time: [n.a.]
Reptilase time: [n.a.]
Ancrod (Arvin) time: [n.a.]

Abnormal subunit? [n.a.]
Abnormal FDPs? [n.a.]

Remarks
[1]Normal amounts of each fibrinopeptide were released; their mobility on RP-HPLC also was normal. Rates of fibrinopeptide release were not determined.

References

1. Henschen, A., Kehl, M., Southan, C., Lottspeich, F. and Georgopoulos, D. Genetically abnormal fibrinogens — some current characterisation strategies. In: *Fibrinogen —Structure, Functional Aspects, Metabolism*, F. Haverkate, A. Henschen, W. Nieuwenhuizen and P.W. Straub (eds.), Walter de Gruyter, Berlin. pp. 125-144, **1983**.

FIBRINOGEN POITIERS I

Last update [1 December 1990]
Alphacode [POITIE01]
Ref. type [Article]

Structural defect [n.a.]
Mutation [n.a.]

Family studies

Homozygote?	[n.a.]
Pedigree published?	[Yes]

Functional defect(s)

FpA release:	[Abnormal]
FpB release:	[n.a.]
Polymerization:	[n.a.]
Stabilization:	[n.a.]

Clinical manifestation(s) Bleeding? [No] Thrombosis? [Yes[1]]

Clinical laboratory results

Plasma fibrinogen concentration (mg/dL)

Chronometric:	[100/(150-300)]
Rate-indep'nt:	[500/(150-300)]
Immunologic:	[n.a.]

*Hypo*dysfibrinogen? [No]

Thrombin time:	[105s/(18-20s)]
Reptilase (batroxobin) time:	[60s/(18-25s)]
Prothrombin time:	[13.9s/(11-13s)]
Partial thromboplastin time:	[60s/(28-32s)]
Euglobulin lysis time:	[n.a.]
Bleeding time:	[n.a.]
Immunoelectrophoresis:	[n.a.]
Platelet aggregation:	[Normal]

Other results with patient plasma

Ancrod (Arvin) time:	[n.a.]	Inhib. normal plasma?	[n.a.]
Recalcification time:	[n.a.]	In vivo synthesis:	[n.a.]
Calcium corrects c.t.?	[No]	In vivo catabolism:	[n.a.]

Evaluation of isolated patient fibrinogen

Thrombin time:	[>500s/(45s)[3]]	Abnormal subunit?	[n.a.]
Reptilase time:	[>500s/(58s)]	Abnormal FDPs?	[Yes[2]]
Ancrod (Arvin) time:	[n.a.]		

Remarks

[1]The propositus died following infection and cerebrovascular accident at age 49 yrs. This is the first report of combined dysfibrinogenemia and protein C deficiency (Compare with fibrinogen Argenteuil I).

[2]A reduced *rate* of FDP formation was reported.

[3]Reduced binding of thrombin to fibrin was reported.

References

1. Gandrille, S., Priollet, P., Capron, L., Roncato, M., Fiessinger, J.N. and Aiach, M. Association of inherited dysfibrinogenaemia and protein C deficiency in two unrelated families. *Brit. J. Haematol.* **68**:329-337, **1988**.

FIBRINOGEN PONTOISE I

Last update	[10 January 1994]	**Structural defect**	[Bβ(335) Ala → Thr[1]]
Alphacode	[PONTOI01]	**Mutation**	[n.a.]
Ref. type	[Article]		

Family studies
Homozygote? [No]
Pedigree published? [No]

Functional defect(s)
FpA release: [Normal]
FpB release: [Normal]
Polymerization: [Abnormal]
Stabilization: [Normal]

Clinical manifestation(s) Bleeding? [n.a.] Thrombosis? [n.a.]

Clinical laboratory results
Plasma fibrinogen concentration (mg/dL)
Chronometric: [n.a.]
Rate-indep'nt: [n.a.]
Immunologic: [n.a.]

*Hypo*dysfibrinogen? [n.a.]

Thrombin time:	[88s/(20s)]
Reptilase (batroxobin) time:	[n.a.]
Prothrombin time:	[n.a.]
Partial thromboplastin time:	[n.a.]
Euglobulin lysis time:	[n.a.]
Bleeding time:	[n.a.]
Immunoelectrophoresis:	[n.a.]
Platelet aggregation:	[n.a.]

Other results with patient plasma

Ancrod (Arvin) time:	[n.a.]	Inhib. normal plasma?	[n.a.]
Recalcification time:	[n.a.]	In vivo synthesis:	[n.a.]
Calcium corrects c.t.?	[n.a.]	In vivo catabolism:	[n.a.]

Evaluation of isolated patient fibrinogen

Thrombin time:	[n.a.]	Abnormal subunit?	[Yes[2]]
Reptilase time:	[n.a.]	Abnormal FDPs?	[Yes[3]]
Ancrod (Arvin) time:	[n.a.]		

Remarks
[1]This substitution yields a new glycosylation site. Carbohydrate at this site accounts for the increased (3,000 Da) m.w. of the Bβ-chain and FDP's derived therefrom. See also ASAHI I CARACAS II, and LIMA I.
[2]An abnormal Bβ-chain was detected by RP-HPLC.
[3]Fragment D with a higher-than-normal m.w. was reported.

References

1. Kaudewitz, H., Henschen, A., Soria, J. and Soria, C. Fibrinogen Pontoise — a genetically abnormal fibrinogen with defective fibrin polymerisation but normal fibrinopeptide release. In: *Fibrinogen, Fibrin Formation and Fibrinolysis*, D.A. Lane, A. Henschen and M.K. Jasani (eds.), W. de Gruyter, Berlin. pp. 91-96, **1986**.

2. Henschen, A., Kehl, M., Southan, C., Lottspeich, F. and Georgopoulos, D. Genetically abnormal fibrinogens — some current characterisation strategies. In: *Fibrinogen —Structure, Functional Aspects, Metabolism*, F. Haverkate, A. Henschen, W. Nieuwenhuizen and P.W. Straub (eds.), Walter de Gruyter, Berlin. pp. 125-144, **1983**.

3. Haverkate, F., Timan, G., Soria, J., Soria, C. and Samama, M.M. Studies on the structure of the fragment D moiety of abnormal fibrinogens: Influence of calcium ions. *Thromb. Res.* **13**:689-692, **1978**.

FIBRINOGEN PRAHRAN I[1]

Last update [1 December 1990]
Alphacode [PRAHRA01]
Ref. type [Article]

Family studies
Homozygote? [n.a.]
Pedigree published? [No]

Structural defect [n.a.]
Mutation [n.a.]

Functional defect(s)
FpA release: [n.a.]
FpB release: [n.a.]
Polymerization: [n.a.]
Stabilization: [n.a.]

Clinical manifestation(s) Bleeding? [Yes[2]] Thrombosis? [No[2]]

Clinical laboratory results
Plasma fibrinogen concentration (mg/dL)
Chronometric: [n.a.]
Rate-indep'nt: [85/(246-550)] *Hypo*dysfibrinogen? [Yes]
Immunologic: [n.a.]

Thrombin time:	[114s/(4s)]
Reptilase (batroxobin) time:	[n.a.]
Prothrombin time:	[Normal[3]]
Partial thromboplastin time:	[Normal[3]]
Euglobulin lysis time:	[Abnormal[4]]
Bleeding time:	[n.a.]
Immunoelectrophoresis:	[Cathodal]
Platelet aggregation:	[n.a.]

Other results with patient plasma
Ancrod (Arvin) time: [n.a.]
Recalcification time: [Normal]
Calcium corrects c.t.? [n.a.]

Inhib. normal plasma? [No]
In vivo synthesis: [n.a.]
In vivo catabolism: [n.a.]

Evaluation of isolated patient fibrinogen
Thrombin time: [n.a.]
Reptilase time: [n.a.]
Ancrod (Arvin) time: [n.a.]

Abnormal subunit? [n.a.]
Abnormal FDPs? [n.a.]

Remarks
[1]Also known (incorrectly) as fibrinogen PARNHAM I [See Bithell, *Clin. Chem.* **31**:509, **1985**].
[2]Excessive post-surgical bleeding was reported. Excessive fibrinolysis (not corrected by Trasylol) also was reported. There was no excessive bleeding during prostatectomy when the patient was pre-treated with fibrinogen and ε-aminocaproic acid.
[3]Data not reported.
[4]Clot lysis was faster than normal.

References

1. Fantl, P. Hypofibrinogenemia with a possibly defective fibrinogen associated with fibrinolysis. *Aust. Ann. Med.* **18**:43, **1969**.

FIBRINOGEN QUEBEC I

Last update [10 January 1994]
Alphacode [QUEBEC01]
Ref. type [Article]

Structural defect [n.a.]
Mutation [n.a.]

Family studies
Homozygote? [n.a.]
Pedigree published? [No]

Functional defect(s)
FpA release: [Normal[1]]
FpB release: [Normal[1]]
Polymerization: [Abnormal]
Stabilization: [n.a.]

Clinical manifestation(s) Bleeding? [No] Thrombosis? [No]

Clinical laboratory results

Plasma fibrinogen concentration (mg/dL)
Chronometric: [174/(175-375)]
Rate-indep'nt: [265/(200-400)]
Immunologic: [254/(200-400)]

*Hypo*dysfibrinogen? [No]

Thrombin time:	[25s/(15-19s)]
Reptilase (batroxobin) time:	[21.5s/(14-16s)]
Prothrombin time:	[10.5s/(9.5-11.5s)]
Partial thromboplastin time:	[36s/(32-45s)]
Euglobulin lysis time:	[Normal[2]]
Bleeding time:	[Normal[2]]
Immunoelectrophoresis:	[Normal]
Platelet aggregation:	[Normal[2]]

Other results with patient plasma
Ancrod (Arvin) time: [n.a.]
Recalcification time: [n.a.]
Calcium corrects c.t.? [Yes[2]]

Inhib. normal plasma? [No]
In vivo synthesis: [n.a.]
In vivo catabolism: [n.a.]

Evaluation of isolated patient fibrinogen
Thrombin time: [n.a.]
Reptilase time: [n.a.]
Ancrod (Arvin) time: [n.a.]

Abnormal subunit? [n.a.]
Abnormal FDPs? [n.a.]

Remarks
[1]The rate of *total* fibrinopeptide release was normal.
[2]F. Jobin, L. Vu, & J.M. Delage, personal communication.

References

1. Jobin, F., Vu, L. and Delage, J.M. [Fibrinogen Quebec I and Quebec II: two new families of dysfibrinogenemia]. *Acta Haematol. (Basel)* **59**:119-127, **1978**.

FIBRINOGEN QUEBEC II

Last update	[1 December 1990]	**Structural defect**	[n.a.]
Alphacode	[QUEBEC02]	**Mutation**	[n.a.]
Ref. type	[Article]		

Functional defect(s)

FpA release:	[n.a.[1]]
FpB release:	[n.a.[1]]
Polymerization:	[Abnormal]
Stabilization:	[n.a.]

Family studies

Homozygote?	[n.a.]
Pedigree published?	[No]

Clinical manifestation(s) Bleeding? [Yes[2]] Thrombosis? [No]

Clinical laboratory results

Plasma fibrinogen concentration (mg/dL)

Chronometric: [130/(175-375)]
Rate-indep'nt: [280/(200-400)]
Immunologic: [311/(200-400)]

*Hypo*dysfibrinogen? [No]

Thrombin time:	[24s/(15-19s)]
Reptilase (batroxobin) time:	[23s/(14-16s)]
Prothrombin time:	[14s/(9.5-11.5s)]
Partial thromboplastin time:	[47s/(32-45s)]
Euglobulin lysis time:	[Normal[2]]
Bleeding time:	[Normal[2]]
Immunoelectrophoresis:	[Normal]
Platelet aggregation:	[Normal[2]]

Other results with patient plasma

Ancrod (Arvin) time:	[n.a.]	Inhib. normal plasma?	[No]
Recalcification time:	[n.a.]	In vivo synthesis:	[n.a.]
Calcium corrects c.t.?	[Yes[2]]	In vivo catabolism:	[n.a.]

Evaluation of isolated patient fibrinogen

Thrombin time:	[n.a.]	Abnormal subunit?	[n.a.]
Reptilase time:	[n.a.]	Abnormal FDPs?	[n.a.]
Ancrod (Arvin) time:	[n.a.]		

Remarks

[1]The rate of *total* fibrinopeptide release was reduced, and only about half the normal amount was released. Individual fibrinopeptide release was not reported.

[2]F. Jobin, L. Vu, & J.M. Delage, personal communication.

References

1. Jobin, F., Vu, L. and Delage, J.M. [Fibrinogen Quebec I and Quebec II: two new families of dysfibrinogenemia]. *Acta Haematol. (Basel)* **59**:119-127, **1978**.

FIBRINOGEN RICHFIELD I^{Abs}

Last update [1 December 1990]
Alphacode [RICHFI01]
Ref. type [Abstract]

Family studies
Homozygote? [n.a.]
Pedigree published? [No]

Structural defect [n.a.]
Mutation [n.a.]

Functional defect(s)
FpA release: [Normal]
FpB release: [n.a.]
Polymerization: [Abnormal]
Stabilization: [n.a.]

Clinical manifestation(s) Bleeding? [No] Thrombosis? [Yes[1]]

Clinical laboratory results
Plasma fibrinogen concentration (mg/dL)
Chronometric: [32/(190-440)]
Rate-indep'nt: [n.a.]
Immunologic: [189/(200-450)]

*Hypo*dysfibrinogen? [No]

Thrombin time:	[28.6s/(11.5-16.5s)]
Reptilase (batroxobin) time:	[35s/(13-17s)]
Prothrombin time:	[n.a.]
Partial thromboplastin time:	[n.a.]
Euglobulin lysis time:	[Abnormal]
Bleeding time:	[Normal]
Immunoelectrophoresis:	[n.a.]
Platelet aggregation:	[n.a.]

Other results with patient plasma
Ancrod (Arvin) time: [n.a.]
Recalcification time: [n.a.]
Calcium corrects c.t.? [n.a.]

Inhib. normal plasma? [n.a.]
In vivo synthesis: [n.a.]
In vivo catabolism: [n.a.]

Evaluation of isolated patient fibrinogen
Thrombin time: [n.a.]
Reptilase time: [n.a.]
Ancrod (Arvin) time: [n.a.]

Abnormal subunit? [Yes[2]]
Abnormal FDPs? [Yes[3]]

Remarks

[1]The 68 year-old propositus experienced deep vein thrombosis at age 28, and myocardial infarction at ages 41 and 63. His mother and sister died from "blood clots" at ages 26 and 42, respectively.

[2]An abnormal γ-chain was detected by reversed-phase HPLC; SDS-PAGE did not disclose any abnormality.

[3]Patient fibrinogen failed to accelerate tPA-mediated plasminogen activation. Abnormal FDP's were detected by SDS-PAGE.

References

1. Schorer, A.E. and Basara, M.L. Fibrinogen Richfield: a congenital dysfibrinogenemia with a thrombotic tendency. *Blood* **76 Suppl. 1**:437a, **1990** ABSTRACT

FIBRINOGEN RIYADH I

Last update	[10 January 1994]	**Structural defect**	[n.a.]
Alphacode	[RIYADH01]	**Mutation**	[n.a.]
Ref. type	[Article]		
		Functional defect(s)	
Family studies		FpA release:	[n.a.]
Homozygote?	[n.a.]	FpB release:	[n.a.]
Pedigree published?	[No[1]]	Polymerization:	[Abnormal]
		Stabilization:	[Normal]

Clinical manifestation(s) Bleeding? [Yes[2]] Thrombosis? [No]

Clinical laboratory results

Plasma fibrinogen concentration (mg/dL)

Chronometric: [<50[3]]

Rate-indep'nt: [n.a.] *Hypo*dysfibrinogen? [No[4]]

Immunologic: [n.a.]

Thrombin time:	[49.7s/(13.8s)]
Reptilase (batroxobin) time:	[>50.5s/(15s)]
Prothrombin time:	[41.4s/(11.4s)]
Partial thromboplastin time:	[90s/(53.1s)]
Euglobulin lysis time:	[n.a.]
Bleeding time:	[n.a.]
Immunoelectrophoresis:	[n.a.]
Platelet aggregation:	[n.a.]

Other results with patient plasma

Ancrod (Arvin) time:	[n.a.]	Inhib. normal plasma?	[No]
Recalcification time:	[n.a.]	In vivo synthesis:	[n.a.]
Calcium corrects c.t.?	[n.a.]	In vivo catabolism:	[n.a.]

Evaluation of isolated patient fibrinogen

Thrombin time:	[n.a.]	Abnormal subunit?	[n.a.]
Reptilase time:	[n.a.]	Abnormal FDPs?	[n.a.]
Ancrod (Arvin) time:	[n.a.]		

Remarks

[1]There is evidence of consanguinity.

[2]The 2 year-old propositus presented with a lifelong bleeding problem, including abnormal umbilical and post-traumatic bleeding, and intracranial hemorrhages with severe neurological complications. Bleeding episodes were successfully managed with cryoprecipitate.

[3]Abnormal clots were observed; normal range not reported.

[4]Based on the results of a turbidometric assay.

References

1. Al-Fawaz, I.M. and Gader, A.M.A. Severe congenital dysfibrinogenemia (fibrinogen-Riyadh): A family study. *Acta Haematol.* **88**:194-197, **1992**.

FIBRINOGEN ROUEN I

Last update [1 December 1990]
Alphacode [ROUEN01]
Ref. type [Article]

Family studies
Homozygote? [No]
Pedigree published? [No]

Structural defect [Aα(12) Gly → Val]
Mutation [n.a.]

Functional defect(s)
FpA release: [Abnormal]
FpB release: [Normal]
Polymerization: [Normal]
Stabilization: [n.a.]

Clinical manifestation(s) Bleeding? [n.a.] Thrombosis? [n.a.]

Clinical laboratory results
Plasma fibrinogen concentration (mg/dL)
Chronometric: [n.a.]
Rate-indep'nt: [n.a.]
Immunologic: [n.a.]

*Hypo*dysfibrinogen? [n.a.]

Thrombin time: [n.a.]
Reptilase (batroxobin) time: [n.a.]
Prothrombin time: [n.a.]
Partial thromboplastin time: [n.a.]
Euglobulin lysis time: [n.a.]
Bleeding time: [n.a.]
Immunoelectrophoresis: [n.a.]
Platelet aggregation: [n.a.]

Other results with patient plasma
Ancrod (Arvin) time: [n.a.]
Recalcification time: [n.a.]
Calcium corrects c.t.? [n.a.]

Inhib. normal plasma? [n.a.]
In vivo synthesis: [n.a.]
In vivo catabolism: [n.a.]

Evaluation of isolated patient fibrinogen
Thrombin time: [n.a.]
Reptilase time: [n.a.]
Ancrod (Arvin) time: [n.a.]

Abnormal subunit? [n.a.]
Abnormal FDPs? [n.a.]

Remarks

References

1. Ni, F., Konishi, Y., Bullock, L.D., Rivetna, M.N. and Scheraga, H.A. High-resolution NMR studies of fibrinogen-like peptides in solution: Structural basis for the bleeding disorder caused by a single mutation of Gly(12) to Val(12) in the Aα chain of human fibrinogen Rouen. *Biochem.* **28**:3106-3119, **1989**.

2. Henschen, A., Kehl, M., Southan, C., Lottspeich, F. and Georgopoulos, D. Genetically abnormal fibrinogens — some current characterisation strategies. In: *Fibrinogen —Structure, Functional Aspects, Metabolism*, F. Haverkate, A. Henschen, W. Nieuwenhuizen and P.W. Straub (eds.), Walter de Gruyter, Berlin. pp. 125-144, **1983**.

3. Kehl, M., Lottspeich, F. and Henschen, A. Genetically abnormal fibrinogens releasing abnormal fibrinopeptides as characterised by high-performance liquid chromatography. In: *Fibrinogen — Structure, Functional Aspects, Metabolism*, F. Haverkate, A. Henschen, W. Nieuwenhuizen and P.W. Straub (eds.), Walter de Gruyter, Berlin. pp. 183-193, **1983**.

FIBRINOGEN SAGA I

Last update [1 December 1990]
Alphacode [SAGA01]
Ref. type [Article]

Structural defect [γ(275) Arg → His]
Mutation [n.a.]

Family studies
Homozygote? [No]
Pedigree published? [No]

Functional defect(s)
FpA release: [Normal]
FpB release: [Normal]
Polymerization: [Abnormal]
Stabilization: [Normal]

Clinical manifestation(s) Bleeding? [Yes[1]] Thrombosis? [No]

Clinical laboratory results
Plasma fibrinogen concentration (mg/dL)
Chronometric: [<40/(150-350)]
Rate-indep'nt: [345[2]]
Immunologic: [245[2]]
*Hypo*dysfibrinogen? [No]

Thrombin time:	[23.4s/(9.4s)]
Reptilase (batroxobin) time:	[n.a.]
Prothrombin time:	[n.a.]
Partial thromboplastin time:	[n.a.]
Euglobulin lysis time:	[n.a.]
Bleeding time:	[n.a.]
Immunoelectrophoresis:	[n.a.]
Platelet aggregation:	[n.a.]

Other results with patient plasma
Ancrod (Arvin) time: [82.4s/(11.3s)]
Recalcification time: [n.a.]
Calcium corrects c.t.? [Yes]
Inhib. normal plasma? [n.a.]
In vivo synthesis: [n.a.]
In vivo catabolism: [n.a.]

Evaluation of isolated patient fibrinogen
Thrombin time: [114s/(14.7s)]
Reptilase time: [n.a.]
Ancrod (Arvin) time: [>180s/(11.3s)]
Abnormal subunit? [No]
Abnormal FDPs? [Yes[3]]

Remarks
[1]The index patient presented with hematuria, but no other bleeding diathesis was noted.
[2]Normal range not reported.
[3]An abnormal fragment D was detected by chromatofocusing.

References

1. Matsuda, M., Yamazumi, K., Terukina, S., Onohara, S. and Ohta, Y. An abnormal fibrinogen with a γ Arg-275 to His substitution found in a Japanese family — fibrinogen Saga. In: *Fibrinogen 3. Biochemistry, Biological Functions, Gene Regulation and Expression*, M.W. Mosesson, D.L. Amrani, K.R. Siebenlist and J.P. DiOrio (eds.), Elsevier Science Publ., B.V., Amsterdam. pp. 267-267, **1988**.

2. Yamazumi, K., Terukina, S., Onohara, S. and Matsuda, M. Normal plasmic cleavage of the γ-chain variant of "fibrinogen Saga" with an Arg-275 to His substitution. *Thromb. Haemostas.* **60**:476-480, **1988**.

FIBRINOGEN SAINT LOUIS I

Last update	[10 January 1994]	**Structural defect**	[n.a.]
Alphacode	[STLOUI01]	**Mutation**	[n.a.]
Ref. type	[Article]		

Functional defect(s)
FpA release: [Normal[1]]
FpB release: [Normal[1]]
Polymerization: [Abnormal]
Stabilization: [n.a.]

Family studies
Homozygote? [n.a.]
Pedigree published? [Yes]

Clinical manifestation(s) Bleeding? [Yes[2]] Thrombosis? [No]

Clinical laboratory results

Plasma fibrinogen concentration (mg/dL)
Chronometric: [n.a.]
Rate-indep'nt: [177/(200-400)[3]]
Immunologic: [n.a.]

*Hypo*dysfibrinogen? [No[3]]

Thrombin time:	[34.7s/(12-18s)[4]]
Reptilase (batroxobin) time:	[n.a.]
Prothrombin time:	[25.6s/(14-16s)]
Partial thromboplastin time:	[114s/(35-53s)]
Euglobulin lysis time:	[n.a.]
Bleeding time:	[Abnormal]
Immunoelectrophoresis:	[Normal]
Platelet aggregation:	[Normal]

Other results with patient plasma

Ancrod (Arvin) time:	[n.a.]	Inhib. normal plasma?	[No]
Recalcification time:	[n.a.]	In vivo synthesis:	[n.a.]
Calcium corrects c.t.?	[No]	In vivo catabolism:	[n.a.]

Evaluation of isolated patient fibrinogen

Thrombin time:	[n.a.[4]]	Abnormal subunit?	[n.a.]
Reptilase time:	[n.a.]	Abnormal FDPs?	[n.a.]
Ancrod (Arvin) time:	[n.a.]		

Remarks

[1]The rate of *total* fibrinopeptide release was normal.

[2]Affected relatives of the propositus who did not have hemophilia A failed to exhibit bleeding diathesis or thrombosis. Successful spleno-renal shunt, cholecystectomy, and appendectomy were performed on the index patient.

[3]Periodic subnormal plasma fibrinogen was attributable to concomitant liver disease.

[4]Thrombin time was unusually dependent on pH.

References

1. Sherman, L.A., Gaston, L.W., Kaplan, M.E. and Spivack, A.R. Fibrinogen St. Louis: a new inherited fibrinogen variant, coincidentally associated with hemophilia A. *J. Clin. Invest.* **51**:590-597, **1972**.

2. Gaston, L.W., Baue, A.E., Pfaff, D.A. and Wise, L. Spleno-renal shunt, cholecystectomy, and appendectomy in a patient with hemophilia A, and abnormal fibrinogen, and thrombocytopenia. *Ann. Surg.* **173**:234-237, **1971**.

3. Sherman, L.A., Gaston, L.W. and Spivack, A.R. Studies on a patient with a fibrinogen variant and hemophilia A. *J. Lab. Clin. Med.* **72**:1017, **1968**. ABSTRACT

FIBRINOGEN SAINT MANDE I

Last update [10 January 1994]
Alphacode [STMAND01]
Ref. type [Article]

Structural defect [n.a.]
Mutation [n.a.]

Family studies
Homozygote? [n.a.]
Pedigree published? [No]

Functional defect(s)
FpA release: [n.a.]
FpB release: [n.a.]
Polymerization: [Abnormal]
Stabilization: [n.a.]

Clinical manifestation(s) Bleeding? [Yes] Thrombosis? [No]

Clinical laboratory results

Plasma fibrinogen concentration (mg/dL)
Chronometric: [334/(>150)[1]]
Rate-indep'nt: [320/(>150)]
Immunologic: [n.a.]

*Hypo*dysfibrinogen? [No]

Thrombin time:	[Abnormal]
Reptilase (batroxobin) time:	[Abnormal[2]]
Prothrombin time:	[Normal]
Partial thromboplastin time:	[Normal]
Euglobulin lysis time:	[n.a.]
Bleeding time:	[Normal]
Immunoelectrophoresis:	[n.a.]
Platelet aggregation:	[n.a.]

Other results with patient plasma
Ancrod (Arvin) time: [n.a.]
Recalcification time: [n.a.]
Calcium corrects c.t.? [n.a.]

Inhib. normal plasma? [Yes]
In vivo synthesis: [n.a.]
In vivo catabolism: [n.a.]

Evaluation of isolated patient fibrinogen
Thrombin time: [n.a.]
Reptilase time: [n.a.]
Ancrod (Arvin) time: [n.a.]

Abnormal subunit? [n.a.]
Abnormal FDPs? [n.a.]

Remarks

[1]Classification of St. Mande I as a dysfibrinogen is questionable in view of the "normal" plasma fibrinogen concentration obtained with a chronometric method.

[2]The Reptilase time was only slightly prolonged.

References

1. Thabaut, A., Durosoir, J.L., Voinesson, A., Laverdant, C. and Essioux, H. [Congenital dysfibrinogenemia: Two new cases]. *Med. Armees* **4**:677-680, **1976**.

FIBRINOGEN SAINT MANDE II

Last update [10 January 1994]
Alphacode [STMAND02]
Ref. type [Article]

Structural defect [n.a.]
Mutation [n.a.]

Family studies
Homozygote? [n.a.]
Pedigree published? [No]

Functional defect(s)
FpA release: [n.a.]
FpB release: [n.a.]
Polymerization: [Abnormal]
Stabilization: [n.a.]

Clinical manifestation(s) Bleeding? [No] Thrombosis? [No]

Clinical laboratory results

Plasma fibrinogen concentration (mg/dL)
Chronometric: [35/(>150)]
Rate-indep'nt: [180/(>150)]
Immunologic: [n.a.]

*Hypo*dysfibrinogen? [No]

Thrombin time:	[Abnormal]
Reptilase (batroxobin) time:	[Abnormal]
Prothrombin time:	[Abnormal]
Partial thromboplastin time:	[Abnormal]
Euglobulin lysis time:	[n.a.]
Bleeding time:	[Normal]
Immunoelectrophoresis:	[n.a.]
Platelet aggregation:	[n.a.]

Other results with patient plasma
Ancrod (Arvin) time: [n.a.]
Recalcification time: [n.a.]
Calcium corrects c.t.? [n.a.]

Inhib. normal plasma? [Yes]
In vivo synthesis: [n.a.]
In vivo catabolism: [n.a.]

Evaluation of isolated patient fibrinogen
Thrombin time: [n.a.]
Reptilase time: [n.a.]
Ancrod (Arvin) time: [n.a.]

Abnormal subunit? [n.a.]
Abnormal FDPs? [n.a.]

Remarks

References

1. Thabaut, A., Durosoir, J.L., Voinesson, A., Laverdant, C. and Essioux, H. [Congenital dysfibrinogenemia: two new cases]. *Med. Armees* **4**:677-680, **1976.**

FIBRINOGEN SALAMANCA I^Abs

Last update [1 December 1990]
Alphacode [SALAMA01]
Ref. type [Abstract]

Family studies
Homozygote? [n.a.]
Pedigree published? [No]

Structural defect [n.a.]
Mutation [n.a.]

Functional defect(s)
FpA release: [Normal]
FpB release: [Normal]
Polymerization: [Abnormal]
Stabilization: [Normal]

Clinical manifestation(s) Bleeding? [n.a.] Thrombosis? [n.a.]

Clinical laboratory results
Plasma fibrinogen concentration (mg/dL)
Chronometric: [Subnormal[1]]
Rate-indep'nt: [n.a.]
Immunologic: [Normal[1]]

*Hypo*dysfibrinogen? [No]

Thrombin time:	[Abnormal[1]]
Reptilase (batroxobin) time:	[Abnormal[1]]
Prothrombin time:	[n.a.]
Partial thromboplastin time:	[n.a.]
Euglobulin lysis time:	[n.a.]
Bleeding time:	[n.a.]
Immunoelectrophoresis:	[Normal]
Platelet aggregation:	[n.a.]

Other results with patient plasma
Ancrod (Arvin) time: [n.a.]
Recalcification time: [n.a.]
Calcium corrects c.t.? [Yes]

Inhib. normal plasma? [Yes]
In vivo synthesis: [n.a.]
In vivo catabolism: [n.a.]

Evaluation of isolated patient fibrinogen
Thrombin time: [Abnormal[1]]
Reptilase time: [n.a.]
Ancrod (Arvin) time: [n.a.]

Abnormal subunit? [No]
Abnormal FDPs? [n.a.]

Remarks
[1]Data not reported.

References

1. Fernández, J., Noguerol, P., Losada, G., Alberca, I., Sosa, R., Martin-Villar, J., Vicente, V. and Rocha, E. Three new cases of congenital dysfibrinogenemia: fibrinogens Sevilla, Madrid and Salamanca. *Thromb. Haemostas.* **54**:160, **1985**. ABSTRACT

FIBRINOGEN SAN FRANCISCO I[Abs1]

Last update	[1 December 1990]	**Structural defect**	[n.a.]
Alphacode	[SANFRA01]	**Mutation**	[n.a.]
Ref. type	[Abstract]		

Family studies
Homozygote? [No]
Pedigree published? [No]

Functional defect(s)
FpA release: [n.a.]
FpB release: [n.a.]
Polymerization: [Abnormal]
Stabilization: [n.a.]

Clinical manifestation(s) Bleeding? [No] Thrombosis? [No]

Clinical laboratory results

Plasma fibrinogen concentration (mg/dL)
Chronometric: [n.a.]
Rate-indep'nt: [n.a.]
Immunologic: [n.a.]

*Hypo*dysfibrinogen? [n.a.]

Thrombin time:	[45s/(7s)]
Reptilase (batroxobin) time:	[n.a.]
Prothrombin time:	[n.a.]
Partial thromboplastin time:	[n.a.]
Euglobulin lysis time:	[n.a.]
Bleeding time:	[n.a.]
Immunoelectrophoresis:	[Normal]
Platelet aggregation:	[n.a.]

Other results with patient plasma

Ancrod (Arvin) time:	[n.a.]	Inhib. normal plasma?	[Yes]
Recalcification time:	[n.a.]	In vivo synthesis:	[n.a.]
Calcium corrects c.t.?	[n.a.]	In vivo catabolism:	[n.a.]

Evaluation of isolated patient fibrinogen

Thrombin time:	[n.a.]	Abnormal subunit?	[n.a.]
Reptilase time:	[n.a.]	Abnormal FDPs?	[n.a.]
Ancrod (Arvin) time:	[n.a.]		

Remarks

[1]The index patient was from Manila, but the variant was studied in San Francisco. In some reviews this is described as fibrinogen Manila.

References

1. Wohl, R.C. and Bradley, T.B. Impaired monomer aggregation in congenital dysfibrinogenemia. *Blood* **44**:935, **1974**. ABSTRACT

FIBRINOGEN SAN JUAN I

Last update [1 December 1990]
Alphacode [SANJUA01]
Ref. type [Article]

Family studies
Homozygote? [n.a.]
Pedigree published? [Yes]

Structural defect [n.a.]
Mutation [n.a.]

Functional defect(s)
FpA release: [n.a.]
FpB release: [n.a.]
Polymerization: [n.a.]
Stabilization: [n.a.]

Clinical manifestation(s) Bleeding? [Yes[1]] Thrombosis? [No]

Clinical laboratory results
Plasma fibrinogen concentration (mg/dL)
Chronometric: [50/(190-365)[2]]
Rate-indep'nt: [n.a.]
Immunologic: [n.a.]
*Hypo*dysfibrinogen? [n.a.[2]]

Thrombin time:	[n.a.[3]]
Reptilase (batroxobin) time:	[n.a.[4]]
Prothrombin time:	[n.a.]
Partial thromboplastin time:	[n.a.]
Euglobulin lysis time:	[n.a.]
Bleeding time:	[Abnormal]
Immunoelectrophoresis:	[n.a.]
Platelet aggregation:	[n.a.]

Other results with patient plasma
Ancrod (Arvin) time: [n.a.]
Recalcification time: [n.a.]
Calcium corrects c.t.? [n.a.]
Inhib. normal plasma? [n.a.]
In vivo synthesis: [n.a.]
In vivo catabolism: [n.a.]

Evaluation of isolated patient fibrinogen
Thrombin time: [21s/(16s)]
Reptilase time: [n.a.]
Ancrod (Arvin) time: [n.a.]
Abnormal subunit? [n.a.]
Abnormal FDPs? [n.a.]

Remarks
[1]The 30 year-old propositus exhibited epistaxis and excessive bleeding after dental extraction.
[2]The method used to determine fibrinogen concentration was not specified; diagnosis of hypodysfibrinogenemia cannot be confirmed.
[3]Thrombin time was "22s" longer than normal; data not reported.
[4]Reptilase time was "17s" longer than normal; data not reported.

In view of the failure to determine the functional defect, the conclusion that San Juan I represents a case of dysfibrinogenemia is open to question.

References

1. Owen, C.A., Jr., Bowie, E.J., Fass, D.N., Perez, R.A., Cole, T.L. and Stewart, M. Hypofibrinogenemia-dysfibrinogenemia and von Willebrand's disease in the same family. *Mayo. Clin. Proc.* **54**:375-380, **1979**.

FIBRINOGEN SANTIAGO I

Last update	[10 January 1994]	**Structural defect**	[n.a.]
Alphacode	[SANTIA01]	**Mutation**	[n.a.]
Ref. type	[Article]		

Family studies
Homozygote? [n.a.]
Pedigree published? [No]

Functional defect(s)
FpA release: [Abnormal]
FpB release: [Abnormal]
Polymerization: [Abnormal]
Stabilization: [n.a.]

Clinical manifestation(s) Bleeding? [Yes[1]] Thrombosis? [No]

Clinical laboratory results

Plasma fibrinogen concentration (mg/dL)
Chronometric: [80[2]]
Rate-indep'nt: [185[2]]
Immunologic: [200[2]]

*Hypo*dysfibrinogen? [No]

Thrombin time:	[24s/(12-15s)[3]]
Reptilase (batroxobin) time:	[Abnormal[4]]
Prothrombin time:	[n.a.]
Partial thromboplastin time:	[n.a.]
Euglobulin lysis time:	[n.a.]
Bleeding time:	[n.a.]
Immunoelectrophoresis:	[Normal]
Platelet aggregation:	[n.a.]

Other results with patient plasma

Ancrod (Arvin) time:	[n.a.]	Inhib. normal plasma?	[No]
Recalcification time:	[n.a.]	In vivo synthesis:	[n.a.]
Calcium corrects c.t.?	[n.a.]	In vivo catabolism:	[n.a.]

Evaluation of isolated patient fibrinogen

Thrombin time:	[n.a.]	Abnormal subunit?	[No]
Reptilase time:	[n.a.]	Abnormal FDPs?	[No[5]]
Ancrod (Arvin) time:	[n.a.]		

Remarks

[1]"Severe" bleeding was reported; details were not provided.
[2]Normal range not reported.
[3]C.L. Arocha-Piñango & N.B. de Bosch, personal communication.
[4]Data not reported; Reptilase time was 15s longer than normal.
[5]An increased *rate* of FDP formation was reported.

Electron microscopy of patient fibrinogen and fibrin (Marchi et al., 1990) disclosed no differences from normal.

References

1. Arocha-Piñango, C.L., Bosch, N., Torres, A., Caires-Tronchoni, D., Marchi, R., Vidal, H. and Rizzo, M.G. Dysfibrinogenemias in Latin America. A cooperative study group. *Rev. Iberoamer. Tromb. Hemostasia* **3**:110-122, **1990**.

2. Marchi, R., Arocha-Piñango, C.L. and Gil, F. Electron microscopy studies of 7 patients with dysfibrinogenemia and some of their relatives. *Rev. Iberoamer. Tromb. Hemostasia* **3**:185-190, **1990**.

FIBRINOGEN SAPPORO I

Last update [1 December 1990]
Alphacode [SAPPOR01]
Ref. type [Article]

Structural defect [Aα(16) Arg → His[1]]
Mutation [n.a.]

Family studies
Homozygote? [No]
Pedigree published? [Yes]

Functional defect(s)
FpA release: [Abnormal]
FpB release: [Abnormal]
Polymerization: [Normal]
Stabilization: [Normal]

Clinical manifestation(s) Bleeding? [No] Thrombosis? [No]

Clinical laboratory results

Plasma fibrinogen concentration (mg/dL)
Chronometric: [64/(243)]
Rate-indep'nt: [186/(176)]
Immunologic: [n.a.]

*Hypo*dysfibrinogen? [No]

Thrombin time:	[57.3s/(11.3s)]
Reptilase (batroxobin) time:	[47.4s/(11.1s)]
Prothrombin time:	[14.3s/(11s)]
Partial thromboplastin time:	[25.4s/(25s)]
Euglobulin lysis time:	[n.a.]
Bleeding time:	[n.a.]
Immunoelectrophoresis:	[n.a.]
Platelet aggregation:	[n.a.]

Other results with patient plasma
Ancrod (Arvin) time: [n.a.]
Recalcification time: [n.a.]
Calcium corrects c.t.? [No]

Inhib. normal plasma? [Yes]
In vivo synthesis: [n.a.]
In vivo catabolism: [n.a.]

Evaluation of isolated patient fibrinogen
Thrombin time: [101s/(20.1s)]
Reptilase time: [n.a.]
Ancrod (Arvin) time: [>200s/(28.3s)]

Abnormal subunit? [No]
Abnormal FDPs? [n.a.]

Remarks

[1]This is the first Japanese patient with an Aα(16) Arg → His substitution to be reported.

References

1. Asakura, S., Terukina, S., Yamazumi, K., Matsuda, M., Murayama, H., Higuchi, A., Musashi, M., Sakurada, K. and Miyazaki, T. Fibrinogen Sapporo: dysfibrinogenemia characterized by the replacement of Aα arginine-16 by histidine resulting in the delayed release of fibrinopeptide A by thrombin. *Nippon Ketsueki Gakkai Zasshi* **52**:1094-1104, **1989**.

FIBRINOGEN SCHWARZACH I

Last update [1 December 1990]
Alphacode [SCHWAR01]
Ref. type [Article]

Family studies
Homozygote? [No]
Pedigree published? [No]

Structural defect [Aα(16) Arg → Cys]
Mutation [n.a.]

Functional defect(s)
FpA release: [Abnormal[1]]
FpB release: [n.a.]
Polymerization: [Abnormal]
Stabilization: [n.a.]

Clinical manifestation(s) Bleeding? [No] Thrombosis? [No]

Clinical laboratory results
Plasma fibrinogen concentration (mg/dL)
Chronometric: [57/(200-400)]
Rate-indep'nt: [n.a.]
Immunologic: [404/(200-400)]

*Hypo*dysfibrinogen? [No]

Thrombin time:	[30s/(12-18s)]
Reptilase (batroxobin) time:	[71s/(12-16s)]
Prothrombin time:	[48%/(75-110%)]
Partial thromboplastin time:	[39s/(35-45s)]
Euglobulin lysis time:	[n.a.]
Bleeding time:	[n.a.]
Immunoelectrophoresis:	[Normal]
Platelet aggregation:	[n.a.]

Other results with patient plasma
Ancrod (Arvin) time: [n.a.]
Recalcification time: [n.a.]
Calcium corrects c.t.? [No]

Inhib. normal plasma? [No]
In vivo synthesis: [n.a.]
In vivo catabolism: [n.a.]

Evaluation of isolated patient fibrinogen
Thrombin time: [n.a.]
Reptilase time: [n.a.]
Ancrod (Arvin) time: [n.a.]

Abnormal subunit? [No]
Abnormal FDPs? [n.a.]

Remarks
[1]Only half the normal amount of fibrinopeptide A was released. Henschen et al. (ref. 3) have shown that the *abnormal* fibrinopeptide A can be released by thrombin after S-aminoethylation.

References

1. Deutsch, E., Dudczak, R., Henschen, A., Mannhalter, Ch. and Pils, P. [Dysfibrinogen "Schwarzach"]. *Med. Welt* **36**:655-661, **1985**.

2. Henschen, A., Kehl, M., Southan, C., Lottspeich, F. and Georgopoulos, D. Genetically abnormal fibrinogens — some current characterisation strategies. In: *Fibrinogen —Structure, Functional Aspects, Metabolism*, F. Haverkate, A. Henschen, W. Nieuwenhuizen and P.W. Straub (eds.), Walter de Gruyter, Berlin. pp. 125-144, **1983**.

3. Henschen, A., Kehl, M. and Deutsch, E. Novel structure elucidation strategy for genetically abnormal fibrinogens with incomplete fibrinopeptide release as applied to fibrinogen Schwarzach. *Hoppe. Seylers. Z. Physiol. Chem.* **364**:1747-1751, **1983**.

FIBRINOGEN SEATTLE I

Last update	[1 December 1990]	**Structural defect**	[Bβ(14) Arg → Cys]
Alphacode	[SEATTL01]	**Mutation**	[n.a.]
Ref. type	[Article]		

Family studies
Homozygote? [No]
Pedigree published? [Yes]

Functional defect(s)
FpA release: [Normal]
FpB release: [Abnormal[1]]
Polymerization: [Abnormal]
Stabilization: [Normal]

Clinical manifestation(s) Bleeding? [No[2]] Thrombosis? [No[2]]

Clinical laboratory results
Plasma fibrinogen concentration (mg/dL)
Chronometric: [57/(200-300)]
Rate-indep'nt: [215/(200-300)]
Immunologic: [n.a.]

*Hypo*dysfibrinogen? [No]

Thrombin time:	[50s/(17s)]
Reptilase (batroxobin) time:	[n.a.]
Prothrombin time:	[13.3s/(12s)]
Partial thromboplastin time:	[35s/(39s)]
Euglobulin lysis time:	[n.a.]
Bleeding time:	[9.5m/(4-8m)]
Immunoelectrophoresis:	[Normal]
Platelet aggregation:	[n.a.]

Other results with patient plasma

Ancrod (Arvin) time:	[n.a.]	Inhib. normal plasma?	[No]
Recalcification time:	[n.a.]	In vivo synthesis:	[n.a.]
Calcium corrects c.t.?	[No]	In vivo catabolism:	[n.a.]

Evaluation of isolated patient fibrinogen

Thrombin time:	[n.a.]	Abnormal subunit?	[No]
Reptilase time:	[n.a.]	Abnormal FDPs?	[n.a.]
Ancrod (Arvin) time:	[n.a.]		

Remarks
[1]Only half the normal amount of fibrinopeptide B was released.
[2]The patient presented with tetralogy of Fallot and underwent open heart surgery without excessive blood loss.

The additional cysteine sulfhydryl was found to form a disulfide bond with the corresponding Bβ(16) Cys in the homodimeric variant fibrinogen.

References

1. Pirkle, H., Kaudewitz, H., Henschen, A., Theodor, I. and Simmons, G. Substitution of Bβ-14 arginine by Cyst(e)ine in fibrinogen Seattle I. In: *Fibrinogen 2. Biochemistry, Physiology and Clinical Relevance*, G.D.O. Lowe, J.T. Douglas, C.D. Forbes and A. Henschen (eds.), Elsevier, Amsterdam. pp. 49-52, **1987**.

2. Branson, H.E., Schmer, G., Theodor, I. and Pirkle, H. Fibrinogen Seattle releases half the normal amount of fibrinopeptide B. *Acta Haematol. (Basel)* **70**:257-263, **1983**.

3. Branson, H.E., Schmer, G. and Dillard, D.H. Fibrinogen Seattle: a qualitatively abnormal fibrinogen in a patient with tetralogy of Fallot. *Am. J. Clin. Pathol.* **67**:236-240, **1977**.

FIBRINOGEN SEATTLE II

Last update	[1 December 1990]	**Structural defect**	[Aα(16) Arg → His]
Alphacode	[SEATTL02]	**Mutation**	[n.a.]
Ref. type	[Article]		

Family studies
Homozygote? [No]
Pedigree published? [No]

Functional defect(s)
FpA release: [Abnormal[1]]
FpB release: [Abnormal]
Polymerization: [Abnormal]
Stabilization: [Normal]

Clinical manifestation(s) Bleeding? [No] Thrombosis? [No]

Clinical laboratory results

Plasma fibrinogen concentration (mg/dL)
Chronometric: [57/(200-400)]
Rate-indep'nt: [297/(200-400)]
Immunologic: [n.a.]

*Hypo*dysfibrinogen? [No]

Thrombin time:	[37s/(20-25s)]
Reptilase (batroxobin) time:	[47s/(18-22s)]
Prothrombin time:	[Normal[2]]
Partial thromboplastin time:	[Normal[2]]
Euglobulin lysis time:	[n.a.]
Bleeding time:	[n.a.]
Immunoelectrophoresis:	[n.a.]
Platelet aggregation:	[n.a.]

Other results with patient plasma

Ancrod (Arvin) time:	[n.a.]	Inhib. normal plasma?	[n.a.]
Recalcification time:	[n.a.]	In vivo synthesis:	[n.a.]
Calcium corrects c.t.?	[n.a.]	In vivo catabolism:	[n.a.]

Evaluation of isolated patient fibrinogen

Thrombin time:	[n.a.]	Abnormal subunit?	[No]
Reptilase time:	[n.a.]	Abnormal FDPs?	[n.a.]
Ancrod (Arvin) time:	[n.a.]		

Remarks

[1]Only half the normal amount of fibrinopeptide A was released.
[2]Data not reported.

References

1. Ebert, R.F., Schreiber, W.E. and Bell, W.R. Fibrinogen Seattle II: congenital dysfibrinogenemia with an Arg (Aα-16) → His substitution. *Thromb. Res.* **43**:7-13, **1986**.

2. Schreiber, W.E. and Schmer, G. Fibrinogen Seattle II: defective release of fibrinopeptide A in a slow clotting fibrinogen. *Thromb. Res.* **37**:45-52, **1985**.

FIBRINOGEN SEVILLA I

Last update	[1 December 1990]	**Structural defect**	[n.a.]
Alphacode	[SEVILL01]	**Mutation**	[n.a.]
Ref. type	[Article]		

Functional defect(s)

FpA release:	[Normal[1]]
FpB release:	[Normal[1]]
Polymerization:	[Abnormal]
Stabilization:	[Normal]

Family studies

Homozygote?	[No[2]]
Pedigree published?	[No]

Clinical manifestation(s) Bleeding? [No] Thrombosis? [No]

Clinical laboratory results

Plasma fibrinogen concentration (mg/dL)

Chronometric:	[49/(200-400)]
Rate-indep'nt:	[123/(200-400)]
Immunologic:	[280/(200-400)]

*Hypo*dysfibrinogen? [No]

Thrombin time:	[38s/(18-20s)]
Reptilase (batroxobin) time:	[41s/(15-18s)]
Prothrombin time:	[12s/(11-13s)]
Partial thromboplastin time:	[56s/(35-40s)]
Euglobulin lysis time:	[180m/(>180m)]
Bleeding time:	[n.a.]
Immunoelectrophoresis:	[Normal]
Platelet aggregation:	[n.a.]

Other results with patient plasma

Ancrod (Arvin) time:	[n.a.]	Inhib. normal plasma?	[No]
Recalcification time:	[n.a.]	In vivo synthesis:	[n.a.]
Calcium corrects c.t.?	[Yes]	In vivo catabolism:	[n.a.]

Evaluation of isolated patient fibrinogen

Thrombin time:	[n.a.]	Abnormal subunit?	[No]
Reptilase time:	[n.a.]	Abnormal FDPs?	[No[3]]
Ancrod (Arvin) time:	[n.a.]		

Remarks

[1]The rate of *total* fibrinopeptide release was normal.
[2]F.J. Fernández, personal communication.
[3]A reduced *rate* of FDP formation was reported.

References

1. Fernández, F.J., Noguerol, P., Sosa, R., Cuesta, B., Paramo, J.A. and Rocha, E. Fibrinogen Sevilla, a congenital dysfibrinogenemia characterized by an abnormal monomer aggregation and a defective plasmin lysis. *Clin. Chim. Acta* **179**:239-250, **1989**.

FIBRINOGEN SHEFFIELD I

Last update [1 December 1990]
Alphacode [SHEFFI01]
Ref. type [Article]

Family studies
Homozygote? [No]
Pedigree published? [No]

Structural defect [Aα(16) Arg → His]
Mutation [n.a.]

Functional defect(s)
FpA release: [n.a.[1]]
FpB release: [n.a.[1]]
Polymerization: [n.a.[1]]
Stabilization: [n.a.]

Clinical manifestation(s) Bleeding? [Yes[2]] Thrombosis? [No]

Clinical laboratory results
Plasma fibrinogen concentration (mg/dL)
Chronometric: [n.a.]
Rate-indep'nt: [210[3]]
Immunologic: [n.a.]

*Hypo*dysfibrinogen? [No]

Thrombin time:	[36s/(10s)]
Reptilase (batroxobin) time:	[32s/(15s)]
Prothrombin time:	[n.a.]
Partial thromboplastin time:	[n.a.]
Euglobulin lysis time:	[n.a.]
Bleeding time:	[n.a.]
Immunoelectrophoresis:	[n.a.]
Platelet aggregation:	[n.a.]

Other results with patient plasma
Ancrod (Arvin) time: [n.a.]
Recalcification time: [n.a.]
Calcium corrects c.t.? [n.a.]

Inhib. normal plasma? [n.a.]
In vivo synthesis: [n.a.]
In vivo catabolism: [n.a.]

Evaluation of isolated patient fibrinogen
Thrombin time: [n.a.]
Reptilase time: [n.a.]
Ancrod (Arvin) time: [n.a.]

Abnormal subunit? [n.a.]
Abnormal FDPs? [n.a.]

Remarks
[1]Rates of fibrinopeptide release and fibrin monomer polymerization were not reported. Other dysfibrinogens with this molecular defect exhibit delayed fibrinopeptide A and B release plus delayed polymerization of fibrin monomers.
[2]Menorrhagia, spontaneous abortion, and excessive bleeding after dental extraction were reported.
[3]Normal range not reported.

References

1. Southan, C., Thompson, E. and Lane, D.A. Direct analysis of plasma fibrinogen-derived fibrinopeptides by high-performance liquid chromatography: investigation of nine congenital fibrinogen abnormalities. *Br. J. Haematol.* **65**:469-473, **1987**.

FIBRINOGEN STONY BROOK I

Last update [1 December 1990]
Alphacode [STONYB01]
Ref. type [Article]

Structural defect [Aα(16) Arg → Cys]
Mutation [n.a.]

Family studies
Homozygote? [No]
Pedigree published? [No]

Functional defect(s)
FpA release: [Abnormal]
FpB release: [n.a.]
Polymerization: [Abnormal]
Stabilization: [n.a.]

Clinical manifestation(s) Bleeding? [No] Thrombosis? [No]

Clinical laboratory results

Plasma fibrinogen concentration (mg/dL)
Chronometric: [56[1]]
Rate-indep'nt: [160[1]]
Immunologic: [210[1]]

*Hypo*dysfibrinogen? [No]

Thrombin time:	[65s/(18s)]
Reptilase (batroxobin) time:	[88s/(21s)]
Prothrombin time:	[18s/(9-11s)]
Partial thromboplastin time:	[56s/(26-37s)]
Euglobulin lysis time:	[Normal[2]]
Bleeding time:	[Normal]
Immunoelectrophoresis:	[n.a.]
Platelet aggregation:	[Normal[3]]

Other results with patient plasma

Ancrod (Arvin) time:	[n.a.]	Inhib. normal plasma?	[Yes]
Recalcification time:	[n.a.]	In vivo synthesis:	[n.a.]
Calcium corrects c.t.?	[n.a.]	In vivo catabolism:	[n.a.]

Evaluation of isolated patient fibrinogen

Thrombin time:	[n.a.]	Abnormal subunit?	[Yes[4]]
Reptilase time:	[n.a.]	Abnormal FDPs?	[n.a.]
Ancrod (Arvin) time:	[n.a.]		

Remarks
[1]Normal range not reported.
[2]Data not reported.
[3]Diminished *support* of platelet aggregation was reported (Galanakis et al., 1988)
[4]Thrombin pre-treatment yielded an α-chain doublet on SDS-PAGE.

FIBRINOGEN STONY BROOK I

References

1. Galanakis, D.K., Henschen, A., Peerschke, E.I.B. and Kehl, M. Fibrinogen Stony Brook, a heterozygous Aα16Arg → Cys dysfibrinogenemia. Evaluation of diminished platelet aggregation support and of enhanced inhibition of fibrin assembly. *J. Clin. Invest.* **84**:295-304, **1989**.

2. Galanakis, D.K., Henschen, A., Peerschke, E.I. and Kehl, M. Fibrinogen Stony Brook I, an heterozygous Aα-16 Arg → Cys dysfibrinogenemia: implication of diminished platelet aggregation support. In: *Fibrinogen 3. Biochemistry, Biological Functions, Gene Regulation and Expression*, M.W. Mosesson, D.L. Amrani, K.R. Siebenlist and J.P. DiOrio (eds.), Elsevier Science Publ., B.V., Amsterdam. pp. 251-254, **1988**.

3. Galanakis, D.K. Aspects of evaluation of fibrinogen Stony Brook. A defect resulting in failure to release fibrinopeptide A. In: *Fibrinogen —Structural Variants and Interactions*, A. Henschen, B. Hessel, J. McDonagh and T. Saldeen (eds.), Walter de Gruyter, Berlin. pp. 207-212, **1985**.

4. Peerschke, E.I.B. and Galanakis, D.K. Binding of fibrinogen to ADP-treated platelets: importance of the Aα-chain. In: *Fibrinogen —Structural Variants and Interactions*, A. Henschen, B. Hessel, J. McDonagh and T. Saldeen (eds.), Walter de Gruyter, New York. pp. 369-377, **1985**.

5. Henschen, A., Kehl, M., Southan, C., Lottspeich, F. and Georgopoulos, D. Genetically abnormal fibrinogens — some current characterisation strategies. In: *Fibrinogen —Structure, Functional Aspects, Metabolism*, F. Haverkate, A. Henschen, W. Nieuwenhuizen and P.W. Straub (eds.), Walter de Gruyter, Berlin. pp. 125-144, **1983**.

FIBRINOGEN STONY BROOK II

Last update [10 January 1994]
Alphacode [STONYB02]
Ref. type [Article]

Structural defect [Aα(16) Arg → His[1]]
Mutation [n.a.]

Family studies
Homozygote? [No]
Pedigree published? [No[2]]

Functional defect(s)
FpA release: [Abnormal]
FpB release: [n.a.]
Polymerization: [Abnormal]
Stabilization: [n.a.]

Clinical manifestation(s) Bleeding? [Yes[3]] Thrombosis? [No]

Clinical laboratory results
Plasma fibrinogen concentration (mg/dL)
Chronometric: [77[4]]
Rate-indep'nt: [n.a.]
Immunologic: [408[4]]

*Hypo*dysfibrinogen? [No]

Thrombin time:	[n.a.]
Reptilase (batroxobin) time:	[n.a.]
Prothrombin time:	[n.a.]
Partial thromboplastin time:	[n.a.]
Euglobulin lysis time:	[Normal]
Bleeding time:	[n.a.]
Immunoelectrophoresis:	[n.a.]
Platelet aggregation:	[n.a.]

Other results with patient plasma
Ancrod (Arvin) time: [n.a.]
Recalcification time: [n.a.]
Calcium corrects c.t.? [n.a.]

Inhib. normal plasma? [Yes]
In vivo synthesis: [n.a.]
In vivo catabolism: [n.a.]

Evaluation of isolated patient fibrinogen
Thrombin time: [Abnormal]
Reptilase time: [Abnormal]
Ancrod (Arvin) time: [n.a.]

Abnormal subunit? [No]
Abnormal FDPs? [n.a.]

Remarks
[1]D.K. Galanakis, personal communication.
[2]The mother of the propositus also was affected.
[3]Recurrent post-traumatic hemarthroses and "inappropriately large muscle hematomas and subcutaneous ecchymoses" were reported.
[4]Normal range not reported.

References

1. Galanakis, D.K., and Hultin, M. Fibrinogen Stony Brook II: partial characterization of a heterozygously transmitted peptide A anomaly. *Blood Coag. & Fibrinol.* **1**:567-570, **1990**.

2. Galanakis, D.K. and Hultin, M. Fibrinogen Stony Brook II: a heterozygously transmitted peptide A defect. Evidence that most mutant molecules are homodimers. *Blood* **76 Suppl. 1**:421a, **1990** ABSTRACT

FIBRINOGEN STRASBOURG I[Abs]

Last update [10 January 1994]
Alphacode [STRASB01]
Ref. type [Abstract]

Family studies
Homozygote? [n.a.]
Pedigree published? [n.a.]

Structural defect [n.a.]
Mutation [n.a.]

Functional defect(s)
FpA release: [n.a.]
FpB release: [n.a.]
Polymerization: [Abnormal[1]]
Stabilization: [n.a.]

Clinical manifestation(s) Bleeding? [No] Thrombosis? [Yes[2]]

Clinical laboratory results
Plasma fibrinogen concentration (mg/dL)
Chronometric: [n.a.]
Rate-indep'nt: [n.a.]
Immunologic: [n.a.]

*Hypo*dysfibrinogen? [n.a.]

Thrombin time:	[n.a.]
Reptilase (batroxobin) time:	[n.a.]
Prothrombin time:	[n.a.]
Partial thromboplastin time:	[n.a.]
Euglobulin lysis time:	[n.a.]
Bleeding time:	[n.a.]
Immunoelectrophoresis:	[n.a.]
Platelet aggregation:	[n.a.]

Other results with patient plasma
Ancrod (Arvin) time: [n.a.]
Recalcification time: [n.a.]
Calcium corrects c.t.? [n.a.]

Inhib. normal plasma? [n.a.]
In vivo synthesis: [n.a.]
In vivo catabolism: [n.a.]

Evaluation of isolated patient fibrinogen
Thrombin time: [n.a.]
Reptilase time: [n.a.]
Ancrod (Arvin) time: [n.a.]

Abnormal subunit? [n.a.]
Abnormal FDPs? [n.a.]

Remarks
[1]An *accelerated* rate of fibrin monomer polymerization was reported. Compare with fibrinogens Chapel Hill VI and Oslo I.
[2]Only a preliminary description has been published. Severe venous thrombosis beginning at age 18 resulted in death of the propositus at age 26.

References

1. Wiesel, M.-L, Grunebaum, L., Freyssinet, J.-M. and Cazenave, J.-P Biological causes of familial thrombosis. *Fibrinolys.* **2** **(Suppl. 2)**:14-15, **1988**.

FIBRINOGEN STRASBOURG II^{Abs}

Last update [10 January 1994]
Alphacode [STRASB02]
Ref. type [Abstract]

Structural defect [n.a.]
Mutation [n.a.]

Family studies
Homozygote? [n.a.]
Pedigree published? [n.a.]

Functional defect(s)
FpA release: [n.a.]
FpB release: [n.a.]
Polymerization: [n.a.]
Stabilization: [n.a.]

Clinical manifestation(s) Bleeding? [No] Thrombosis? [Yes[1]]

Clinical laboratory results
Plasma fibrinogen concentration (mg/dL)
Chronometric: [n.a.]
Rate-indep'nt: [n.a.]
Immunologic: [n.a.]

*Hypo*dysfibrinogen? [n.a.]

Thrombin time:	[n.a.]
Reptilase (batroxobin) time:	[n.a.]
Prothrombin time:	[n.a.]
Partial thromboplastin time:	[n.a.]
Euglobulin lysis time:	[n.a.]
Bleeding time:	[n.a.]
Immunoelectrophoresis:	[n.a.]
Platelet aggregation:	[n.a.]

Other results with patient plasma
Ancrod (Arvin) time: [n.a.]
Recalcification time: [n.a.]
Calcium corrects c.t.? [n.a.]

Inhib. normal plasma? [n.a.]
In vivo synthesis: [n.a.]
In vivo catabolism: [n.a.]

Evaluation of isolated patient fibrinogen
Thrombin time: [n.a.]
Reptilase time: [n.a.]
Ancrod (Arvin) time: [n.a.]

Abnormal subunit? [n.a.]
Abnormal FDPs? [n.a.]

Remarks
[1]Only a preliminary description has been published. Venous thrombosis at age 79 was reported (F. Haverkate, personal communication).

References

1. Wiesel, M.-L, Grunebaum, L., Freyssinet, J.-M. and Cazenave, J.-P Biological causes of familial thrombosis. *Fibrinolys.* 2 (**Suppl.** 2):14-15, **1988**.

FIBRINOGEN SYDNEY I

Last update [1 December 1990]
Alphacode [SYDNEY01]
Ref. type [Article]

Family studies
Homozygote? [No]
Pedigree published? [No]

Structural defect [Aα(16) Arg → His]
Mutation [n.a.]

Functional defect(s)
FpA release: [Abnormal]
FpB release: [Abnormal[1]]
Polymerization: [Abnormal]
Stabilization: [n.a.]

Clinical manifestation(s) Bleeding? [No] Thrombosis? [No]

Clinical laboratory results

Plasma fibrinogen concentration (mg/dL)
Chronometric: [n.a.]
Rate-indep'nt: [n.a.]
Immunologic: [Normal[2]]

*Hypo*dysfibrinogen? [No]

Thrombin time:	[85s/(20s)]
Reptilase (batroxobin) time:	[n.a.]
Prothrombin time:	[n.a.]
Partial thromboplastin time:	[n.a.]
Euglobulin lysis time:	[n.a.]
Bleeding time:	[n.a.]
Immunoelectrophoresis:	[n.a.]
Platelet aggregation:	[n.a.]

Other results with patient plasma
Ancrod (Arvin) time: [n.a.]
Recalcification time: [n.a.]
Calcium corrects c.t.? [n.a.]

Inhib. normal plasma? [n.a.]
In vivo synthesis: [n.a.]
In vivo catabolism: [n.a.]

Evaluation of isolated patient fibrinogen
Thrombin time: [n.a.]
Reptilase time: [n.a.]
Ancrod (Arvin) time: [n.a.]

Abnormal subunit? [No]
Abnormal FDPs? [n.a.]

Remarks

[1]Fibrinopeptide B release was delayed in this heterozygous variant only at low thrombin concentrations (Southan, Henschen & Lane 1985; Southan, Lane et al., 1985).

[2]Plasma fibrinogen concentration was within normal limits when determined by an immunologic method; data not reported.

FIBRINOGEN SYDNEY I

References

1. Lane, D.A., Ireland, H., Thompson, E., Southan, C. and Henschen, A. Fibrinogens London I - IV, Manchester, Sydney I and II. Cleavage of fibrinopeptides by thrombin and expression of their polymerisation abnormalities. In: *Fibrinogen —Structural Variants and Interactions*, A. Henschen, B. Hessel, J. McDonagh and T. Saldeen (eds.), W. de Gruyter, Berlin. pp. 197-206, **1985**.

2. Southan, C., Henschen, A. and Lane, D.A. Fibrinogens Sydney I and II: a kinetic study of (His-16) FPA cleavage and its effect on FPB cleavage. In: *Fibrinogen —Structural Variants and Interactions*, A. Henschen, B. Hessel, J. McDonagh and T. Saldeen (eds.), Walter de Gruyter, Berlin. pp. 185-206, **1985**.

3. Southan, C., Lane, D.A., Bode, W. and Henschen, A. Thrombin-induced fibrinopeptide release from a fibrinogen variant (fibrinogen Sydney I) with an Aα Arg-16 → His substitution. *Eur. J. Biochem.* **147**:593-600, **1985**.

4. Henschen, A., Kehl, M., Southan, C., Lottspeich, F. and Georgopoulos, D. Genetically abnormal fibrinogens — some current characterisation strategies. In: *Fibrinogen —Structure, Functional Aspects, Metabolism*, F. Haverkate, A. Henschen, W. Nieuwenhuizen and P.W. Straub (eds.), Walter de Gruyter, Berlin. pp. 125-144, **1983**.

5. Lane, D.A., Ireland, H., Thompson, E., Frost, T.J. and Cuddigan, B. Two more abnormal fibrinogens (London III and Sydney) with impaired fibrinopeptide release. *Thromb. Res.* **28**:821-824, **1982**.

FIBRINOGEN SYDNEY II

Last update [1 December 1990]
Alphacode [SYDNEY02]
Ref. type [Article]

Family studies
Homozygote? [No]
Pedigree published? [No]

Structural defect [Aα(16) Arg → His]
Mutation [n.a.]

Functional defect(s)
FpA release: [Abnormal]
FpB release: [Abnormal]
Polymerization: [n.a.[1]]
Stabilization: [n.a.]

Clinical manifestation(s) Bleeding? [n.a.] Thrombosis? [n.a.]

Clinical laboratory results
Plasma fibrinogen concentration (mg/dL)
Chronometric: [n.a.]
Rate-indep'nt: [n.a.]
Immunologic: [n.a.]

*Hypo*dysfibrinogen? [n.a.]

Thrombin time:	[n.a.]
Reptilase (batroxobin) time:	[n.a.]
Prothrombin time:	[n.a.]
Partial thromboplastin time:	[n.a.]
Euglobulin lysis time:	[n.a.]
Bleeding time:	[n.a.]
Immunoelectrophoresis:	[n.a.]
Platelet aggregation:	[n.a.]

Other results with patient plasma
Ancrod (Arvin) time: [n.a.]
Recalcification time: [n.a.]
Calcium corrects c.t.? [n.a.]

Inhib. normal plasma? [n.a.]
In vivo synthesis: [n.a.]
In vivo catabolism: [n.a.]

Evaluation of isolated patient fibrinogen
Thrombin time: [n.a.]
Reptilase time: [n.a.]
Ancrod (Arvin) time: [n.a.]

Abnormal subunit? [n.a.]
Abnormal FDPs? [n.a.]

Remarks
[1]Fibrin monomer polymerization was not evaluated. Other variants with this molecular defect exhibit delayed fibrinopeptide A and B release plus delayed polymerization of fibrin monomers.

References

1. Lane, D.A., Ireland, H., Thompson, E., Southan, C. and Henschen, A. Fibrinogens London I - IV, Manchester, Sydney I and II. Cleavage of fibrinopeptides by thrombin and expression of their polymerisation abnormalities. In: *Fibrinogen —Structural Variants and Interactions*, A. Henschen, B. Hessel, J. McDonagh and T. Saldeen (eds.), W. de Gruyter, Berlin. pp. 197-206, **1985**.

2. Southan, C., Henschen, A. and Lane, D.A. Fibrinogens Sydney I and II, A kinetic study of (His-16) FPA Cleavage and its effect on FPB cleavage. In: *Fibrinogen —Structural Variants and Interactions*, A. Henschen, B. Hessel, J. McDonagh and T. Saldeen (eds.), Walter de Gruyter, Berlin. pp. 185-206, **1985**.

3. Henschen, A., Kehl, M., Southan, C., Lottspeich, F. and Georgopoulos, D. Genetically abnormal fibrinogens — some current characterisation strategies. In: *Fibrinogen —Structure, Functional Aspects, Metabolism*, F. Haverkate, A. Henschen, W. Nieuwenhuizen and P.W. Straub (eds.), Walter de Gruyter, Berlin. pp. 125-144, **1983**.

FIBRINOGEN TAMPERE I

Last update [10 January 1994]
Alphacode [TAMPER01]
Ref. type [Article]

Structural defect [n.a.]
Mutation [n.a.]

Family studies
Homozygote? [n.a.]
Pedigree published? [No]

Functional defect(s)
FpA release: [n.a.]
FpB release: [n.a.]
Polymerization: [n.a.]
Stabilization: [n.a.]

Clinical manifestation(s) Bleeding? [No] Thrombosis? [Yes[1]]

Clinical laboratory results
Plasma fibrinogen concentration (mg/dL)
Chronometric: [140-180/(170-360)]
Rate-indep'nt: [n.a.]
Immunologic: [250/(200-450)]

*Hypo*dysfibrinogen? [No]

Thrombin time:	[>90s/(<18s)]
Reptilase (batroxobin) time:	[64s/(<11.5s)]
Prothrombin time:	[98%/(70-120%)]
Partial thromboplastin time:	[41.4s/(32-42s)]
Euglobulin lysis time:	[n.a.]
Bleeding time:	[n.a.]
Immunoelectrophoresis:	[n.a.]
Platelet aggregation:	[n.a.]

Other results with patient plasma
Ancrod (Arvin) time: [n.a.]
Recalcification time: [112s/(<113s)]
Calcium corrects c.t.? [n.a.]

Inhib. normal plasma? [n.a.]
In vivo synthesis: [n.a.]
In vivo catabolism: [n.a.]

Evaluation of isolated patient fibrinogen
Thrombin time: [n.a.]
Reptilase time: [n.a.]
Ancrod (Arvin) time: [n.a.]

Abnormal subunit? [n.a.]
Abnormal FDPs? [n.a.]

Remarks
[1]Post-surgical pulmonary embolism, pregnancy-associated thrombophlebitis (9th week), vaginal hemorrhage (35th week), and placental abruption were reported.

References

1. Takala, T., Oksa, H., Rasi, V. and Tuimala, R. Dysfibrinogenemia associated with thrombosis and third-trimester fetal loss: a case report. *J. Reprod. Med.* **36**:410-412, **1991**.

2. Blombäck, B., Banerjee, D., Carlsson, K., Hamsten, A., Hessel, B., Procyk, R., Silveira, A. and Zacharski, L. Native fibrin gel networks and factors influencing their formation in health and disease. *Adv. Exp. Med. Biol.* **281**:1-23, **1990**.

FIBRINOGEN TEMPLE I

Last update [1 December 1990]
Alphacode [TEMPLE01]
Ref. type [Article]

Family studies
Homozygote? [n.a.]
Pedigree published? [No]

Structural defect [n.a.]
Mutation [n.a.]

Functional defect(s)
FpA release: [n.a.[1]]
FpB release: [n.a.[1]]
Polymerization: [n.a.]
Stabilization: [n.a.]

Clinical manifestation(s) Bleeding? [n.a.] Thrombosis? [n.a.]

Clinical laboratory results
Plasma fibrinogen concentration (mg/dL)
Chronometric: [n.a.]
Rate-indep'nt: [n.a.]
Immunologic: [n.a.]

*Hypo*dysfibrinogen? [n.a.]

Thrombin time:	[n.a.]
Reptilase (batroxobin) time:	[n.a.]
Prothrombin time:	[n.a.]
Partial thromboplastin time:	[n.a.]
Euglobulin lysis time:	[n.a.]
Bleeding time:	[n.a.]
Immunoelectrophoresis:	[n.a.]
Platelet aggregation:	[n.a.]

Other results with patient plasma
Ancrod (Arvin) time: [n.a.]
Recalcification time: [n.a.]
Calcium corrects c.t.? [n.a.]

Inhib. normal plasma? [n.a.]
In vivo synthesis: [n.a.]
In vivo catabolism: [n.a.]

Evaluation of isolated patient fibrinogen
Thrombin time: [n.a.]
Reptilase time: [n.a.]
Ancrod (Arvin) time: [n.a.]

Abnormal subunit? [n.a.]
Abnormal FDPs? [n.a.]

Remarks
[1]The normal *amount* of fibrinopeptides A and B was released; the *rate* of fibrinopeptide release was not reported.

References

1. Henschen, A., Kehl, M., Southan, C., Lottspeich, F. and Georgopoulos, D. Genetically abnormal fibrinogens — some current characterisation strategies. In: *Fibrinogen —Structure, Functional Aspects, Metabolism*, F. Haverkate, A. Henschen, W. Nieuwenhuizen and P.W. Straub (eds.), Walter de Gruyter, Berlin. pp. 125-144, **1983**.

FIBRINOGEN TEMPLE II

Last update [1 December 1990]
Alphacode [TEMPLE02]
Ref. type [Article]

Family studies
Homozygote? [n.a.]
Pedigree published? [No]

Structural defect [n.a.]
Mutation [n.a.]

Functional defect(s)
FpA release: [n.a.[1]]
FpB release: [n.a.[1]]
Polymerization: [n.a.]
Stabilization: [n.a.]

Clinical manifestation(s) Bleeding? [n.a.] Thrombosis? [n.a.]

Clinical laboratory results
Plasma fibrinogen concentration (mg/dL)
Chronometric: [n.a.]
Rate-indep'nt: [n.a.]
Immunologic: [n.a.]

*Hypo*dysfibrinogen? [n.a.]

Thrombin time:	[n.a.]
Reptilase (batroxobin) time:	[n.a.]
Prothrombin time:	[n.a.]
Partial thromboplastin time:	[n.a.]
Euglobulin lysis time:	[n.a.]
Bleeding time:	[n.a.]
Immunoelectrophoresis:	[n.a.]
Platelet aggregation:	[n.a.]

Other results with patient plasma
Ancrod (Arvin) time: [n.a.]
Recalcification time: [n.a.]
Calcium corrects c.t.? [n.a.]

Inhib. normal plasma? [n.a.]
In vivo synthesis: [n.a.]
In vivo catabolism: [n.a.]

Evaluation of isolated patient fibrinogen
Thrombin time: [n.a.]
Reptilase time: [n.a.]
Ancrod (Arvin) time: [n.a.]

Abnormal subunit? [n.a.]
Abnormal FDPs? [n.a.]

Remarks
[1]The normal *amount* of fibrinopeptides A and B was released; the *rate* of fibrinopeptide release was not reported.

References

1. Henschen, A., Kehl, M., Southan, C., Lottspeich, F. and Georgopoulos, D. Genetically abnormal fibrinogens — some current characterisation strategies. In: *Fibrinogen —Structure, Functional Aspects, Metabolism*, F. Haverkate, A. Henschen, W. Nieuwenhuizen and P.W. Straub (eds.), Walter de Gruyter, Berlin. pp. 125-144, **1983**.

FIBRINOGEN TOCHIGI I

Last update [1 December 1990]
Alphacode [TOCHIG01]
Ref. type [Article]

Structural defect [γ(275) Arg → Cys]
Mutation [n.a.]

Family studies
Homozygote? [No]
Pedigree published? [No]

Functional defect(s)
FpA release: [Normal]
FpB release: [Normal]
Polymerization: [Abnormal]
Stabilization: [Normal]

Clinical manifestation(s) Bleeding? [No] Thrombosis? [No]

Clinical laboratory results
Plasma fibrinogen concentration (mg/dL)
Chronometric: [44/(150-350)]
Rate-indep'nt: [142/(150-350)]
Immunologic: [210/(150-350)]
*Hypo*dysfibrinogen? [No]

Thrombin time:	[>150s/(8-12s)]
Reptilase (batroxobin) time:	[>150s/(13-18s)]
Prothrombin time:	[Normal[1]]
Partial thromboplastin time:	[Normal]
Euglobulin lysis time:	[n.a.]
Bleeding time:	[n.a.]
Immunoelectrophoresis:	[Normal]
Platelet aggregation:	[n.a.]

Other results with patient plasma
Ancrod (Arvin) time: [n.a.]
Recalcification time: [n.a.]
Calcium corrects c.t.? [Yes]
Inhib. normal plasma? [n.a.]
In vivo synthesis: [n.a.]
In vivo catabolism: [n.a.]

Evaluation of isolated patient fibrinogen
Thrombin time: [>150s/(15-17s)]
Reptilase time: [>150s/(12-14s)]
Ancrod (Arvin) time: [n.a.]
Abnormal subunit? [Yes[2]]
Abnormal FDPs? [Yes[3]]

Remarks
[1]Data not reported.
[2]An abnormal γ-chain (approx. 500 Da larger than normal) was detected by SDS-PAGE.
[3]The size heterogeneity of the γ-chain persisted in fragments D_1 and D_2, and γ-chain remnants thereof.

References

1. Yoshida, N., Ota, K., Moroi, M. and Matsuda, M. An apparently higher molecular weight γ-chain variant in a new congenital abnormal fibrinogen Tochigi characterized by the replacement of γ arginine-275 by cysteine. *Blood* **71**:480-487, **1988**.

FIBRINOGEN TOKUSHIMA I

Last update [1 December 1990]
Alphacode [TOKUSH01]
Ref. type [Article]

Structural defect [n.a.]
Mutation [n.a.]

Family studies
Homozygote? [n.a.]
Pedigree published? [Yes]

Functional defect(s)
FpA release: [Normal[1]]
FpB release: [Normal[1]]
Polymerization: [Abnormal]
Stabilization: [Normal]

Clinical manifestation(s) Bleeding? [No] Thrombosis? [No]

Clinical laboratory results

Plasma fibrinogen concentration (mg/dL)
Chronometric: [105[2]]
Rate-indep'nt: [627[2]]
Immunologic: [581[2]]

*Hypo*dysfibrinogen? [No]

Thrombin time:	[58s/(11s)]
Reptilase (batroxobin) time:	[86.2s/(19.5s)]
Prothrombin time:	[15.2s/(11.4s)]
Partial thromboplastin time:	[51.4s/(40.2s)]
Euglobulin lysis time:	[10h/(9.5h)]
Bleeding time:	[Normal]
Immunoelectrophoresis:	[n.a.]
Platelet aggregation:	[Normal]

Other results with patient plasma
Ancrod (Arvin) time: [n.a.]
Recalcification time: [n.a.]
Calcium corrects c.t.? [n.a.]

Inhib. normal plasma? [n.a.]
In vivo synthesis: [n.a.]
In vivo catabolism: [n.a.]

Evaluation of isolated patient fibrinogen
Thrombin time: [188s/(30.8s)]
Reptilase time: [>1800s/(78.6s)]
Ancrod (Arvin) time: [n.a.]

Abnormal subunit? [No]
Abnormal FDPs? [n.a.]

Remarks
[1]The rate of *total* fibrinopeptide release was normal.
[2]Normal range not reported.

References

1. Shigekiyo, T., Shirakami, A., Kawauchi, S., Hirai, Y., Takeichi, T., Inomoto, T., Inoue, T., Shintani, Y., Takada, Y., Mizuguchi, Y. and Masuda, K. [Dysfibrinogenemia and nephrotic syndrome: a case report]. *Rinsho Ketsueki* **26**:761-765, **1985**.

FIBRINOGEN TOKYO I

Last update [1 December 1990]
Alphacode [TOKYO01]
Ref. type [Article]

Family studies
Homozygote? [n.a.]
Pedigree published? [No[1]]

Structural defect [n.a.]
Mutation [n.a.]

Functional defect(s)
FpA release: [n.a.]
FpB release: [n.a.]
Polymerization: [n.a.]
Stabilization: [Abnormal]

Clinical manifestation(s) Bleeding? [Yes[2]] Thrombosis? [No]

Clinical laboratory results
Plasma fibrinogen concentration (mg/dL)
Chronometric: [n.a.]
Rate-indep'nt: [163-320/(150-350)]
Immunologic: [182-263/(200-400)]

*Hypo*dysfibrinogen? [No]

Thrombin time:	[11s/(10-11s)]
Reptilase (batroxobin) time:	[Normal[3]]
Prothrombin time:	[12.5s/(11-13s)]
Partial thromboplastin time:	[64s/(55-75s)]
Euglobulin lysis time:	[Normal[3]]
Bleeding time:	[Normal]
Immunoelectrophoresis:	[Anodal]
Platelet aggregation:	[Normal]

Other results with patient plasma
Ancrod (Arvin) time: [n.a.]
Recalcification time: [Normal[3]]
Calcium corrects c.t.? [n.a.]

Inhib. normal plasma? [No]
In vivo synthesis: [n.a.]
In vivo catabolism: [n.a.]

Evaluation of isolated patient fibrinogen
Thrombin time: [n.a.]
Reptilase time: [n.a.]
Ancrod (Arvin) time: [n.a.]

Abnormal subunit? [Yes]
Abnormal FDPs? [Yes[4]]

Remarks
[1]Pedigree is on file (T. Samori, personal communication); autosomal dominant inheritance pattern is evident.
[2]Subnormal factor XIII levels were reported. Propositus and affected family members have a mild to moderate bleeding tendency, especially following trauma or surgery (T. Samori, personal communication).
[3]Data not reported.
[4]Immunoelectrophoresis disclosed an abnormal fragment D.

References

1. Samori, T. Studies on fibrinogen Tokyo (dysfibrinogenemia) with special reference to the analysis of FDP-D fragment. *J. Tokyo Med. Coll.* **36**:583-594, **1978**.

2. Samori, T., Konishi, S., Itoh, O., Kato, M., Ikematsu, S., Yatabe, M., Fujimaki, M. and Fukutake, K. A new type of congenital dysfibrinogenemia with defective stabilization of fibrin polymers — fibrinogen Tokyo. *Blood & Vessel* **8**:628-632, **1977**.

3. Samori, T., Yatabe, M., Ukita, M., Fujimaki, M. and Fukutake, K. Proceedings: A new type of congenital dysfibrinogenemia (fibrinogen Tokyo) with defective stabilization of fibrin polymers. *Thromb. Diath. Haemorrh.* **34**:329, **1975**. ABSTRACT

FIBRINOGEN TOKYO II

Last update	[1 December 1990]	**Structural defect**	[γ(275) Arg → Cys[1]]
Alphacode	[TOKYO02]	**Mutation**	[n.a.]
Ref. type	[Article]		

Family studies

Homozygote?	[No]
Pedigree published?	[Yes]

Functional defect(s)

FpA release:	[Normal[2]]
FpB release:	[Normal[2]]
Polymerization:	[Abnormal]
Stabilization:	[Normal]

Clinical manifestation(s) Bleeding? [No] Thrombosis? [No]

Clinical laboratory results

Plasma fibrinogen concentration (mg/dL)

Chronometric:	[27/(200-400)]
Rate-indep'nt:	[197/(200-350)]
Immunologic:	[378/(200-400)]

*Hypo*dysfibrinogen? [No]

Thrombin time:	[155s/(11.8s)]
Reptilase (batroxobin) time:	[172s/(18.7s)]
Prothrombin time:	[15.8s/(11.3s)]
Partial thromboplastin time:	[37.9s/(21.3s)]
Euglobulin lysis time:	[n.a.]
Bleeding time:	[Normal]
Immunoelectrophoresis:	[Normal]
Platelet aggregation:	[Normal]

Other results with patient plasma

Ancrod (Arvin) time:	[n.a.]	Inhib. normal plasma?	[n.a.]
Recalcification time:	[n.a.]	In vivo synthesis:	[n.a.]
Calcium corrects c.t.?	[Yes]	In vivo catabolism:	[n.a.]

Evaluation of isolated patient fibrinogen

Thrombin time:	[n.a.]	Abnormal subunit?	[No]
Reptilase time:	[n.a.]	Abnormal FDPs?	[n.a.]
Ancrod (Arvin) time:	[n.a.]		

Remarks

[1]M. Matsuda, personal communication.

[2]The rate of *total* fibrinopeptide release was normal; individual fibrinopeptide release was not reported.

References

1. Matsuda, M., Nakamikawa, C., Baba, M. and Morimoto, K. Fibrinogen Tokyo II: an abnormal fibrinogen with an impaired polymerization site on the aligned DD domain of fibrin molecules. In: *Fibrinogen —Structural Variants and Interactions*, A. Henschen, B. Hessel, J. McDonagh and T. Saldeen (eds.), Walter de Gruyter, Berlin. pp. 213-222, **1985**.

2. Matsuda, M., Baba, M., Morimoto, K. and Nakamikawa, C. "Fibrinogen Tokyo II:" an abnormal fibrinogen with an impaired polymerization site on the aligned DD domain of fibrin molecules. *J. Clin. Invest.* **72**:1034-1041, **1983**.

FIBRINOGEN TORINO I

Last update	[1 December 1990]	**Structural defect**	[Aα(16) Arg → Cys]
Alphacode	[TORINO01]	**Mutation**	[n.a.]
Ref. type	[Article]		

Family studies
Homozygote? [No]
Pedigree published? [No]

Functional defect(s)
FpA release: [n.a.[1]]
FpB release: [n.a.[1]]
Polymerization: [Abnormal]
Stabilization: [n.a.]

Clinical manifestation(s) Bleeding? [No] Thrombosis? [No]

Clinical laboratory results

Plasma fibrinogen concentration (mg/dL)
Chronometric: [20/(200)]
Rate-indep'nt: [270/(200)]
Immunologic: [230/(200)]

*Hypo*dysfibrinogen? [No]

Thrombin time:	[40s/(18s)]
Reptilase (batroxobin) time:	[53s/(20s)]
Prothrombin time:	[n.a.]
Partial thromboplastin time:	[n.a.]
Euglobulin lysis time:	[n.a.]
Bleeding time:	[n.a.]
Immunoelectrophoresis:	[n.a.]
Platelet aggregation:	[n.a.]

Other results with patient plasma

Ancrod (Arvin) time:	[n.a.]	Inhib. normal plasma?	[n.a.]
Recalcification time:	[n.a.]	In vivo synthesis:	[n.a.]
Calcium corrects c.t.?	[n.a.]	In vivo catabolism:	[n.a.]

Evaluation of isolated patient fibrinogen

Thrombin time:	[n.a.]	Abnormal subunit?	[n.a.]
Reptilase time:	[n.a.]	Abnormal FDPs?	[n.a.]
Ancrod (Arvin) time:	[n.a.]		

Remarks

[1]Rates of fibrinopeptide release were not reported. Other dysfibrinogens with this molecular defect exhibit delayed fibrinopeptide A and B release plus delayed polymerization of fibrin monomers.

References

1. Reber, P., Furlan, M., Beck, E.A. and Barbui, T. Fibrinogen Bergamo III and fibrinogen Torino: two further variants with hereditary molecular defects in fibrinopeptide A. *Thromb. Res.* **46**:163-167, **1987**.

FIBRINOGEN TROYES I

Last update	[1 December 1990]	**Structural defect**	[n.a.]
Alphacode	[TROYES01]	**Mutation**	[n.a.]
Ref. type	[Article]		

Functional defect(s)

FpA release:	[Normal]
FpB release:	[Normal]
Polymerization:	[Abnormal]
Stabilization:	[n.a.]

Family studies

Homozygote?	[n.a.]
Pedigree published?	[Yes]

Clinical manifestation(s) Bleeding? [No] Thrombosis? [No]

Clinical laboratory results

Plasma fibrinogen concentration (mg/dL)

Chronometric:	[55/(300-450)]
Rate-indep'nt:	[250/(300-450)]
Immunologic:	[360/(240-480)]

*Hypo*dysfibrinogen? [No]

Thrombin time:	[60s/(19s)]
Reptilase (batroxobin) time:	[98s/(22s)]
Prothrombin time:	[18s/(12s)]
Partial thromboplastin time:	[n.a.]
Euglobulin lysis time:	[240m/(240m)]
Bleeding time:	[Normal]
Immunoelectrophoresis:	[Normal]
Platelet aggregation:	[Abnormal]

Other results with patient plasma

Ancrod (Arvin) time:	[n.a.]	Inhib. normal plasma?	[n.a.]
Recalcification time:	[n.a.]	In vivo synthesis:	[n.a.]
Calcium corrects c.t.?	[No]	In vivo catabolism:	[n.a.]

Evaluation of isolated patient fibrinogen

Thrombin time:	[n.a.]	Abnormal subunit?	[No]
Reptilase time:	[n.a.]	Abnormal FDPs?	[n.a.]
Ancrod (Arvin) time:	[n.a.]		

Remarks

References

1. Corrihons, G., Soria, J., Soria, C., Conard, J., Horellou, M.H. and Samama, M. [Congenital dysfibrinogenemia. Apropos of 13 cases]. *Sem. Hop. Paris* **59**:2517-2523, **1983**.

2. Soria, J., Soria, C., Durand, G. and Feger, J. [Electrofocusing of abnormal fibrinogens in polyacrylamide gel]. *Ann. Biol. Clin. (Paris)* **30**:161-165, **1972**.

3. Soria, J., Soria, C., Samama, M., Poirot, E. and Kling, C. Fibrinogen Troyes — fibrinogen Metz. Two new cases of congenital dysfibrinogenemia. *Thromb. Diath. Haemorrh.* **27**:619-633, **1972**.

FIBRINOGEN VALENCIA I

Last update [1 December 1990]
Alphacode [VALENC01]
Ref. type [Article]

Family studies
Homozygote? [n.a.]
Pedigree published? [Yes[1]]

Structural defect [n.a.]
Mutation [n.a.]

Functional defect(s)
FpA release: [n.a.]
FpB release: [n.a.]
Polymerization: [Normal]
Stabilization: [Abnormal[6]]

Clinical manifestation(s) Bleeding? [Yes[2]] Thrombosis? [No]

Clinical laboratory results
Plasma fibrinogen concentration (mg/dL)
Chronometric: [n.a.]
Rate-indep'nt: [76-80/(250)[3]]
Immunologic: [n.a.]

*Hypo*dysfibrinogen? [Yes]

Thrombin time:	[No clot]
Reptilase (batroxobin) time:	[No clot]
Prothrombin time:	[n.a.]
Partial thromboplastin time:	[<5%[4]]
Euglobulin lysis time:	[n.a.[5]]
Bleeding time:	[Abnormal]
Immunoelectrophoresis:	[n.a.]
Platelet aggregation:	[n.a.]

Other results with patient plasma
Ancrod (Arvin) time: [n.a.]
Recalcification time: [n.a.]
Calcium corrects c.t.? [No]

Inhib. normal plasma? [No]
In vivo synthesis: [n.a.]
In vivo catabolism: [n.a.]

Evaluation of isolated patient fibrinogen
Thrombin time: [n.a.]
Reptilase time: [n.a.]
Ancrod (Arvin) time: [n.a.]

Abnormal subunit? [No]
Abnormal FDPs? [n.a.[5]]

Remarks
[1]The family history was positive for consanguinity.
[2]The propositus was an infant with cephalohematoma and hemorrhage at injection sites.
[3]A second rate-independent method yielded 87-90 mg/dL (control: 283 mg/dL).
[4]Normal range not reported; this result is abnormal.
[5]A "shortened" euglobulin lysis time was reported. There also is evidence for an increased rate of plasmin degradation.
[6]E. Regañon, personal communication.

References

1. Aznar, J., Fernández-Pavon, A., Regañon, E., Vila, V. and Orellana, F. Fibrinogen Valencia. A new case of congenital dysfibrinogenemia. *Thromb. Diath. Haemorrh.* **32**:564-577, **1974**.

FIBRINOGEN VALHALLA I[Abs]

Last update [1 December 1990]
Alphacode [VALHAL01]
Ref. type [Abstract]

Family studies
Homozygote? [No]
Pedigree published? [No]

Structural defect [n.a.]
Mutation [n.a.]

Functional defect(s)
FpA release: [Normal]
FpB release: [Abnormal[1]]
Polymerization: [Abnormal]
Stabilization: [n.a.]

Clinical manifestation(s) Bleeding? [Yes[2]] Thrombosis? [No]

Clinical laboratory results
Plasma fibrinogen concentration (mg/dL)
Chronometric: [n.a.]
Rate-indep'nt: [n.a.]
Immunologic: [n.a.]

*Hypo*dysfibrinogen? [n.a.]

Thrombin time:	[Normal[3]]
Reptilase (batroxobin) time:	[n.a.]
Prothrombin time:	[Normal[3]]
Partial thromboplastin time:	[Normal[3]]
Euglobulin lysis time:	[Normal]
Bleeding time:	[Abnormal]
Immunoelectrophoresis:	[n.a.]
Platelet aggregation:	[n.a.]

Other results with patient plasma
Ancrod (Arvin) time: [n.a.]
Recalcification time: [n.a.]
Calcium corrects c.t.? [n.a.]

Inhib. normal plasma? [n.a.]
In vivo synthesis: [n.a.]
In vivo catabolism: [n.a.]

Evaluation of isolated patient fibrinogen
Thrombin time: [73s/(45s)]
Reptilase time: [n.a.]
Ancrod (Arvin) time: [n.a.]

Abnormal subunit? [No]
Abnormal FDPs? [n.a.]

Remarks
[1]Only half the normal amount of fibrinopeptide B was released.
[2]Postpartum bleeding was reported.
[3]Data not reported.

References

1. Lerner, R.G., Galanakis, D.K., Nelson, J.C. and Franco, P. Fibrinogen Valhalla: a bleeding disorder with defective fibrinopeptide B release. *Blood* **68 (Suppl. 1)**:336a, **1986**. ABSTRACT

FIBRINOGEN VANCOUVER I

Last update [10 January 1994]
Alphacode [VANCOU01]
Ref. type [Article]

Family studies
Homozygote? [n.a.]
Pedigree published? [Yes]

Structural defect [n.a.]
Mutation [n.a.]

Functional defect(s)
FpA release: [n.a.]
FpB release: [n.a.]
Polymerization: [n.a.]
Stabilization: [n.a.]

Clinical manifestation(s) Bleeding? [Yes[1]] Thrombosis? [No]

Clinical laboratory results
Plasma fibrinogen concentration (mg/dL)
Chronometric: [n.a.]
Rate-indep'nt: [76[2]]
Immunologic: [n.a.]

*Hypo*dysfibrinogen? [Yes[3]]

Thrombin time:	[Abnormal[4]]
Reptilase (batroxobin) time:	[n.a.]
Prothrombin time:	[63%[2]]
Partial thromboplastin time:	[n.a.]
Euglobulin lysis time:	[n.a.]
Bleeding time:	[Normal]
Immunoelectrophoresis:	[n.a.]
Platelet aggregation:	[n.a.]

Other results with patient plasma
Ancrod (Arvin) time: [n.a.]
Recalcification time: [n.a.]
Calcium corrects c.t.? [n.a.]

Inhib. normal plasma? [n.a.]
In vivo synthesis: [n.a.]
In vivo catabolism: [n.a.]

Evaluation of isolated patient fibrinogen
Thrombin time: [n.a.]
Reptilase time: [n.a.]
Ancrod (Arvin) time: [n.a.]

Abnormal subunit? [n.a.]
Abnormal FDPs? [n.a.]

Remarks
[1]The 27 year-old proposita exhibied easy bruising, excessive postpartum bleeding, and excessive bleeding after dental extraction.
[2]Normal range not reported.
[3]Since neither a functional nor structural defect has been identified, the possibility that fibrinogen Vancouver represents only hypofibrinogenemia has not been excluded.
[4]Data not reported.

References

1. Hasselback, R., Marion, R.B. and Thomas, J.W. Congenital hypofibrinogenemia in five members of a family. *Canad. Med. Assoc. J.* **88**:19-22, **1963**.

FIBRINOGEN VERSAILLES I

Last update	[1 December 1990]	**Structural defect**	[n.a.]
Alphacode	[VERSAI01]	**Mutation**	[n.a.]
Ref. type	[Article]		

Family studies
Homozygote? [n.a.]
Pedigree published? [Yes]

Functional defect(s)
FpA release: [n.a.]
FpB release: [n.a.]
Polymerization: [Abnormal]
Stabilization: [n.a.]

Clinical manifestation(s) Bleeding? [No] Thrombosis? [No]

Clinical laboratory results
Plasma fibrinogen concentration (mg/dL)
Chronometric: [40/(200-400)]
Rate-indep'nt: [240[1]]
Immunologic: [180[1]]
*Hypo*dysfibrinogen? [No]

Thrombin time:	[62s/(23.5s)]
Reptilase (batroxobin) time:	[36.5s/(19s)]
Prothrombin time:	[50%[1]]
Partial thromboplastin time:	[38s/(34s)]
Euglobulin lysis time:	[>3h/(>3h)]
Bleeding time:	[Normal]
Immunoelectrophoresis:	[Normal]
Platelet aggregation:	[n.a.]

Other results with patient plasma

Ancrod (Arvin) time:	[n.a.]	Inhib. normal plasma?	[n.a.]
Recalcification time:	[n.a.]	In vivo synthesis:	[n.a.]
Calcium corrects c.t.?	[No]	In vivo catabolism:	[n.a.]

Evaluation of isolated patient fibrinogen

Thrombin time:	[n.a.]	Abnormal subunit?	[n.a.]
Reptilase time:	[n.a.]	Abnormal FDPs?	[n.a.]
Ancrod (Arvin) time:	[n.a.]		

Remarks
[1]Normal range not reported.

References

1. Voinnesson, A. and Salaün, M. [Hereditary dysfibrinogenaemia. Study of a family]. *Sem. Hop. Paris* **55**:1507-1512, **1979**.

FIBRINOGEN VICENZA I

Last update [1 December 1990]
Alphacode [VICENZ01]
Ref. type [Article]

Structural defect [n.a.]
Mutation [n.a.]

Family studies
Homozygote? [No]
Pedigree published? [No]

Functional defect(s)
FpA release: [Normal[1]]
FpB release: [Normal[1]]
Polymerization: [Abnormal]
Stabilization: [Normal]

Clinical manifestation(s) Bleeding? [Yes[2]] Thrombosis? [No]

Clinical laboratory results

Plasma fibrinogen concentration (mg/dL)
Chronometric: [84/(200-400)]
Rate-indep'nt: [240/(180-400)]
Immunologic: [280/(200-450)]

*Hypo*dysfibrinogen? [No]

Thrombin time:	[58s/(13-17s)]
Reptilase (batroxobin) time:	[67s/(15-20s)]
Prothrombin time:	[17.4s/(12-14s)]
Partial thromboplastin time:	[34s/(27-33s)]
Euglobulin lysis time:	[Normal]
Bleeding time:	[Normal]
Immunoelectrophoresis:	[Normal]
Platelet aggregation:	[Normal]

Other results with patient plasma
Ancrod (Arvin) time: [41s/(12-18s)]
Recalcification time: [n.a.]
Calcium corrects c.t.? [No]

Inhib. normal plasma? [Yes]
In vivo synthesis: [n.a.]
In vivo catabolism: [n.a.]

Evaluation of isolated patient fibrinogen
Thrombin time: [48s/(15-20s)]
Reptilase time: [n.a.]
Ancrod (Arvin) time: [n.a.]

Abnormal subunit? [No]
Abnormal FDPs? [No]

Remarks

[1]The rate of *total* fibrinopeptide release was normal. The rate of fibrinopeptide A release also was determined by radioimmunoassay and found to be normal.

[2]The 24 year-old propositus exhibited easy bruising, epistaxis, and gingival bleeding.

References

1. Rodeghiero, F., Castaman, G.C., Dal Belin Peruffo, A., Dini, E., Galletti, A., Barone, E. and Gastaldi, G. Fibrinogen Vicenza and Genova II: two new cases of congenital dysfibrinogenemia with isolated defect of fibrin monomer polymerization and inhibitory activity on normal coagulation. *Thromb. Haemostas.* **57**:252-258, **1987**.

FIBRINOGEN VIENNA I[Abs]

Last update [1 December 1990]
Alphacode [VIENNA01]
Ref. type [Abstract]

Structural defect [n.a.]
Mutation [n.a.]

Family studies
Homozygote? [n.a.]
Pedigree published? [No]

Functional defect(s)
FpA release: [n.a.]
FpB release: [n.a.]
Polymerization: [Abnormal]
Stabilization: [n.a.]

Clinical manifestation(s) Bleeding? [Yes[1]] Thrombosis? [No]

Clinical laboratory results

Plasma fibrinogen concentration (mg/dL)
Chronometric: [Subnormal[2]]
Rate-indep'nt: [n.a.]
Immunologic: [Normal[2]]

*Hypo*dysfibrinogen? [No]

Thrombin time:	[Abnormal[2]]
Reptilase (batroxobin) time:	[Abnormal[2]]
Prothrombin time:	[Abnormal[2]]
Partial thromboplastin time:	[n.a.]
Euglobulin lysis time:	[n.a.]
Bleeding time:	[n.a.]
Immunoelectrophoresis:	[Normal]
Platelet aggregation:	[Normal]

Other results with patient plasma
Ancrod (Arvin) time: [n.a.]
Recalcification time: [n.a.]
Calcium corrects c.t.? [n.a.]

Inhib. normal plasma? [n.a.]
In vivo synthesis: [n.a.]
In vivo catabolism: [n.a.]

Evaluation of isolated patient fibrinogen
Thrombin time: [n.a.]
Reptilase time: [n.a.]
Ancrod (Arvin) time: [n.a.]

Abnormal subunit? [No]
Abnormal FDPs? [n.a.]

Remarks
[1]Postpartum bleeding and spontaneous abortions were reported.
[2]Data not reported.

References

1. Thaler, E., Niessner, H. and Lechner, K. Fibrinogen Vienna I: Gerinnungsphysiologische und biochemische studien. *Acta Med. Austr.* 3:148-149, **1976**.

FIBRINOGEN VILLEPARISIS I

Last update [1 December 1990]
Alphacode [VILLEP01]
Ref. type [Article]

Family studies

Homozygote?	[n.a.]
Pedigree published?	[No]

Structural defect [n.a.]
Mutation [n.a.]

Functional defect(s)

FpA release:	[n.a.]
FpB release:	[n.a.]
Polymerization:	[n.a.]
Stabilization:	[n.a.]

Clinical manifestation(s) Bleeding? [n.a.] Thrombosis? [n.a.]

Clinical laboratory results

Plasma fibrinogen concentration (mg/dL)

Chronometric:	[55[1]]
Rate-indep'nt:	[90[1]]
Immunologic:	[90[1]]

*Hypo*dysfibrinogen? [Yes[2]]

Thrombin time:	[33s/(20s)]
Reptilase (batroxobin) time:	[23s/(15s)]
Prothrombin time:	[39%/(>70%)]
Partial thromboplastin time:	[41s/(37s)]
Euglobulin lysis time:	[n.a.]
Bleeding time:	[n.a.]
Immunoelectrophoresis:	[n.a.]
Platelet aggregation:	[n.a.]

Other results with patient plasma

Ancrod (Arvin) time:	[n.a.]	Inhib. normal plasma?	[No]
Recalcification time:	[n.a.]	In vivo synthesis:	[n.a.]
Calcium corrects c.t.?	[n.a.]	In vivo catabolism:	[n.a.]

Evaluation of isolated patient fibrinogen

Thrombin time:	[n.a.]	Abnormal subunit?	[n.a.]
Reptilase time:	[n.a.]	Abnormal FDPs?	[n.a.]
Ancrod (Arvin) time:	[n.a.]		

Remarks

[1]Normal range not reported.

[2]Since neither the functional nor the structural defect has been identified, the possibility that this variant represents only hypofibrinogenemia has not been excluded.

References

1. Corrihons, G., Soria, J., Soria, C., Conard, J., Horellou, M.H. and Samama, M. [Congenital dysfibrinogenemia. Apropos of 13 cases]. *Sem. Hop. Paris* **59**:2517-2523, **1983**.

FIBRINOGEN VILLIERS-SUR-MARNE I

Last update	[10 January 1994]	**Structural defect**	[n.a.]
Alphacode	[VILLIE01]	**Mutation**	[n.a.]
Ref. type	[Article]		

Family studies
Homozygote? [n.a.]
Pedigree published? [No]

Functional defect(s)
FpA release: [n.a.]
FpB release: [n.a.]
Polymerization: [n.a.]
Stabilization: [n.a.]

Clinical manifestation(s) Bleeding? [n.a.] Thrombosis? [n.a.]

Clinical laboratory results
Plasma fibrinogen concentration (mg/dL)
Chronometric: [45[1]]
Rate-indep'nt: [215[1]]
Immunologic: [350[1]]

*Hypo*dysfibrinogen? [No]

Thrombin time:	[>60s/(21s)]
Reptilase (batroxobin) time:	[>60s/(21s)]
Prothrombin time:	[44%/(>70%)]
Partial thromboplastin time:	[39s/(32s)]
Euglobulin lysis time:	[n.a.]
Bleeding time:	[n.a.]
Immunoelectrophoresis:	[n.a.]
Platelet aggregation:	[n.a.]

Other results with patient plasma

Ancrod (Arvin) time:	[n.a.]	Inhib. normal plasma?	[n.a.]
Recalcification time:	[n.a.]	In vivo synthesis:	[n.a.]
Calcium corrects c.t.?	[n.a.]	In vivo catabolism:	[n.a.]

Evaluation of isolated patient fibrinogen

Thrombin time:	[n.a.]	Abnormal subunit?	[n.a.]
Reptilase time:	[n.a.]	Abnormal FDPs?	[n.a.]
Ancrod (Arvin) time:	[n.a.]		

Remarks
[1]Normal range not reported.

References

1. Corrihons, G., Soria, J., Soria, C., Conard, J., Horellou, M.H. and Samama, M. [Congenital dysfibrinogenemia. Apropos of 13 cases]. *Sem. Hop. Paris* **59**:2517-2523, **1983**.

FIBRINOGEN VITRY-SUR-SEINE I

Last update [10 January 1994]
Alphacode [VITRYS01]
Ref. type [Article]

Family studies
Homozygote? [n.a.]
Pedigree published? [No]

Structural defect [n.a.]
Mutation [n.a.]

Functional defect(s)
FpA release: [n.a.]
FpB release: [n.a.]
Polymerization: [n.a.]
Stabilization: [n.a.]

Clinical manifestation(s) Bleeding? [n.a.] Thrombosis? [n.a.]

Clinical laboratory results
Plasma fibrinogen concentration (mg/dL)
Chronometric: [170[1]]
Rate-indep'nt: [500[1]]
Immunologic: [550[1]]

*Hypo*dysfibrinogen? [No]

Thrombin time:	[>60s/(20s)]
Reptilase (batroxobin) time:	[38s/(18s)]
Prothrombin time:	[44%/(>70%)]
Partial thromboplastin time:	[38s/(35s)]
Euglobulin lysis time:	[n.a.]
Bleeding time:	[n.a.]
Immunoelectrophoresis:	[n.a.]
Platelet aggregation:	[n.a.]

Other results with patient plasma
Ancrod (Arvin) time: [n.a.]
Recalcification time: [n.a.]
Calcium corrects c.t.? [n.a.]

Inhib. normal plasma? [n.a.]
In vivo synthesis: [n.a.]
In vivo catabolism: [n.a.]

Evaluation of isolated patient fibrinogen
Thrombin time: [n.a.]
Reptilase time: [n.a.]
Ancrod (Arvin) time: [n.a.]

Abnormal subunit? [n.a.]
Abnormal FDPs? [n.a.]

Remarks
[1]Normal range not reported.

References

1. Corrihons, G., Soria, J., Soria, C., Conard, J., Horellou, M.H. and Samama, M. [Congenital dysfibrinogenemia. Apropos of 13 cases]. *Sem. Hop. Paris* **59**:2517-2523, **1983**.

FIBRINOGEN VLISSINGEN I

Last update [10 January 1994]
Alphacode [VLISSI01]
Ref. type [Article]

Structural defect [γ(319-320) deletion[1]]
Mutation [AATGAT deletion[1]]

Family studies
Homozygote? [No]
Pedigree published? [No]

Functional defect(s)
FpA release: [Normal]
FpB release: [Normal]
Polymerization: [Abnormal]
Stabilization: [n.a.]

Clinical manifestation(s) Bleeding? [No] Thrombosis? [Yes[2]]

Clinical laboratory results

Plasma fibrinogen concentration (mg/dL)
Chronometric: [40/(200-400)]
Rate-indep'nt: [180/(200-400)]
Immunologic: [310/(200-400)]

*Hypo*dysfibrinogen? [No]

Thrombin time:	[57.5s/(18.6s)]
Reptilase (batroxobin) time:	[41.3s/(20.1s)]
Prothrombin time:	[n.a.]
Partial thromboplastin time:	[n.a.]
Euglobulin lysis time:	[n.a.]
Bleeding time:	[n.a.]
Immunoelectrophoresis:	[n.a.]
Platelet aggregation:	[n.a.]

Other results with patient plasma

Ancrod (Arvin) time:	[n.a.]	Inhib. normal plasma?	[n.a.]
Recalcification time:	[n.a.]	In vivo synthesis:	[n.a.]
Calcium corrects c.t.?	[n.a.]	In vivo catabolism:	[n.a.]

Evaluation of isolated patient fibrinogen

Thrombin time:	[n.a.]	Abnormal subunit?	[Yes[3]]
Reptilase time:	[n.a.]	Abnormal FDPs?	[Yes[4]]
Ancrod (Arvin) time:	[n.a.]		

Remarks

[1]The structural defect was determined with the PCR method. A six-nucleotide deletion at codons γ(319-320) was reported.
[2]Massive pulmonary embolism in the 23 year-old proposita was reported.
[3]A γ-chain with subnormal molecular weight was reported.
[4]In the presence of calcium, plasmin degrades the abnormal γ-chain to a size that is smaller than normal.

References

1. Koopman, J., Haverkate, F., Briët, E. and Lord, S.T. A congenitally abnormal fibrinogen (Vlissingen) with a 6-base deletion in the γ-chain gene, causing defective calcium binding and impaired fibrin polymerization. *J. Biol. Chem.* **266**:13456-13461, **1991**.

2. Koopman, J. and Haverkate, F. Structure-function relationships in abnormal fibrinogens. Defects at the DNA level. In: *Fibrinogen 4. Current Basic and Clinical Aspects*, M. Matsuda, S. Iwanaga, A. Takada and A. Henschen (eds.), Elsevier Science Publ., B.V., Amsterdam. pp. 179-183, **1990**.

3. Koopman, J., Haverkate, F., Lord, S., Caekebeke-Peerlinck, K., Brommer, E. and Briet, E. A six base deletion in the γ-chain gene of dysfibrinogen Vlissingen, coding for Asn-319 and Asp-320, resulting in defective interaction with calcium. *Thromb. Haemostas.* **62**:158, **1989**. ABSTRACT

FIBRINOGEN WHITE MARSH I

Last update [10 January 1994]
Alphacode [WHITEM01]
Ref. type [Article]

Structural defect [Aα(16) Arg → His]
Mutation [n.a.]

Family studies
Homozygote? [No]
Pedigree published? [No]

Functional defect(s)
FpA release: [Abnormal]
FpB release: [Abnormal]
Polymerization: [Abnormal]
Stabilization: [n.a.[1]]

Clinical manifestation(s) Bleeding? [n.a.] Thrombosis? [n.a.]

Clinical laboratory results
Plasma fibrinogen concentration (mg/dL)
Chronometric: [79[2]]
Rate-indep'nt: [n.a.]
Immunologic: [384[2]]

*Hypo*dysfibrinogen? [No]

Thrombin time:	[44s/(19s)]
Reptilase (batroxobin) time:	[34s/(13s)]
Prothrombin time:	[14s/(12s)]
Partial thromboplastin time:	[26s/(25s)]
Euglobulin lysis time:	[n.a.]
Bleeding time:	[n.a.]
Immunoelectrophoresis:	[n.a.]
Platelet aggregation:	[n.a.]

Other results with patient plasma
Ancrod (Arvin) time: [n.a.]
Recalcification time: [n.a.]
Calcium corrects c.t.? [n.a.]

Inhib. normal plasma? [n.a.]
In vivo synthesis: [n.a.]
In vivo catabolism: [n.a.]

Evaluation of isolated patient fibrinogen
Thrombin time: [n.a.]
Reptilase time: [n.a.]
Ancrod (Arvin) time: [n.a.]

Abnormal subunit? [No]
Abnormal FDPs? [n.a.]

Remarks
[1]Other variants with this amino acid substitution exhibit normal stabilization of fibrin polymers.
[2]Normal range not reported.

White Marsh is located in Virginia (USA).

References

1. Carr, M.E., Jr. and Qureshi, G.D. The impact of delayed fibrinopeptide-A release on fibrin structure. *J. Biol. Chem.* **262**:15568-15574, **1987**.

2. Qureshi, G.D., Evans, H.J., Vennart, R.M., Magnant, J.P., Sabau, J.M., Willoughby, J.B. and Koehn, J.A. Fibrinogen White Marsh - A new human variant with α-chain defect. *Clin. Res.* **31**:321A, **1983**. ABSTRACT

FIBRINOGEN WIESBADEN I

Last update [1 December 1990]
Alphacode [WIESBA01]
Ref. type [Article]

Family studies
Homozygote? [n.a.]
Pedigree published? [No]

Structural defect [n.a.]
Mutation [n.a.]

Functional defect(s)
FpA release: [n.a.]
FpB release: [n.a.]
Polymerization: [n.a.]
Stabilization: [Abnormal[1]]

Clinical manifestation(s) Bleeding? [Yes] Thrombosis? [Yes]

Clinical laboratory results
Plasma fibrinogen concentration (mg/dL)
Chronometric: [38/(280)]
Rate-indep'nt: [91/(334)]
Immunologic: [440/(240)]

*Hypo*dysfibrinogen? [No]

Thrombin time:	[No clot]
Reptilase (batroxobin) time:	[No clot]
Prothrombin time:	[23.5s/(11.6s)]
Partial thromboplastin time:	[40.6s/(34.5s)]
Euglobulin lysis time:	[n.a.]
Bleeding time:	[n.a.]
Immunoelectrophoresis:	[Normal]
Platelet aggregation:	[n.a.]

Other results with patient plasma
Ancrod (Arvin) time: [n.a.]
Recalcification time: [n.a.]
Calcium corrects c.t.? [n.a.]

Inhib. normal plasma? [Yes]
In vivo synthesis: [n.a.]
In vivo catabolism: [n.a.]

Evaluation of isolated patient fibrinogen
Thrombin time: [n.a.]
Reptilase time: [n.a.]
Ancrod (Arvin) time: [n.a.]

Abnormal subunit? [n.a.]
Abnormal FDPs? [n.a.]

Remarks
[1]Increased clot solubility in urea was reported.

References

1. Winckelmann, G. [Congenital dysfibrinogenemia. Report on a new family (fibrinogen "Wiesbaden")]. *Thromb. Diath. Haemorrh.* **Suppl. 55**:345-356, **1973**.

FIBRINOGEN YERRES I

Last update [1 December 1990]
Alphacode [YERRES01]
Ref. type [Article]

Family studies
Homozygote? [n.a.]
Pedigree published? [No]

Structural defect [n.a.]
Mutation [n.a.]

Functional defect(s)
FpA release: [n.a.]
FpB release: [n.a.]
Polymerization: [n.a.]
Stabilization: [n.a.]

Clinical manifestation(s) Bleeding? [n.a.] Thrombosis? [n.a.]

Clinical laboratory results
Plasma fibrinogen concentration (mg/dL)
Chronometric: [45[1]]
Rate-indep'nt: [175[1]]
Immunologic: [200[1]]

*Hypo*dysfibrinogen? [No]

Thrombin time:	[43s/(20s)]
Reptilase (batroxobin) time:	[55s/(22s)]
Prothrombin time:	[64%/(>70%)]
Partial thromboplastin time:	[48s/(42s)]
Euglobulin lysis time:	[n.a.]
Bleeding time:	[n.a.]
Immunoelectrophoresis:	[n.a.]
Platelet aggregation:	[n.a.]

Other results with patient plasma
Ancrod (Arvin) time: [n.a.]
Recalcification time: [n.a.]
Calcium corrects c.t.? [n.a.]

Inhib. normal plasma? [No]
In vivo synthesis: [n.a.]
In vivo catabolism: [n.a.]

Evaluation of isolated patient fibrinogen
Thrombin time: [n.a.]
Reptilase time: [n.a.]
Ancrod (Arvin) time: [n.a.]

Abnormal subunit? [n.a.]
Abnormal FDPs? [n.a.]

Remarks
[1]Normal range not reported.

References

1. Corrihons, G., Soria, J., Soria, C., Conard, J., Horellou, M.H. and Samama, M. [Congenital dysfibrinogenemia. Apropos of 13 cases]. *Sem. Hop. Paris* **59**:2517-2523, **1983**.

FIBRINOGEN ZÜRICH I

Last update	[1 December 1990]	**Structural defect**	[Aα(16) Arg → Cys]
Alphacode	[ZURICH01]	**Mutation**	[n.a.]
Ref. type	[Article]		

Family studies
Homozygote? [No]
Pedigree published? [No]

Functional defect(s)
FpA release: [Abnormal[1]]
FpB release: [n.a.]
Polymerization: [Abnormal]
Stabilization: [Normal]

Clinical manifestation(s) Bleeding? [No] Thrombosis? [No]

Clinical laboratory results

Plasma fibrinogen concentration (mg/dL)
Chronometric: [20-50/(150-500)]
Rate-indep'nt: [400/(200-400)]
Immunologic: [n.a.]

*Hypo*dysfibrinogen? [No]

Thrombin time:	[38s/(15s)]
Reptilase (batroxobin) time:	[n.a.]
Prothrombin time:	[17s/(12s)]
Partial thromboplastin time:	[n.a.]
Euglobulin lysis time:	[n.a.]
Bleeding time:	[Normal]
Immunoelectrophoresis:	[Normal]
Platelet aggregation:	[n.a.]

Other results with patient plasma

Ancrod (Arvin) time:	[n.a.]	Inhib. normal plasma?	[Yes]
Recalcification time:	[105s/(<120s)]	In vivo synthesis:	[n.a.]
Calcium corrects c.t.?	[Yes]	In vivo catabolism:	[n.a.]

Evaluation of isolated patient fibrinogen

Thrombin time:	[n.a.]	Abnormal subunit?	[No]
Reptilase time:	[n.a.]	Abnormal FDPs?	[n.a.]
Ancrod (Arvin) time:	[n.a.]		

Remarks
[1]Only half the normal amount of fibrinopeptide A was released.

A brief discussion of fibrinogen Zürich I is published in *Thromb. Diath. Haemorrh.* **39**:331-338 (1970).

FIBRINOGEN ZÜRICH I

References

1. Hofmann, V., Gati, W.P. and Straub, P.W. Fibrinogen Zürich I: Impaired release of fibrinopeptide A. *Thromb. Haemostas.* **41**:709-713, **1979**.

2. Hofmann, V., Gati, W.P. and Straub, P.W. [Fibrinogen Zürich I: Defective fibrinopeptide-A release]. *Schweiz. Med. Wochenschr.* **107**:1468, **1977**. ABSTRACT

3. Henschen, A., Kehl, M., Southan, C., Lottspeich, F. and Georgopoulos, D. Genetically abnormal fibrinogens — some current characterisation strategies. In: *Fibrinogen —Structure, Functional Aspects, Metabolism*, F. Haverkate, A. Henschen, W. Nieuwenhuizen and P.W. Straub (eds.), Walter de Gruyter, Berlin. pp. 125-144, **1983**.

4. Southan, C., Henschen, A. and Lottspeich, F. The search for molecular defects in abnormal fibrinogens. In: *Fibrinogen —Recent Biochemical and Medical Aspects*, A. Henschen, H. Graeff and F. Lottspeich (eds.), W. de Gruyter, Berlin. pp. 153-166, **1982**.

5. Felten, A.von, Duckert, F. and Frick, P.G. Gerinnungsstorung ohne hamorrhagische diathese infolge verzogerter aggregation der fibrinmolekule. *Schweiz. Med. Wschr.* **95**:1453-1456, **1965**.

6. Felten, A.von, Frick, P.G. and Straub, P.W. Familial disturbance of fibrin monomer aggregation. *Br. J. Haematol.* **12**:667-677, **1966**.

7. Felten, A.von, Frick, P.G. and Straub, P.W. Studies on fibrin monomer aggregation in congenital dysfibrinogenemia: separation of a pathological from a normal fibrin fraction. *Br. J. Haematol.* **16**:353-361, **1969**.

FIBRINOGEN ZÜRICH II

Last update [10 January 1994]
Alphacode [ZURICH02]
Ref. type [Article]

Structural defect [n.a.]
Mutation [n.a.]

Family studies
Homozygote? [n.a.]
Pedigree published? [No]

Functional defect(s)
FpA release: [Normal[1]]
FpB release: [Normal[1]]
Polymerization: [Abnormal]
Stabilization: [Normal]

Clinical manifestation(s) Bleeding? [No[2]] Thrombosis? [No[2]]

Clinical laboratory results
Plasma fibrinogen concentration (mg/dL)
Chronometric: [Subnormal[1]]
Rate-indep'nt: [Normal[1]]
Immunologic: [Normal[1]]

*Hypo*dysfibrinogen? [No]

Thrombin time:	[Abnormal[1]]
Reptilase (batroxobin) time:	[n.a.]
Prothrombin time:	[Abnormal[1]]
Partial thromboplastin time:	[n.a.]
Euglobulin lysis time:	[n.a.]
Bleeding time:	[n.a.]
Immunoelectrophoresis:	[Anodal[3]]
Platelet aggregation:	[n.a.]

Other results with patient plasma
Ancrod (Arvin) time: [n.a.]
Recalcification time: [n.a.]
Calcium corrects c.t.? [n.a.]

Inhib. normal plasma? [Yes]
In vivo synthesis: [n.a.]
In vivo catabolism: [n.a.]

Evaluation of isolated patient fibrinogen
Thrombin time: [n.a.]
Reptilase time: [n.a.]
Ancrod (Arvin) time: [n.a.]

Abnormal subunit? [No[3]]
Abnormal FDPs? [n.a.]

Remarks
[1]Data not reported.
[2]The index patient presented with tetralogy of fallot (compare with SEATTLE I).
[3]Increased sialic acid in the Bβ- ad γ-chains was reported.

References

1. Straub, P.W. and Gati, W.P. Increase of the sialic acid-rich variants of the Bβ- and γ-chains of fibrinogen Zürich II. *Thromb. Haemostas.* **41**:714-717, **1979**.

2. Gati, W.P. and Straub, P.W. Separation of both the Bβ- and the γ-polypeptide chains of human fibrinogen into two main types which differ in sialic acid content. *J. Biol. Chem.* **253**:1315-1321, **1978**.

3. Gati, W.P. and Straub, P.W. [Resolution of Bβ- and γ-chains from normal human fibrinogen Zürich II into 2 variants with each differing sialic acid content]. *Schweiz. Med. Wochenschr.* **106**:1379, **1976**.

SECTION 4

BIBLIOGRAPHY

The literature on dysfibrinogenemia is listed by year and alphabetically within each year.

1. Yoshida, N., Hirata, H., Imaoka, S., Matsuda, M., Yamazumi, K. and Asakura, S. Effect of calcium on the mobility of γ-chain from fibrinogen Osaka V on sodium dodecyl sulfate-polyacrylamide gel electrophoresis. *Thromb. Res.* **73**:79-82, **1994**.

2. Uemichi, T., Liepnieks, J.J. and Benson, M.D. Hereditary renal amyloidosis with a novel variant fibrinogen. *J. Clin. Invest.* **93**:731-736, **1994**.

3. Baumann, R.E. and Henschen, A.H. Human fibrinogen polymorphic site analysis by restriction endonuclease digestion and allele-specific polymerase chain reaction amplification: identification of polymorphisms at positions Aα312 and Bβ448. *Blood* **82**:2117-2124, **1993**.

4. Benson, M.D., Liepnieks, J., Uemichi, T., Wheeler, G. and Correa, R. Hereditary renal amyloidosis associated with a mutant fibrinogen α-chain. *Nature Genet.* **3**:252-255, **1993**.

5. Borrell, M., Valivé, C., Coll, I., Garí, M. and Fontcuberta, J. Abnormal fibrin polymerization is frequently associated with impaired t-PA-mediated plasminogen activation. *Thromb. Haemostas.* **69**:820, **1993**. ABSTRACT

6. Collet, J.P., Soria, J., Mirshahi, M., Hirsch, M., Dagonnet, F.B., Caen, J. and Soria, C. Dusart syndrome: a new concept of the relationship between fibrin clot architecture and fibrin clot degradability: hypofibrinolysis related to an abnormal clot structure. *Blood* **82**:2462-2469, **1993**.

7. Egbring, R., Seitz, R., Koopman, J., Haverkate, F., Fuchs, G., Appel, D. and Lerch, L. Bleeding complications in homozygous and heterozygous patients with hypodysfibrinogenemia (H-DF) Marburg (M). *Blood Coag. & Fibrinol.* **4**:821, **1993**. ABSTRACT

8. Galanakis, D., Spitzer, S. and Scharrer, I. Unusual Aα 16 Arg → Cys dysfibrinogenaemic family: absence of normal Aα-chains in fibrinogen from two of four heterozygous siblings. *Blood Coag. & Fibrinol.* **4**:67-71, **1993**.

9. Galanakis, D.K. Inherited dysfibrinogenemia: emerging abnormal structure associations with pathologic and non-pathologic dysfunction. *Sem. Thromb. Haemostas.* **19**:386-395, **1993**.

10. Grailhe, P., Boyer-Neumann, C., Haverkate, F., Grimbergen, J., Larrieu, M.J. and Anglés-Cano, E. The mutation in fibrinogen Bicêtre II (γ Asn308 → Lys) does not affect the binding of t-PA and plasminogen to fibrin. *Blood Coag. & Fibrinol.* **4**:679-687, **1993**.

11. Henschen, A.H. Human fibrinogen — structural variants and functional sites. *Thromb. Haemost.* **70**:42-47, **1993**.

12. Koopman, J., Haverkate, F., Grimbergen, J., Lord, S.T., Mosesson, M.W., DiOrio, J.P., Siebenlist, K.S., Legrand, C., Soria, J., Soria, C. and Caen, J.P. Molecular basis for fibrinogen Dusart (Aα 554 Arg → Cys) and its association with abnormal fibrin polymerization and thrombophilia. *J. Clin. Invest.* **91**:1637-1643, **1993**.

13. Niwa, K., Yaginuma, A., Nakanishi, M., Wada, Y., Sugo, T., Asakura, S., Watanabe, N. and Matsuda, M. Fibrinogen Mitaka II: a hereditary dysfibrinogen with defective thrombin binding caused by an Aα Glu-11 to Gly substitution. *Blood* **82**:3658-3663, **1993**.

14. Niwa, K., Wada, Y., Asakura, S., Yaginuma, A., Watanabe, N. and Matsuda, M. Fibrinogen Mitaka II: a new type of hereditary abnormal fibrinogen with an Aα Glu-11 to Gly substitution characterized by impaired binding with thrombin. *Blood Coag. & Fibrinol.* **4**:819-820, **1993**. ABSTRACT

15. Rosenberg, J.B., Newman, P.J., Mosesson, M.W., Guillin, M.-C. and Amrani, D.L. Paris I dysfibrinogenemia: a point mutation in intron 8 results in insertion of a 15 amino acid sequence in the fibrinogen γ-chain. *Thromb. Haemost.* **69**:217-220, **1993**.

16. Siebenlist, K.R., Mosesson, M.W., DiOrio, J.P., Soria, J., Soria, C. and Caen, J.P. The polymerization of fibrinogen Dusart (Aα 554 Arg → Cys) after removal of carboxy terminal regions of the Aα-chains. *Blood Coag. & Fibrinol.* **4**:61-65, **1993**.

17. Sobel, J., Wu, H.Q., Trakht, I., Haverkate, F. and Egbring, R. Alpha chain crosslinking in fibrinogen Marburg (Aα #1-461). *Blood Coag. & Fibrinol.* **4**:812-813, **1993**. ABSTRACT

18. Soria, J., Lu, H., Mirshahi, M., Vasse, M., Mirshahi, S.S., Woimant, F., Favier, J.P., Desvignes, P., Bonnet, P., Schved, J.F. and Soria, C. Defective fibrin polymerization: a risk for stroke at young age. The case of fibrinogen Alès. *Blood Coag. & Fibrinol.* **4**:820-821, **1993**. ABSTRACT

19. Steinmann, C., Reber, P., Jungo, M., Lämmle, B., Heinemann, G., Wermuth, B. and Furlan, M. Fibrinogen Bern I: substitution γ 337 Asn → Lys is responsible for defective fibrin monomer polymerization. *Blood* **82**:2104-2108, **1993**.

20. Steinmann, C., Bögli, C., Iungo, M., Lämmle, B., Heinemann, G., Wermuth, B., Redaelli, R., Baudo, F. and Furlan, M. A new substitution, γ-358 Ser → Cys, in fibrinogen Milano VII causes defective fibrin polymerization. *Thromb. Haemostas.* **69**:962, **1993**. ABSTRACT

21. Wada, Y., Niwa, K., Maekawa, H., Asakura, S., Sugo, T., Nakanishi, M., Auerswald, G., Popp, M. and Matsuda, M. A new type of congenital dysfibrinogen, fibrinogen Bremen, with an Aα Gly-17 to Val substitution associated with hemorrhagic diathesis and delayed wound healing. *Thromb. Haemost.* **70**:397-403, **1993**.

22. Yamazumi, K., Terukina, S., Matsuda, M., Kanbayashi, J., Sakon, M. and Tsujinaka, T. Fibrinogen Osaka IV: a congenital dysfibrinogenemia found in a patient originally reported in relation to surgery, now defined to have an Aα arginine-16 to histidine substitution. *Jpn. J. Surg.* **23**:45-50, **1993**.

23. Al-Fawaz, I.M. and Gader, A.M.A. Severe congenital dysfibrinogenemia (fibrinogen-Riyadh): a family study. *Acta Haematol.* **88**:194-197, **1992**.

24. Auerswald, G., Popp, M. and Matsuda, M. Clinical aspects combined with a new fibrinogen (fibrinogen Bremen) with an Aα Gly-17 to Val substitution. *Proc. XI Int'l. F'gen. Wkshop.* 9, **1992**. ABSTRACT

25. Bögli, C., Hofer, A., Baudo, F., Redaelli, R. and Furlan, M. Fibrinogen Milano IV, another case of congenital dysfibrinogenemia with an abnormal fibrinopeptide A release (Aα 16 Arg → His). *Haemostas.* **22**:7-11, **1992**.

26. Connor, J.M., Fowkes, F.G.R., Wood, J., Smith, F.B., Donnan, P.T. and Lowe, G.D.O. Genetic variation at fibrinogen loci and plasma fibrinogen levels. *J. Med. Genet.* **29**:480-482, **1992**.

27. Galanakis, D.K. Fibrinogen anomalies and disease: a clinical update. *Hematol. Oncol. Clin. North Am.* **6**:1171-1187, **1992**.

28. Koopman, J., Haverkate, F., Grimbergen, J., Engesser, L., Nováková, I., Kerst, A.F.J.A. and Lord, S.T. Abnormal fibrinogens IJmuiden (BβArg_{14} → Cys) and Nijmegen (BβArg_{44} → Cys) form disulfide-linked fibrinogen-albumin complexes. *Proc. Natl. Acad. Sci. USA* **89**:3478-3482, **1992**.

29. Koopman, J., Haverkate, F., Lord, S.T., Grimbergen, J. and Mannucci, P.M. Molecular basis of fibrinogen Naples associated with defective thrombin binding and thrombophilia. Homozygous substitution of Bβ 68 Ala → Thr. *J. Clin. Invest.* **90**:238-244, **1992**.

30. Koopman, J., Haverkate, F., Grimbergen, J., Egbring, R. and Lord, S.T. Fibrinogen Marburg: a homozygous case of dysfibrinogenemia, lacking amino acids Aα 461-610 (Lys 461 AAA → Stop TAA). *Blood* **80**:1972-1979, **1992**.

31. Maekawa, H., Yamazumi, K., Muramatsu, S., Kaneko, M., Hirata, H., Takahashi, N., Arocha-Piñango, C.L., Rodríguez, S., Nagy, H., Perez-Requejo, J.L. and Matsuda, M. Fibrinogen Lima: a homozygous dysfibrinogen with an Aα-arginine-141 to serine substitution associated with extra *N*-glycosylation at Aα-asparagine-139. Impaired fibrin gel formation but normal fibrin-facilitated plasminogen activation catalyzed by tissue-type plasminogen activator. *J. Clin. Invest.* **90**:67-76, **1992**.

32. Mimuro, J., Muramatsu, S., Maekawa, H., Sakata, Y., Kaneko, M., Yoshitake, S., Okuma, M., Ito, Y., Takeda, Y. and Matsuda, M. Gene analyses of abnormal fibrinogens with a mutation in the γ chain. *Intl. J. Hematol.* **56**:129-134, **1992**.

33. Rodgers, G.M. and Chandler, W.L. Laboratory and clinical aspects of inherited thrombotic disorders. *Am. J. Hematol.* **41**:113-122, **1992**.

34. Rodgers, G.M. and Garr, S.B. Comparison of functional and antigenic fibrinogen values from a normal population. *Thromb. Res.* **68**:207-210, **1992**.

35. Steinmann, C., Lämmle, B., Heinemann, G., Wermuth, B. and Furlan, M. Fibrinogen Bern I: substitution γ 337 Asn → Lys is responsible for defective fibrin monomer polymerization and impaired interactions with calcium. *Proc. XI Int'l. F'gen. Wkshop.* 2, **1992**. ABSTRACT

36. Steinmann, C., Bögli, C., Lämmle, B., Heinemann, G., Wermuth, B., Baudo, F., Redaelli, R. and Furlan, M. A new substitution γ 358 Ser → Cys in fibrinogen Milano VII causes defective fibrin monomer polymerization. *Proc. XI Int'l. F'gen. Wkshop.* 7, **1992**. ABSTRACT

37. Wada, Y., Niwa, K., Maekawa, H., Nakanishi, M., Auerswald, G., Popp, M. and Matsuda, M. Fibrinogen Bremen with an Aα Gly-17 to Val substitution: normal fibrin monomer polymerization despite the structural alteration in the "A" polymerization site. *Proc. XI Int'l. F'gen. Wkshop.* 10, **1992**. ABSTRACT

38. Webb, C.D., Hantgan, R.R., Byeff, P.D. and Owen, J. Fibrinogen New Britain: an Aα16 Arg → His substitution also showing abnormal polymerization. *Proc. XI Int'l. F'gen. Wkshop.* 11, **1992**. ABSTRACT

39. Yoshida, N., Hirata, H., Asakura, S., Yamazumi, K., Matsuda, M., Wada, H., Shirakawa, S. and Okuma, M. Calcium binding to abnormal fibrinogens with a single amino acid replacement in the NH2-terminal region of fibrin α- or β-chain. *Thromb. Res.* **67**:613-618, **1992**.

40. Yoshida, N., Imaoka, S., Hirata, H., Matsuda, M. and Asakura, S. Heterozygous abnormal fibrinogen Osaka III with the replacement of γ arginine-275 by histidine has an apparently higher molecular weight γ-chain variant. *Thromb. Haemost.* **68**:534-538, **1992**.

41. Yoshida, N., Hirata, H., Morigami, Y., Imaoka, S., Matsuda, M., Yamazumi, K. and Asakura, S. Characterization of an abnormal fibrinogen Osaka V with the replacement of γ-arginine 375 by glycine. The lack of high affinity calcium binding to D-domains and the lack of protective effect of calcium on fibrinolysis. *J. Biol. Chem.* **267**:2753-2759, **1992**.

42. Zheng, Z., Ashton, R.W., Ni, F. and Scheraga, H.A. Thrombin hydrolysis of an N-terminal peptide from fibrinogen Lille: kinetic and NMR studies. *Biochemistry* **31**:4426-4431, **1992**.

43. Furlan, M., Leupin, L., Biasiutti, F.D. and Lämmle, B. Fibrinogen Bern III: a further case of the hereditary fibrinogen variant with substitution Aα 16 Arg → Cys. *Schweiz. Med. Wochenschr.* **121**:1068-1071, **1991**.

44. Ieko, M., Sawada, K.-I., Sakurama, S., Yamagishi, I., Isogawa, S., Nakagawa, S., Satoh, M., Yasukouchi, T. and Matsuda, M. Fibrinogen Date: congenital hypodysfibrinogenemia associated with decreased binding of tissue-plasminogen activator. *Am. J. Hematol.* **37**:228-233, **1991**.

45. Koopman, J., Haverkate, F., Briët, E. and Lord, S.T. A congenitally abnormal fibrinogen (Vlissingen) with a 6-base deletion in the γ-chain gene, causing defective calcium binding and impaired fibrin polymerization. *J. Biol. Chem.* **266**:13456-13461, **1991**.

46. Lee, M.H., Kaczmarek, E., Chin, D.T., Oda, A., McIntosh, S., Bauer, K.A., Clyne, L.P. and McDonagh, J. Fibrinogen Ledyard (AαArg$_{16}$ → Cys): biochemical and physiologic characterization. *Blood* **78**:1744-1752, **1991**.

47. Maekawa, H., Yamazumi, K., Muramatsu, S., Kaneko, M., Hirata, H., Takahashi, N., de Bosch, N.B., Carvajal, Z., Ojeda, A., Arocha-Piñango, C.L. and Matsuda, M. An Aα Ser-434 to *N*-glycosylated Asn substitution in a dysfibrinogen, fibrinogen Caracas II, characterized by impaired fibrin gel formation. *J. Biol. Chem.* **266**:11575-11581, **1991**.

48. Martinez, J. Quantitative and qualitative disorders of fibrinogen. In: *Hematology — Basic Principles and Practice*, R. Hoffman, E.J. Benz Jr., S.J. Shattil, B. Furie and H.J. Cohen (eds.). Churchill Livingstone, New York; pp. 1342-1354, **1991**.

49. Matsuda, M. Abnormal fibrinogens: the present status of structure elucidation. *Biomed. Prog.* **4**:51-54, **1991**.

50. Meyer, M., Lutze, G. and Gromnica-Ilhe, E. Dysfibrinogenemia: abnormalities in the Bβ chains of fibrinogens Berlin II and Magdeburg II. *Thromb. Haemostas.* **65**:903, **1991**. ABSTRACT

51. Muramatsu, S., Mimuro, J., Maekawa, H., Sakata, Y., Matsuda, M., Yoshitake, S. and Okuma, M. Gene analysis of abnormal fibrinogens characterized by a mutation in the γ chain. *Thromb. Haemostas.* **65**:821, **1991**. ABSTRACT

52. Seydewitz, H.H, Gram, J., Bruhn, H.D. and Witt, I. Fibrinogen Kiel: a congenital dysfibrinogenaemia with (Aα-16 Arg → His) substitution characterized by HPLC without prior isolation of fibrinogen. *Blood Coag. & Fibrinol.* **2**:501-506, **1991**.

53. Tabernero, M.D., Tomas, J.F., Alberca, I., Orfao, A., Borrasca, A.L. and Vicente, V. Incidence and clinical characteristics of hereditary disorders associated with venous thrombosis. *Am. J. Hematol.* **36**:249-254, **1991**.

54. Takala, T., Oksa, H., Rasi, V. and Tuimala, R. Dysfibrinogenemia associated with thrombosis and third-trimester fetal loss: a case report. *J. Reprod. Med.* **36**:410-412, **1991**.

55. Uotani, C., Miyata, T., Kumabashiri, I., Asakura, H., Saito, M., Matsuda, T., Kajiyama, S. and Iwanaga, S. Fibrinogen Kanazawa: a congenital dysfibrinogenaemia with delayed polymerization having a replacement of proline-18 by leucine in the Aα-chain. *Blood Coag. & Fibrinol.* **2**:413-417, **1991**.

56. Warnock, L.J. The application of molecular biology techniques to haemostasis and thrombosis. *Blood Coag. & Fibrinol.* **2**:529-538, **1991**.

57. Yoshida, N., Okuma, M., Hirata, H., Matsuda, M., Yamazumi, K. and Asakura, S. Fibrinogen Kyoto II, a new congenitally abnormal molecule, characterized by the replacement of Aα proline-18 by leucine. *Blood* **78**:149-153, **1991**.

58. Yoshida, N., Wada, H., Morita, K., Hirata, H., Matsuda, M., Yamazumi, K., Asakura, S. and Shirakawa, S. A new congenital abnormal fibrinogen Ise characterized by the replacement of Bβ Glycine-15 by cysteine. *Blood* **77**:1958-1963, **1991**.

59. Arocha-Piñango, C.L., Rodríguez, S., Naggy, H. and Perez-Requejo, J.L. Fibrinogen Lima. A new dysfibrinogenaemia with a high-molecular-weight α-chain and effective polymerization. *Blood Coag. & Fibrinol.* **1**:561-565, **1990**.

60. Arocha-Piñango, C.L., Bosch, N., Torres, A., Caires-Tronchoni, D., Marchi, R., Vidal, H. and Rizzo, M.G. Dysfibrinogenemias in Latin America. A cooperative study group. *Rev. Iberoamer. Tromb. Hemostasia* **3**:110-122, **1990**.

61. Arocha-Piñango, C.L., Marchi, R. and Tronchoni, D.C. Dysfibrogenemias. A puzzle. A critical review. *Rev. Iberoamer. Tromb. Hemostasia* **3**:75-94, **1990**.

62. Arocha-Piñango, C.L., Rodríguez, S., Naggy, H. and Perez-Requejo, J.L. Fibrinogen Lima. A new dysfibrinogenemia with abnormal polymerization and slow plasmin degradation. *Fibrinogen Workshop (Rouen)* **1990**. ABSTRACT

63. Bantia, S., Bell, W.R. and Dang, C.V. Polymerization defect of fibrinogen Baltimore III due to a γ Asn^{308} → Ile mutation. *Blood* **75**:1659-1663, **1990**.

64. Bantia, S., Dang, C.V. and Bell, W.R. Γ Asn308 → Ile substitution in fibrinogen Baltimore III with impaired fibrin monomer polymerization. In: *Fibrinogen 4. Current Basic and Clinical Aspects*, M. Matsuda, S. Iwanaga, A. Takada and A. Henschen (eds.). Elsevier Science Publ. B.V., Amsterdam; pp. 167-170, **1990**.

65. Bantia, S., Mane, S.M., Bell, W.R. and Dang, C.V. Fibrinogen Baltimore I: polymerization defect associated with a γ 292 Gly → Val (GGC → GTC) mutation. *Blood* **76**:2279-2283, **1990**.

66. Blombäck, B., Banerjee, D., Carlsson, K., Hamsten, A., Hessel, B., Procyk, R., Silveira, A. and Zacharski, L. Native fibrin gel networks and factors influencing their formation in health and disease. *Adv. Exp. Med. Biol.* **281**:1-23, **1990**.

67. Borrell, M., Vila, L., Solá, J., Coll, I. and Fontcuberta, J. Fibrinogen Barcelona II: a new case of Aα 16 Arg → His substitution. *Haemostas.* **20**:1-7, **1990**.

68. Bögli, C., Cofrancesco, E., Cortellaro, M., Della Volpe, A., Hofer, A., Furlan, M. and Zanussi, C. Fibrinogen Milano. VI: a heterozygous dysfibrinogenemia (Aα 16 Arg → His) with bleeding tendency. *Eur. J. Haematol.* **45**:26-30, **1990.**

69. Caen, J. Dusard syndrome in 1990. *Fibrinogen Workshop (Rouen)* **1990**. ABSTRACT

70. Chung, D.W., Harris, J.E. and Davie, E.W. Nucleotide sequences of the three genes coding for human fibrinogen. In: *Fibrinogen, Thrombosis, Coagulation, and Fibrinolysis*, C.Y. Liu and S. Chien (eds.). Plenum Press, NY; pp. 39-48, **1990.**

71. Dempfle, C.E.H. and Henschen, A. Fibrinogen Mannheim I — identification of an Aα 19 Arg → Gly substitution in dysfibrinogenaemia associated with bleeding tendency. In: *Fibrinogen 4. Current Basic and Clinical Aspects*, M. Matsuda, S. Iwanaga, A. Takada and A. Henschen (eds.). Elsevier Science Publ. B.V., Amsterdam; pp. 159-166, **1990.**

72. Fernández, F.J., Rodriguez Pinto, C., Páramo, J., Cuesta, B., Collado, M. and Rocha, E. Fibrinogen Oviedo I. A new Spanish dysfibrinogenaemia. *Blood Coag. & Fibrinol.* **1**:571-575, **1990.**

73. Furlan, M., Bögli, C., Hofer, A., Bouvier, C.A. and de Moerloose, P. Fibrinogen Geneva, a new case of Aα 16 Arg → Cys dysfibrinogenaemia. *Blood Coag. & Fibrinol.* **1**:139-144, **1990.**

74. Galanakis, D.K., Henschen, A., Schubach, W., Lord, S. and Al-Mondhiry, H. Determination of abnormal structure and heterozygosity by amplification of genomic DNA using the polymerase chain reaction and by amino acid sequence analyses. In: *Fibrinogen 4. Current Basic and Clinical Aspects*, M. Matsuda, S. Iwanaga, A. Takada and A. Henschen (eds.). Elsevier Science Publ., B.V., Amsterdam; pp. 173-178, **1990.**

75. Galanakis, D.K. and Hultin, M. Fibrinogen Stony Brook II: a heterozygously transmitted peptide A defect. Evidence that most mutant molecules are homodimers. *Blood* **76 Suppl. 1**:421a, **1990**. ABSTRACT

76. Galanakis, D.K. and Hultin, M. Fibrinogen Stony Brook II: partial characterization of a heterozygously transmitted peptide A anomaly. *Blood Coag. & Fibrinol.* **1**:567-570, **1990.**

77. Gralnick, H.R. Congenital abnormalities of fibrinogen. In: *Hematology*, W.J. Williams, E. Beutler, A.J. Erslev and M.A. Lichtman (eds.). McGraw-Hill, New York; pp. 1474-1490, **1990.**

78. Heidegger, H., Spannagel, M. and Schramm, W. [Obstetrical management in dysfibrinogenemia]. *Geburtshilfe. Frauenheilkd.* **50**:365-367, **1990.**

79. Koopman, J. and Haverkate, F. Structure-function relationships in abnormal fibrinogens. Defects at the DNA level. In: *Fibrinogen 4. Current Basic and Clinical Aspects*, M. Matsuda, S. Iwanaga, A. Takada and A. Henschen (eds.). Elsevier Science Publ., B.V., Amsterdam; pp. 179-183, **1990.**

80. Koopman, J., Grimbergen, J., Lord, S.T., Haverkate, F. and Mannucci, P.M. The functional and structural defect of fibrinogen Naples and its relation with thrombosis. *Fibrinogen Workshop (Rouen)* **1990**. ABSTRACT

81. Koopman, J., Haverkate, F., Lord, S.T. and Grimbergen, J. Identification of structural defects in abnormal fibrinogens using the polymerase chain reaction. *Fibrinogen Workshop (Rouen)* **1990**. ABSTRACT

82. Lee, M.H., Kaczmarek, E. and McDonagh, J. Fibrinogen Ledyard (Aα 16 Arg → Cys): biochemical and physiological characterization. *Circ.* **(Suppl. III) 82**:III-368, **1990**. ABSTRACT

83. Lord, S.T., Byrd, P.A., Hede, K.L., Wei, C. and Colby, T.J. Analysis of fibrinogen Aα-fusion proteins. Mutants which inhibit thrombin equivalently are not equally good substrates. *J. Biol. Chem.* **265**:838-843, **1990.**

84. Maekawa, H., Yamazumi, K., Muramatsu, S., Arocha-Piñango, C.L., Rodríguez, S., Naggy, H. and Perez-Requejo, J.L. Fibrinogen Lima with a replacement of Aα Arg 141 by Ser identified in the Aα chain part of the D-domain. *Fibrinogen Workshop (Rouen)* **1990**. ABSTRACT

85. Marchi, R., Arocha-Piñango, C.L. and Gil, F. Electron microscopy studies of 7 patients with dysfibrinogenemia and some of their relatives. *Rev. Iberoamer. Tromb. Hemostasia* **3**:185-190, **1990.**

86. Matsuda, M., Terukina, S., Yoshida, N., Yamazumi, K. and Maekawa, H. Abnormal fibrinogens with two structural defects. *Adv. Exp. Med. Biol.* **281**:63-72, **1990**.

87. Matsuda, M., Yoshida, N., Terukina, S., Yamazumi, K. and Maekawa, H. Molecular abnormalities of fibrinogen — the present status of structure elucidation. In: *Fibrinogen 4. Current Basic and Clinical Aspects*, M. Matsuda, S. Iwanaga, A. Takada and A. Henschen (eds.). Elsevier Science Publ. B.V., Amsterdam; pp. 139-152, **1990**.

88. Mimuro, J., Yamazumi, K., Terukina, S. and Matsuda, M. A T → C exchange in exon VIII of the fibrinogen γ chain gene defined by the polymerase chain reaction for fibrinogen Asahi with a γ Met-310 to Thr substitution and *N*-glycosylated Asn-308. *Fibrinogen Workshop (Rouen)* **1990**. ABSTRACT

89. Schorer, A.E. and Basara, M.L. Fibrinogen Richfield: a congenital dysfibrinogenemia with a thrombotic tendency. *Blood* **76 Suppl. 1**:437a, **1990**. ABSTRACT

90. Terukina, S., Yamazumi, K., Maekawa, H., Okamoto, K., Akasaka, K., Yamashita, H., Ito, Y. and Matsuda, M. Fibrinogen Kyoto III: a replacement of γ Asp-330 by Tyr. In: *Fibrinogen 4. Current Basic and Clinical Aspects*, M. Matsuda, S. Iwanaga, A. Takada and A. Henschen (eds.). Elsevier Science Publ., B.V., Amsterdam; pp. 171, **1990**.

91. Wenzel, E., Seyfert, U.T., Weier, B., Bohnerth, St., Pindur, G., Gu, L., Jung, F., Mrowietz, Ch., Harbauer, G. and Kotitschke, R. Clinical, rheological and haemostaseological aspects of dysfibrinogenemia. In: *Fibrinogen 4. Current Basic and Clinical Aspects*, M. Matsuda, S. Iwanaga, A. Takada and A. Henschen (eds.). Elsevier Science Publ., B.V., Amsterdam; pp. 153-158, **1990**.

92. Yamazumi, K., Shimura, K., Maekawa, H., Muramatsu, S., Terukina, S. and Matsuda, M. Delayed intermolecular γ-chain cross-linking by factor XIIIa in fibrinogen Asahi characterized by a γ-Met-310 to Thr substitution with an *N*-glycosylated γ-Asn-308. *Blood Coag. & Fibrinol.* **1**:557-559, **1990**.

93. Yoshida, N. and Matsuda, M. Fibrinogen Osaka V with a γ Arg-375 to gly substitution is defective in the high-affinity but normal in the low-affinity calcium binding sites. *Fibrinogen Workshop (Rouen)* **1990**. ABSTRACT

94. Asakura, S., Terukina, S., Yamazumi, K., Matsuda, M., Murayama, H., Higuchi, A., Musashi, M., Sakurada, K. and Miyazaki, T. Fibrinogen Sapporo: dysfibrinogenemia characterized by the replacement of Aα arginine-16 by histidine resulting in the delayed release of fibrinopeptide A by thrombin. *Nippon Ketsueki. Gakkai Zasshi.* **52**:1094-1104, **1989**.

95. Bantia, S. Γ Asn 308 → Ile substitution in fibrinogen Baltimore III with impaired fibrin monomer polymerization. *Fibrinogen Workshop (Kyoto)* 35, **1989**. ABSTRACT

96. Dang, C.V., Bell, W.R. and Shuman, M. The normal and morbid biology of fibrinogen. *Am. J. Med.* **87**:567-576, **1989**.

97. Dempfle, C.E. and Henschen, A. Fibrinogen Mannheim I — identification of an Aα 19 Arg → Gly substitution in dysfibrinogenaemia associated with bleeding tendency. *Fibrinogen Workshop (Kyoto)* 38, **1989**. ABSTRACT

98. Dempfle, C.E., Kirschstein, W., Watzlawick, H., Brossmer, R., Simianer, S., Harenberg, J. and Heene, D.L. Hypodysfibrinogenaemia with impaired fibrin polymerization associated with excessive postpartum bleeding: fibrinogen Mannheim II. *Thromb. Haemostas.* **62**:159, **1989**. ABSTRACT

99. Fernández, F.J., Noguerol, P., Sosa, R., Cuesta, B., Páramo, J.A. and Rocha, E. Fibrinogen Sevilla, a congenital dysfibrinogenemia characterized by an abnormal monomer aggregation and a defective plasmin lysis. *Clin. Chim. Acta* **179**:239-250, **1989**.

100. Galanakis, D., Henschen, A., Schubach, W., Lord, S. and Al-Mondhiry, H. Two new and structurally identical dysfibrinogens, Hershey II and Leogan. Determination of Aα 16 Arg → Cys substitution and of heterozygosity by amplification of genomic DNA using the polymerase chain reaction (PCR). *Fibrinogen Workshop (Kyoto)* 37, **1989**. ABSTRACT

101. Galanakis, D.K., Henschen, A., Peerschke, E.I.B. and Kehl, M. Fibrinogen Stony Brook, a heterozygous Aα16 Arg → Cys dysfibrinogenemia. Evaluation of diminished platelet aggregation support and of enhanced inhibition of fibrin assembly. *J. Clin. Invest.* **84**:295-304, **1989**.

102. Heene, D.L., Dempfle, C.E., Borck, P., Kirschstein, W., Harenberg, J. and Brossmer, R. Dysfibrinogenaemia with impaired release of fibrinopeptide A and t-PA-induced plasminogen activation: fibrinogen Mannheim I. *Thromb. Haemostas.* **62**:75, **1989**. ABSTRACT

103. Hortin, G.L. Sulfation of a γ-chain variant of human fibrinogen. *Biochem. Int.* **19**:1355-1362, **1989**.

104. Koopman, J., Haverkate, F., Lord, S., Caekebeke-Peerlinck, K., Brommer, E. and Briet, E. A six base deletion in the γ-chain gene of dysfibrinogen Vlissingen, coding for Asn-319 and Asp-320, resulting in defective interaction with calcium. *Thromb. Haemostas.* **62**:158, **1989**. ABSTRACT

105. Miyata, T., Furukawa, K., Iwanaga, S., Takamatsu, J. and Saito, H. Fibrinogen Nagoya, a replacement of glutamine-329 by arginine in the γ-chain that impairs the polymerization of fibrin monomer. *J. Biochem. (Tokyo)* **105**:10-14, **1989**.

106. Ni, F., Konishi, Y., Bullock, L.D., Rivetna, M.N. and Scheraga, H.A. High-resolution NMR studies of fibrinogen-like peptides in solution: structural basis for the bleeding disorder caused by a single mutation of Gly(12) to Val(12) in the Aα chain of human fibrinogen Rouen. *Biochemistry* **28**:3106-3119, **1989**.

107. Schmelzer, C.H., Ebert, R.F. and Bell, W.R. Fibrinogen Baltimore IV: congenital dysfibrinogenemia with a γ(275) (Arg → Cys) substitution. *Thromb. Res.* **56**:307-316, **1989**.

108. Siebenlist, K.R., Mosesson, M.W., Di Orio, J.P., Tavori, S., Tatarsky, I. and Rimon, A. The polymerization of fibrin prepared from fibrinogen Haifa (γ 275 Arg → His). *Thromb. Haemostas.* **62**:875-879, **1989**.

109. Terukina, S., Yamazumi, K., Okamoto, K., Yamashita, H., Ito, Y. and Matsuda, M. Fibrinogen Kyoto III: a congenital dysfibrinogen with a γ aspartic acid-330 to tyrosine substitution. *Blood* **74**:2681-2687, **1989**.

110. Tripodi, A. Screening for congenital coagulation disorders. *Res. Clin. Lab.* **19**:327-332, **1989**.

111. Yamazumi, K., Shimura, K., Terukina, S., Takahashi, N. and Matsuda, M. A γ methionine-310 to threonine substitution and consequent *N*-glycosylation at γ asparagine-308 identified in a congenital dysfibrinogenemia associated with posttraumatic bleeding, fibrinogen Asahi. *J. Clin. Invest.* **83**:1590-1597, **1989**.

112. Blombäck, B., Hessel, B., Fields, R. and Procyk, R. Fibrinogen Aarhus: an abnormal fibrinogen with Aα 19 Arg → Gly substitution. In: *Fibrinogen 3. Biochemistry, Biological Functions, Gene Regulation and Expression*, M.W. Mosesson, D.L. Amrani, K.R. Siebenlist and J.P. DiOrio (eds.). Elsevier, Amsterdam; pp. 263-266, **1988**.

113. Ebert, R.F. and Schmelzer, C.H. Isolation and comparative peptide mapping of fibrinogen subunits by reversed-phase high-performance liquid chromatography. *J. Chromatogr.* **443**:309-316, **1988**.

114. Ebert, R.F. and Bell, W.R. Fibrinogen Baltimore III: congenital dysfibrinogenemia with a shortened γ-subunit. *Thromb. Res.* **51**:251-258, **1988**.

115. Engesser, L., Koopman, J., de Munk, G., Haverkate, F., Novakova, I., Verheijen, J.H., Briet, E. and Brommer, E.J.P. Fibrinogen Nijmegen: congenital dysfibrinogenemia associated with impaired t-PA mediated plasminogen activation and decreased binding of t-PA. *Thromb. Haemostas.* **60**:113-120, **1988**.

116. Engesser, L., Koopman, J., de Munk, G., Haverkate, F., Novakova, I., Verheijen, J.H., Briet, E. and Brommer, E.J.P. An abnormal fibrinogen (Fibrinogen Nijmegen) with a decreased binding of t-PA and a reduced acceleration of t-PA induced plasminogen activation. In: *Fibrinogen 3. Biochemistry, Biological Functions, Gene Regulation and Expression*, M.W. Mosesson, D.L. Amrani, K.R. Siebenlist and J.P. DiOrio (eds.). Elsevier Science Publ., B.V., Amsterdam; pp. 259-262, **1988**.

117. Fernández, J., de la Torre, S., Losada, G., Villar, J.M., Páramo, J.A., Cuesta, B. and Rocha, E. Two cases of congenital dysfibrinogenemia. Fibrinogens Madrid III and Malaga. In: *Fibrinogen 3. Biochemistry, Biological Functions, Gene Regulation and Expression*, M.W. Mosesson, D.L. Amrani, K.R. Siebenlist and J.P. DiOrio (eds.). Elsevier Science Publ., B.V., Amsterdam; pp. 255-258, **1988**.

118. Galanakis, D.K., Henschen, A., Peerschke, E.I. and Kehl, M. Fibrinogen Stony Brook I, an heterozygous Aα 16 Arg → Cys dysfibrinogenemia: implication of diminished platelet aggregation support. In: *Fibrinogen 3. Biochemistry, Biological Functions, Gene Regulation and Expression*, M.W. Mosesson, D.L. Amrani, K.R. Siebenlist and J.P. DiOrio (eds.). Elsevier Science Publ., B.V., Amsterdam; pp. 251-254, **1988**.

119. Gandrille, S., Priollet, P., Capron, L., Roncato, M., Fiessinger, J.N. and Aiach, M. Association of inherited dysfibrinogenaemia and protein C deficiency in two unrelated families. *Brit. J. Haematol.* **68**:329-337, **1988**.

120. Koopman, J., Haverkate, F., Lane, D.A. and Lord, S.T. Sequence analysis of the fibrinogen Manchester Aα chain gene after amplification of genomic DNA using the polymerase chain reaction (PCR). In: *Fibrinogen 3. Biochemistry, Biological Functions, Gene Regulation and Expression*, M.W. Mosesson, D.L. Amrani, K.R. Siebenlist and J.P. DiOrio (eds.). Elsevier Science Publ., B.V., Amsterdam; pp. 275-278, **1988**.

121. Köther, M., Egbring, R., Fuchs, G. and Henschen, A. Bleeding and thrombotic events related to structural variants of fibrinogen. In: *Fibrinogen 3. Biochemistry, Biological Functions, Gene Regulation and Expression*, M.W. Mosesson, D.L. Amrani, K.R. Siebenlist and J.P. DiOrio (eds.). Elsevier Science Publishers B.V., Amsterdam; pp. 333-335, **1988**.

122. Maak, B. Hereditary dysfibrinogenaemia (fibrinogen Jena) — report of a family study. *Folia Haematol. (Leipz.)* **115**:519-522, **1988**.

123. Matsuda, M., Yamazumi, K., Terukina, S., Onohara, S. and Ohta, Y. An abnormal fibrinogen with a γ Arg-275 to His substitution found in a Japanese family — fibrinogen Saga. *Elsevier Science Publ. ,B. V.* 267, **1988**. ABSTRACT

124. Meyer, M., Vogel, G., Gromnica-Ihle, E., Schellenberg, I. and Ostermann, G. Hereditary dysfibrinogenaemia: structural and functional studies on three fibrinogen variants. *Folia Haematol. (Leipz.)* **115**:499-502, **1988**.

125. Meyer, M., Schellenberg, I., Vogel, G. and Bischoff, I. A new genetic fibrinogen variant (Fibrinogen Erfurt I) structurally characterized by an abnormal Bβ-chain and present both in plasma and platelets. *Thromb. Haemostas.* **59**:138-142, **1988**.

126. Miyata, T. and Iwanaga, S. [Dysfibrinogenemia and dysprothrombinemia]. *Tanpakushitsu. Kakusan. Koso.* **33**:959-963, **1988**.

127. Muller, E. and Henschen, A. Isolation and characterization of human plasma fibrinogen molecular-size-variants by high-performance liquid chromatography and amino acid sequence analysis. In: *Fibrinogen 3. Biochemistry, Biological Functions, Gene Regulation and Expression*, M.W. Mosesson, D.L. Amrani, K.R. Siebenlist and J.P. DiOrio (eds.). Elsevier Science Publ., B.V., Amsterdam; pp. 279-282, **1988**.

128. Ruf, W., Bender, A., Lane, D.A., Preissner, K.T., Selmayr, E. and Müller-Berghaus, G. Thrombin-induced fibrinopeptide B release from normal and variant fibrinogens: influence of inhibitors of fibrin polymerization. *Biochim. Biophys. Acta* **965**:169-175, **1988**.

129. Samama, M., Conard, J. and Soria, J. Congenital dysfibrinogenemia and thrombosis. *Fibrinolys.* **2, Suppl. 2**:18-23, **1988**.

130. Schmelzer, C.H., Ebert, R.F. and Bell, W.R. A polymorphism at Bβ 448 of fibrinogen identified during structural studies of fibrinogen Baltimore II. *Thromb. Res.* **52**:173-177, **1988**.

131. Siebenlist, K.R., Prchal, J.T. and Mosesson, M.W. Fibrinogen Birmingham: a heterozygous dysfibrinogenemia (Aα 16 Arg → His) containing heterodimeric molecules. *Blood* **71**:613-618, **1988**.

132. Siebenlist, K.R., Mosesson, M.W., DiOrio, J.P., Tavori, S., Tatarsky, I. and Rimon, A. Studies on the polymerization of fibrin Haifa (γ 275 Arg → His). In: *Fibrinogen 3. Biochemistry, Biological Functions, Gene Regulation and Expression*, M.W. Mosesson, D.L. Amrani, K.R. Siebenlist and J.P. DiOrio (eds.). Elsevier Science Publ., B.V., Amsterdam; pp. 271-274, **1988**.

133. Southan, C. Molecular and genetic abnormalities of fibrinogen. In: *Fibrinogen, Fibrin Stabilisation, and Fibrinolysis*, J.L. Francis (ed.). Ellis Horwood Ltd., Chichester; pp. 65-99, **1988**.

134. Southan, C. The elucidation of molecular defects in congenital dysfibrinogenaemia. In: *Fibrinogen, Fibrin Stabilisation, and Fibrinolysis*, J.L. Francis (ed.). Ellis Horwood Ltd., Chichester; pp. 100-127, **1988**.

135. Terukina, S., Matsuda, M., Hirata, H., Takeda, Y., Miyata, T., Takao, T. and Shimonishi, Y. Substitution of γ Arg-275 by Cys in an abnormal fibrinogen, "fibrinogen Osaka II:" evidence for a unique solitary cystine structure at the mutation site. *J. Biol. Chem.* **263**:13579-13587, **1988**.

136. Tsujinaka, T., Kambayashi, J., Kang, J., Sakon, M. and Mori, T. Intraoperative management of a dysfibrinogenemic patient with gastric cancer. *Jpn. J. Surg.* **18**:43-46, **1988**.

137. Vander Woude, J.C., Milam, J.D., Walker, W.E., Houchin, D.P., Weiland, A.P. and Cooley, D.A. Cardiovascular surgery in patients with congenital plasma coagulopathies. *Ann. Thorac. Surg.* **46**:283-288, **1988**.

138. Wiesel, M.-L, Grunebaum, L., Freyssinet, J.-M. and Cazenave, J.-P Biological causes of familial thrombosis. *Fibrinolysis* **2 (Suppl. 2)**:14-15, **1988**.

139. Yamazumi, K., Terukina, S., Shimura, K., Matsuda, M. and Takahashi, N. A substitution of γ Met-310 to Thr and an extra glycosylation at γ Asn-308 in an abnormal fibrinogen "Asahi." In: *Fibrinogen 3. Biochemistry, Biological Functions, Gene Regulation and Expression*, M.W. Mosesson, D.L. Amrani, K.R. Siebenlist and J.P. DiOrio (eds.). Elsevier Science Publ., B.V., Amsterdam; pp. 269, **1988**.

140. Yamazumi, K., Terukina, S., Onohara, S. and Matsuda, M. Normal plasmic cleavage of the γ-chain variant of "fibrinogen Saga" with an Arg-275 to His substitution. *Thromb. Haemostas.* **60**:476-480, **1988**.

141. Yoshida, N., Ota, K., Moroi, M. and Matsuda, M. An apparently higher molecular weight γ-chain variant in a new congenital abnormal fibrinogen Tochigi characterized by the replacement of γ arginine-275 by cysteine. *Blood* **71**:480-487, **1988**.

142. Yoshida, N., Terukina, S., Okuma, M., Moroi, M., Aoki, N. and Matsuda, M. Characterization of an apparently lower molecular weight γ-chain variant in fibrinogen Kyoto I. The replacement of γ-asparagine 308 by lysine which causes accelerated cleavage of fragment D1 by plasmin and the generation of a new plasmin cleavage site. *J. Biol. Chem.* **263**:13848-13856, **1988**.

143. Al-Mondhiry, H. and Galanakis, D. Dysfibrinogenemia and lupus anticoagulant in a patient with recurrent thrombosis. *J. Lab. Clin. Med.* **110**:726-733, **1987**.

144. Alving, B.M. and Henschen, A.H. Fibrinogen Giessen I: a congenital homozygously expressed dysfibrinogenemia with Aα 16 Arg → His substitution. *Am. J. Hematol.* **25**:479-482, **1987**.

145. Arocha-Piñango, C.L., Torres, A., Marchi, R., Rodríguez, S., Camarillo, H., Muller-Soyano, A. and Bosch, N.B. A new thrombotic dysfibrinogenemia present in several members of a venezuelan family. *Thromb. Haemostas.* **58**:149, **1987**. ABSTRACT

146. Borrell, M., Vila, L., Solá, J., Coll, I., Gómez, N., González, N. and Rutllant, M.L. Two cases of dysfibrinogenemia characterized by abnormal FPB release: fibrinogen Madrid I & II. *Thromb. Res.* **45**:591-599, **1987**.

147. Bögli, C., Hofer, A., Furlan, M., Beck, E.A., Baudo, F. and Redaelli, R. Fibrinogen Milano III, a new abnormal hereditary fibrinogen variant with a defect in the Aα chain. *Thromb. Haemostas.* **58**:515, **1987**. ABSTRACT

148. Carr, M.E., Jr. and Qureshi, G.D. The impact of delayed fibrinopeptide-A release on fibrin structure. *J. Biol. Chem.* **262**:15568-15574, **1987**.

149. Castaman, G., Rodeghiero, F., Galletti, A., Barone, E. and Gastaldi, G. Fibrinogen Genova III: a new congenital dysfibrinogenemia with bleeding diathesis and defective lysis by plasmin. *Thromb. Haemostas.* **58**:149, **1987**. ABSTRACT

150. Di Minno, G., Cerbone, A.M., Cirillo, F., Colucci, M., Semeraro, N., Di Santo, G., Mattioli, P.L., Mancini, M. and Quattrone, A. Abnormal fibrinogen (fibrinogen Naples) characterized by defective interaction with thrombin and plasmin in two young siblings with arterial thrombosis. *Thromb. Haemostas.* **58**:514, **1987**. ABSTRACT

151. Hamulyak, K., Muller, A.D. and Hemker, H.C. A new case of congenital combined hypo-dysfibrinogenemia? *Thromb. Haemostas.* **58**:148, **1987**. ABSTRACT

152. Haverkate, F., Koopman, J., Kluft, C., D'Angelo, A., Cattaneo, M. and Mannucci, P.M. Fibrinogens "Milano II" and "Naples." *Thromb. Haemostas.* **57**:375, **1987**.

153. Karp, G. and Liu, C.Y. Fibrinogens New York II, III, and IV: relationship between abnormal fibrin monomer polymerization, bleeding tendency, and thrombotic tendency. *Thromb. Haemostas.* **58**:148, **1987**. ABSTRACT

154. Köther, M., Egbring, R., Fuchs, G. and Henschen, A. Bleeding and thrombosis in individuals with structurally elucidated genetically abnormal fibrinogens. In: *Fibrinogen 2. Biochemistry, Physiology, and Clinical Relevance*, G.D.O. Lowe, J.T. Douglas, C.D. Forbes and A. Henschen (eds.). Elsevier, Amsterdam; pp. 45-48, **1987**.

155. Lane, D.A., Thompson, E. and Southan, C. Rapid screening method of fibrinopeptide analysis applied to congenital dysfibrinogenaemia: summary of 23 cases. In: *Fibrinogen 2. Biochemistry, Physiology and Clinical Relevance*, G.D.O. Lowe, J.T. Douglas, C.D. Forbes and A. Henschen (eds.). Elsevier, Amsterdam; pp. 71-74, **1987**.

156. Lane, D.A. and Southan, C. Inherited abnormalities of fibrinogen synthesis and structure. In: *Haemostasis and Thrombosis*, A.L. Bloom and D.P. Thomas (eds.). Churchill Livingstone, Edinburgh; pp. 442-451, **1987**.

157. Liu, C.Y. and Karp, G. Fibrinogen New York II, III, and IV: relationship between abnormal fibrin monomer polymerization, bleeding tendency, and thrombotic tendency. In: *Fibrinogen 2. Biochemistry, Physiology and Clinical Relevance*, G.D.O. Lowe, J.T. Douglas, C.D. Forbes and A. Henschen (eds.). Elsevier, Amsterdam; pp. 53-56, **1987**.

158. Matsuo, T. [Congenital dysfibrinogenemia and thrombosis]. *Rinsho Byori* **35**:493-496, **1987**.

159. Matsuo, T., Okuno, S., Mukaida, T., Ueshima, S., Okada, K. and Matsuo, O. A hereditary dysfibrinogenemia: fibrinogen Awaji. *Haemostasis* **17**:89-97, **1987**.

160. Miyata, T., Terukina, S., Matsuda, M., Kasamatsu, A., Takeda, Y., Murakami, T. and Iwanaga, S. Fibrinogens Kawaguchi and Osaka: an amino acid substitution of Aα arginine-16 to cysteine which forms an extra interchain disulfide bridge between the two Aα chains. *J. Biochem. (Tokyo)* **102**:93-101, **1987**.

161. Mosesson, M.W., DiOrio, J.P., Muller, M.F., Shainoff, J.R., Siebenlist, K.R., Amrani, D.L., Homandberg, G.A., Soria, J., Soria, C. and Samama, M. Studies on the ultrastructure of fibrin lacking fibrinopeptide B (β-fibrin). *Blood* **69**:1073-1081, **1987**.

162. Pirkle, H., Kaudewitz, H., Henschen, A., Theodor, I. and Simmons, G. Substitution of Bβ 14 arginine by Cyst(e)ine in fibrinogen Seattle I. In: *Fibrinogen 2. Biochemistry, Physiology and Clinical Relevance*, G.D.O. Lowe, J.T. Douglas, C.D. Forbes and A. Henschen (eds.). Elsevier, Amsterdam; pp. 49-52, **1987**.

163. Pirkle, H., Theodor, I., Vukasin, P., Nandi, B., Miyada, D., Baker, J. and Dukes, M. Fibrinogen Long Beach. *Thromb. Haemostas.* **58**:148, **1987**. ABSTRACT

164. Reber, P., Furlan, M., Beck, E.A. and Barbui, T. Fibrinogen Bergamo III and fibrinogen Torino: two further variants with hereditary molecular defects in fibrinopeptide A. *Thromb. Res.* **46**:163-167, **1987**.

165. Rodeghiero, F., Castaman, G.C., Dal Belin Peruffo, A., Dini, E., Galletti, A., Barone, E. and Gastaldi, G. Fibrinogen Vicenza and Genova II: two new cases of congenital dysfibrinogenemia with isolated defect of fibrin monomer polymerization and inhibitory activity on normal coagulation. *Thromb. Haemostas.* **57**:252-258, **1987**.

166. Ruf, W., Preissner, K.T., Lane, D.A. and Müller-Berghaus, G. Decreased rate of fibrinopeptide B release from fibrinogen London I. In: *Fibrinogen 2. Biochemistry, Physiology and Clinical Relevance*, G.D.O. Lowe, J.T. Douglas, C.D. Forbes and A. Henschen (eds.). Elsevier, Amsterdam; pp. 67-70, **1987**.

167. Siebenlist, K.R., Prchal, J.T. and Mosesson, M.W. Fibrinogen Birmingham: a new heterodimeric dysfibrinogenemia with defective fibrinopeptide A release (Aα 16 Arg → His). In: *Fibrinogen 2. Biochemistry, Physiology and Clinical Relevance*, G.D.O. Lowe, J.T. Douglas, C.D. Forbes and A. Henschen (eds.). Elsevier, Amsterdam; pp. 63-66, **1987**.

168. Soria, C., Soria, J., Mirshahi, M., Desvignes, P., Bonnet, P. and Caen, J.P. [Importance of the structure of the clot in thrombolysis]. *Ann. Biol. Clin. (Paris)* **45**:207-211, **1987**.

169. Soria, J., Soria, C., Samama, M., Tabori, S., Kehl, M., Henschen, A., Nieuwenhuizen, W., Rimon, A. and Tatarski, I. Fibrinogen Haifa: fibrinogen variant with absence of protective effect of calcium on plasmin degradation of γ chains. *Thromb. Haemostas.* **57**:310-313, **1987**.

170. Soria, J., Soria, C., Bertrand, O., Roussel, B., Dieval, J., Vendrely, C. and Delobel, J. Molecular basis for the Aα chain substitutions in dysfibrinogenemia with a description of two new cases of the disorder: fibrinogen Amiens I and fibrinogen Amiens II. In: *Fibrinogen 2. Biochemistry, Physiology and Clinical Relevance*, G.D.O. Lowe, J.T. Douglas, C.D. Forbes and A. Henschen (eds.). Elsevier, Amsterdam; pp. 57-62, **1987**.

171. Southan, C., Thompson, E. and Lane, D.A. Direct analysis of plasma fibrinogen-derived fibrinopeptides by high-performance liquid chromatography: investigation of nine congenital fibrinogen abnormalities. *Br. J. Haematol.* **65**:469-473, **1987**.

172. Terukina, S., Matsuda, M., Yoshida, N., Yamazumi, K., Takeda, Y. and Takano, T. Two abnormal fibrinogens designated as Osaka II and Morioka with a hitherto unidentified amino acid substitution; γ Arg-275 by Cys. *Thromb. Haemostas.* **58**:515, **1987**. ABSTRACT

173. Verstraete, M. and Vermylen, J. [Molecular defects of coagulation factors and of the fibrinolytic system associated with thromboembolism]. *J. Mal. Vasc.* **12**:3-13, **1987**.

174. Vila, V., Regañon, E., Aznar, J., Navarro, G. and Salas, M. Fibrinogen Barcelona I. Congenital dysfibrinogenemia characterized by defective release of fibrinopeptide A and fibrinogen degradation products. *Thromb. Res.* **45**:437-449, **1987**.

175. Ebert, R.F., Schreiber, W.E. and Bell, W.R. Fibrinogen Seattle II: congenital dysfibrinogenemia with an Arg (Aα 16) → His substitution. *Thromb. Res.* **43**:7-13, **1986**.

176. Fernández, J., Páramo, J.A., Cuesta, B., Aranda, A. and Rocha, E. Fibrinogen Pamplona II. A new congenital dysfibrinogenemia with abnormal fibrin-enhanced plasminogen activation and defective binding of thrombin to fibrin. In: *Fibrinogen and Its Derivatives. Biochemistry, Physiology and Pathophysiology*, G. Muller-Berghaus, U. Scheefers-Borchel, E. Selmayr and A. Henschen (eds.). Excerpta Medica, Amsterdam; pp. 25-30, **1986**.

177. Haverkate, F., Koopman, J., Kluft, C., D'Angelo, A., Cattaneo, M. and Mannucci, P.M. Fibrinogen Milano II: a congenital dysfibrinogenaemia associated with juvenile arterial and venous thrombosis. *Thromb. Haemostas.* **55**:131-135, **1986**.

178. Henschen, A. and McDonagh, J. Fibrinogen, fibrin and factor XIII. In: *New Comprehensive Biochemistry vol. 13: Blood Coagulation*, A. Neuberger and L.L.M. van Deenen (eds.). Elsevier, Amsterdam; pp. 171-241, **1986**.

179. Henschen, A. and Alving, B. Fibrinogen Giessen I, a classical dysfibrinogen: the molecular defect. In: *Fibrinogen and Its Derivatives. Biochemistry, Physiology, and Pathophysiology*, G. Muller-Berghaus, U. Scheefers-Borchel, E. Selmayr and A. Henschen (eds.). Excerpta Medica, Amsterdam; pp. 23-24, **1986**.

180. Hessel, B., Stenbjerg, S., Dyr, J., Kudryk, B., Therkildsen, L. and Blombäck, B. Fibrinogen Aarhus — a new case of dysfibrinogenemia. *Thromb. Res.* **42**:21-37, **1986**.

181. Kaudewitz, H., Henschen, A., Soria, J. and Soria, C. Fibrinogen Pontoise — a genetically abnormal fibrinogen with defective fibrin polymerisation but normal fibrinopeptide release. In: *Fibrinogen — Fibrin Formation and Fibrinolysis*, D.A. Lane, A. Henschen and M.K. Jasani (eds.). W. de Gruyter, Berlin; pp. 91-96, **1986**.

182. Kaudewitz, H., Henschen, A., Soria, C., Soria, J., Bertrand, O. and Heaton, D. The molecular defect of the genetically abnormal fibrinogen Christchurch II. In: *Fibrinogen and Its Derivatives*, G. Muller-Berghaus, V. Scheefers-Borchel, E. Selmayr and A. Henschen (eds.). Elsevier, Amsterdam; pp. 31-36, **1986**.

183. Kobayashi, H., Sakaguchi, Y. and Matsuo, T. [Serum FDP in patients with congenital dysfibrinogenemia]. *Rinsho Byori* **34**:973-976, **1986**.

184. Koopman, J., Engesser, L., Nieveen, M., Haverkate, F. and Brommer, E.J.P. Fibrin polymerization associated with tissue-type plasminogen activator (t-PA) induced glu-plasminogen activation. In: *Fibrinogen and Its Derivatives*, G. Muller-Berghaus, U. Scheefers-Borchel, E. Selmayr and A. Henschen (eds.). Excerpta Medica, Amsterdam; pp. 315-318, **1986**.

185. Lerner, R.G., Galanakis, D.K., Nelson, J.C. and Franco, P. Fibrinogen Valhalla: a bleeding disorder with defective fibrinopeptide B release. *Blood* **68 (Suppl. 1)**:336a, **1986**. ABSTRACT

186. Liu, C.Y., Wallen, P. and Handley, D.A. Fibrinogen New York I: the structural, functional, and genetic defects and an hypothesis of the role of fibrin in the regulation of coagulation and fibrinolysis. In: *Fibrinogen — Fibrin Formation and Fibrinolysis*, D.A. Lane, A. Henschen and M.K. Jasani (eds.). W. de Gruyter, Berlin; pp. 79-90, **1986**.

187. Matsuda, M., Terukina, S., Miyata, T. and Iwanaga, S. Defective release of fibrinopeptide A due to substitution of Aα arginine-16 by cysteine in two abnormal fibrinogens Kawaguchi and Osaka. In: *Fibrinogen and Its Derivatives; Biochemistry, Physiology, and Pathophysiology*, Excerpta Medica, Amsterdam, New York, Oxford; pp. 37-40, **1986**.

188. Matsuo, T., Mukaida, T., Mori, E. and Matsuo, O. [Congenital dysfibrinogenemia in a patient with left internal carotid artery occlusion]. *Nippon Naika Gakkai Zasshi* **75**:51-56, **1986**.

189. Mosesson, M.W., Siebenlist, K.R., DiOrio, J.P., Hainfeld, J.F, Wall, J.S., Soria, J., Soria, C. and Samama, M. Evidence that proximal NH2-terminal portions of fibrinogen Metz (Aα 16 Arg → Cys) Aα chains are oriented in the same direction. In: *Fibrinogen and Its Derivatives. Biochemistry, Physiology, and Pathophysiology*, G. Muller-Berghaus, U. Scheefers-Borchel, E. Selmayr and A. Henschen (eds.). Excerpta Medica, Amsterdam; pp. 3-15, **1986**.

190. Reber, P., Furlan, M., Rupp, C., Kehl, M., Henschen, A., Manucci, P.M. and Beck, E.A. Fibrinogen Milano I: abnormal fibrin polymerization related to a carboxy-terminal defect of the γ-chain (γ-330 Asp → Val). In: *Fibrinogen — Fibrin Formation and Fibrinolysis*, D.A. Lane, A. Henschen and M.K. Jasani (eds.). W. de Gruyter, Berlin; pp. 97-102, **1986**.

191. Reber, P., Furlan, M., Rupp, C., Kehl, M., Henschen, A., Mannucci, P.M. and Beck, E.A. Characterization of fibrinogen Milano I: amino acid exchange γ 330 Asp → Val impairs fibrin polymerization. *Blood* **67**;1751-1756, **1986**.

192. Reber, P., Furlan, M., Henschen, A. and Beck, E.A. Three new fibrinogen variants with defective polymerization site in the γ chain. In: *Fibrinogen and Its Derivatives. Biochemistry, Physiology and Pathophysiology*, G. Muller-Berghaus, U. Scheefers-Borchel, E. Selmayr and A. Henschen (eds.). Excerpta Medica, Amsterdam; pp. 41-42, **1986**.

193. Reber, P., Furlan, M. and Beck, E.A. Fibrinogen "Bergamo I" (Aα 16 Arg → Cys): alternative methods for structure elucidation. In: *Fibrinogen — Fibrin Formation and Fibrinolysis*, D.A. Lane, A. Henschen and M.K. Jasani (eds.). W. de Gruyter, Berlin; pp. 103-110, **1986**.

194. Reber, P., Furlan, M., Henschen, A., Kaudewitz, H., Barbui, T., Hilgard, P., Nenci, G.G., Berrettini, M. and Beck, E.A. Three abnormal fibrinogen variants with the same amino acid substitution (γ 275 Arg → His): fibrinogens Bergamo II, Essen and Perugia. *Thromb. Haemostas.* **56**:401-406, **1986**.

195. Southan, C., Thompson, E. and Lane, D.A. Direct analysis of plasma fibrinogen-derived fibrinopeptides by high performance liquid chromatography: investigation of Aα-chain N-terminal heterogeneity. *Thromb. Haemostas.* **56**:193-197, **1986**.

196. Southan, C. and Lane, D.A. Screening small plasma samples by HPLC for abnormalities of fibrinopeptide release. In: *Fibrinogen — Fibrin Formation and Fibrinolysis*, D.A. Lane, A. Henschen and M.K. Jasani (eds.). W. de Gruyter, Berlin; pp. 111-120, **1986**.

197. Southan, C., Thompson, E. and Lane, D.A. Direct analysis of plasma fibrinogen-derived fibrinopeptides by high-performance liquid chromatography. *Thromb. Res.* **43**:195-204, **1986**.

198. Thorsen, L.I., Brosstad, F., Solum, N.O. and Stormorken, H. Increased binding to ADP-stimulated platelets and aggregation effect of the dysfibrinogen Oslo I as compared with normal fibrinogen. *Scand. J. Haematol.* **36**:203-210, **1986**.

199. Yoshida, N., Okuma, M., Moroi, M. and Matsuda, M. A lower molecular weight γ-chain variant in a congenital abnormal fibrinogen (Kyoto). *Blood* **68**:703-707, **1986**.

200. Bithell, T.C. Hereditary dysfibrinogenemia. *Clin. Chem.* **31**:509-516, **1985**.

201. Carrell, N. Functional defects in abnormal fibrinogens. In: *Fibrinogen — Structural Variants and Interactions*, A. Henschen, B. Hessel, J. McDonagh and T. Saldeen (eds.). Walter de Gruyter, Berlin; pp. 155-164, **1985**.

202. Deutsch, E., Dudczak, R., Henschen, A., Mannhalter, Ch. and Pils, P. [Dysfibrinogen "Schwarzach"]. *Med. Welt* **36**:655-661, **1985**.

203. Ebert, R.F. and Bell, W.R. Assay of human fibrinopeptides by high-performance liquid chromatography. *Anal. Biochem.* **148**:70-78, **1985**.

204. Ebert, R.F. and Bell, W.R. Fibrinogen Baltimore IV: congenital dysfibrinogenemia with delayed fibrin monomer polymerization. *Thromb. Res.* **38**:121-128, **1985**.

205. Fernández, J., Noguerol, P., Losada, G., Alberca, I., Sosa, R., Martin-Villar, J., Vicente, V. and Rocha, E. Three new cases of congenital dysfibrinogenemia: fibrinogens Sevilla, Madrid and Salamanca. *Thromb. Haemostas.* **54**:160, **1985**. ABSTRACT

206. Fernández, J., Rodriguez Pinto, C., Rocha, E., Fernández Urgelles, M., Páramo, J.A. and Romo, M. Fibrinogens Oviedo I, Oviedo II and Oviedo III: three new cases of dysfibrinogenemia with abnormal fibrin aggregation. *Thromb. Haemostas.* **54**:159, **1985**. ABSTRACT

207. Galanakis, D.K. Aspects of evaluation of fibrinogen Stony Brook. A defect resulting in failure to release fibrinopeptide A. In: *Fibrinogen — Structural Variants and Interactions*, A. Henschen, B. Hessel, J. McDonagh and T. Saldeen (eds.). Walter de Gruyter, Berlin; pp. 207-212, **1985**.

208. Girolami, A., De Marco, L., Dal Bo Zanon, R., Patrassi, G. and Capellato, M.G. Rarer quantitative and qualitative abnormalities of coagulation. In: *Clinics in Haematology 14*, Z.M. Ruggeri (ed.). W.B. Saunders Co., London; pp. 385-411, **1985**.

209. Haverkate, F., Koopman, J. and Kluft, C. Fibrinogen Milan II: a congenital dysfibrinogenaemia with a defective clotting by thrombin, normal clotting by arvin, reptilase and prothrombin-staphylocoagulase complex, associated with thrombotic episodes. In: *Fibrinogen — Structural Variants and Interactions*, A. Henschen, B. Hessel, J. McDonagh and T. Saldeen (eds.). Walter de Gruyter, Berlin; pp. 223-236, **1985**.

210. Henschen, A. Genetically abnormal fibrinogens — a summary of 32 structurally elucidated variants. *Prot. Biol. Fluid.* **33**:107-110, **1985**.

211. Lane, D.A., Ireland, H., Thompson, E., Southan, C. and Henschen, A. Fibrinogens London I—IV, Manchester, Sydney I and II. Cleavage of fibrinopeptides by thrombin and expression of their polymerisation abnormalities. In: *Fibrinogen — Structural Variants and Interactions*, A. Henschen, B. Hessel, J. McDonagh and T. Saldeen (eds.). W. de Gruyter, Berlin; pp. 197-206, **1985**.

212. Lehmer, R.R., Elias, A.N., Capdeville, M.J., Brown, D.R. and Branson, H.E. Fibrinogen Irvine: a qualitatively abnormal fibrinogen associated with the predisposition to recurrent visceral and peripheral venous thrombosis. *J. Natl. Med. Assoc.* **78**:561-565, **1985**.

213. Liu, C.Y., Koehn, J.A. and Morgan, F.J. Characterization of fibrinogen New York I. A dysfunctional fibrinogen with a deletion of Bβ(9-72) corresponding exactly to exon 2 of the gene. *J. Biol. Chem.* **260**:4390-4396, **1985**.

214. Matsuda, M., Saeki, E., Kasamatsu, A., Nakamikawa, C., Manabe, S. and Samejima, Y. Fibrinogen Kawaguchi: an abnormal fibrinogen characterized by defective release of fibrinopeptide A. *Thromb. Res.* **37**:379-390, **1985**.

215. Matsuda, M., Nakamikawa, C., Baba, M. and Morimoto, K. Fibrinogen Tokyo II: an abnormal fibrinogen with an impaired polymerization site on the aligned DD domain of fibrin molecules. In: *Fibrinogen — Structural Variants and Interactions*, A. Henschen, B. Hessel, J. McDonagh and T. Saldeen (eds.). Walter de Gruyter, Berlin; pp. 213-222, **1985**.

216. Matsuo, T., Okuno, S., Mukaida, T. and Matsuo, O. [Fibrinogen Awaji: a congenital dysfibrinogenemia characterized by abnormal fibrin monomer polymerization]. *Nippon Ketsueki Gakkai Zasshi* **48**:1594-1597, **1985**.

217. Miyashita, C., Schwamborn, J., von Blohn, G., Wenzel, E. and Hellstern, P. Preliminary report concerning two new cases of congenital dysfibrinogenemia (Homburg II and Homburg III). In: *Fibrinogen — Structural Variants and Interactions*, A. Henschen, B. Hessel, J. McDonagh and T. Saldeen (eds.). Walter de Gruyter, Berlin; pp. 237-246, **1985**.

218. Peerschke, E.I.B. and Galanakis, D.K. Binding of fibrinogen to ADP-treated platelets: importance of the Aα chain. In: *Fibrinogen — Structural Variants and Interactions*, A. Henschen, B. Hessel, J. McDonagh and T. Saldeen (eds.). Walter de Gruyter, New York; pp. 369-377, **1985**.

219. Reber, P., Furlan, M., Beck, E.A., Finazzi, G., Buelli, M. and Barbui, T. Fibrinogen Bergamo I (Aα 16 Arg → Cys): susceptibility towards thrombin following aminoethylation, methylation or carboxamidomethylation of cysteine residues. *Thromb. Haemostas.* **54**:390-393, **1985**.

220. Rocha, E., Páramo, J.A., Aranda, A., Cuesta, B. and Fernández, J. Congenital dysfibrinogenemias. A review. *Ric. Clin. Lab.* **15**:205-229, **1985**.

221. Saeki, E., Matsuda, M., Ichinose, A., Samejima, Y., Kasamatsu, A., Ara, R., Mitsuno, K., Kihara, T. and Hara, Y. ["Fibrinogen Kawaguchi:" a hereditary dysfibrinogenemia characterized by defective release of fibrinopeptide A associated with altered polymerization of fibrin monomers]. *Nippon Ketsueki Gakkai Zasshi* **48**:1229-1235, **1985**.

222. Schreiber, W.E. and Schmer, G. Fibrinogen Seattle II: defective release of fibrinopeptide A in a slow clotting fibrinogen. *Thromb. Res.* **37**:45-52, **1985**.

223. Shigekiyo, T., Shirakami, A., Kawauchi, S., Hirai, Y., Takeichi, T., Inomoto, T., Inoue, T., Shintani, Y., Takada, Y., Mizuguchi, Y. and Masuda, K. [Dysfibrinogenemia and nephrotic syndrome: a case report]. *Rinsho Ketsueki* **26**:761-765, **1985**.

224. Soria, J., Soria, C., Hedner, U., Nilsson, I.M., Bergqvist, D. and Samama, M. Episodes of increased fibronectin level observed in a patient suffering from recurrent thrombosis related to congenital hypodysfibrinogenaemia (fibrinogen Malmöe). *Br. J. Haematol.* **61**:727-738, **1985**.

225. Soria, J., Soria, C., Samama, M. and Caen, J. Study of ten cases of congenital dysfibrinogenemia. Clinical and molecular biological aspects. In: *Fibrinogen — Structural Variants and Interactions*, A. Henschen, B. Hessel, J. McDonagh and T. Saldeen (eds.). Walter de Gruyter, — Berlin; pp. 165-183, **1985**.

226. Southan, C., Lane, D.A., Knight, I., Ireland, H. and Bottomley, J. Fibrinogen Manchester. Detection of a heterozygous phenotype in the intraplatelet pool. *Biochem. J.* **229**:723-730, **1985**.

227. Southan, C., Lane, D.A., Bode, W. and Henschen, A. Thrombin-induced fibrinopeptide release from a fibrinogen variant (fibrinogen Sydney I) with an Aα Arg-16 → His substitution. *Eur. J. Biochem.* **147**:593-600, **1985**.

228. Southan, C., Henschen, A. and Lane, D.A. Fibrinogens Sydney I and II: a kinetic study of (His-16) FPA cleavage and its effect on FPB cleavage. In: *Fibrinogen — Structural Variants and Interactions*, A. Henschen, B. Hessel, J. McDonagh and T. Saldeen (eds.). Walter de Gruyter, Berlin; pp. 185-206, **1985**.

229. Southan, C., Thompson, E., Panico, M., Etienne, T., Morris, H.R. and Lane, D.A. Characterization of peptides cleaved by plasmin from the C-terminal polymerization domain of human fibrinogen. *J. Biol. Chem.* **260**:13095-13101, **1985**.

230. Bithell, T.C. Hereditary dysfibrinogenemia — the first 25 years. *Acta Haematol. (Basel)* **71**:145-149, **1984**.

231. Exner, T., Barber, S., Sage, R.E. and Kronenberg, H. Fibrinogen Adelaide: a familial hypodysfibrinogenaemia associated with abnormal α chains. *Br. J. Haematol.* **56**:95-106, **1984**.

232. Galanakis, D.K. Dysfibrinogenemia. A current perspective. *Clin. Lab. Med.* **4**:395-418, **1984**.

233. Hansen, M.S. and Schousboe, I. An abnormal fibrinogen (Copenhagen II) with increased sialic acid content associated with thrombotic tendency and normal liver function. *Scand. J. Haematol.* **33**:9-14, **1984**.

234. Henschen, A., Kehl, M. and Southan, C. Genetically abnormal fibrinogens — strategies for structure elucidation, including fibrinopeptide analysis. *Curr. Probl. Clin. Biochem.* **14**:273-320, **1984**.

235. Henschen, A., Kehl, M. and Southan, C. Genetically abnormal fibrinogens — strategies for structure elucidation, including fibrinopeptide analysis. In: *Variants of Human Fibrinogen*, E.A. Beck and M. Furlan (eds.). Hans Huber Publ., Berne; pp. 273-320, **1984**.

236. Laugen, R.H. and Bithell, T.C. Hereditary dysfibrinogenemia characterized by slow fibrinopeptide release and competitive inhibition of thrombin. *Acta Haematol. (Basel)* **71**:150-157, **1984**.

237. Lijnen, H.R., Soria, J., Soria, C., Collen, D. and Caen, J.P. Dysfibrinogenemia (fibrinogen Dusard) associated with impaired fibrin-enhanced plasminogen activation. *Thromb. Haemostas.* **51**:108-109, **1984**.

238. Mihalyi, E. Physicochemical studies of variants of human fibrinogen. In: *Variants of Human Fibrinogen*, E.A. Beck and M. Furlan (eds.). Hans Huber Publ., Berne; pp. 146-178, **1984**.

239. Perret, B.A. Electrophoretic procedures. In: *Variants of Human Fibrinogen*, E.A. Beck and M. Furlan (eds.). Hans Huber Publ., Berne; pp. 179-224, **1984**.

240. Polack, B., Valiron, O., Concord, E., Freyssinet, J.M. and Hudry-Clergeon, G. Molecular characterization of an abnormal fibrinogen by two-dimensional electrophoresis. *Clin. Chem.* **30**:2093-2097, **1984**.

241. Rocha, E., Lasierra, J., Narvaiza, M.J., Vilades, E., Palacios, E. and Fernández, J. Fibrinogen Logroño. A new case of congenital dysfibrinogenemia. *Ric. Clin. Lab.* **14**:663-672, **1984**.

242. Rupp, C. and Beck, E.A. Congenital dysfibrinogenemia. In: *Variants of Human Fibrinogen*, E.A. Beck and M. Furlan (eds.). Hans Huber Publ., Berne; pp. 65-130, **1984**.

243. Schreiber, W.E. and Schmer, G. Application of mechanical impedance measurements to the study of dysfibrinogens. *J. Lab. Clin. Med.* **104**:494-500, **1984**.

244. Soria, J., Soria, C., Mirshahi, M., Desvignes, P., Dunn, F. and Bonnet, P. Homozygous dysfibrinogen variant characterized by an absence of reactivity of the polymerizing site 'a' located in the γ-chain: fibrinogen Ales. *Proc. VIII Int. Congr. Thrombos.* 81, **1984**. ABSTRACT

245. Vila, V., Regañon, E., Fernández-Pavon, A. and Aznar, J. Dysfibrinogenaemia associated with a defect in the aggregation of the fibrin monomers (Alméria I fibrinogen). A preliminary study. *Scand. J. Haematol.* **33**:460-465, **1984**.

246. Andes, W.A. Fibrinogen New Orleans II: a new dysfibrinogenemia with venous thrombosis. *Thromb. Haemostas.* **50**:337, **1983**. ABSTRACT

247. Branson, H.E., Schmer, G., Theodor, I. and Pirkle, H. Fibrinogen Seattle releases half the normal amount of fibrinopeptide B. *Acta Haematol. (Basel)* **70**:257-263, **1983**.

248. Brook, J.G., Tabori, S., Tatarsky, I., Hashmonai, M. and Schramek, A. Fibrinogen "Haifa:" — a new fibrinogen variant. A case report. *Haemostasis* **13**:277-281, **1983**.

249. Brosstad, F., Teige, B., Olaisen, B., Gravem, K., Godal, H.C. and Stormorken, H. Two-dimensional electrophoretic characterization (iso-dalt) of fibrinogen and fibrin subunit chains from four different genetic dysfibrinogen variants. In: *Fibrinogen — Structure, Functional Aspects, Metabolism*, F. Haverkate, A. Henschen, W. Nieuwenhuizen and P.W. Straub (eds.). Walter de Gruyter, Berlin; pp. 145-154, **1983**.

250. Carrell, N., Gabriel, D.A., Blatt, P.M., Carr, M.E. and McDonagh, J. Hereditary dysfibrinogenemia in a patient with thrombotic disease. *Blood* **62**:439-447, **1983**.

251. Corrihons, G., Soria, J., Soria, C., Conard, J., Horellou, M.H. and Samama, M. [Congenital dysfibrinogenemia. Apropos of 13 cases]. *Sem. Hop. Paris* **59**:2517-2523, **1983**.

252. Dupuy, E., Tobelem, G., Soria, C., Pellerin, A., Drouet, L., Bellucci, S. and Caen, J. [Molecular abnormalities in recurrent thromboembolic disease]. *Presse. Med.* **12**:95-98, **1983**.

253. Ebert, R.F. and Bell, W.R. Fibrinogen Baltimore II: congenital hypodysfibrinogenemia with delayed release of fibrinopeptide B and decreased rate of fibrinogen synthesis. *Proc. Natl. Acad. Sci. U. S. A.* **80**:7318-7322, **1983**.

254. Finlayson, J.S. "Fibrinogen Oklahoma:" A study of interactions. *Ann. N. Y. Acad. Sci.* **408**:577-582, **1983**.

255. Galanakis, D.K., Henschen, A., Keeling, M., Kehl, M., Dismore, R. and Peerschke, E.I. Fibrinogen Louisville: an Aα 16 Arg → His defect that forms no hybrid molecules in heterozygous individuals and inhibits aggregation of normal fibrin monomers. *Ann. N. Y. Acad. Sci.* **408**:644-648, **1983**.

256. Henschen, A., Kehl, M., Southan, C., Lottspeich, F. and Georgopoulos, D. Genetically abnormal fibrinogens — some current characterisation strategies. In: *Fibrinogen — Structure, Functional Aspects, Metabolism*, F. Haverkate, A. Henschen, W. Nieuwenhuizen and P.W. Straub (eds.). Walter de Gruyter, Berlin; pp. 125-144, **1983**.

257. Henschen, A., Kehl, M. and Deutsch, E. Novel structure elucidation strategy for genetically abnormal fibrinogens with incomplete fibrinopeptide release as applied to fibrinogen Schwarzach. *Hoppe Seylers Z. Physiol. Chem.* **364**:1747-1751, **1983**.

258. Kehl, M., Lottspeich, F. and Henschen, A. Genetically abnormal fibrinogens releasing abnormal fibrinopeptides as characterised by high-performance liquid chromatography. In: *Fibrinogen — Structure, Functional Aspects, Metabolism*, F. Haverkate, A. Henschen, W. Nieuwenhuizen and P.W. Straub (eds.). Walter de Gruyter, Berlin; pp. 183-193, **1983**.

259. Lane, D.A., Ireland, H., Southan, C., Kehl, M. and Henschen, A. The molecular abnormality of fibrinogen Manchester. In: *Fibrinogen — Structure, Functional Aspects, Metabolism*, F. Haverkate, A. Henschen, W. Nieuwenhuizen and P.W. Straub (eds.). Walter de Gruyter, Berlin; pp. 155-166, **1983**.

260. Lane, D.A., Southan, C., Ireland, H., Thompson, E., Kehl, M. and Henschen, A. Delayed release of an abnormal fibrinopeptide A from fibrinogen Manchester: effect of the Aα 16 Arg leads to His substitution upon fibrin monomer polymerization and the immunological crossreactivity of the peptide. *Br. J. Haematol.* **53**:587-597, **1983**.

261. Matsuda, M., Baba, M., Morimoto, K. and Nakamikawa, C. "Fibrinogen Tokyo II." An abnormal fibrinogen with an impaired polymerization site on the aligned DD domain of fibrin molecules. *J. Clin. Invest.* **72**:1034-1041, **1983**.

262. Ménaché, D. Congenital fibrinogen abnormalities. In: *Molecular Biology of Fibrinogen and Fibrin*, M.W. Mosesson and R.F. Doolittle (eds.). The New York Academy of Sciences, New York; pp. 121-130, **1983**.

263. Neidhardt, B., Schricker, K.T. and Weniger, J. [Aortocoronary venous bypass in dysfibrinogenemia]. *Med. Welt* **34**:119-122, **1983**.

264. Quattrone, A., Colucci, M., Donati, M.B., Meduri, M., Mussoni, L., Roncaglioni, M.C., Semeraro, N., Carlomagno, S. and Bonavita, V. Stroke in two young siblings with congenital dysfibrinogenemia. *Ital. J. Neurol. Sci.* **4**:229-232, **1983**.

265. Qureshi, G.D., Evans, H.J., Vennart, R.M., Magnant, J.P., Sabau, J.M., Willoughby, J.B. and Koehn, J.A. Fibrinogen White Marsh — A new human variant with α-chain defect. *Clin. Res.* **31**:321A, **1983**. ABSTRACT

266. Rupp, C., Sievi, R., Furlan, M. and Beck, E.A. [Fibrinogen Bern II: hereditary fibrinogen variant with amino acid substitution of arginine replaced by histidine in position 16 of the Aα chain]. *Schweiz. Med. Wochenschr.* **113**:1460-1462, **1983**.

267. Soria, J., Soria, C. and Caen, P. A new type of congenital dysfibrinogenaemia with defective fibrin lysis — Dusard syndrome: possible relation to thrombosis. *Br. J. Haematol.* **53**:575-586, **1983**.

268. Southan, C., Lane, D.A. and Henschen, A. Functional characterisation and protein chemical analysis of two new cases of dysfibrinogenemia, London III and IV. In: *Fibrinogen — Structure, Functional Aspects, Metabolism*, F. Haverkate, A. Henschen, W. Nieuwenhuizen and P.W. Straub (eds.). Walter de Gruyter, Berlin; pp. 167-182, **1983**.

269. Southan, C., Kehl, M., Henschen, A. and Lane, D.A. Fibrinogen Manchester: identification of an abnormal fibrinopeptide A with a C-terminal arginine leads to histidine substitution. *Br. J. Haematol.* **54**:143-151, **1983**.

270. Stormorken, H., Brosstad, F. and Seim, H. A new dysfibrinogenemia: fibrinogen Oslo IV. *Thromb. Haemostas.* **49**:120-122, **1983**.

271. Vaugier, G.L., Maze, A., Griffault, J., Vacher, J. and Plutino, C. [Fibrinogen Orleans. A new case of congenital dysfibrinogenemia (letter)]. *Presse. Med.* **12**:1079-1080, **1983**. ABSTRACT

272. Andes, W.A. Fibrinogen New Orleans II: a new dysfibrinogenemia with venous thrombosis. *Blood* **60 (Suppl. 1)**:206a, **1982**. ABSTRACT

273. Andes, W.A., Chavin, S.I., Beltran, G. and Stuckey, W.J. Fibrinogen New Orleans: hereditary dysfibrinogenemia with an Aα chain abnormality. *Thromb. Res.* **25**:41-50, **1982**.

274. Beck, E.A. Congenital disorders of fibrin formation and stabilization. In: *Hemostasis and Thrombosis – Basic Principles and Clinical Practice*, R.W. Colman, J. Hirsch, V.J. Marder and E.W. Salzmann (eds.). Lippincott, Philadelphia; pp. 185-209, **1982**.

275. Caen, J.P., Soria, J. and Soria, C. [Structural anomaly of the fibrin clot with reduction of lys-plasminogen binding, as a cause of familial thrombosis]. *C. R. Seances. Acad. Sci. [III]* **294**:695-697, **1982**.

276. Capel, P., Bosson, D., Heriga-Muller, Ch., Mandelbaum, I.M., Vertongen, F. and Fondu, P. Investigation of an inherited defect in fibrinogen polymerization, with special emphasis on ultrastructural disturbances (fibrinogen Brussels). *Haemostas.* **12**:186, **1982**. ABSTRACT

277. Carrell, N. and McDonagh, J. Fibrinogen Chapel Hill II: defective in reactions with thrombin, factor XIIIa and plasmin. *Br. J. Haematol.* **52**:35-47, **1982**.

278. Hassan, H.J., Orlando, M., Tonini, G.P., Casalbore, P., Sarti, A., Boeri, E., Giacchino, R., Tentori, L. and Mori, P.G. An abnormal inherited fibrinogen (fibrinogen Genova) with delayed fibrin aggregation. *Scand. J. Haematol.* **29**:287-294, **1982**.

279. Higgins, D.L., Lewis, S.D., Penner, J.A. and Shafer, J.A. A kinetic method for characterization of heterogenous fibrinogen and its application to fibrinogen Grand Rapids, a congenital dysfibrinogenemia. *Thromb. Haemostas.* **48**:182-186, **1982**.

280. Jandrot-Perrus, M., Aurousseau, M.H., Rabiet, M.J. and Josso, F. Fibrinogen Bondy: a new case of dysfibrinogenemia. Isolation of the abnormal fibrinogen molecules. *Thromb. Res.* **27**:659-670, **1982**.

281. Kehl, M., Lottspeich, F. and Henschen, A. High-performance liquid chromatography of proteins as applied to fibrinogen chains. *Hoppe Seylers Z. Physiol. Chem.* **363**:1501-1505, **1982**.

282. Ladure, P., Ricordel, Y., Soria, J., Soria, C. and Samama, M. Binding of citrate to normal fibrinogen and to Metz fibrinogen. In: *Fibrinogen — Recent Biochemical and Medical Aspects*, A. Henschen, H. Graeff and F. Lottspeich (eds.). W. de Gruyter, Berlin; pp. 145-152, **1982**.

283. Lane, D.A., Ireland, H., Thompson, E., Frost, T.J. and Cuddigan, B. Two more abnormal fibrinogens (London III and Sydney) with impaired fibrinopeptide release. *Thromb. Res.* **28**:821-824, **1982**.

284. Lane, D.A., Allen, A.K., Markwick, J., Thompson, E. and Mackie, I. Carbohydrate in abnormal fibrinogens. In: *Fibrinogen — Recent Biochemical and Medical Aspects*, A. Henschen, H. Graeff and F. Lottspeich (eds.). W. deGruyter, Berlin; pp. 183-192, **1982**.

285. Marx, R. and Schramm, W. On dysfibrinogenemia. In: *Fibrinogen — Recent Biochemical and Medical Aspects*, A. Henschen, H. Graeff and F. Lottspeich (eds.). W. de Gruyter, Berlin; pp. 123-128, **1982**.

286. Miyashita, C., Nienhaus, K.-H., Wenzel, E., Kohler, M. and Hellstern, P. Observation on a new variant of hereditary dysfibrinogenemia (Homburg I) with delayed fibrin polymerisation and without clinical abnormality. In: *Fibrinogen — Recent Biochemical and Medical Aspects*, A. Henschen, H. Graeff and F. Lottspeich (eds.). W. de Gruyter, Berlin; pp. 193-200, **1982**.

287. Mizuochi, T., Taniguchi, T., Asami, Y., Takamatsu, J., Okude, M., Iwanaga, S. and Kobata, A. Comparative studies on the structures of the carbohydrate moieties of human fibrinogen and abnormal fibrinogen Nagoya. *J. Biochem. (Tokyo)* **92**:283-293, **1982**.

288. Rupp, C., Kuyas, C., Häberli, A., Furlan, M., Perret, B.A. and Beck, E.A. Fibrinogen Bern I: a hereditary fibrinogen variant with defective conformational stabilization by calcium ions. In: *Fibrinogen — Recent Biochemical and Medical Aspects*, A. Henschen, H. Graeff and F. Lottspeich (eds.). W. de Gruyter, Berlin; pp. 167-182, **1982**.

289. Soria, J., Soria, C., Samama, M., Henschen, A. and Southan, C. Detection of fibrinogen abnormality in dysfibrinogenemia: special report on fibrinogen Metz characterized by an amino acid substitution located at the peptide bond cleaved by thrombin. In: *Fibrinogen — Recent Biochemical and Medical Aspects*, A. Henschen, H. Graeff and F. Lottspeich (eds.). W. de Gruyter, Berlin; pp. 129-144, **1982**.

290. Southan, C., Henschen, A. and Lottspeich, F. The search for molecular defects in abnormal fibrinogens. In: *Fibrinogen — Recent Biochemical and Medical Aspects*, A. Henschen, H. Graeff and F. Lottspeich (eds.). W. de Gruyter, Berlin; pp. 153-166, **1982**.

291. Tavori, S., Brook, J.G., Hashmonai, M. and Tatarsky, I. A new variant of hereditary dysfibrinogenemia: a possible causal relationship to arterial thrombosis. *Adv. Pathol.* **1**:407-411, **1982**.

292. Bloom, A.L. Inherited disorders of blood coagulation. In: *Haemostasis and Thrombosis*, A.L. Bloom and D.P. Thomas (eds.). Churchill Livingstone, Edinburgh; pp. 321-370, **1981**.

293. Gastearena, J., Rocha, E., Orue, M.T., Narvaiza, M.J., Perez Equiza, E. and Fernández, J. [Fibrinogen Pamplona. A new molecular variant]. *Sangre. (Barc.)* **26**:575-587, **1981**.

294. Henschen, A., Southan, C., Soria, J., Soria, C. and Samama, M. Structure abnormality of fibrinogen Metz and its relationship to the clotting defect. *Thromb. Haemostas.* **46**:103, **1981**. ABSTRACT

295. Hensen, A., Brommer, E.J., Gravesen, M. and Haverkate, F. [Familial dysfibrinogenemia; fibrinogen Haarlem I and II]. *Ned. Tijdschr. Geneeskd.* **125**:734-737, **1981**.

296. Higgins, D.L. and Shafer, J.A. Fibrinogen Petoskey, a dysfibrinogenemia characterized by replacement of Arg-Aα 16 by a histidyl residue. *J. Biol. Chem.* **256**:12013-12017, **1981**.

297. Higgins, D.L., Penner, J.A. and Shafer, J.A. Fibrinogen Petoskey: identification of a new dysfibrinogenemia characterized by altered release of fibrinopeptide A. *Thromb. Res.* **23**:491-504, **1981**.

298. Kehl, M., Lottspeich, F. and Henschen, A. Analysis of human fibrinopeptides by high-performance liquid chromatography. *Hoppe Seylers Z. Physiol. Chem.* **362**:1661-1664, **1981**.

299. Ménaché, D. Congenital abnormal fibrinogens. In: *Hemophilia and Hemostasis*, Alan R. Liss, Inc., New York; pp. 205-220, **1981**.

300. Morris, S., Denninger, M.H., Finlayson, J.S. and Ménaché, D. Fibrinogen Lille: Aα 7 ASP → ASN. *Thromb. Haemostas.* **46**:104, **1981**. ABSTRACT

301. Papp, A.C., Snopko, R.M., Cole, E.R., Sassetti, R.J. and Wu, K.K. Recurrent venous thrombosis related to a hereditary dysfibrinogen with abnormal crossed immunoelectrophoretic pattern. *Thromb. Haemostas.* **46**:360, **1981**. ABSTRACT

302. Rupp, C., Kuyas, C., Häberli, A., Furlan, M., von Fliedner, V. and Beck, E.A. [Fibrinogen Bern I and fibrinogen Bern II: 2 hereditary fibrinogen variants with diverse biochemical properties]. *Schweiz. Med. Wochenschr.* **111**:1543-1545, **1981**.

303. Finlayson, J.S., Reamer, L.A., Mosesson, M.W. and Ménaché, D. Fibrinopeptide release from fibrinogen Paris I. *Thromb. Res.* **17**:577-579, **1980**.

304. Hansen, S.M., Clemmensen, I. and Wither, D. Fibrinogen Copenhagen; an abnormal fibrinogen with defective polymerization and release of fibrinopeptide A, but normal adsorption of plasminogen. *Scand. J. Clin. Lab. Invest.* **40**:221-226, **1980**.

305. Hasler, K., Böttcher, D., Köttgen, E. and Neumann, H. [Defective stabilization of fibrin in a family with hypodysfibrinogenemia]. In: *Fibrinolyse, Thrombose, Hamostase*, E. Deutsch and K. Lechner (eds.). F.K. Schattauer, Stuttgart, New York; pp. 538-541, **1980**.

306. Lagier, R., Bouvier, C.A. and Van Strijthem, N. Skeletal changes in congenital fibrinogen abnormalities. *Skeletal. Radiol.* **5**:233-239, **1980**.

307. Lane, D.A., VanRoss, M., Kakkar, V.V., Bottomley, K.J., Dhir, K., Holt, L.P. and MacIver, J.E. An abnormal fibrinogen with delayed fibrinopeptide A release. *Br. J. Haematol.* **46**:89-98, **1980**.

308. Lane, D.A., Cuddigan, B., VanRoss, M. and Kakkar, V.V. Dysfibrinogenaemia characterized by abnormal fibrin monomer polymerization and normal fibrinopeptide A release. *Br. J. Haematol.* **44**:483-494, **1980**.

309. Marx, R. and Schramm, W. Diskussionsbeitrag zum Thema 'Fibrinogenopathien'. In: *Fibrinogen, Fibrin und Fibrinkleber*, K.I. Schimpf (ed.). F.K. Schattauer, Stuttgart; pp. 195-197, **1980**.

310. McDonagh, R.P., Carrell, N.A., Roberts, H.R., Blatt, P.M. and McDonagh, J. Fibrinogen Chapel Hill: hypodysfibrinogenemia with a tertiary polymerization defect. *Am. J. Hematol.* **9**:23-38, **1980**.

311. Morse, E.E. Fibrinogen and dysfibrinogenemia. *Ann. Clin. Lab. Sci.* **10**:351-355, **1980**.

312. Mosesson, M.W., Feldmann, G. and Ménaché, D. Electron microscopy of fibrin Paris I. *Blood* **56**:80-83, **1980**.

313. Nienhaus, K.H., Wenzel, E., Taubert, W., Vief, B., Podolsak, B., Dreher, B., Giannitsis, D., Hoffsymmer, B. and Hess, H. [A clinically asymptomatic, new form of dysfibrinogenemia, fibrinogen 'Homburg']. In: *Fibrinogen, Fibrin, und Fibrinkleber*, K.I. Schimpf (ed.). F.K. Schattauer, Stuttgart, New York; pp. 185-190, **1980**.

314. Scharrer, I., Kirchmaier, C. and Maas, C. [Experimental study of congenital dysfibrinogenemia ("fibrinogen Frankfurt")]. In: *Fibrinogen, Fibrin und Fibrinkleber*, K.I. Schimpf (ed.). F.K. Schattauer, Stuttgart, New York; pp. 165-173, **1980**.

315. Soria, J., Soria, C., Juhan, I., Perrimond, H., Haverkate, F. and Orsini, A. Fibrinogen Marseille. A new case of congenital dysfibrinogenaemia. *Haemostas.* **9**:214-225, **1980**.

316. Takamatsu, J. and Iwanaga, S. [Studies on abnormal fibrinogen]. *Nippon Ketsueki Gakkai Zasshi* **43**:1203-1211, **1980**.

317. Weinger, R.S., Rudy, C., Moake, J.L., Conlon, C.L. and Cimo, P.L. Fibrinogen Houston: a dysfibrinogen exhibiting defective fibrin monomer aggregation and α-chain cross-linkages. *Am. J. Hematol.* **9**:237-248, **1980**.

318. Beck, E.A. Congenital abnormalities of fibrinogen. *Clin. Haematol.* **8**:169-181, **1979**.

319. Böttcher, D., Hasler, K., Köttgen, E. and Maurath, J. Hereditary hypodysfibrinogenemia with defective release of fibrinogenopeptide A (Fibrinogen Freiburg). *Thromb. Haemostas.* **42**:78, **1979**. ABSTRACT

320. Denninger, M.H., Finlayson, J.S., Reamer, L.A., Parquet-Gernez, A., Goudemand, M. and Ménaché, D. Congenital dysfibrinogenemia: fibrinogen Lille (Errata). *Thromb. Res.* **15**:291-293, **1979**.

321. Gralnick, H.R., Coller, B.S., Fratantoni, J.C. and Martinez, J. Fibrinogen Bethesda III: a hypodysfibrinogenemia. *Blood* **53**:28-46, **1979**.

322. Hofmann, V., Gati, W.P. and Straub, P.W. Fibrinogen Zürich I: impaired release of fibrinopeptide A. *Thromb. Haemostas.* **41**:709-713, **1979**.

323. Jandrot-Perrus, M., Mosesson, M.W., Denninger, M.H. and Ménaché, D. Studies of platelet fibrinogen from a subject with a congenital plasma fibrinogen abnormality (fibrinogen Paris I). *Blood* **54**:1109-1116, **1979**.

324. Owen, C.A., Jr., Bowie, E.J., Fass, D.N., Perez, R.A., Cole, T.L. and Stewart, M. Hypofibrinogenemia-dysfibrinogenemia and von Willebrand's disease in the same family. *Mayo. Clin. Proc.* **54**:375-380, **1979**.

325. Quattrone, A., Colucci, M., Donati, M.B., Mussoni, L., Roncaglioni, M.C., Semararo, N., Carlomagno, S. and Bonavita, V. Cerebral thrombosis in two young siblings with dysfibrinogenemia. *Neurosci. Lett.* **Suppl. 3**:S54, **1979**. ABSTRACT

326. Scharrer, I., Kirchmaier, C. and Maas, C. [Experimental study of congenital dysfibrinogenemia ("Fibrinogen Frankfurt")]. *Blut* **38**:62, **1979**. ABSTRACT

327. Stein, I.D., Poskitt, T.R., Arkel, Y. and Wu, H.V. Minimal dysfibrinogenemia. *Blood* **54 (Suppl. 1)**:196, **1979**.

328. Straub, P.W. and Gati, W.P. Increase of the sialic acid-rich variants of the Bβ- and γ-chains of fibrinogen Zürich II. *Thromb. Haemostas.* **41**:714-717, **1979**.

329. Takamatsu, J., Ogata, K., Kamiya, T. and Koie, K. A novel dysfibrinogenemia with abnormal γ chain (Fibrinogen Nagoya). *Thromb. Haemostas.* **42**:78, **1979**. ABSTRACT

330. Voinnesson, A. and Salaün, M. [Hereditary dysfibrinogenaemia. Study of a family]. *Sem. Hop. Paris* **55**:1507-1512, **1979**.

331. Amsellem, M., Samama, M., Conard, J., Levyne, S. and Ohlgiesser, C. [Congenital dysfibrinogenaemia. Two new cases]. *Nouv. Presse Med.* **7**:3745-3748, **1978**.

332. Denninger, M.H., Finlayson, J.S., Reamer, L.A., Parquet-Gernez, A., Goudemand, M. and Ménaché, D. Congenital dysfibrinogenemia: fibrinogen Lille. *Thromb. Res.* **13**:453-466, **1978**.

333. Gati, W.P. and Straub, P.W. Separation of both the Bβ- and the γ-polypeptide chains of human fibrinogen into two main types which differ in sialic acid content. *J. Biol. Chem.* **253**:1315-1321, **1978**.

334. Godal, H.C., Brosstad, F. and Kierulf, P. Three new cases of an inborn qualitative fibrinogen defect (fibrinogen Oslo II). *Scand. J. Haematol.* **20**:57-62, **1978**.

335. Gonzales-Llaven, J., Vargas-Linares, M.E., Azaola-Espinoza, P., Gonzales-Angulo, A. and Watanabe, C. An abnormal fibrinogen identified in a Mexican Family. *Proc. XVII Congr. Int. Soc. Hematol.* 938, **1978**. ABSTRACT

336. Haverkate, F., Timan, G., Soria, J., Soria, C. and Samama, M.M. Studies on the structure of the fragment D moiety of abnormal fibrinogens: influence of calcium ions. *Thromb. Res.* **13**:689-692, **1978**.

337. Hawiger, J., Hammond, D.K., Timmons, S. and Budzynski, A.Z. Interaction of human fibrinogen with Staphylococci: presence of a binding region on normal and abnormal fibrinogen variants and fibrinogen derivatives. *Blood* **51**:799-812, **1978**.

338. Jobin, F., Vu, L. and Delage, J.M. [Fibrinogen Quebec I and Quebec II: two new families of dysfibrinogenemia]. *Acta Haematol. (Basel)* **59**:119-127, **1978**.

339. Morse, E.E. The fibrinogenopathies. *Ann. Clin. Lab. Sci.* **8**:234-238, **1978**.

340. Mosesson, M.W., Natale, P.D., Amrani, D.L., Sherman, L.A., Joist, J.H. and Krause, W.H. Comparison of plasmic hydrolysis of normal fibrinogen and fibrinogen Giessen I. *Thromb. Res.* **12**:693-696, **1978**.

341. Samori, T. Studies on fibrinogen Tokyo (dysfibrinogenemia) with special reference to the analysis of FDP-D fragment. *J. Tokyo Med. Coll.* **36**:583-594, **1978**.

342. Barthels, M. and Sandvoss, G. [Fibrinogen "Hannover:, a further abnormal fibrinogen]. *Blut* **34**:99-106, **1977**.

343. Bosch, N.B., Arocha-Piñango, C.L., Rodriguez, A., Ojeda, A. and Carvajal, Z. Another inherited abnormality in plasma fibrinogen. *Thromb. Haemostas.* **38**:100, **1977**.

344. Branson, H.E., Schmer, G. and Dillard, D.H. Fibrinogen Seattle: a qualitatively abnormal fibrinogen in a patient with tetralogy of Fallot. *Am. J. Clin. Pathol.* **67**:236-240, **1977**.

345. Crum, E.D. Abnormal fibrinogens. In: *Haemostasis: Biochemistry, Physiology and Pathology*, D. Ogston and B. Bennett (eds.). Wiley & Sons, London; pp. 424-445, **1977**.

346. de Bosch, N.B., Arocha-Piñango, C.L., Soria, J., Soria, C., Rodriguez, A. and Rodríguez, S. An abnormal fibrinogen in a Venezuelan family. *Thromb. Res.* **10**:253-265, **1977**.

347. Denninger, M.H., Parquet-Gernez, A., Goudemand, M. and Ménaché, D. [A new case of dysfibrinogenemia: fibrinogen Lille]. *Nouv. Rev. Fr. Hematol.* **18**:519, **1977**. ABSTRACT

348. Flute, P.T. Disorders of plasma fibrinogen synthesis. *Br. Med. Bull.* **33**:253-259, **1977**.

349. Forman, W.B. and Kraus, J. Transurethral resection in a patient with a dysfibrinogen: fibrinogen Cleveland I. *J. Urol.* **118**:885, **1977**.

350. Fuchs, G., Egbring, R. and Havemann, K. Fibrinogen Marburg. A new genetic variant of fibrinogen. *Blut* **34**:107-118, **1977**.

351. Hofmann, V., Gati, W.P. and Straub, P.W. [Fibrinogen Zürich I: defective fibrinopeptide-A release]. *Schweiz. Med. Wochenschr.* **107**:1468, **1977**. ABSTRACT

352. Matthias, F.R., Krause, W.H., Ganssert, S., Mueller, K. and Lasch, H.G. [Dysfibrinogenemia. A new case: dysfibrinogenemia Giessen III]. *Klin. Wochenschr.* **55**:539-543, **1977**.

353. Samama, M., Soria, J. and Soria, C. Congenital and acquired dysfibrinogenaemia. In: *Recent Advances In Blood Coagulation*, L. Poller (ed.). Churchill Livingston, Edinburgh; pp. 313-335, **1977**.

354. Samori, T., Konishi, S., Itoh, O., Kato, M., Ikematsu, S., Yatabe, M., Fujimaki, M. and Fukutake, K. A new type of congenital dysfibrinogenemia with defective stabilization of fibrin polymers — fibrinogen Tokyo. *Blood & Vessel* **8**:628-632, **1977**.

355. Bleyl, H. and Krause, W.H. Studies on the degradation of fibrinogen Giessen I. *Thromb. Res.* **9**:329-334, **1976**.

356. Budzynski, A.Z. and Marder, V.J. Plasmic degradation of fibrinogen Paris I. *J. Lab. Clin. Med.* **88**:817-825, **1976**.

357. Forman, W.B. and Hadady, M. A simplified method for isolation of the S-carboxymethyl derivative chains of normal fibrinogen and fibrinogen Cleveland I. *Thromb. Res.* **8**:731-736, **1976**.

358. Gati, W.P. and Straub, P.W. [Resolution of Bβ and γ chains from normal human fibrinogen Zürich II into 2 variants with each differing sialic acid content]. *Schweiz. Med. Wochenschr.* **106**:1379, **1976**.

359. Krantz, S. and Lober, M. [Congenital and acquired variants of plasma fibrinogen]. *Folia Haematol. (Leipz.)* **103**:793-806, **1976**.

360. Krause, W.H., Heene, D.L., Lasch, H.G. and Huth, K. [Congenital dysfibrinogenemia: fibrinogen Giessen II]. *Verh. Dtsch. Ges. Inn. Med.* **82**:1646-1649, **1976**.

361. Kudryk, B., Blombäck, B. and Blombäck, M. Fibrinogen Detroit — an abnormal fibrinogen with non-functional NH2-terminal polymerization domain. *Thromb. Res.* **9**:25-36, **1976**.

362. Laurin, S. and Capet-Antonini, F.C. Evaluation of a non-hemorrhagic dysfibrinogenemia: fibrinogen "Montreal III". *Proc. XVI Cong. Int. Soc. Hematol.* 310-311, **1976**. ABSTRACT

363. Mammen, E.F. Congenital dysfibrinogenemias: molecular abnormalities of fibrinogen. *Blut* **33**:229-234, **1976**.

364. Marder, V.J. The functional defects of hereditary dysfibrinogens. *Thromb. Haemostas.* **36**:1-8, **1976**.

365. Mosesson, M.W., Amrani, D.L. and Ménaché, D. Studies on the structural abnormality of fibrinogen Paris I. *J. Clin. Invest.* **57**:782-790, **1976**.

366. Mosesson, M.W., Denninger, M.H. and Ménaché, D. Hydrolysis of fibrinogen Paris I by plasmin. *Thromb. Res.* **9**:115-121, **1976**.

367. Muraki, H., Ando, Y., Matsuda, S., Kikuchi, M., Hasegawa, M., Ono, F., Yamamoto, M., Suzuki, M., Nakamura, S. and Iwanaga, S. Fibrinogen 'Mitaka': a hereditary hypodysfibrinogenemia. *Proc. XVI Cong. Int. Soc. Hematol.* 310, **1976**. ABSTRACT

368. Ratnoff, O.D. and Forman, W.B. Criteria for the differentiation of dysfibrinogenemic states. *Semin. Hematol.* **13**:141-157, **1976**.

369. Soria, J., Soria, C., Samama, M., Poirot, E. and Kling, C. Human platelet fibrinogen: a protein different from plasma fibrinogen. *Pathol. Biol. (Paris.)* **24**:15-17, **1976**.

370. Thabaut, A., Durosoir, J.L., Voinesson, A., Laverdant, C. and Essioux, H. [Congenital dysfibrinogenemia: two new cases]. *Med. Armees* **4**:677-680, **1976**.

371. Thaler, E., Niessner, H. and Lechner, K. Fibrinogen Vienna I: Gerinnungsphysiologische und biochemische studien. *Acta Med. Austr.* **3**:148-149, **1976**.

372. Ulutin, O.N. *The Platelets. Fundamentals and Clinical Applications*, pp. 288-289, **1976**.

373. Al-Mondhiry, H., Bilezikian, S.B. and Nossel, H.L. Fibrinogen "New York" — an abnormal fibrinogen associated with thromboembolism: functional evaluation. *Blood* **45**:607-619, **1975**.

374. Brown, C.H. and Crowe, M.F. Defective α-polymerization in the conversion of fibrinogen Baltimore to fibrin. *J. Clin. Invest.* **55**:1190-1194, **1975**.

375. Budzynski, A.Z., Marder, V.J., Ménaché, D. and Guillin, M.C. Proceedings: Structural abnormality in the γ polypeptide chain of Paris I fibrinogen. *Thromb. Diath. Haemorrh.* **34**:329, **1975**. ABSTRACT

376. Buraschi, J.A., Sack, E.S., Quiroga, E. and Hendler, H. A new fibrinogen anomaly: fibrinogen Buenos Aires. *Thromb. Diath. Haemorrh.* **34**:570-571, **1975**. ABSTRACT

377. D'Angelo, G., Lacombe, M., Lemay, J., Lavallée, R., Bonny, Y. and Boileau, J. A new congenital dysfibrinogenemia with hemorrhagic diathesis (fibrinogen Montreal II). *Thromb. Diath. Haemorrh.* **39**:570, **1975**. ABSTRACT

378. Krause, W.H., Huth, K., Heene, D.L. and Lasch, H.G. [Hypodysfibrinogenemia: fibrinogen Giessen II]. *Klin. Wochenschr.* **53**:781-782, **1975**.

379. Samori, T., Yatabe, M., Ukita, M., Fujimaki, M. and Fukutake, K. Proceedings: A new type of congenital dysfibrinogenemia (fibrinogen Tokyo) with defective stabilization of fibrin polymers. *Thromb. Diath. Haemorrh.* **34**:329, **1975**. ABSTRACT

380. Soria, C., Soria, J., Samama, M., Poirot, E. and Kling, C. Proceedings: Role of trisodium citrate in the unclottability by thrombin of fibrinogen Metz. *Thromb. Diath. Haemorrh.* **34**:571, **1975**. ABSTRACT

381. Soria, J., Soria, C., Houbouyan, L. and Goguel, A. Fibrinogen Boulogne. A congenital abnormality in the aggregation of fibrin monomers. *Proc. III Congr. Europ. Afr. Div. Int. Soc. Haematol.* 23, **1975**. ABSTRACT

382. Soria, J., Soria, C., Bezou, M.J., Picot, J., Bernard-Griffiths, I. and Coulet, M. [Dysfibrinogenemia with defective aggregation of fibrin monomers: fibrinogen Clermont-Ferrand]. *Proc. I Congr. Franc. Hematol.* 66, **1975**. ABSTRACT

383. Aznar, J., Fernández-Pavon, A., Regañon, E., Vila, V. and Orellana, F. Fibrinogen Valencia. A new case of congenital dysfibrinogenemia. *Thromb. Diath. Haemorrh.* **32**:564-577, **1974**.

384. Budzynski, A.Z., Marder, V.J., Ménaché, D. and Guillin, M.C. Defect in the γ polypeptide chain of a congenital abnormal fibrinogen (Paris I). *Nature* **252**:66-68, **1974**.

385. Crum, E.D., Shainoff, J.R., Graham, R.C. and Ratnoff, O.D. Fibrinogen Cleveland II. An abnormal fibrinogen with defective release of fibrinopeptide A. *J. Clin. Invest.* **53**:1308-1319, **1974**.

386. Mammen, E.F. Congenital abnormalities of the fibrinogen molecule. *Sem. Thromb. Haemostas.* **1**:184-201, **1974**.

387. Martinez, J., Holburn, R.R., Shapiro, S.S. and Erslev, A.J. Fibrinogen Philadelphia. A hereditary hypodysfibrinogenemia characterized by fibrinogen hypercatabolism. *J. Clin. Invest.* **53**:600-611, **1974**.

388. Soria, J. and Soria, C. [Familial dysfibrinogenemia with abnormal monomer aggregation Paris III fibrinogen]. *Pathol. Biol. (Paris.)* **22**:72-79, **1974**.

389. Verhaeghe, R., Verstraete, M., Vermylen, J. and Vermylen, C. Fibrinogen 'Leuven', another genetic variant. *Br. J. Haematol.* **26**:421-433, **1974**.

390. Wohl, R.C. and Bradley, T.B. Impaired monomer aggregation in congenital dysfibrinogenemia. *Blood* **44**:935, **1974**. ABSTRACT

391. Aguercif, M., Soria, J., Soria, C., Ritschard, J., Samama, M. and Bouvier, C. A new family with dysfibrinogenaemia, fibrinogen Alba/Geneva. *Proc. IV Int. Congr. Thrombos. Haemost.* 38, **1973**. ABSTRACT

392. Beck, E.A. and Duckert, F. Congenital dysfibrinogenemia: fibrinogen Aarau. *Proc. II Congr. Europ. Afr. Div. Int. Soc. Haematol.* 253, **1973**. ABSTRACT

393. Biggs, R. Dysfibrinogenemia. *Thromb. Diath. Haemorrh.* **29**:523-524, **1973**.

394. Crum, E.D., Shainoff, J.R. and Ratnoff, O.D. Fibrinogen Cleveland II. *Clin. Res.* **21**:550, **1973**. ABSTRACT

395. Gajdos, A. [Fibrinogen. Hereditary hypo- and dysfibrinogenemia]. *Nouv. Presse. Med.* **2**:1067-1071, **1973**.

396. Graham, J.B., Barrett, D.A., Blombäck, B., Cann, H.M., Hardisty, R.M., Larrieu, M.J. and Renwick, J.H. A genetic nomenclature for human blood coagulation. *Thromb. Diath. Haemorrh.* **30**:2-11, **1973**.

397. Gralnick, H.R., Givelber, H.M. and Finlayson, J.S. A new congenital abnormality of human fibrinogen. Fibrinogen Bethesda II. *Thromb. Diath. Haemorrh.* **29**:562-571, **1973**.

398. Guillin, M.-C. and Ménaché, D. Fetal fibrinogen and fibrinogen Paris I: comparative fibrin monomers aggregation studies. *Thromb. Res.* **3**:117-135, **1973**.

399. Jacobsen, C.D. and Hoak, J.C. Fibrinogen Iowa City: an abnormal fibrinogen with no clinical symptoms. *Thromb. Res.* **2**:261-270, **1973**.

400. Krause, W.H. and Bleyl, H. Investigation on plasmin-proteolysis of abnormal fibrinogen (fibrinogen Giessen). *Thromb. Res.* **2**:361-364, **1973**.

401. Krause, W.H., Heene, D.L. and Lasch, H.G. Congenital dysfibrinogenemia (fibrinogen Giessen). *Thromb. Diath. Haemorrh.* **29**:547-561, **1973**.

402. Lacombe, M., Soria, J., Soria, C., D'Angelo, G., Lavallée, R. and Bonny, Y. Fibrinogen Montreal. A new case of congenital dysfibrinogenemia with defective aggregation of monomers. *Thromb. Diath. Haemorrh.* **29**:536-546, **1973**.

403. Ménaché, D. Abnormal fibrinogens. A review. *Thromb. Diath. Haemorrh.* **29**:525-535, **1973**.

404. Ratnoff, O.D. and Bennett, B. The genetics of hereditary disorders of blood coagulation. *Science* **179**:1291-1298, **1973**.

405. Soria, J., Soria, C., Samama, M. and Bousser, J. [Congenital dysfibrinogenemia]. *Nouv. Presse. Med.* **2**:1792, **1973**.

406. Thaler, E., Lechner, K. and Deutsch, E. Fibrinogen Wien. Verhandlungen der Deutschen arbeitsgemeinschaft fur blutgerinnungsforschung. In: *Tagung in Munster 15-17 February*, F.K. Schattauer Verlag, Stuttgart (im Druck); **1973**.

407. Ulutin, O.N. and Ulutin, S.B. Fibrinogen Istanbul — a new case of dysfibrinogenemia. *Second Meeting of the European and African Division of the International Society of Haematology* 252, **1973**. ABSTRACT

408. Winckelmann, G. [Congenital dysfibrinogenemia. Report on a new family (fibrinogen "Wiesbaden")]. *Thromb. Diath. Haemorrh.* **Suppl. 55**:345-356, **1973**.

409. Aguercif, M., Anner, R., Ritschard, J., Nydegger, U., Soria, J. and Bouvier, C.A. [Syndromes of congenital and familial disfibrinogenemia. Apropos of 2 additional families]. *Pediatrie* **27**:317-323, **1972**.

410. Gralnick, H.R. and Finlayson, J.S. Congenital dysfibrinogenemias. *Ann. Intern. Med.* **77**:471-473, **1972**.

411. Henschen, A. and Edman, P. Large scale preparation of S-carboxymethylated chains of human fibrin and fibrinogen and the occurrence of γ-chain variants. *Biochim. Biophys. Acta* **263**:351-367, **1972**.

412. Krause, W.H., Heene, D., Heinrich, D., Roka, L. and Lasch, H.G. [A new case of dysfibrinogenemia]. *Verh. Dtsch. Ges. Inn. Med.* **78**:1651-1653, **1972**.

413. Krause, W.H. and Zimmermann, P. [Quantitative electron microscopic studies on fibrin structure in dysfibrinogenemia]. *Klin. Wochenschr.* **50**:557-561, **1972**.

414. Philippe, N. [Dysfibrinogenemia]. *Phlebologie* **27**:93-100, **1972**.

415. Sherman, L.A., Gaston, L.W., Kaplan, M.E. and Spivack, A.R. Fibrinogen St. Louis: a new inherited fibrinogen variant, coincidentally associated with hemophilia A. *J. Clin. Invest.* **51**:590-597, **1972**.

416. Soria, J., Soria, C. and Boulard, C. [Structural anomaly of Metz fibrinogen, localized on the (A) chain of the molecule]. *Biochimie* **54**:415-417, **1972**.

417. Soria, J., Soria, C., Durand, G. and Feger, J. [Electrofocusing of abnormal fibrinogens in polyacrylamide gel]. *Ann. Biol. Clin. (Paris)* **30**:161-165, **1972**.

418. Soria, J., Soria, C., Samama, M., Poirot, E. and Kling, C. Fibrinogen Troyes — fibrinogen Metz. Two new cases of congenital dysfibrinogenemia. *Thromb. Diath. Haemorrh.* **27**:619-633, **1972**.

419. Beck, E.A., Shainoff, J.R., Vogel, A. and Jackson, D.P. Functional evaluation of an inherited abnormal fibrinogen: fibrinogen "Baltimore." *J. Clin. Invest.* **50**:1874-1884, **1971**.

420. Bouvier, C.A. and Aguercif, M. [Congenital dysfibrinogenemia]. *Ther. Umsch.* **28**:617-624, **1971**.

421. Gaston, L.W., Baue, A.E., Pfaff, D.A. and Wise, L. Spleno-renal shunt, cholecystectomy, and appendectomy in a patient with hemophilia A, and abnormal fibrinogen, and thrombocytopenia. *Ann. Surg.* **173**:234-237, **1971**.

422. Gralnick, H.R., Givelber, H.M., Shainoff, J.R. and Finlayson, J.S. Fibrinogen Bethesda: a congenital dysfibrinogenemia with delayed fibrinopeptide release. *J. Clin. Invest.* **50**:1819-1830, **1971**.

423. Janssen, C.L. and Vreeken, J. Fibrinogen Amsterdam, another hereditary abnormality of fibrinogen. *Br. J. Haematol.* **20**:287-298, **1971**.

424. Krause, W.H., Heene, D. and Lasch, H.G. [A new case of dysfibrinogenemia]. *Klin. Wochenschr.* **49**:806-808, **1971**.

425. Smith, E.B. and Holder, W.R. Stasis ulcer and "fibrinogen Baltimore." *Arch. Dermatol.* **104**:221-222, **1971**.

426. Streiff, F., Alexandre, P., Vigneron, C., Soria, J., Soria, C. and Mester, L. [A new case of Congenital and familial dysfibrinogenemia without Hemorrhagic Diathesis]. *Thromb. Diath. Haemorrh.* **26**:565-576, **1971**.

427. Beck, E.A. Diagnosis of structural abnormalities of human fibrinogen. *Thromb. Diath. Haemorrh.* **Suppl. 39**:323-329, **1970**.

428. Blombäck, B. and Blombäck, M. Molecular defects and variants of fibrinogen. *Nouv. Rev. Fr. Hematol.* **10**:671-678, **1970**.

429. Blombäck, M. and Blombäck, B. Fibrinogen Detroit — a molecular defect in the N-terminal disulphide knot. In: *Hemophilia and New Hemorrhagic States*, K.M. Brinkhous (ed.). Univ. of North Carolina Press, Chapel Hill; pp. 242-246, **1970**.

430. Fukui, H. [Afibrinogenemia and dysfibrinogenemia]. *Nippon Rinsho.* **28**:2086-2091, **1970**.

431. Funk, C. and Straub, P.W. Hereditary abnormality of fibrin monomer aggregation (Fibrinogen Zürich II). *Eur. J. Clin. Invest.* **1**:131, **1970**. ABSTRACT

432. Hampton, J.W. Fibrinogen abnormality with defective cross-linkage. *Fed. Proc.* **29**:647, **1970**. ABSTRACT

433. Jackson, D.P. Hereditary disorders of blood coagulation due to defective and deficient synthesis of protein. *Trans. Am. Clin. Hematol. Assoc.* **82**:114-123, **1970**.

434. Mammen, E.F., Prasad, A.S., Barnhart, M.I. and Au, C.C. Fibrinogen Detroit. In: *Hemophilia and New Hemorrhagic States*, K.M. Brinkhous (ed.). University of North Carolina Press, Chapel Hill; pp. 233-241, **1970**.

435. Ménaché, D. Congenitally abnormal fibrinogens. *Thromb. Diath. Haemorrh.* **Suppl. 39**:307-321, **1970**.

436. Ménaché, D. [Congenital dysfibrinogenemias]. *Nouv. Rev. Fr. Hematol.* **10**:653-665, **1970**.

437. Morton, R.O. and Hampton, J.W. Fibrinogen Oklahoma — characterization of a familial bleeding diathesis. *Clin. Res.* **18**:533, **1970**. ABSTRACT

438. Mosesson, M.W. Fibrinogen Baltimore: physiochemical characterization. In: *Hemophilia and New Hemorrhagic States*, K.M. Brinkhous (ed.). University of North Carolina Press, Chapel Hill; pp. 247-253, **1970**.

439. Ulutin, O.N. and Ulutin, S.B. [Fibrinogen Istanbul]. *Hematoloji, Turkey* **1**:153-167, **1970**.

440. Zietz, B.H. and Scott, J.L. An inherited defect in fibrinogen polymerization: fibrinogen Los Angeles. *Clin. Res.* **18**:179, **1970**. ABSTRACT

441. Fantl, P. Hypofibrinogenemia with a possibly defective fibrinogen associated with fibrinolysis. *Aust. Ann. Med.* **18**:43-49, **1969**.

442. Felten, A.von, Frick, P.G. and Straub, P.W. Studies on fibrin monomer aggregation in congenital dysfibrinogenemia: separation of a pathological from a normal fibrin fraction. *Br. J. Haematol.* **16**:353-361, **1969**.

443. Mammen, E.F., Prasad, A.S., Barnhart, M.I. and Au, C.C. Congenital dysfibrinogenemia: fibrinogen Detroit. *J. Clin. Invest.* **48**:235-249, **1969**.

444. Mosesson, M.W. and Beck, E.A. Chromatographic, ultracentrifugal, and related studies of fibrinogen "Baltimore." *J. Clin. Invest.* **48**:1656-1662, **1969**.

445. Samama, M., Soria, J., Soria, C. and Bousser, J. [Congenital and familial dysfibrinogenemia without hemorrhagic tendency]. *Nouv. Rev. Fr. Hematol.* 9:817-832, **1969**.

446. Blombäck, M., Blombäck, B., Mammen, E.F. and Prasad, A.S. Fibrinogen Detroit — a molecular defect in the N-terminal disulphide knot of human fibrinogen. *Nature* **218**:134-137, **1968**.

447. Forman, W.B., Ratnoff, O.D. and Boyer, M.H. An inherited qualitative abnormality in plasma fibrinogen: fibrinogen Cleveland. *J. Lab. Clin. Med.* **72**:455-472, **1968**.

448. Hampton, J.W. and Bird, R.M. Qualitative fibrinogen defect associated with abnormal fibrin stabilization. *J. Lab. Clin. Med.* **72**:882, **1968**. ABSTRACT

449. Mammen, E.F. and Prasad, A.S. [Familial dysfibrinogenemia — "Detroit fibrinogen"]. *Verh. Dtsch. Ges. Inn. Med.* **74**:140-144, **1968**.

450. Mammen, E.F., Prasad, A.S. and Au, C.C. Studies on a family with dysfibrinogenemia. *Thromb. Diath. Haemorrh.* **19**:603-604, **1968**.

451. Mester, L. and Szabados, L. Differences constitutionneles et fonctionnelles entre les fragments glucidiques du fibrinogene humain normal et d'un fibrinogene humaine anormal. *Bull. Soc. Chim. Biol.* **50**:2561-2566, **1968**.

452. Sherman, L.A., Gaston, L.W. and Spivack, A.R. Studies on a patient with a fibrinogen variant and hemophilia A. *J. Lab. Clin. Med.* **72**:1017, **1968**. ABSTRACT

453. Vogel, A. and Beck, E.A. [Qualitative electromicroscopic study on the fibrin structure originating from Baltimore fibrinogen]. *Schweiz. Med. Wochenschr.* **98**:1651-1653, **1968**.

454. Egeberg, O. Inherited fibrinogen abnormality causing thrombophilia. *Thromb. Diath. Haemorrh.* **17**:176-187, **1967**.

455. Forman, W.B., Boyer, M.H. and Ratnoff, O.D. A hereditary defect in the coagulation of fibrinogen by thrombin: studies in a family with fibrinogen Cleveland. *Blood* **30**:863, **1967**. ABSTRACT

456. Beck, E.A., Mosesson, M.W., Charache, P. and Jackson, D.P. [Hemorrhagic diathesis with dominant heredity, caused by an abnormal fibrinogen (fibrinogen Baltimore)]. *Schweiz. Med. Wochenschr.* **96**:1196-1199, **1966**.

457. Felten, A.von, Frick, P.G. and Straub, P.W. Familial disturbance of fibrin monomer aggregation. *Br. J. Haematol.* **12**:667-677, **1966**.

458. Hampton, J.W., Cunningham, G.R. and Bird, R.M. The pattern of inheritance of defective fibrinase (Factor XIII). *J. Lab. Clin. Med.* **67**:914-921, **1966**.

459. Beck, E.A., Charache, P. and Jackson, D.P. A new inherited coagulation disorder caused by an abnormal fibrinogen ('fibrinogen Baltimore'). *Nature* **208**:143-145, **1965**.

460. Felten, A.von, Duckert, F. and Frick, P.G. Gerinnungsstorung ohne hamorrhagische diathese infolge verzogerter aggregation der fibrinmolekule. *Schweiz. Med. Wschr.* **95**:1453-1456, **1965**.

461. Hampton, J.W., Bird, R.M. and Hammarsten, D.M. Defective fibrinase activity in two brothers. *J. Lab. Clin. Med.* **65**:469-474, **1965**.

462. Jackson, D.P., Beck, E.A. and Charache, P. Congenital disorders of fibrinogen. *Fed. Proc.* **24**:816-821, **1965**.

463. Beck, E. Abnormal fibrinogen (fibrinogen 'Baltimore') as a cause of a familial hemorrhagic disorder. *Blood* **24**:853-854, **1964**.

464. Ménaché, D. Constitutional and familial abnormal fibrinogen. *Thromb. Diath. Haemorrh.* **Suppl. 13**:173-185, **1964**.

465. Hasselback, R., Marion, R.B. and Thomas, J.W. Congenital hypofibrinogenemia in five members of a family. *Canad. Med. Assoc. J.* **88**:19-22, **1963**.

466. Ménaché, D. Dysfibrinogenemie constitutionnelle at familiale. In: *Proc. 9th Congr. Europ. Soc. Haemat., Lisbon 1963*, R. Fauvert and J.P. Soulier (eds.). S. Karger, New York; pp. 1255-1259, **1963**.

467. Imperato, C. and Dettori, A.G. Ipofibrinogenemia congenita con fibroastenia. *Helvet. Paediat. Acta* **13**:380-399, **1958**.